Essentials of
Biochemistry
for BDS and Allied Life Sciences Students

Essentials of
Biochemistry
for BDS and Allied Life Sciences Students

Purvi Purohit
MSc (Med) Biochemistry PhD (Med) Biochemistry
Assistant Professor
Department of Biochemistry
All India Institute of Medical Sciences
Jodhpur, Rajasthan, India

Foreword
Praveen Sharma

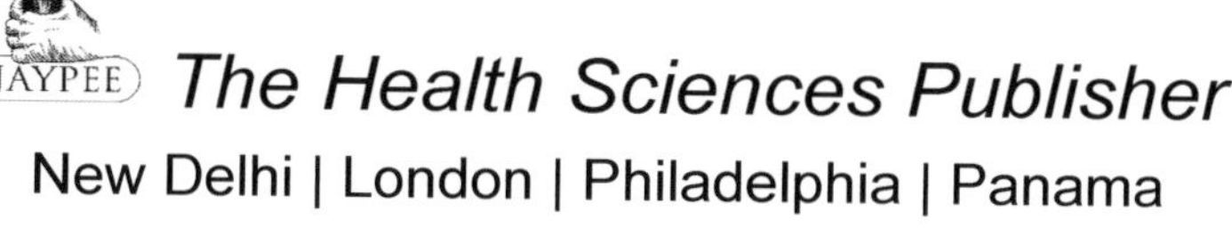
The Health Sciences Publisher
New Delhi | London | Philadelphia | Panama

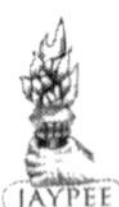

Jaypee Brothers Medical Publishers (P) Ltd

Headquarters

Jaypee Brothers Medical Publishers (P) Ltd
4838/24, Ansari Road, Daryaganj
New Delhi 110 002, India
Phone: +91-11-43574357
Fax: +91-11-43574314
Email: jaypee@jaypeebrothers.com

Overseas Offices

J.P. Medical Ltd
83 Victoria Street, London
SW1H 0HW (UK)
Phone: +44 20 3170 8910
Fax: +44 (0)20 3008 6180
Email: info@jpmedpub.com

Jaypee-Highlights Medical Publishers Inc
City of Knowledge, Bld. 237, Clayton
Panama City, Panama
Phone: +1 507-301-0496
Fax: +1 507-301-0499
Email: cservice@jphmedical.com

Jaypee Medical Inc
325 Chestnut Street
Suite 412, Philadelphia, PA 19106, USA
Phone: +1 267-519-9789
Email: jpmed.us@gmail.com

Jaypee Brothers Medical Publishers (P) Ltd
17/1-B Babar Road, Block-B, Shaymali
Mohammadpur, Dhaka-1207
Bangladesh
Phone: +08801912003485
Email: jaypeedhaka@gmail.com

Jaypee Brothers Medical Publishers (P) Ltd
Bhotahity, Kathmandu, Nepal
Phone: +977-9741283608
Email: kathmandu@jaypeebrothers.com

Website: www.jaypeebrothers.com
Website: www.jaypeedigital.com

Inquiries for bulk sales may be solicited at: jaypee@jaypeebrothers.com

Essentials of Biochemistry for BDS and Allied Life Sciences Students

First Edition: **2016**

ISBN 978-93-5250-146-5

Printed at Sanat Printers

Dedicated to

My father—Shri RC Purohit, and my mother—Smt Tara Purohit,
who inspired and encouraged me at every step of writing this book.
Not the least my sister—Pragna, whose excellent inputs and comments made writing a pleasure

Foreword

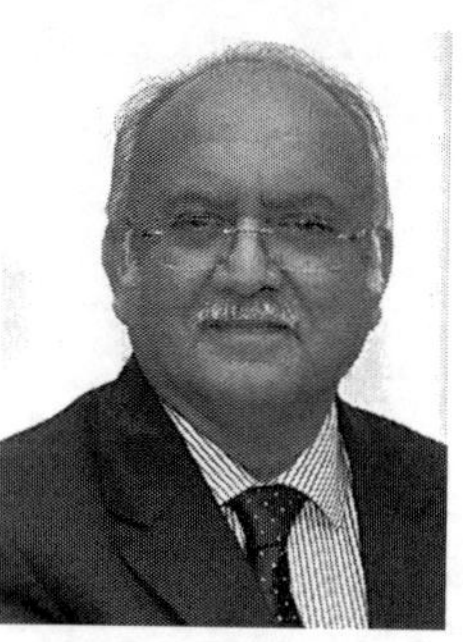

Science is objective, but human intelligence and endeavor has discovered and created interesting new substances. To date, we have discovered or created more than thirty million structurally well-defined compounds. Medical biochemistry is a branch of science that blends chemistry, biology and medicine and it explains in simple language the various biomolecules structure, scientific concepts that are necessary for the understanding of various biochemical processes that make life happen!

The world over, in the last decade, especially in the developed Western countries, there is integration, both horizontal and vertical directions in the handling of the teaching of health care concepts to the learners in medicine, dentistry and its allied sciences. Today, the teaching of the basic science subjects, like biochemistry, is no longer separate but a part of an integrated curriculum.

Biochemistry as it is taught today in the contemporary textbooks for dental and allied health sciences stream pays little attention to its role in health and disease. Biochemistry should be taught as a disease-oriented subject, rather than being an esoteric-related subject.

It is thus gratifying to see a book being written by young and dynamic teacher of All India Institute of Medical Sciences (AIIMS), Jodhpur. Dr Purvi Purohit, apart from her active involvement in research, over the years, visualized the need of students and thus the concept of teaching of biochemistry according to their requirement. I am sure the book contributed by her would be a boon to all those associated with dental and allied health sciences. The lucid and easily understandable presentation in the book aptly reaches the needs of the readers. The book encompasses all the biochemistry basics, necessary for the students of medicine and gives complete, in-depth information of theory, practical and clinical applications of biochemistry.

Indeed, the book is much-needed addition to the existing textbooks for understanding the subject and the student's need for performance in an examination system.

Praveen Sharma
MSc Biochemistry PhD Biochemistry FACBI
Professor and Head
Department of Biochemistry
All India Institute of Medical Sciences
Jodhpur, Rajasthan, India

Preface

I am pleased to present the *Essentials of Biochemistry for BDS and Allied Life Sciences Students.* This book has been comprehensively written in a lucid manner that is easy to understand and includes the theory as well as the practical sections essential for the undergraduate students.

The whole manuscript has been categorized into seven sections with the first six sections addressing the theory part of biochemistry and the last section deals with the practical exercises for the undergraduate students.

Every chapter has been designed in a way that it just suffices the needs for the BDS and allied health sciences students without overburdening them with loads of information. The practical section has been added with some viva-voce questions at the end of the chapters that would help the students to prepare for the practical viva-voce questions.

The book is well illustrated and has 60 plus figures, flowcharts and tables making reading and learning fun and interesting. The end of the book has some useful data that includes preparation of common reagents, common units, and glossary of important terms.

This is one of its kind book for the undergraduate students which conglomerates theory and practical in a single book. This makes the reading easy and the students can correlate the theory part with the practical exercises simultaneously just by turning the pages!!

I hope this book is able to more than satisfy its target audience and also prove a handy reference text for the faculties teaching this strata of the students.

The whole manuscript has been painstakingly read and re-read to avoid any kind of errors, however, to err is human! I regret any errors in the text and would be more than pleased to be informed about these errors so as to improve my further editions.

Purvi Purohit

Acknowledgments

The timely and accurate preparation of this book required cooperation of veritable people. I take this opportunity to thank them all.

I am indebted to Professor Sanjeev Misra, Director, AIIMS, Jodhpur, for providing an excellent academic environment and encouraging me to venture into various sections of academics from research to academic writing.

I take this opportunity to extend my sincere thanks to Professor Praveen Sharma, Professor and Head, Department of Biochemistry, AIIMS, Jodhpur, for his guidance and unfailing trust in my abilities that I have been able to pen-down this draft.

I am thankful to all my friends and colleagues at Department of Biochemistry, AIIMS, Jodhpur, who are always there to keep me in high spirits and ready to help at odd hours. It is their constant support and encouragement which kept me motivated to complete this daunting task of writing this elaborate draft. I appreciate and extend my thanks to:

- All my teachers—who are the guiding force behind all my academic achievements
- My family—my true strength.

I cannot repay in words the support and motivation extended to me by Dr MCR Vyas, Former Professor and Head, Department of Pathology, Dr SN Medical College and Ex-MCI Inspector, and Dr AK Acharya (Family Physician). I would also like to thank Dr Piyush Karoli, for keeping his team motivated and getting this draft proof checked in record time.

Finally, I would greatly remiss if I do not thank Shri Jitendar P Vij (Group Chairman), Mr Ankit Vij (Group President) and Mr Tarun Duneja (Director-Publishing) of M/s Jaypee Brothers Medical Publishers (P) Ltd, New Delhi, India, for kindly agreeing to publish this book and accomplishing the task in a splendid manner. I would also like to thank Mrs Samina Khan and Mr Rajesh Sharma, whose consistent support, untiring cooperation and time-bound proofreading made it possible for me to come out with this book in the shortest possible time. I am much obliged to my publisher for being extremely helpful and accommodating; without their support it was not possible to bring out this book. I once again thank everybody.

Contents

Section 1

Chemistry of Biomolecules

Section 2

Biocatalysts, Vitamins, Minerals and Nutrition

Section 3

Biological Oxidation and Energy Metabolism

Section 5

Genetics

Section 6

Miscellaneous

Section 7

Practical Biochemistry

Part A Introduction to Practical Biochemistry

Part B Qualitative Exercises

Part C Quantitative Exercises

Part E Applications of Clinical Biochemistry

Part F Demonstrations

An Introduction to Biochemistry

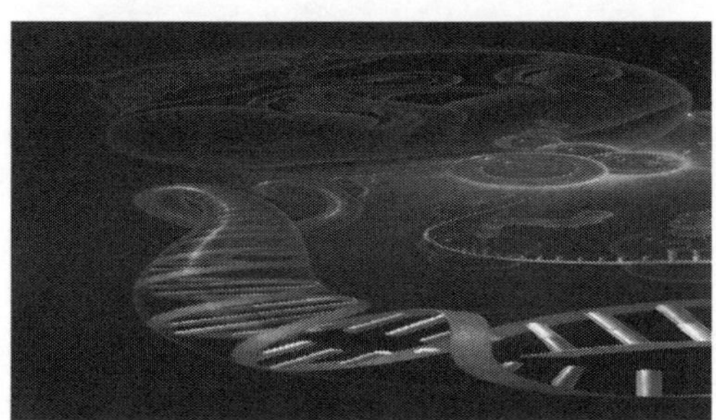

Chapter Framework

- Introduction
- Biochemistry in human life
- All life sciences are associated with biochemistry
- Biochemistry is an important tool in a physician's armour
- Biochemistry in dentistry

Introduction

From the most general point of view that we can take, it must be obvious that no kind of matter, non-living, dead, or alive, can possibly exist outside the realm of the operation of 'the laws of chemical affinity'.

It is intensely true that life is a chemical rather than a physical affair; for is not life dependent in an exceedingly intimate fashion on the chemical affinity between oxygen and hemoglobin!

Biochemistry in Human Life

The human body is composed of trillions of cells. Each cell is composed of a number of biomolecules (carbohydrates, lipids, amino acids, nucleic acids, vitamins, minerals, water, etc.) which are metabolized to liberate their inherent energies that powers all life processes.

Biochemistry is the study of the chemical basis of life. To unravel the mystery of life a sound knowledge of biochemistry is quintessential. It encompasses the study of the structure and function of biomolecules, biochemical reactions they undergo to maintain a normal healthy life. The enzymatic reactions involving various biomolecules are part of the anabolic and catabolic pathways. The study of these metabolic pathways including their regulation, bioenergetics (energy yielded or consumed) and the defects that may be present in these pathways (genetic or acquired), is what biochemistry is all about.

The knowledge of the structure of various biomolecules enhanced our understanding of the functions of these molecules and also helped to understand the basis of many diseases, for example, study of the structure of Hb helped to understand the affinity of Hb for O_2 and also explained the reason of sickle cell anemia due to HbS, i.e. an altered sequence of amino acids in Hb converts it into HbS (β-6-Glu-by-Val).

Optimally good health is a pre-requisite for a long life. The health, vigor and vitality of any individual are maintained by the nutrients present in the diet. The biochemical composition and functions of various nutritional components is studied as nutritional biochemistry. Various nutritional disorders like anorexia nervosa, obesity, night blindness, iron deficiency anemia, etc. are explained by their biochemical correlation and can be managed appropriately with a thorough knowledge of biochemistry.

All Life Sciences are Associated with Biochemistry

The study of biochemistry gives a foundation for the study all life sciences including physiology, pharmacology, pathology, microbiology, immunology, toxicology, and medicine. All these need the support of biochemistry for complete and thorough understanding. Physiology, the study of organ system functioning, completely overlaps with biochemistry. The effects of various drugs, their metabolism using various enzymes and clearance from the body are fully elucidated with the knowledge of biochemistry. Pathology of the tissues leads to biochemical alterations in these tissues, which are mirrored in the patients' serum profile of the biochemical parameters and will help in the diagnosis and treatment of the various diseases. Biochemical knowledge of the structure of bacterial cell wall and their released toxins help treat bacterial infections; in fact the knowledge of bacterial cell division and its need of folate have helped deduce the action of sulfa drugs as antibacterial agents. Biochemistry attenuates the understanding of effects of various poisons on the enzymatic reactions, which is the study of toxicology. Immunology has been incorporated as an important principle of many biochemical techniques like ELISA, RIA, chemiluminescence techniques for identifying and evaluating the presence of various biochemical markers.

Biochemistry is an Important Tool in a Physician's Armour

Biochemical analysis of the body fluids like whole blood, serum, plasma, CSF, amniotic fluid, etc. has greatly enhanced the knowledge regarding important diseases afflicting the humans. The biochemical parameters like sugar, urea, creatinine, cholesterol, triglycerides (TGs), various hormones, etc. can be evaluated using different biochemical techniques, the evaluation of serum total cholesterol, TGs and lipoproteins helps assess the potential risk of cardiovascular disorders (CVDs), or the evaluation of serum urea and creatinine would give an idea about the renal function.

The prime concern of the physicians today is not just to treat various diseases but also to make an early diagnosis of the diseases and effective management. This would help reduce morbid complications, improve the quality of patient's life and also ensure longevity.

Biochemistry in Dentistry

A sound knowledge of clinical biochemistry is of paramount importance in the field of dentistry. A dental physician has to be well versed with all the basic life sciences. Since, biochemistry is associated profoundly with all the fundamental life sciences, a sound knowledge of this subject would truly enhance the potentialities of a dental physician. A dentist should be capable of identifying and managing the medical problems that may be present in a patient prior to giving a dental treatment. This would help prevent development of a complication that may arise if not checked, for example, a diabetic patient with uncontrolled blood sugar may not be a suitable case for a dental surgical procedure, unless the blood sugar is managed. A simple blood test recommended prior to a dental surgical procedure for blood sugar level would be of great help to a dentist to infer the presence of DM and treat the patient accordingly.

Dentistry is an important branch of medicine as it incorporates the maintenance of the good oral hygiene and oral health of not just an individual but the community at large.

Section – 1

Chemistry of Biomolecules

- Chemistry of Carbohydrates
- Chemistry of Lipids
- Chemistry of Amino Acids and Proteins
- Chemistry of Nucleic Acids

CHAPTER

1

Chemistry of Carbohydrates

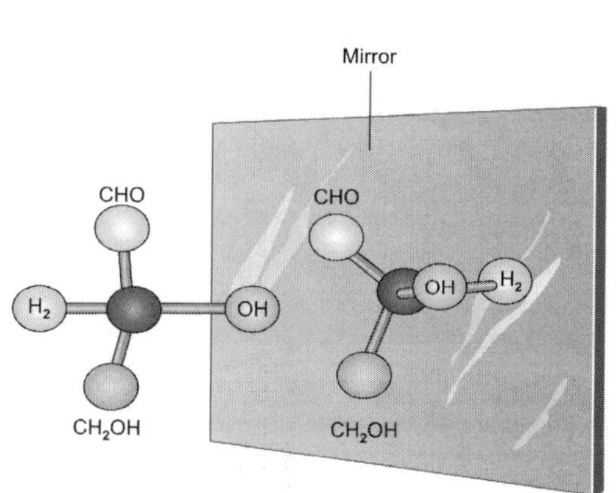

Chapter Framework

Introduction

Carbohydrates are the most abundantly found biomolecules. Plants synthesize carbohydrates using CO_2, H_2O and sunlight by photosynthesis. These carbohydrates synthesized by the plants are an important source of energy for the plants and almost all heterotrophs, including mammals. Humans are dependent upon the carbohydrates as the principal source of energy.

Chemical Composition of Carbohydrates

Chemically carbohydrates are composed of C, H and O, with an empirical formula $[CH_2O]_n$.

Definition of Carbohydrate

Carbohydrates can be defined as aldehyde or ketone derivatives of polyhydric alcohol or compounds, which yield the same on hydrolysis.

Classification of Carbohydrates

Carbohydrates can be classified into 4 major classes as shown in Figure 1.1.

1. *Monosaccharides*: These are the simplest carbohydrates that cannot be hydrolyzed into simpler units. For example, Glucose, fructose, galactose, etc. Monosaccharides can be classified further on the basis of functional group and number of carbon atoms (Table 1.1).
2. *Disaccharides:* These have two monosaccharide units linked together by a glycosidic linkage. For example lactose (glucose + galactose), maltose (glucose + glucose), sucrose (glucose + fructose).

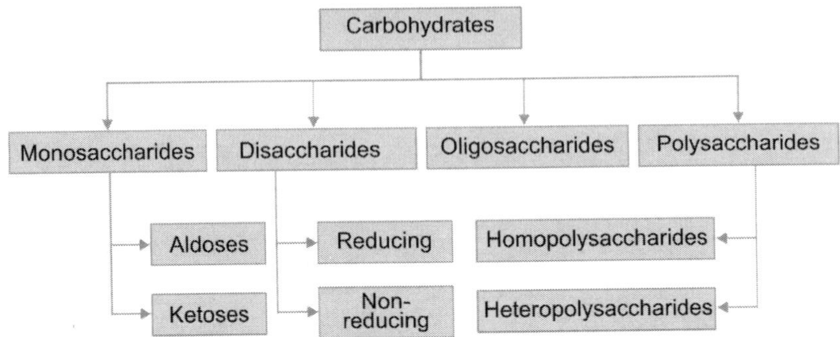

Fig 1.1 Classification of carbohydrates

Table 1.1 Classification of monosaccharides

Carbon atoms	*Aldoses*	*Ketoses*
C3	Glycerose	Dihydroxy acetone
C4	Erythrose	Erythrulose
C5	Ribose	Ribulose
C6	Glucose	Fructose
C7	Glucoheptose	Sedoheptulose

Table 1.2 Classification of disaccharide

Reducing disaccharide	*Nonreducing disaccharide*
Lactose (β1–4)	Sucrose (α1–2)
Maltose (α1–4)	Trehalose (α1–1)

Disaccharides can be further classified as reducing and nonreducing depending upon the presence of a potentially free aldehyde or ketone group (Table 1.2).

- Reducing disaccharides have a potentially-free aldehyde or ketone group.
- Nonreducing disaccharides do not have a potentially-free aldehyde or ketone group.

3. *Oligosaccharides:* These are made up of 3–9 monosaccharide units linked up by glycosidic linkage, e.g. Raffinose (glucose+galactose+fructose).
4. *Polysaccharides:* These are made up of more than 10–1000s of monosaccharide units polymerized by glycosidic linkage. These are of two types—
   - Homopolysaccahrides—Containing similar monosaccharide units, e.g. starch, glycogen, cellulose, inulin, chitin, etc.
   - Heteropolysaccharides—Made up of dissimilar repeating units comprising of uronic acid and amino sugars, e.g. hyaluronic acid, heparin, chondroitin, keratan, blood group substances, etc.

Functions of Carbohydrates

Carbohydrates are synthesized by the plants during photosynthesis. Starch is synthesized during the process. Starch is the chief source of energy in humans. Besides acting as the source of energy, carbohydrates play several other significant roles as shown in the Table 1.3A and B.

Table 1.3A Functions of monosaccharides and disaccharides

Carbohydrate	*Sources*	*Function/Biomedical importance*
Monosaccharides C3: Glyceraldehyde Dihydroxy acetone phosphate (DHAP)	–	Intermediates of glycolysis Intermediates of glycolysis
C4: Erythrose, Erythrulose	–	Intermediates of HMP shunt Intermediates of HMP shunt
C5: Ribose Ribulose	Nucleic acids	Synthesis of RNA, NAD, NADP, FAD, FMN Intermediate of HMP shunt
C6: Glucose	Sweet fruits, honey, sugar	Principle sugar of blood FBS—70–110 mg/dL Exclusive fuel of brain, CNS, RBCs Adds up to BSL by conversion to glucose at liver
Fructose	Honey, fruits	High energy intermediates of glycolysis Adds up to BSL by conversion to glucose at liver
Galactose	Milk and milk products	Component of gangliosides, cerebrosides, thus help in brain development
Disaccharides *Reducing* lactose (Gluc + Galac) (β 1 – 4)	Milk and milk products	Adds up to BSL by conversion to glucose at liver Component of gangliosides, cerebrosides, thus help in brain development
Maltose (α 1 – 4) (Gluc + Gluc)	Germinated cereals, starch hydrolysis	Adds up to BSL by conversion at liver to glucose
Nonreducing disaccharides Sucrose (α 1 – 2) (Gluc + Fruc)	Table sugar, sugar beet, sugar cane, jaggery, fruit juices	Adds up to BSL by conversion to glucose at liver

Abbreviation: HMP, Hexose monophosphote shunt; BSL, Blood sugar level

Table 1.3B Functions of polysaccharides

Carbohydrate	*Sources*	*Function/Biomedical importance*
Homopolysaccahrides Starch (α1–4 and α1–6) [Glucan]	Cereals, legumes, tuberous vegetables	Adds up to BSL
Dextrin (α1–4 and α1–6) [Glucan]	Partial hydrolysis of starch	Adds up to BSL
Glycogen (α1–4 and α1–6 [Glucan]	5% by weight in liver 1% by weight in muscles	Liver glycogen—adds up to BSL Muscle glycogen—provides energy for muscle contraction
Cellulose (β1–4) [Glucan]	All vegetarian food since plant cell wall is made of cellulose	Helps in proper bowl motility Prevents constipation Forms bulk of diet and gives satiety Lowers serum cholesterol Improves glucose tolerance
Inulin (β 1–2) [Fructosan]	Roots of artichoke, dahlia, dandelions	Helps in estimation of GFR

Contd...

Contd...

Chitin (β 1–4) (N-acetylglucoseamine)	Exoskeleton of crustaceans	Protection of crustaceans
Heteropolysaccharides Hyaluronic acid (N-acetylglucosamine + glucuronic acid)	Skin, umbilical cord, synovial fluid	It is the ground cementing substance of mesenchymal tissue
Heparin (N-acetylglucosamine + iduronic acid	Lungs, mast cells, arterial walls, spleen	In-vivo anticoagulant
Chondroitin (N-acetylgalactosamine + glucuronic acid)	Cartilage, bones	Gives compressibility to cartilages
Keratan (N-acetylglucosamine + galactose)	Cornea, cartilage, intervertebral disks	Transparency of cornea
Blood group substances (glucose, fructose, galactose, glucose NH_2)	Membrane of RBCs	Specifies the blood group

Monosaccharides Structure

- The monosaccharides can be represented by a straight chain structure (Fischer projection) and by ring structure (Haworth projections).
- The Haworth projections are thermodynamically more stable and naturally occurring sugars exist in these ring structure forms.
- The rings can be either 5 membered (furanose rings) or 6 membered (pyranose rings).
- Naturally occurring glucose is present as glucopyranose form and fructose as fructofuranose form (Figs 1.2A and B).

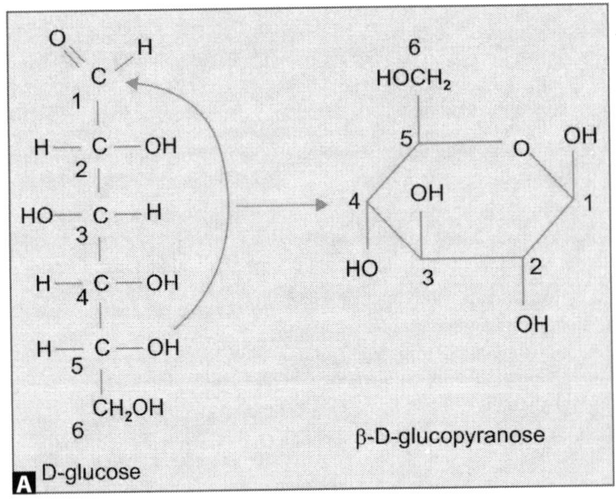

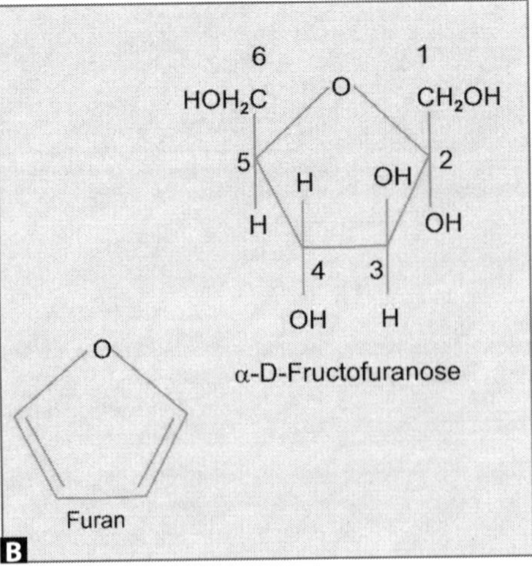

Figs 1.2A and B Fischer projections and Haworth projections

Monosaccharides Show Isomerism

Isomers are compounds having the same molecular formula and different structural formula. This phenomenon is termed as isomerism. Carbohydrates show the following types of isomerism:

- *Aldose-ketose*—Sugars which have the same molecular formula but differ in the functional groups i.e. one isomer has aldehyde group and the other isomer has ketone group. Thus show aldose – ketose isomerism, e.g. Glucose and fructose.
- *Stereoisomerism*—The sugars having same molecular and structural formula but differ in the spatial arrangement of the H and –OH group about the penultimate carbon atom. When the OH group is on right hand side (RHS), it is termed as the 'D' isomer and when on left hand side (LHS), it is termed as 'L' isomer. Such isomers are mirror images of each other, e.g. D – glyceraldehyde and L – glyceraldehyde (Figs 1.3A and B).
- *Penultimate carbon is the carbon just next to the primary alcoholic group of a monosaccharide.*
- *Optical isomerism*—Stereoisomers contain a chiral (asymmetric) C atom, therefore show optical activity i.e. rotate plane of polarized light. The solutions of sugars which rotate the plane of polarized light towards right are termed as dextro rotatory, depicted by (d) or (+). The sugar solutions that rotate the plane of polarised light towards left are termed as levo rotatory, depicted by (l) or (–). An equimolar mixture of (D) and (L) forms do not deviate the plane of polarized light. This is the racemic mixture.
- *Diastereo isomers* are isomers with more than one chiral center. Pairs of isomers that have opposite configurations at one or more of the chiral centers but that are not mirror images of each other.
- *Epimerism*—Epimers are diastereoisomers that differ at only one carbon atom. Epimers are formed due to difference in orientation of the H and OH group about a carbon atom other than the penultimate carbon atom and the phenomenon they show is epimerism, e.g. Glucose and Mannose are C2 epimers and Glucose and Galactose are C4 epimers.
- *Anomerism*—The straight chain structures of the carbohydrates (Fischer projections) are thermodynamically unstable. The stable structures of naturally occurring sugars are cyclic structures (Haworth projections). These cyclic structures are formed by the reaction between

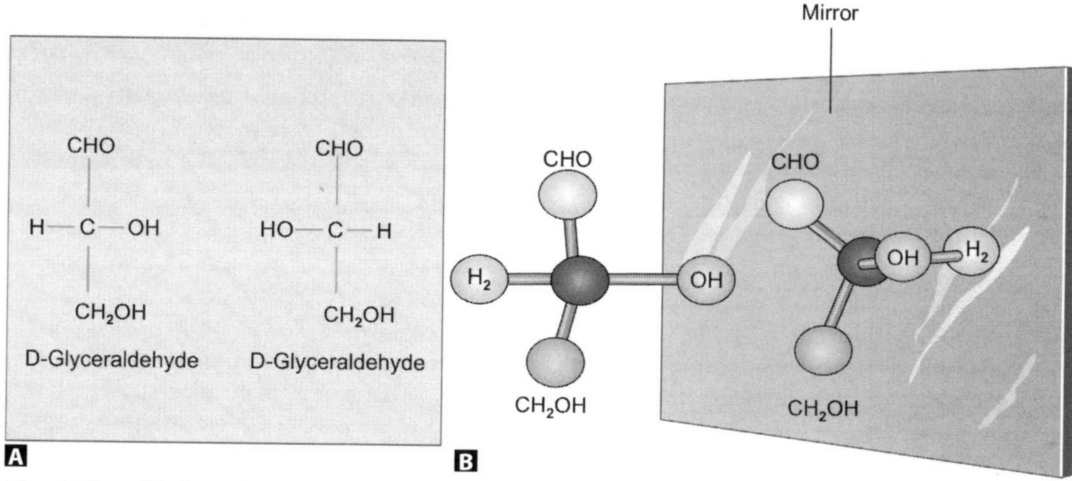

Figs 1.3A and B Stereoisomers of glyceraldehyde

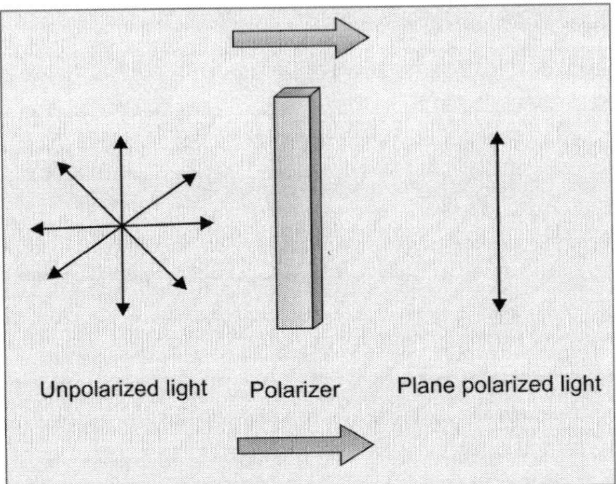

Fig. 1.4 Optical rotation

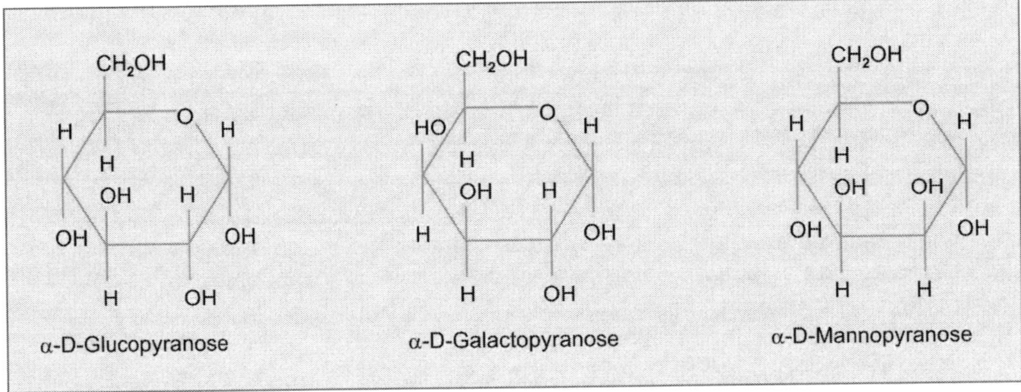

Fig. 1.5 Epimers of glucose

the carbonyl group (-CHO or – C=O) and the –OH group. When the ring structure is formed between –CHO and –OH group, it is termed as the hemiacetal ring (Fig. 1.6). When the linkage is formed between – C=O group and –OH group, it is termed as hemiketal ring. This ring formation gives rise a new chiral carbon atom, i.e. the carbonyl carbon which is now termed as the anomeric carbon. Depending upon the orientation of H and OH group about this anomeric carbon, the sugars maybe either alpha (α) or beta (β) anomers. When the OH group is on the RHS, the sugar is alpha anomer and when on LHS, it is beta anomer. These anomers also rotate the plane of polarized light. This phenomenon is termed as anomerism.

- If the hydroxyl group attached to this carbon atom projects below plane of the ring, it is known as the α-anomer. In the β-anomer, it projects above the plane of the ring. Naturally occurring glucose is mostly β – D Glucopyranose.
- Most common sugars can form either a 5 membered furanose ring or a 6 membered pyranose ring. But the naturally occurring glucose is predominantly a glucopyranose and fructose, the ketosugar is fructofuranose (Figs 1.7 and 1.8).

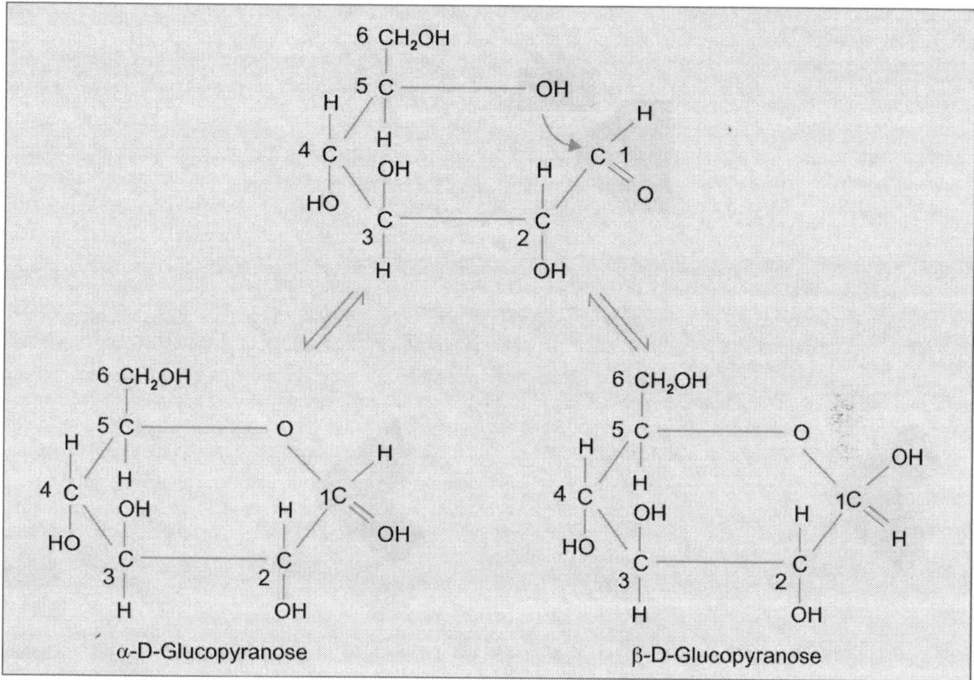

Fig. 1.6 Formation of hemiacetal linkage

- *Mutarotation*—When glucose is crystallized from boiling pyridine and redissolved, the solution shows an optical activity of + 19° i.e. it is the β – D glucose. On keeping this solution overnight, the optical rotation stabilises to + 52.5°. Similarly, on crystallising glucose from alcohol-water mixture, the crystals on redissolving show an optical rotation of +112° i.e. it is α – D glucose, which stabilises to +52.5°, on keeping overnight. This phenomenon of the change in the specific optical rotation of a sugar solution over duration of time due to interconversion of the alpha and the beta anomers through an open chain aldehydo form is termed as mutarotation. At equilibrium 36% is alpha form, 64 % is beta form and less than 0.3% is the open chain form.

Chemical Properties of Monosaccharides

Oxidation

Monosaccharides on oxidation with different oxidizing agents form acids of different types depending upon the strength of oxidizing agent.

a. *Weak oxidizing agents (Br_2 water)*
   - In presence of weak oxidizing agents aldonic acid is formed by oxidation of aldehyde group to carboxylic acid, e.g. Glucose gives gluconic acid.
b. *Strong oxidizing agents (HNO_3)*
   - In presence of strong oxidizing agent saccharic acid is formed by oxidation of both aldehyde and primary alcohol group into – COOH group, e.g. glucose gives glucaric acid.

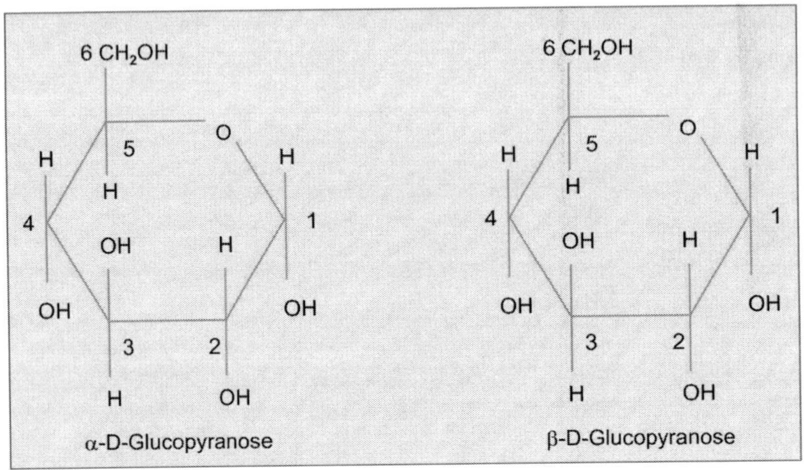

Fig. 1.7 Anomeric forms of glucose

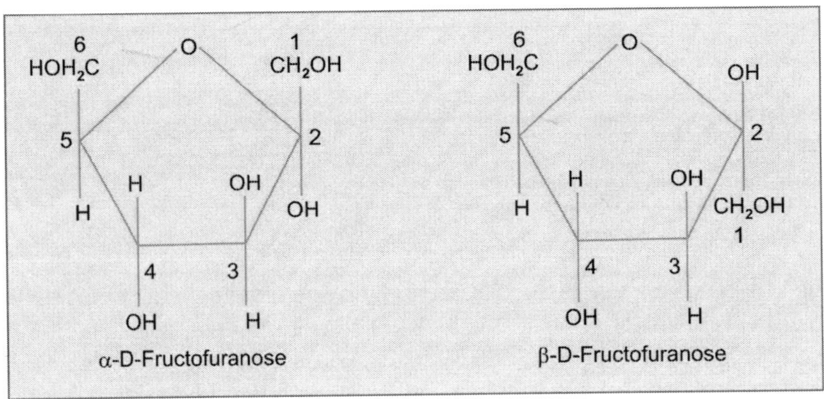

Fig. 1.8 Anomeric forms of fructose

c. *Special conditions (Enzymes of uronic acid pathway)*
   - Uronic acid is formed in presence of oxidative enzymes of uronic acid pathway by first protecting the aldehyde group and then the primary alcoholic group is oxidized, e.g. glucose gives glucuronic acid.
   Importance in Conjugation of – Bilirubin, Steroid hormones, Drugs.

Reduction

Reduction by Na–amalgam gives rise to sugar alcohols.

Glucose → Sorbitol

Mannose → Mannitol

Fructose → Sorbitol and mannitol

Applied significance
- Sorbitol accumulates in lens of eye in diabetes to cause diabetic cataract
- Mannitol is used to reduce intracranial tension by forced diuresis

Action of Strong Acids

Monosaccharides are dehydrated to furfural derivatives in presence of strong acids (H_2SO_4, HCl), which condense with aromatic compounds to give specific color, e.g. Molisch's test—α-naphthol, Selivanoff' test—resorcinol.

Action of Strong Alkali

Strong alkali causes the monosaccharides to caramelize. When carbohydrates are heated at high temperatures, they are converted into a brown colored degradation product, caramel.

Action of Weak Alkali

Enediol is formed (Fig. 1.9). (Interconversion of monosaccharides):

The enediols are strong reducing agents and their formation during the Benedict's test of monosaccharides causes reduction of the Cu^{+2} into Cu^{+} ions, which gives the red precipitate of Cu_2O.

Formation of Osazones (Figs 1.10 and 1.11)

This is another reaction given by carbohydrates that possess a free aldehyde or ketone group. The reaction involves carbon atoms 1 and 2 of the aldoses and ketoses. When the carbohydrate is heated with phenyl hydrazine in a boiling water-bath in the presence of acetate buffer (pH 4.3), a series of reactions occur leading to the formation of osazone of the given carbohydrate.

- Since the differences between carbon atoms 1 and 2 are obliterated in these reactions, those carbohydrates that differ only with respect these two carbon atoms, e.g. glucose, mannose and fructose, will form identical osazones. Crystals of lactose are cotton puff-shaped and maltose is sunflower-shaped.

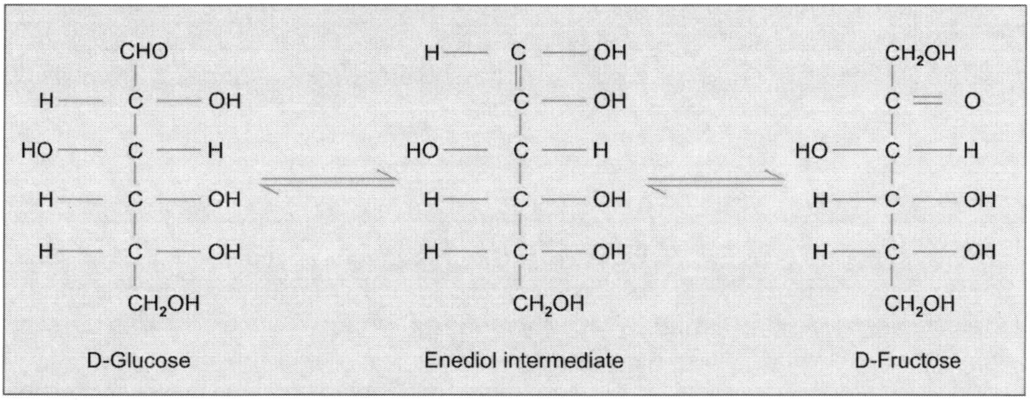

D-Glucose ⇌ Enediol intermediate ⇌ D-Fructose

Fig. 1.9 Enediol formation

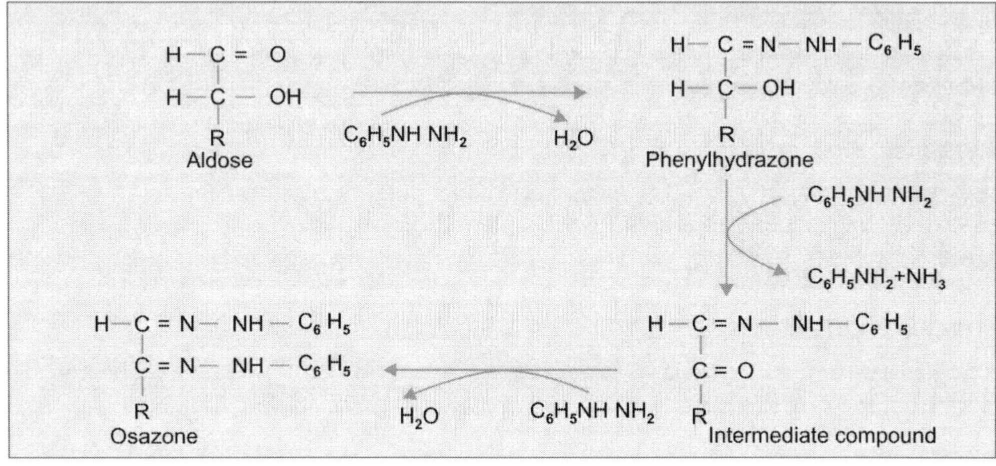

Fig. 1.10 Osazone reaction

Properties due to –OH Groups

Substitution of OH groups on a monosaccharide gives rise to sugar derivatives like amino sugar, e.g. Glucose amine, galactose amine. These sugars maybe further acetylated to form N-acetyl amino sugars, which are important components of heteropolysaccharides (mucoploysaccharides – MPS); antibiotic erythromycin is an amino sugar.

Glycosides

Monosaccharides react with another monosaccharide or noncarbohydrate compound (aglycone) by eliminating a molecule of water between OH groups of the 2 molecules and forms a glycosidic linkage. Such a compound when formed by 2 or more monosaccharide is a disaccharide or trisaccahride and so on. Conversely, if the glycosidic linkage is formed between a monosaccharide and an aglycone, it is termed as a glycoside. An aglycone can be an alcohol, sterol, glycerol, etc. For example, cardiac glycosides – digitonin (aglycone is digitoxin), ouabain (aglycone is sterols).

Deoxy Sugars

Elimination of H atom from an – OH group of a monosaccharide forms a deoxysugar. For example, Ribose deoxysugar is converted into 2–deoxy ribose.

Disaccharides

- Disaccharides are natural sugars presents in fruits and vegetables like maltose, sucrose or milk sugar lactose. They give the sweet taste to the fruits, vegetables, and milk.
- Disaccharides are formed by linking 2 monosaccharide units together by a glycosidic linkage.
- The linkage involves the OH group of the anomeric carbon and an OH group from the second monosaccharide which may or may not be from anomeric carbon atom.
- The disaccharide may be reducing or nonreducing depending upon the presence of a free or potentially free carbonyl group.

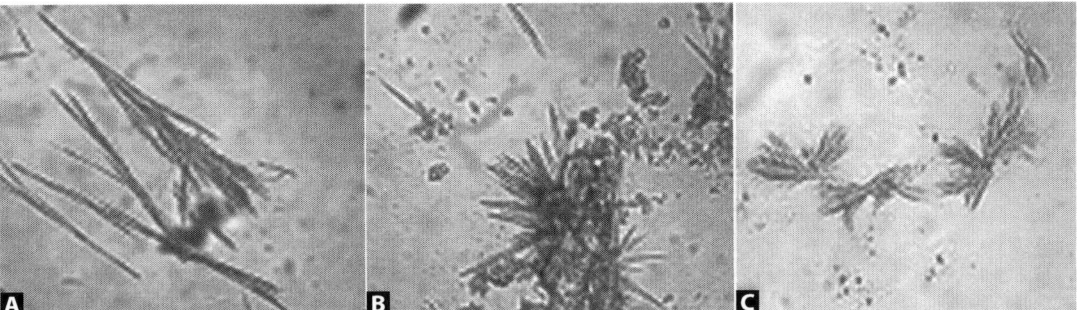

Figs 1.11A to C Osazone of glucose, lactose and maltose

Nonreducing Disaccharides

If both the carbon atoms involved in the glycosidic linkage are anomeric carbon atoms, there is no free or potentially-free carbonyl group, thus the sugar is nonreducing, e.g. sucrose, trehalose.

Reducing Disaccharides

When anomeric carbon of one monosaccharide forms a glycosidic linkage with a nonanomeric carbon of the next monosaccharide, the disaccharide formed has a potentially-free carbonyl group making it reducing in nature, e.g. lactose, maltose.

Lactose (Fig. 1.12)

- It is also termed as the milk sugar since it is present in milk.
- It is secreted by mammary glands during lactation.
- It is the prime source of energy for a new born infant.
- It is reducing in nature and is made up of glucose and galactose, linked up by β–1-4 glycosidic linkage.
- The galactose part of lactose is an important component of brain glycolipids. Thus, lactose is significant for proper brain development.
- Galactose also adds up to the BSL by converting to glucose at liver, using the hepatic enzymes of galactose metabolism.

Maltose (Fig. 1.13)

- It is abundantly present in the germinating cereals, as it is formed by the hydrolysis of starch by the amylase present in these seeds.
- Maltose is also termed as the 'malt sugar'.
- Maltose is a reducing disaccharide, comprising of 2 glucose units linked up by α-1-4 glycosidic linkage.
- The glucose units in maltose if present in beta anomeric form, the linkage formed is beta glycosidic linkage and it is beta maltose.
- Maltose is also synthesized in the gut during the partial hydrolysis of starch and dextrin.
- It gets completely hydrolyzed by a disaccahridases, maltase at the intestinal brush borders into 2 units of glucose, thus adding up to BSL.

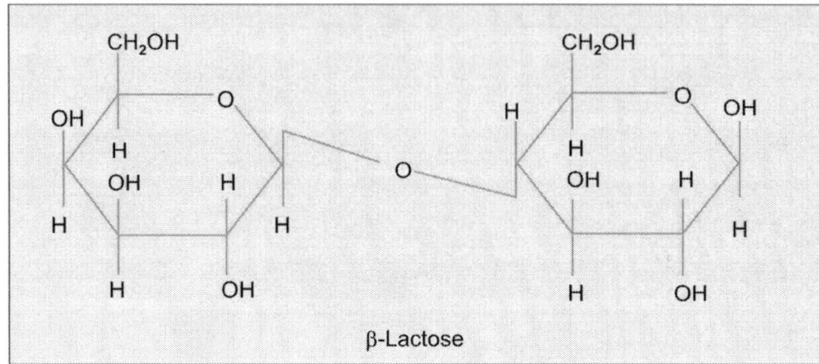

Fig.1.12 Lactose

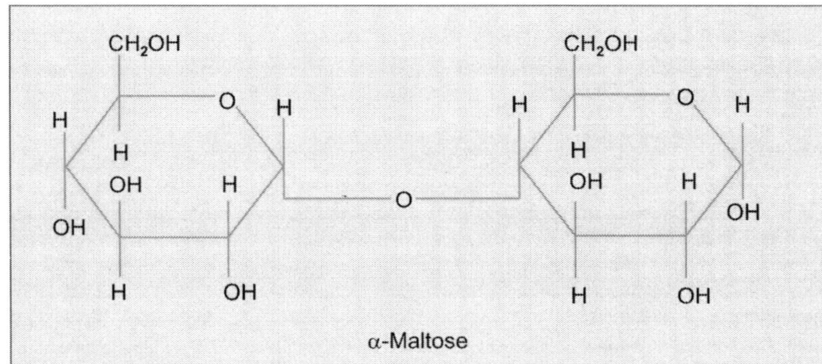

Fig.1.13 Maltose

Sucrose (Fig. 1.14)

- Sucrose is a nonreducing disaccharide constituted of a monosaccharide unit of glucose linked by an alpha 1–2 glycosidic linkage to a fructose unit.
- The linkage involves the aldehyde group of glucose and the keto group of fructose, so that there is no free or potentially-free carbonyl group.
- Sucrose is naturally present in sugar cane, sugar beet, jaggery, fruit juices etc.
- Sucrose has a specific optical rotation of + 66.5° i.e. it is dextrorotatory.
- However, on hydrolysis it gives an equimolar mixture of glucose and fructose which shows an optical rotation of – 92.3°. This is due to the greater levorotation of fructose (– 92.3°) than glucose (+52.5°). Such hydrolysis mixture is termed as invert solution and the process as 'inversion'.
- Invert sugar (equimolar mixture of glucose and fructose) is naturally present in honey.

Chemical Properties of Disaccharides

- Disaccharides react with the strong acids (H_2SO_4) to be dehydrated and form furfural derivatives that condense with aromatic compounds like alpha naphthol to give a positive Molisch's test.
- Like the monosaccharides, reducing disaccharides reduce the metal ions (Cu^{+2} to Cu^{+}) in a mildly alkaline medium. Thus, give a positive Benedict's and Fehling's test.

- Reducing disaccharides react with the phenyl hydrazine hydrochloride in presence of sodium acetate and glacial acetic acid to form osazone crystals of characteristic shape. Lactose—cotton puff-shaped and Maltose—sunflower-shaped.

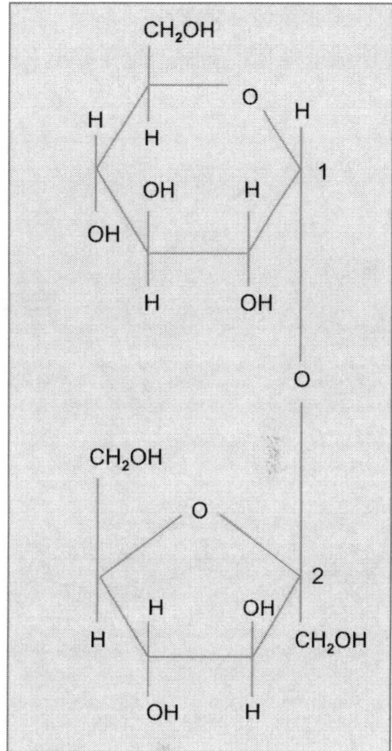

Fig. 1.14 Sucrose

Polysaccharides

- Polysaccharides are polymers of monosaccharides with more than 10 monosaccharide units, linked up by glycosidic linkages. These can be classified further as—
  - *Homopolysaccahrides*
  - *Heteropolysaccharides.*

Homopolysaccahrides

Containing similar monosaccharide units, e.g. Starch, dextrin, glycogen, cellulose, inulin, chitin etc.

Starch (Fig. 1.15)

- Starch is a 'glucan', i.e. it is made up of repeating units of glucose.
- It has 2 components—water-soluble amylose and water-insoluble amylopectin (Table 1.4).
- Starch is present in cereals, legumes, fruits and tuberous vegetables.
- It is the principal dietary carbohydrate and the chief source of energy in vegetarians.
- Starch gets hydrolyzed during digestion by the action of an α 1–4 amylolytic enzyme—amylase. This enzyme hydrolyze the alpha 1–4 glycosidic linkages.
- Two amylases are present in the human body—a salivary amylase that hydrolyses only boiled starch and a pancreatic amylase that hydrolyzes both boiled and unboiled starch.

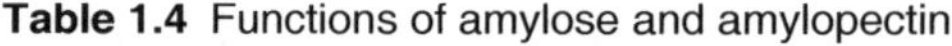

Table 1.4 Functions of amylose and amylopectin

Amylose	*Amylopectin*
Soluble in water	Insoluble in water
80–90% of total starch	10–20% of total starch
Unbranched	Branched
α-1-4 linkage in the straight chain part	α-1–4 linkage in straight chain part and alpha 1–6 at branch points
Low molecular weight	High molecular weight
300 glucose units	1000 glucose units
Gives blue color with iodine solution	Gives violet color with starch

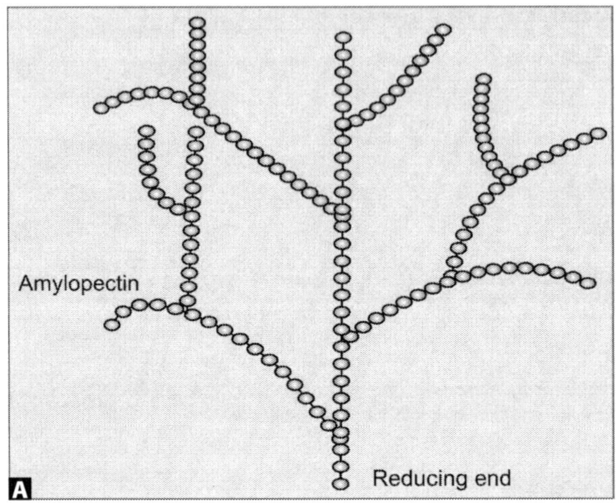

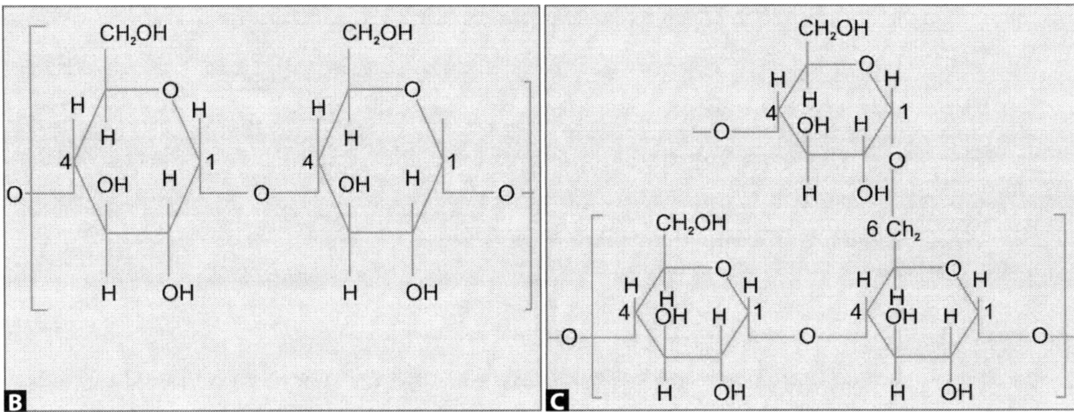

Figs 1.15A to C Starch molecule with α1–4 and α 1–6 linkage

- Starch on hydrolysis gives rise to smaller branched molecules called dextrin, which on further hydrolysis gives maltose and finally maltose is completely hydrolyzed to glucose. Thus the principal role of starch is to add up to the BSL.

Dextrin

- It is a branched 'glucan'.
- The glycosidic linkage is α 1–4 in the straight chain part and α 1–6 at the branch points.
- Dextrin is formed by the partial hydrolysis of starch.
- Depending upon the chain length, dextrins may be erythrodextrin (gives red color with starch), amylodextrin (gives violet color with starch), achrodextrin (gives no color with starch).

Glycogen (Fig. 1.16)

- It is also termed as the 'animal starch'.

- It is a branched 'glucan' with α 1–4 in the straight chain part and α 1–6 at the branch points.
- However, it is more compact in structure as compared with the starch molecule.
- The branching in glycogen molecule is more frequent and branch point is seen every 12–18 glucose units as opposed to that of starch after every 24–30 glucose units.
- This compact nature of the glycogen molecule is important for storing a greater number of glucose units in a smaller area.
- The center of the glycogen molecule has a protein molecule attached, termed as 'glycogenin'.

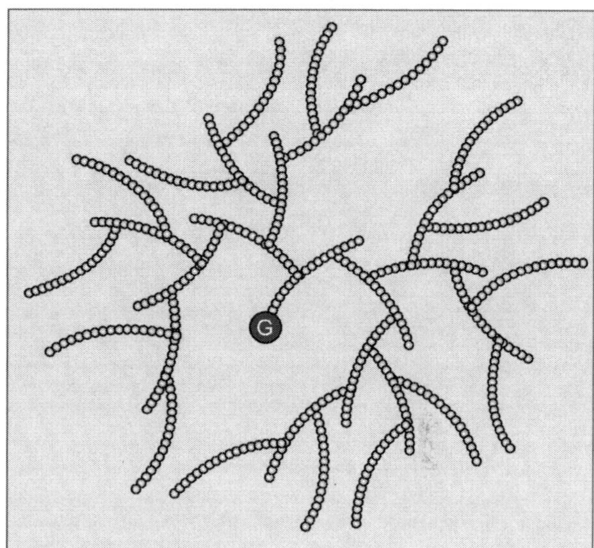

Fig. 1.16 Glycogen

- The glycogenin molecule acts as a primer and a backbone during the process of glycogenesis, on which the new glycogen molecule gets synthesized.
- It is the stored form of carbohydrates in animals and is stored at liver (5% by weight of liver) and at muscles (1% by weight of muscles).
- The liver glycogen breaks down during the process of glycogenolysis and augments the BSL to maintain the BSL during fasting and in between meals.
- The muscle glycogen is used as an energy source during muscle contraction. It cannot add up to the BSL owing to the lack of a key gluconeogenesis enzyme, glucose – 6 – phosphatase.
- Glycogen gives reddish brown color on reacting with iodine.

Cellulose (Fig. 1.17)

- It is an unbranched 'Glucan'.
- The glucose units of cellulose are linked up in a β 1 – 4 glycosidic linkage.
- Cellulose is constituent of plant cell wall, thus is the most abundant carbohydrate.
- It is the dietary insoluble fibers.
- As the dietary fibers, it plays significant role in:
  - Forming the bulk of diet.
  - Giving satiety or a feeling of stomach fullness without consumption of an excess of calories.
  - Improving the bowl motility, thus preventing constipation.
  - Helps maintain normal serum cholesterol. This is due to the adsorption of the dietary cholesterol to these fibers, which reduces the absorption of the dietary cholesterol.
  - Reduce the rate of gastric emptying, thus helps improve the glucose tolerance. This would be of great value to the diabetic patients.

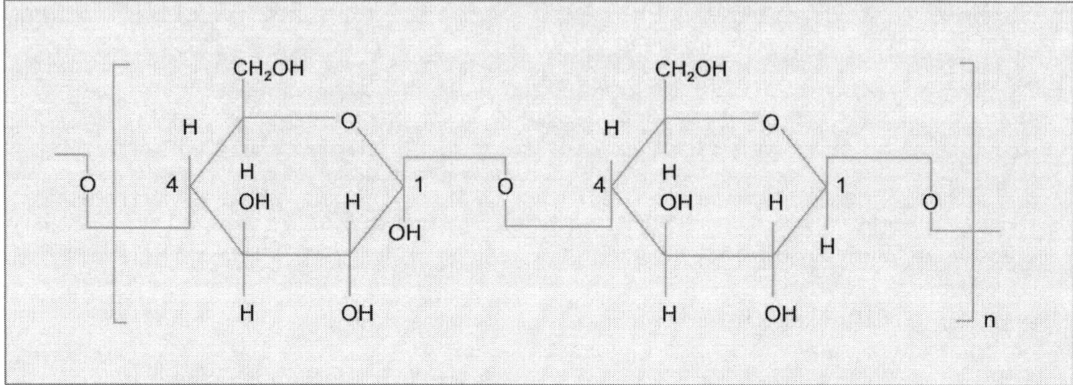

Fig. 1.17 Cellulose

Inulin (Fig. 1.18)

- It is a 'fructan'.
- It is present in the tubers of dahlia, artichoke, dandelions.
- The fructose units are linked by β 1–2 glycosidic linkage.
- It has a unique property that if injected parentally it gets completely excreted by the renal tubules, without getting metabolized.
- Once filtered it is neither reabsorbed by the renal tubules nor further secreted. Thus it gives the true value of the glomerular filtration rate (GFR).

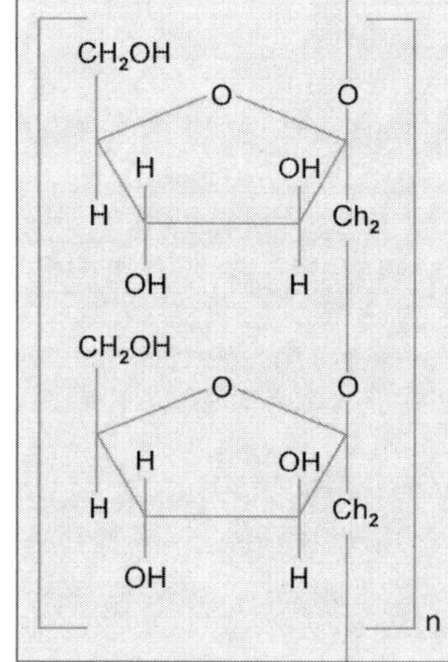

Fig. 1.18 Inulin with β 1 – 2 glycosidic linkage

Heteropolysaccharides

Made up of dissimilar repeating units comprising of uronic acid and amino sugars, e.g. hyaluronic acid, heparin, chondroitin, keratan, blood group substances, etc.

Hyaluronic Acid (Fig. 1.19)

- It is composed of repeating units of [N-acetyl glucose amine and glucuronic acid] N-linked together by a beta 1–3 glycosidic linkage.
- The hyaluronic acid is an important constituent of the ground cementing substance of the mesenchymal tissue. Being hygroscopic it imbibes water and cements the cells together.
- It thus has a wide distribution.
- It also acts as a lubricant and shock absorber in the synovial joint cavities and protects the synovial membrane against the wear n tear.
- Besides, hyaluronic acid is also present in skin and umbilical cord.
- Sperm head secretes the enzyme hyalurinidase, which helps it to penetrate the ovum. Similarly, bacteria possessing this enzyme activity cause infection by hydrolyzing the hyaluronic acid of the ground substance of tissues.

Heparin (Figs 1.20 and 1.21)

- It is composed of repeating units of [sulfated N – acetyl glucose amine and sulfated iduronic acid linked up by α 1–4 glycosidic linkage.
- Iduronic acid is the L isomer of D glucuronic acid.
- It is an important in-vivo anticoagulant.
- It is secreted by mast cells, liver, spleen, lungs, and walls of large arteries.
- Heparin binds with antithrombin III and activates it, which in turn inactivates thrombin, factor IX and factor X. Thus prevent the formation of active fibrin.

Chondroitin (Fig. 1.22)

- It is made up of [glucuronic acid and N-acetyl galactose amine sulfate]$_n$.
- The glycosidic bonds are similar to those in hyaluronic acid β 1–3 linkage.
- There are two types of chondroitin sulfate, chondroitin-4-sulphate and Chondroitin-6-sulphate.
- It is mainly found in cartilages and bones. It is present in some other tissues also but in very small amounts.
- It is responsible for the compressibility of cartilages.

Keratan Sulfate

- It is composed of repeating units of [N – acetyl glucose amine and galactose]$_n$.
- The linkage is β 1–3 glycosidic linkage.
- It is abundantly present in various tissues like—cornea (transparency of cornea), costal cartilages, intervertebral disks, and walls of aorta.

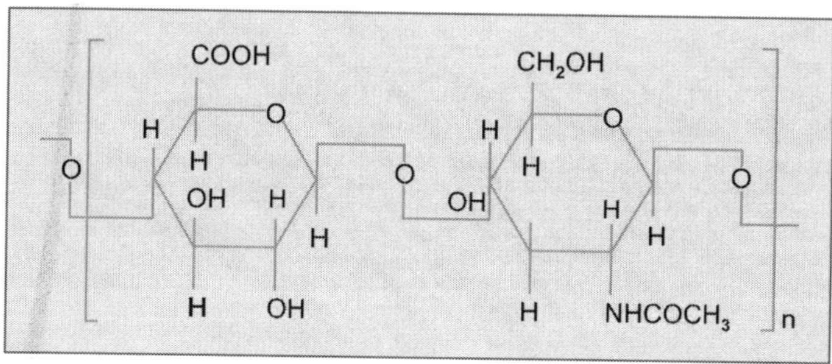

Fig. 1.19 Hyaluronic acid

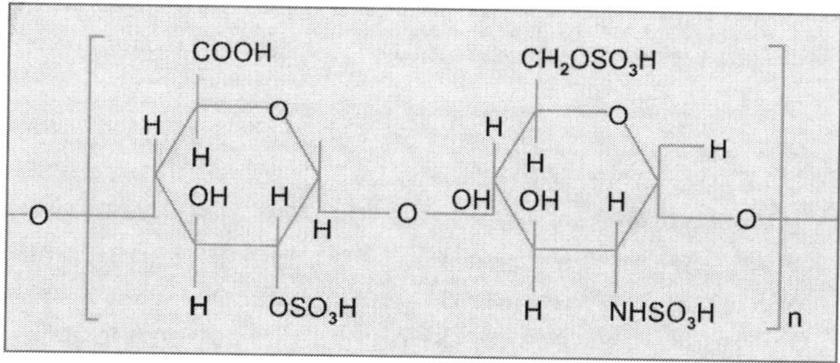

Fig. 1.20 Heparin

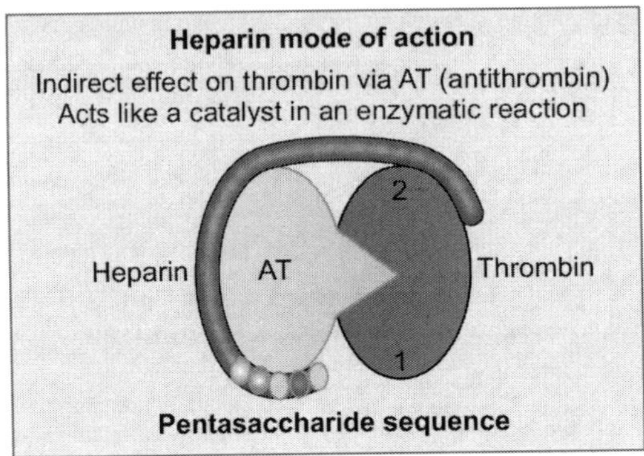

Fig. 1.21 Mode of action of heparin

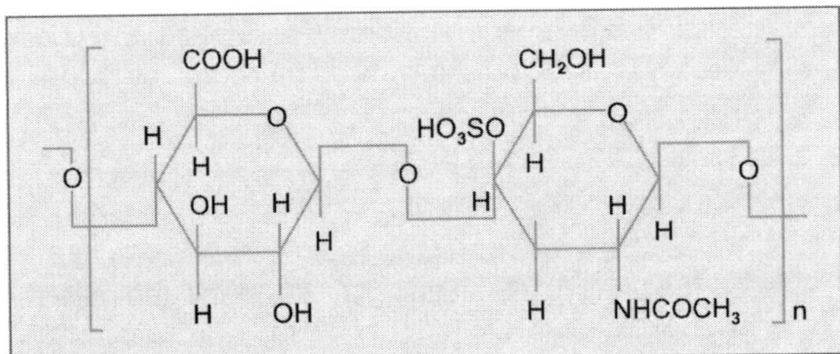

Fig. 1.22 Chondroitin sulfate

Blood Group Substances

- These are glycoproteins present on the RBC membranes.
- The carbohydrate moieties present in these glycoproteins are MPS, made up of repeating units of glucose, fructose, galactose, glucosamine.
- They provide the blood group specificity to the RBCs.

Applied Aspect of Mucopolysaccharides

Mucopolysaccharidoses

- The mucopolysaccharidoses are a group of inherited metabolic diseases caused by the absence or malfunctioning of certain enzymes needed to breakdown glycosaminoglycan.
- Lysosomal enzymes cause the breakdown of MPS. When these enzymes are deficient, MPS accumulate in cells of cornea, cartilages, and bones.
- The mucopolysaccharidoses share many clinical features but have varying degrees of severity.
- Typical symptoms like—bone deformities, deafness, mental retardation and corneal clouding are seen. These features may not be apparent at birth but progress as storage of glycosaminoglycan affects bone, skeletal structure, connective tissues, and organs.
- Neurological complications may include damage to neurons, as well as pain and impaired motor function. This results from compression of nerves or nerve roots in the spinal cord or in the peripheral nervous system.

- *Mental retardation*—Depending on the mucopolysaccharidoses subtype, affected individuals may have normal intellect or may be profoundly *mentally retarded*, may experience developmental delay, or may have *severe behavioral problems*.
- *Deafness*—Many individuals have hearing loss, either conductive, neuro-sensitive, or both.
- *Corneal clouding*—The eye's cornea often becomes cloudy from intracellular storage of MPS and degeneration of the retina. Glaucoma also may affect the patient's vision.
- *Physical symptoms* generally include coarse or rough facial features:
  - Including a flat nasal bridge
  - Thick lips and enlarged mouth and tongue
  - Short stature with disproportionately short trunk (dwarfism)
  - Dysplasia (abnormal bone size and/or shape) and other skeletal irregularities
  - Thickened skin
  - Enlarged organs, such as liver or spleen, hernias, and excessive body hair growth.
- Recurring respiratory infections are common, as are obstructive airway disease and obstructive sleep apnea.
- Many affected individuals also have heart disease, often involving enlarged or diseased heart valves.
- Some typical examples of mucopolysaccharidoses are *Hurler's disease, Hunter's and San filipo's diseases.*

A Quick Look at the Carbohydrates

- Carbohydrates are polyhydric aldehyde or ketones.
- Carbohydrates are classified into 4 major classes—monosaccharides, disaccharides, oligosaccharides and polysaccharides.
- Structurally, carbohydrates are made up of pyranose and furanose rings.
- Carbohydrates show isomerism—stereoisomerism, optical isomerism, epimerism and anomerism.
- Carbohydrates show mutarotation—change in specific optical rotation of sugar solutions over a time period.
- Carbohydrates with free or potentially free aldehyde or ketonic groups are reducing in nature and give reactions based on reducing property positive.
- Monosaccharides and reducing disaccharides form characteristically shaped osazone crystals.
- Homopolysaccahrides are polymers of identical monosaccharide units.
- Starch is the principal source of energy in vegetarians.
- Cellulose forms the dietary insoluble fibers.
- Glycogen is the animal starch.
- Liver glycogen maintains blood sugar level in between meals, and muscle glycogen gives energy for muscle contraction.
- Heteropolysaccharides are polymers of repeating units of [amino sugars + uronic acid].
- MPS storage disorders occur due to defect in the degradation of the MPS by lysosomal enzymes leading to skeletal deformities, corneal clouding, deafness and mental retardedness.

CHAPTER

2

Chemistry of Lipids

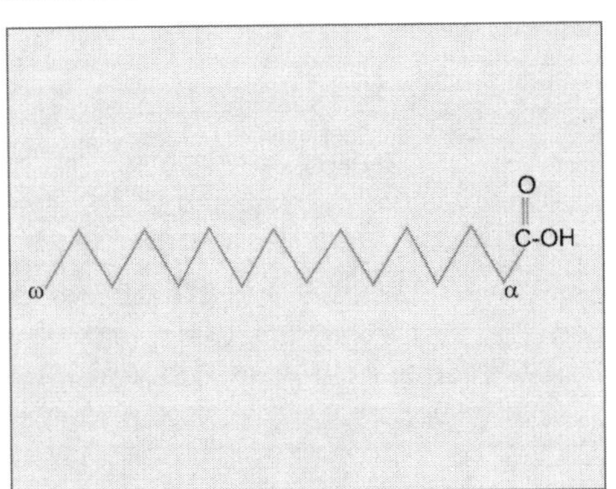

Chapter Framework

Introduction

Lipids are a diverse group of organic compounds. They are grouped together primarily due to their insolubility in water. Functionally the lipids are as diverse as their chemical nature—ranging from storage form of energy to their role as structural component of biologic membranes and as coenzymes for enzymes.

Definition

Lipids are a heterogeneous group of organic compounds characterized by solubility in non – polar solvents and insolubility in polar solvents. Chemically lipids can be defined as esters of fatty acids with certain alcohols.

Distribution

- Lipids are distributed widely in the animal kingdom—from the stored fat in adipose tissue of mammals to the waxy secretion of preen glands of birds that helps to keep their feathers waterproof.
- In the plants, lipids are present as waxy coating on the leaves, preventing the loss of water by transpiration, as stored form in nuts and seeds that acts as a source of energy during germination.
- Humans have lipids as stored form of energy in the adipose tissue. This provides the necessary energy during period of dearth. The calorific value of fat is 9 kcal/g.
- Dietary lipids are found in vegetable seeds, nuts, fish liver oil and eggs.

Functions of Lipids

- Dietary lipids are the cooking medium and give taste and palatability to food.
- Dietary lipids are the source of fat-soluble vitamins.
- Dietary lipids are the source of essential fatty acids.
- Lipids are present in the cell membrane as a phospholipid bilayer and are the provision for the structural integrity of the membrane.
- Excess calories are stored as triglycerides in adipose tissue.
- Lipid around the viscera protects them against shocks.
- Subcutaneous fat acts as an insulating layer against extremes of temperatures.
- Subcutaneous fat also gives shape and contour to body.
- Lipids present in the myelin sheath act as an insulating layer helping in saltatory conduction of nerve impulses.
- Amphipathic lipids like phospholipids help in emulsification of dietary fat during digestion.

Classification of Lipids (Flowchart. 2.1)

Simple Lipids

These are esters of fatty acids with certain alcohols like glycerol or other high molecular weight alcohols, e.g. oils, fats and waxes.

Compound Lipids

These are lipids which contain fatty acids, alcohol (Glycerol/ Sphingol) and other compounds like—phosphoric acid, N_2 base or protein in addition to fatty acids and alcohol, e.g. Phospholipids like—lecithin, sphingomyelin, lipoproteins like—LDLc, HDLc, VLDL, glycolipids like—cerebrosides, gangliosides.

Derived Lipids

These are compounds obtained on hydrolysis of simple and compound lipids but still possess the properties of lipids, e.g. fatty acids, glycerol, sterols like—cholesterol.

Flowchart 2.1 Classification of lipids

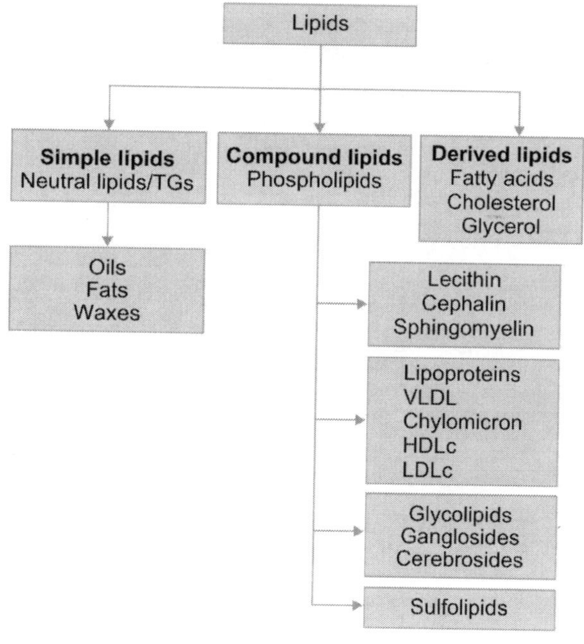

Derived Lipids

Fatty Acids

- Fatty acids are monocarboxylic acids ranging from C_4–C_{24}. These are aliphatic, unbranched and monocarboxylic acids.

Nomenclature (Fig. 2.1)

- They generally contain an even number of carbon atoms because two carbon atoms are added at a time during their synthesis. Each fatty acid possesses a carboxy terminal end and a methyl terminal (ω) end.
- The carbon atoms are numbered from the carboxy terminal, the carboxyl atom being numbered 1. The second, third and fourth carbon atoms are also known as α, β and γ carbon atoms respectively. The position of double bond is shown by sign of Δ.

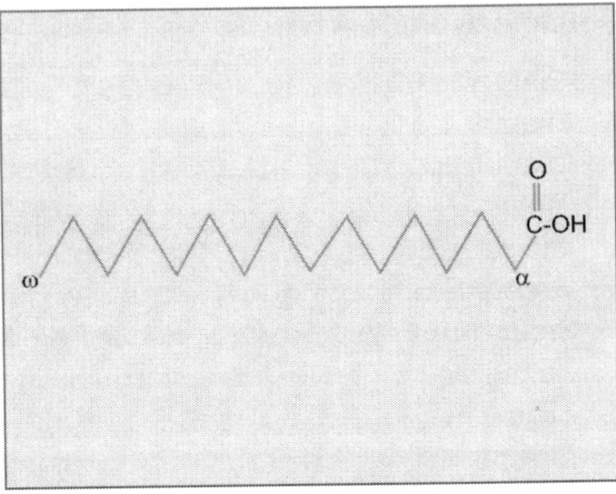

Fig. 2.1 Numbering of a saturated fatty acid

Isomerism

- The unsaturated fatty acids (FAs) show geometric isomerism, i.e. Cis-Trans due to presence of double bond. The naturally occurring fats contain cis-isomer predominately.

Types

- Fatty acids are of 2 types:
  - *Saturated Fatty acids*: The saturated fatty acids have no double bonds and are saturated:
    e.g. C_4 – Butyric – Butter, ghee
    C_6—Caproic—Butter, ghee, vegetables
    C_8—Caprylic—Butter, vegetables
    C_{12}—Lauric—Coconut oil
    C_{14}—Myristic—Coconut oil
    C_{16}—Palmitic—Vegetable oil, animal fat
    C_{18}—Stearic—Vegetable oil, animal fat
    C_{20}—Arachidic—Peanut oil
  - *Unsaturated fatty acids:* They have at least one double bond. Depending upon the number of double bonds unsaturated fatty acids are further of two types:
    MUFA—e.g. Oleic acid, palmitoleic acid (this occur in almost all natural fats and oils).
    PUFA—e.g. Linoleic, linolenic, arachidonic.

    The polyunsaturated fatty acids possess more than one double bond. They are termed as the ***essential fatty acids*** since they are essential for the normal growth and development and they cannot be synthesized in the body. Thus these fatty acids are nutritionally essential and have to be taken in diet.

Linoleic ω6	$C_{18}\Delta_{9,12}$	Soybean oil, peanut oil, cottonseed oil, corn oil
Linolenic ω3	$C_{18}\Delta_{9,\ 12,\ 15}$	Linseed oil, soybean oil, fish liver oil
Arachidonic ω6	$C_{20}\Delta_{5,\ 8,\ 11,\ 14}$	Peanut oil

- Out of these three, linolenic acid is the most important one as the other two can be synthesized from linolenic acid in the body by introduction of a double bond.

Functions/Importance of Essential Fatty Acids (EFAs)

- EFAs are present in the membrane phospholipids in cell membrane and other organelle membranes like mitochondrial membrane. Thus are responsible for the structural integrity of membrane.
- EFAs are present in the membranes of germinal epithelium of gonads.
- EFAs are present in the phospholipids of lipoprotein HDLc. HDLc helps in the transport of cholesterol from tissues to liver. The EFA present at C_2 of peripheral PLs of HDLc esterify the free cholesterol from LDLc and extra hepatic tissues to cholesterol esters (CES), which move to the center of nascent HDLc making it spherical. Now this HDLC transports the CES to liver, where they are oxidized to bile salts and excreted with feces. This is called **reverse cholesterol transport** (Fig. 2.2). This helps in reducing the serum cholesterol level.
- EFAs are needed for the synthesis of lipoprotein particles VLDL at the liver. VLDL transports the endogenously synthesized triglycerides. Thus in EFA deficiency there occurs fatty infiltration of liver—**Fatty liver** (Fig. 2.3).

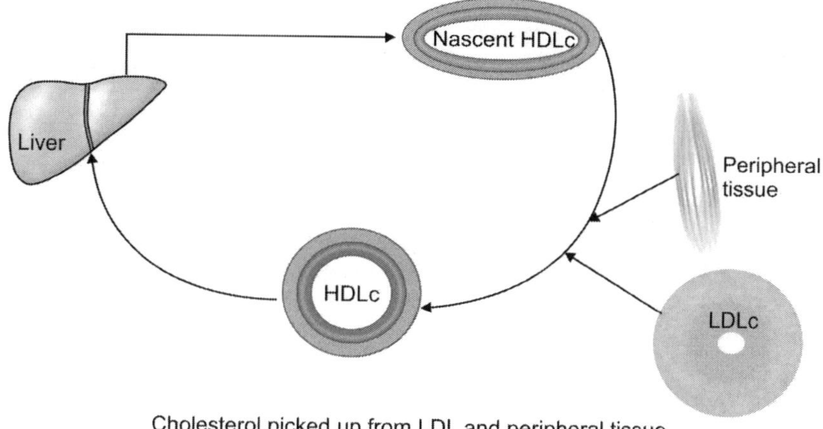

Fig. 2.2 Reverse cholesterol transport

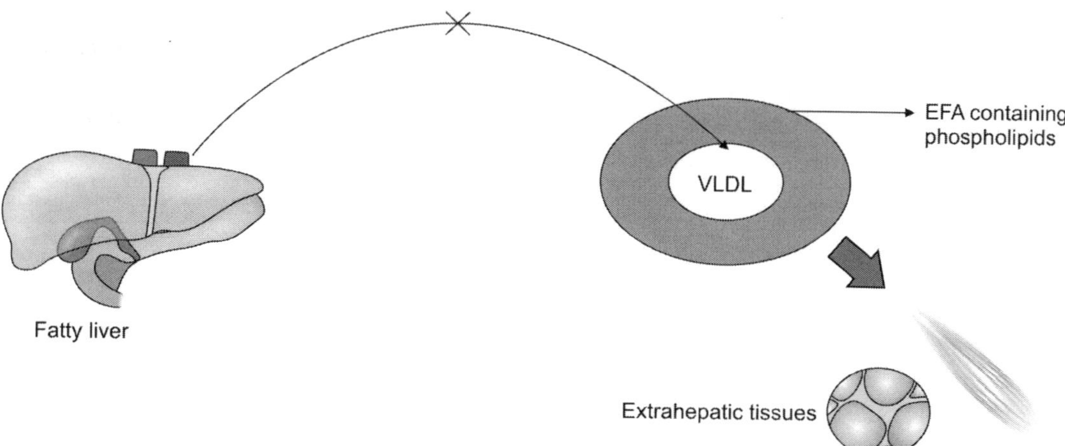

Fig. 2.3 Fatty liver due to EFA deficiency

- EFAs arachidonic acid is the precursor of prostaglandin which acts as local hormone behaving as inflammatory mediators, vasodilators, smooth muscle constrictor, platelet aggregation inhibitors. Prostaglandins are formed by cyclooxygenase pathway and used as pharmacologic agent.
- EFAs arachidonic acid is also precursor of thromboxane. Thromboxanes are formed from prostaglandins. These are also potent physiologically active compounds. They are vasoconstrictor and platelet aggregators.
- Leukotrienes are synthesized from arachidonic acid by lipoxygenase pathway and are activators of leukocytes, vasoconstrictors, smooth muscle constrictors, increase vascular permeability, mediators of allergic reactions.
- Docosahexenoic acid (DHA) is synthesized from linolenic acid. It is present in the photoreceptor cells of eyes and increases their electrical response to illumination.
- DHA also helps in proper brain development in infants and children.

Deficiency of EFAs Leads to Impairment of Normal Health

- Infertility in experimental animals but not seen in humans.
- In humans there are skin lesions like—dermatitis, eczema in skin.
- Degenerative changes in arterial wall.
- Fatty liver progressing to cirrhosis of liver.

Some Unique Fatty Acids

- Branched chain fatty acids found in sebum, and phytanic acid in butter
- Cyclic fatty acids—Chaulmoogric and hydnocarpic acid used for therapy in leprosy.
- Substituted fatty acids—Substituent group like –OH, or – CH_3 group, e.g. Cerebronic acid of glycolipids.

Glycerol (Figs 2.4A and B)

- It is a trihydric alcohol. It is obtained on hydrolysis of TGs in human body (lipolysis) and is converted to glucose at liver.
- Commercially, it is obtained as by product of soap manufacture.
- It is sweet in taste and is used in cosmetics.
- Clinically important preparation is nitroglycerin, which is used as vasodilator.

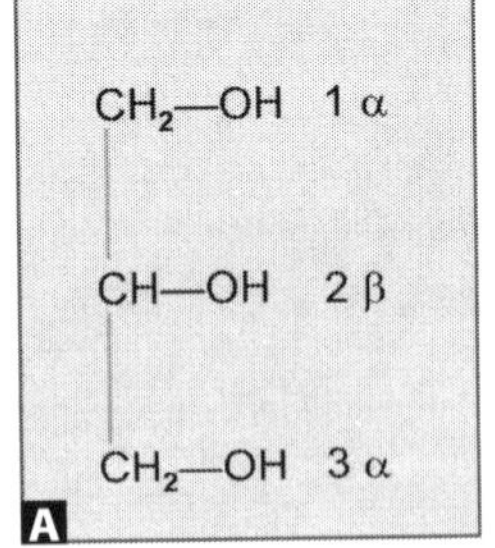

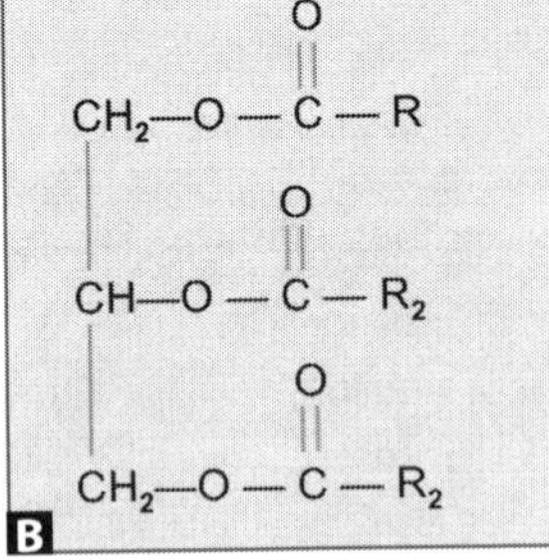

Figs 2.4A and B Glycerol and triglyceride

Cholesterol

Structure (Fig. 2.5)

- Cholesterol is an animal sterol. It has a sterol ring nucleus termed as the CPPP—Cyclo pentano per hydro phenanthrene nucleus. It has 3 cyclohexane rings, 1 cyclo pentane ring, a double bond between C_5 and C_6, an OH group at C_3 which participates in the esterification, a hydrocarbon chain at C_{17}, CH_3 groups at C_{10} and C_{13}.

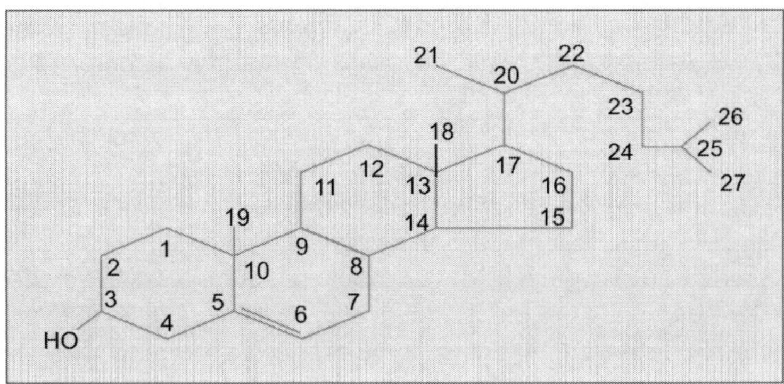

Fig. 2.5 Cholesterol

Occurrence

Cholesterol is abundantly present in brain nervous tissue, liver, adrenal cortex and other tissues. Serum cholesterol level is 150–220 mg/dL, 70% is esterified and 30% is free. Fifty percent of esterification is by linoleic acid. Rest is by oleic, palmitic and arachidonic acid.

Physical Characteristics

It is yellowish white crystalline solid, soluble in nonpolar solvent.

Biomedical Importance of Cholesterol

- Cholesterol is the component of all the biological membrane.
- Cholesterol is precursor of sex hormones of male and female.
- Cholesterol is the precursor of adrenocorticoid hormones, e.g. Glucocorticoids, mineralocorticoids.
- Cholesterol is the precursor of bile acids in liver. The bile acids are needed for the emulsification of dietary lipids.
- Cholesterol is present as 7-dehydrocholesterol in the malphigian layer of skin and it is this 7-dehydrocholesterol that an exposure to sunlight is activated to vitamin-D.
- Cholesterol is the component of myelin sheath of nerves and acts as an insulator thus helps in nerve impulse conduction and prevents leakage of charge.

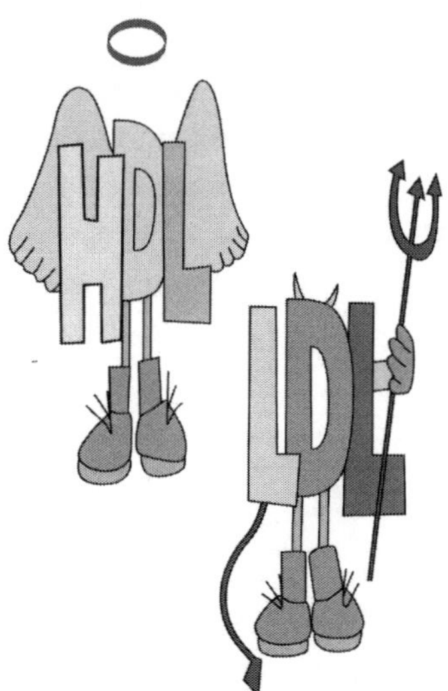

Fig. 2.6 Good and bad cholesterol

Serum Cholesterol and Hypercholesterolemia

- The normal serum cholesterol level is 150–220 mg/dL. This level should be maintained levels higher than 250 mg/dL are harmful and the condition is termed as *hypercholesterolemia.*
  - Dietary and endogenously synthesized cholesterol is transported via the plasma lipoproteins HDLc, LDLc (mainly endogenous), chylomicron (dietary) and chylomicron remnants.

- HDLc is termed as good cholesterol and LDLc as bad cholesterol (Fig. 2.6). HDLc scavenges the free cholesterol (harmful) in the LDLc and carries it to the liver to be oxidized to bile acids which are ultimately excreted out via bile in feces.
- When the serum cholesterol level exceeds the normal value, the cholesterol particularly LDL cholesterol tends to deposit in the intima of blood vessels.
- Oxidized LDLc has a greater tendency to deposit in the intima of medium and large sized arteries, narrowing them leading to formation of atherosclerotic plaques. This phenomenon is called atherosclerosis, which leads to cardiovascular diseases like myocardial infarction and hypertension.
- Primary hypercholesterolemia is seen in some inherited disorders of cholesterol metabolism.
- Secondary hypercholesterolemia occurs secondary to diseases like—diabetes mellitus, nephrotic syndrome, obstructive jaundice, hypothyroidism, etc.
- Management of hypercholesterolemia is discussed with cholesterol metabolism in chapter 11.

Derivatives of Derived Lipids (Eicosanoids)

Prostaglandins

- They are named after the prostate tissue where they were first extracted from.
- These are derived from arachidonic acid of membrane phospholipids.
- Phospholipids in membranes of various tissues like—blood vessel wall, lungs are acted upon by enzymes phospholipases, which hydrolyze and release arachidonic acid.
- Arachidonic acid is then acted upon by cyclooxygenase pathway enzymes—prostaglandin synthase, peroxidase to give prostaglandins.
- Structurally all prostaglandins have a saturated cyclopentane ring and unsaturated hydrocarbon chain.
- They are named as *PG1, PG3* etc. depending upon their position of double bonds.
- Functionally, they act like local hormones, since they affect the local tissue where they are produced and are not transported by blood to different tissues.
- Their important functions are:
  - They are smooth muscle constrictors/relaxation.
  - They are vasodilators.
  - They cause inhibition of platelet aggregation.
  - They act as mediators of inflammation.
    (Aspirin—antiinflammatory—inhibits PG synthesis by blocking enzyme cyclooxygenase)
  - Bronchodilator prostaglandin is PGE, and is used in asthma pumps.

Thromboxanes (TXAs)

- They are derived from PGs.
- They are secreted by platelets, hence the name thromboxanes.
- They cause *platelet aggregation* and *vasoconstriction.*
- Aspirin inhibition of cyclooxygenase completely blocks synthesis of TXA2 as the platelets cannot regenerate cyclooxygenase. Thus it is *helpful in heart attacks.*

Leukotrienes (LTs)

- They are synthesized from arachidonic acid by *lipoxygenase* pathway.
- These are:
  - *Activators of leukocytes*
  - *Vasoconstrictors*
  - *Smooth muscle constrictors*
  - *Bronchoconstrictors*
  - *Increases capillary permeability.*
  - Mediators of *allergic reactions* (hypersensitivity).

Simple Lipids/Neutral Fats

- They are esters of Fatty acid with glycerol. They are present in the adipose tissue as TGs.
- Naturally occurring TGs are mostly mixed TGs, i.e. there are more than one type of fatty acids esterifying the – 3OH groups.
- C1 and C3 are mostly esterified with C16 and C18 Palmitic and Stearic acids respectively.
- C2 is mostly PUFA.
- Oils are neutral lipids that are liquid with one or more fatty acids residues unsaturated at room temperature whereas fats are neutral lipids that are solid or semi-solid at room temperature.

Physical Properties of Simple Lipids

- *Solubility*—The lipids, by definition, are insoluble in water and soluble in organic solvents.
- *Melting point*—Some of them are liquid at room temperature while others are solid. Melting temperature is dependent upon the hydrocarbon chain length of the FAs. If the FAs are unsaturated, the TG will be liquid at room temperature as in vegetable oils. Conversely if it is saturated the TGs will be solid (long chain) or semi-solid (shorter chain) at room temperature as in ghee, butter, or other animal fat.
- *Odor and taste*—They have characteristic odors and tastes.
- *Specific gravity* is less than water.
- *Emulsification*—Lipids get emulsified in presence of surfactants like—detergents and bile salts. Emulsification is the breakdown of a large lipid globule into smaller droplets due to physical agents (vigorous shaking) or chemical agents (bile salts, soap solution) as they reduce the surface tension of water *(also see practical section lipid analysis).*

Chemical Properties of Simple Lipids

- *Hydrolysis*—The ester bonds of lipids can be hydrolyzed by specific enzymes.
- *Saponification*—Hydrolysis of triglycerides by alkalis is known as saponification, and results in the formation of alkali salts of fatty acids (soaps).
- Saponification number is the number of mgs of KOH required to completely saponify 1 g of fat.
- *Hydrogenation*—Double bonds of unsaturated fatty acids can be hydrogenated in the presence of catalysts, e.g. nickel. This process of hydrogenation is used for the commercial preparation of vegetable ghee from vegetable oils.
- *Iodination*—Iodine can also reduce the double bonds of unsaturated fatty acids. Thus can be used to find out adulteration of vegetable oils as oils have a specific number of double bonds to be saturated by iodine.

- Iodine number is the number of gram of iodine taken up by 100 g of the lipid. It gives the degree of unsaturation in oil.
  - *Oxidation*—Unsaturated fatty acids can spontaneously react with atmospheric oxygen to form fatty acid peroxides, fatty acids epoxides and fatty acid aldehydes. Fat which undergoes this type of oxidation becomes rancid.
  - Oxidized fat becomes rancid, i.e. it develops a bad taste, color, odor and is not suitable for use. This process is termed as rancidity. Rancidity can be oxidative and hydrolytic.
  - *Hydrolytic rancidity* is observed in case of vegetable oils kept for a long time in high temperatures, where the naturally occurring lipases of the oils hydrolyze them into free fatty acids which are then oxidized by the atmospheric oxygen in the presence of catalyst like metal containers of Cu.
  - *Oxidative rancidity*—This is seen in vegetable oils exposed to atmospheric oxygen in presence of metallic catalyst like copper. Under such conditions the fatty acids of oil are oxidized to their respective peroxides, epoxides and aldehydes giving characteristic taste and odor to it.
  - Vegetable oils contain vitamin – E which is an antioxidant and prevents the oxidation, increasing shelf life of these oils.

Compound Lipids

These contain some groups in addition to fatty acids and alcohols like—phosphoric acid, protein, or a carbohydrate moiety. They are further classified into:

Phospholipids

- These can be defined as esters of fatty acids with alcohol like glycerol or sphingol and contain an additional group like phosphoric acid and nitrogenous base.
- The former are known as *glycerophospholipids* and the latter are known as *sphingophospholipids.*
- Glycerophospholipids may be considered to be the derivatives of *phosphatidic acid (Fig. 2.7).*
- C_2 is always a PUFA in glycerophospholipid.
  - The phosphate group of phosphatidic acid gets linked with a nitrogenous base by an ester linkage at C_3 phosphoric acid OH group, to form phospholipids, e.g. choline in phosphatidyl choline *(lecithin)*, ethanolamine in phosphatidyl ethanolamine *(cephalin)*, serine in phosphatidyl serine.

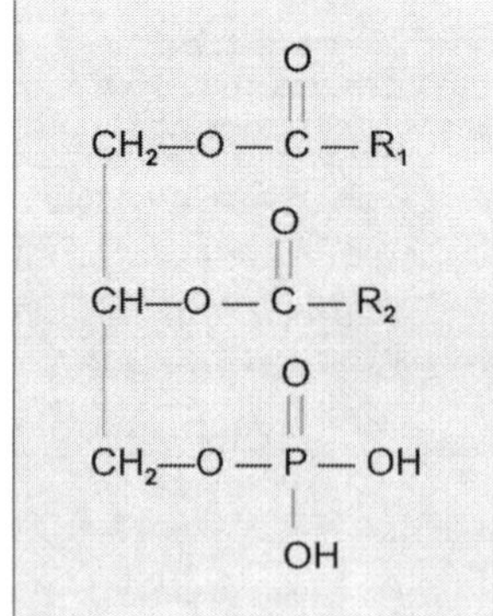

Fig. 2.7 Phosphatidic acid

- Plasmalogens—They are similar to cephalin except that at C_1 instead of a fatty acid in ester linkage, it is an unsaturated aldehyde in ether linkage.
- Sphingolipids—In sphingolipids, the alcohol is a long chain amino alcohol sphingol instead of glycerol of glycerophospholipids (Fig. 2.8).
- The most important sphingophospholipid in our body is sphingomyelin which is a constituent of nervous tissue (Fig. 2.9).
- It is made up of sphingosine, a fatty acid, phosphoric acid and choline.
- It is present in the myelin sheath.

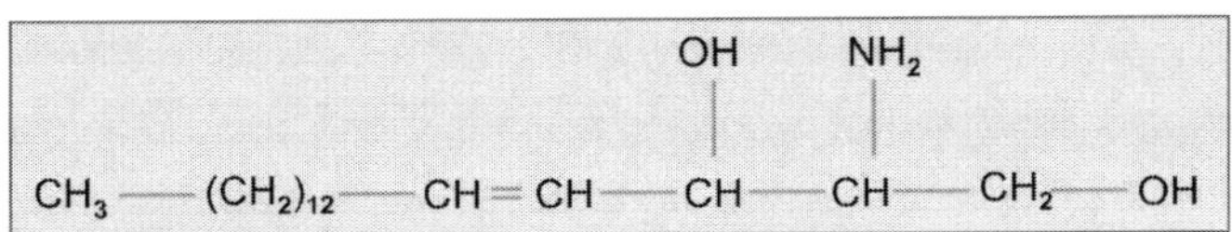

Fig. 2.8 Sphingol

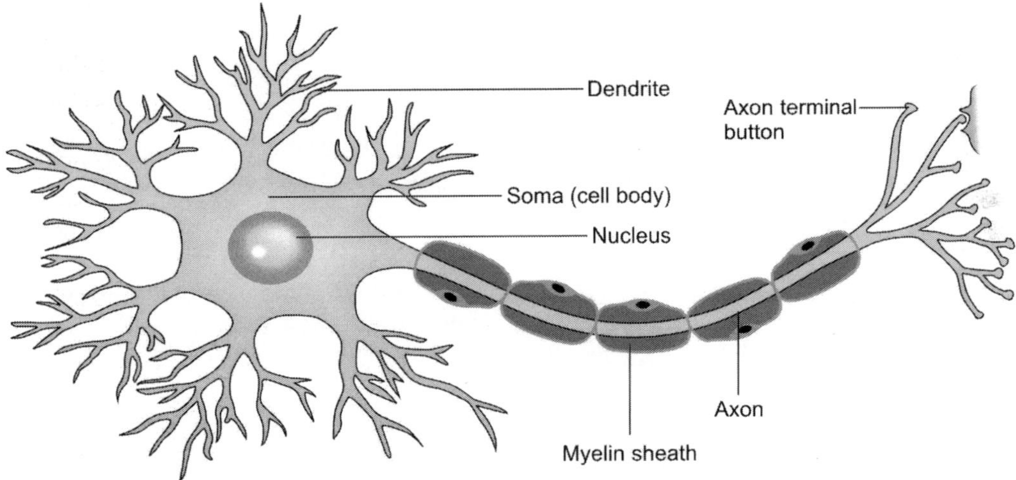

Fig. 2.9 Neuron with myelin sheath

Functions of Phospholipids

- Phospholipids are present in the cell membrane as lipid bilayer and are responsible for the *semipermeability* of cell membrane.
- As component of *mitochondrial membrane,* phospholipids give the structural integrity to mitochondrial membrane and thus a proper site of oxidative phosphorylation.
- Phospholipids are *amphipathic,* thus required for *micellization* during lipids digestion.
- Dipalmitoyl lecithin *(DPL)* is present in alveoli as a surfactant and prevents the collapse of alveoli when they deflate. Its deficiency is seen in an inherited disorder—*Respiratory distress syndrome.*
- Phospholipids are components of *lipoprotein complexes,* therefore necessary for the synthesis of lipoproteins.
- Phospholipids of lipoproteins act like *coenzyme* for enzyme lipoprotein lipase (LPL) during metabolism of lipoproteins.
- Phospholipids like—lecithin, cephalin, plasmalogens are important components of *brain and nervous tissue.*
- *Cardiolipin* is a component of *mitochondrial membrane.*
- *Sphingomyelin* is necessary for the formation of *myelin sheath.*
- *Phospholipids of platelets* help in the process of blood coagulation.

Glycolipids

They contain carbohydrate moiety (glucose/galactose/NANA) in addition to Fatty acid and alcohol sphingosine. They are of 2 types:

Cerebrosides

They contain galactose as carbohydrate moiety

For example,
- Nervon – Nervonic acid
- Kerasin – Lignoceric acid
- Oxy nervon – Oxynervonic acid
- Cerebron – Cerebronic acid

- They are present in white matter of brain. They accumulate in the RE cells of spleen, liver, CNS in Gaucher's disease—an inherited disorder (Lipid storage disease) (Table 2.1).

Gangliosides

- They contain n-acetyl neuraminic acid, sphingosine, fatty acid and 3 carbohydrate moieties glucose/galactose. They are present in gray matter. Accumulate of gangliosides is seen in inherited disease Niemannpick's disease.

Lipoproteins

- Lipids are insoluble in water therefore for the transport of dietary lipids and lipids of endogenous origin lipids complex with proteins to form lipoprotein complexes. These lipoprotein complexes are HDLc, LDLc, VLDL and Chylomicron.
- The protein part is called apo protein. These apo protein have specific roles to play—
  - They help in recognition of the specific lipoprotein by its tissue receptor, i.e. act as ligand.
  - Some of the apo proteins act as a coenzyme and activate certain enzymes of lipid metabolism.
  - Structurally lipoproteins are made up of a central core of hydrophobic nonpolar lipids cholesterol esters and TGs and a peripheral coat of amphipathic lipids like—cholesterol, phospholipids with apo proteins attached either peripherally or integrally (Fig. 2.10).

Table 2.1 Important lipid storage diseases

Gaucher's	Glucosidase	Glucocerebroside	Hepatosplenomegaly, moderate anemia, bone deformities
Niemann Pick	Sphingomyelinase	Sphingomyelin	Mental retardation, hepatosplenomegaly, cherry red spot in macula and fatal in early life
Tay Sach's	Hexoseaminidase	Ganglioside GM2	Mental retardation, blindness, muscle weakness

Types of Lipoproteins

- Lipoproteins are classified based upon their relative densities. Greater the lipid content as compared to apo protein, lesser the density and vice versa.
  - Chylomicron—Transports all dietary lipids to different body tissues and liver.
  - VLDL—Very low density lipoprotein—Transports endogenously synthesized TGs from liver to extra hepatic tissues.
  - IDL—Intermediate density lipoprotein—Formed as an intermediate of metabolism from VLDL to LDL.
  - LDL—Low density lipoprotein—Transports cholesterol from liver to extra hepatic tissues
  - HDL—High density lipoprotein—Transports cholesterol from extra hepatic tissues to liver as cholesterol esters.

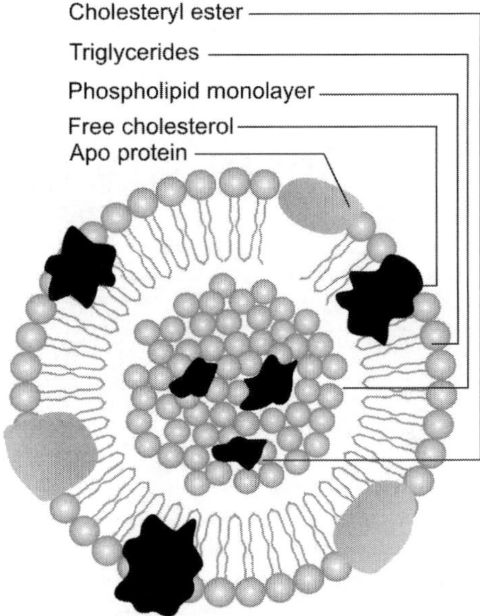

Fig. 2.10 Lipoprotein structure

Sulfolipids

- Sulfated derivatives of glycolipids are sulfolipids. They are abundantly found in the white matter of brain, e.g. Sulfogalactoceremide of myelin sheath.

A Quick Look at the Lipids

- Lipids are esters of fatty acids with alcohols.
- Lipids are classified into Simple, compound and derived lipids.
- Simple lipids are neutral lipids/ triglycerides—esters of fatty acids with glycerol.
- Compound lipids are esters of fatty acids with alcohol that may be glycerol or sphingol with some additional group.
- Derived lipids are derived by hydrolysis of simple and compound lipids and still retain properties of lipids.
- Important derived lipids are—essential fatty acids, cholesterol and glycerol.
- Essential fatty acids are important for normal growth and development and are essential in diet as they cannot be synthesized by the body.
- Deficiency of EFAs causes fatty liver owing to the blockage of VLDL synthesis by liver.
- Cholesterol plays important roles in steroid hormones synthesis, vitamin D synthesis, bile acid synthesis.
- Hypercholestrolemia causes atherosclerosis which is the prime cause of CVDs.
- Compound lipids like phospholipids and glycolipids are important in normal development of nervous system.
- Defects in metabolism of phospho and glycolipids cause lipid storage diseases.
- Oxidation of neutral lipids like oils causes their rancidity.

CHAPTER

3

Chemistry of Amino Acids and Proteins

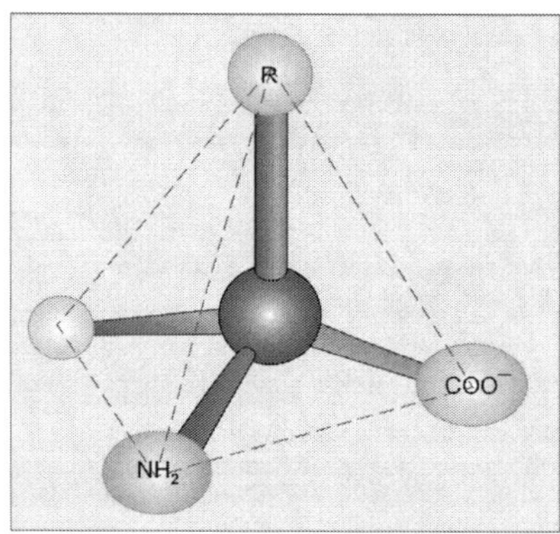

Chapter Framework

- Introduction
- Definition
- Functions
- Chemistry of Proteins
- Classification of Amino Acids
- Physical and Chemical Properties of Amino Acids
- Classification of Proteins
- Structure of Proteins
- Techniques of Protein Sequencing and Isolation

Introduction

Proteins are the most abundant biomolecules. Proteins word has been derived from the Greek word 'Proteios' meaning of paramount importance. All life forms depend upon these biomolecules, be it the simplest unicellular bacteria with the protein capsule around it or a virus requiring the capsid protein or the multicellular organisms, whose body is composed of millions of cells and each cell made of many proteins. Proteins are the fundamental molecules which sustain life. All life processes need proteins.

Functions of Proteins

- *Enzymes* which liberate the energy driving the life.
- *Hemoglobin (Hb) transporting* respiratory gases.
- *Nucleoproteins* for perpetuating genetic information to the next generation.
- *Immunoglobulin* protecting against harmful antigens.
- *Hormones* regulating the cellular functions.
- *Structural proteins* like collagen, dentine, keratin forming the bones, cartilages, teeth, hair, skin, nails, etc.
- *Plasma proteins* maintain the fluid and electrolyte balance by exerting the colloid osmotic pressure.
- *Storage proteins* like ferritin store iron to be used in periods of deficiency.

Chemistry of Proteins

- Chemically proteins are the dehydration biopolymers of amino acids, linked by a peptide linkage.
- Amino acids form the language of proteins, like alphabets form the language of English. Universally all proteins are composed of the same set of 20 amino acids.
- Different proteins differ in the number and sequence of amino acids in them. The differential arrangement of the amino acids determines the 3D structure of the protein and also gives rise to the functional diversity of the proteins.
- The amino acids sequence in turn is determined by the sequence of genes in the genome. Each amino acid is denoted by 3 nucleotide sequence, i.e. triplet codon.
- Each gene is a collection of such codons. Thus the hypothesis '1 gene 1 protein' was proposed.
- Each amino acid can be denoted by a 3 letter abbreviation, using it like shorthand during denoting their sequence in proteins or during biochemical reactions, e.g. Glycine – Gly, Leucine – Leu, Phenylalanine – Phe, etc.

Chemistry of Amino Acids

An amino acid is composed of a central C atom with its 4 valencies saturated by – an alpha amino group, a carboxylic acid group, 'R' group and H atom (Figs 3.1A and B).

Classification of Amino Acids

Chemical Basis of Classification

The 20 amino acids can be broadly classified into the following classes based on their 'R' group structure:

- Aliphatic amino acids—They have an aliphatic chain as the 'R' group, e.g. Glycine, alanine, leucine, isoleucine, valine.
- S-containing amino acids—Cysteine, cystine, methionine.
- Hydroxy amino acids—Serine, threonine.
- Acidic amino acids—Aspertate, glutamate.
- Basic amino acids—Asparagine, glutamine, arginine, lysine.
- Aromatic amino acids—Phenylalanine, tyrosine, histidine.
- Imino acids—Proline

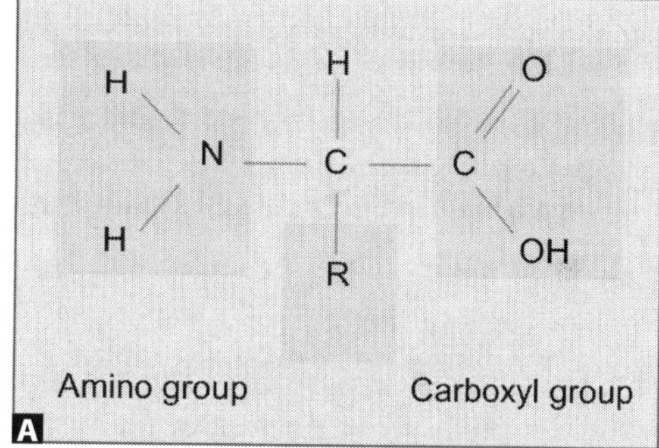

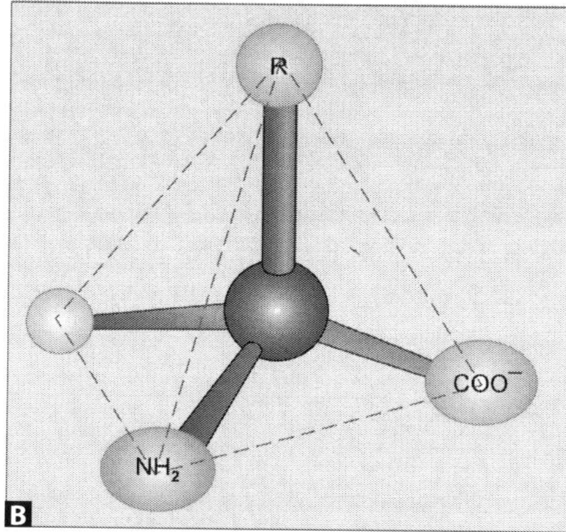

Figs 3.1A and B (A)Structure of amino acid; (B) Ball and stick model showing 3–D structure of amino acid

Nutritional Classification of Amino Acids

The 20 standard amino acids can be classified nutritionally as:

- Essential
- Semiessential
- Nonessential

Essential Amino Acids

These are not synthesized by the body and have to be essentially consumed as a daily nutrient for the maintenance of optimal health, growth and development. There are 8 such amino acids—Val, Leu, Isoleu, Thr, Trp, Phe, Met, and Lys.

Semiessential Amino Acids

They can be synthesized by the body but their requirement exceeds the supply by the body in certain circumstances like pregnancy, lactation, infants and growing children, in puberty. Thus these amino acids become nutritionally essential during these situations and should be consumed in diet, e.g. Arginine and histidine.

Nonessential Amino Acids

They can be synthesized by the body, using the carbon skeletons of the essential amino acids. Thus such amino acids are nutritionally nonessential, e.g. Gly, Ala, Cys, Cyst, Ser, Asp, Asn, Glu, Gln, Pro.

Nutritional Importance of Proteins

- Human beings need to take in their daily dietary proteins containing all essential amino acids, since proteins are the only source of N in our body, for maintaining a state of N balance as they supply N as amino acids.
- The amino acids are not stored in the body rather they are utilized for protein synthesis (tissue and plasma proteins). Amino acids in excess of the protein synthesis would be catabolized and excreted as urea in humans. Depending upon their essential amino acids content, the dietary proteins are—

Excellent Quality (1st class) Proteins

- Containing all essential amino acids in abundance, e.g. animal proteins like organ meat, poultry, fish, etc.

Good Quality Proteins

- Containing all essential amino acids but in just optimum amount, e.g. milk and milk products.

Fair Quality (Complimentary Proteins)

- Deficient in one essential amino acid, e.g. Cereals lack methionine and legumes lack lysine. When cereals and legumes consumed together they give all essential amino acids like a 1st class protein. Such proteins are termed as *Complimentary proteins* since they complement each other's deficiency.

Bad Quality Proteins

- More than one essential amino acid deficient, e.g. Gelatin (derived protein)
- Essential amino acids are necessary for maintenance of N_2 balance in body. Deficiency of these amino acids leads to a state of negative nitrogen balance (intake of N < than excretion), e.g. in chronic debilitating diseases like cancer or when a person is on total parenteral nutrition for a long time or in old age or in starvation, malnutrition in children—Kwashiorkor and Marasmus.

- *Kwashiorkor*—5 years of age
- *Marasmus*—In infants below 1 year of age.

Physical and Chemical Properties of Amino Acids

Physical Properties of Amino Acids

- Amino acids are crystalline solids, soluble in polar solvents, e.g. water and ethanol, and insoluble in nonpolar solvents, e.g. ether, chloroform, etc.
- The aromatic amino acids absorb ultraviolet light.

Isomerism

- Amino acids show stereo isomerism. Like the carbohydrates they can exist in D-form and L-form. The amino group is present on the righthand side of the asymmetric α -carbon in D-amino acids, and on the left hand side in L-amino acids (Fig. 3.2).
- Naturally occurring amino acids are L isomers as the enzymes have asymmetric active sites causing the reactions they catalyse to be stereospecific.
- Glycine is the only amino acid that has no asymmetric carbon atom and, hence, no stereoisomers.

Chemical Properties of Amino Acids

Amphoteric Nature

- Amino acids can act as ampholytes i.e. they act as acids (proton donors) as well as bases (proton acceptors), as they possess 2 ionisable/titrable groups –COOH and –NH_2 groups.
- Whether they will behave as acids or bases at a given time depends on the pH of the medium in which they are present.
- In an acidic medium, the amino group is ionized as it accepts a proton while ionization of the carboxyl group is suppressed. Thus, the amino acid acts as a proton acceptor (base) in an acidic medium.
- In alkaline medium carboxyl group ionizes by donating proton and the amino acid acts as an acid.
- Between these two extremes, there is a certain pH at which both carboxyl and amino groups are ionized—*Isoelectric pH (Fig. 3.3).*

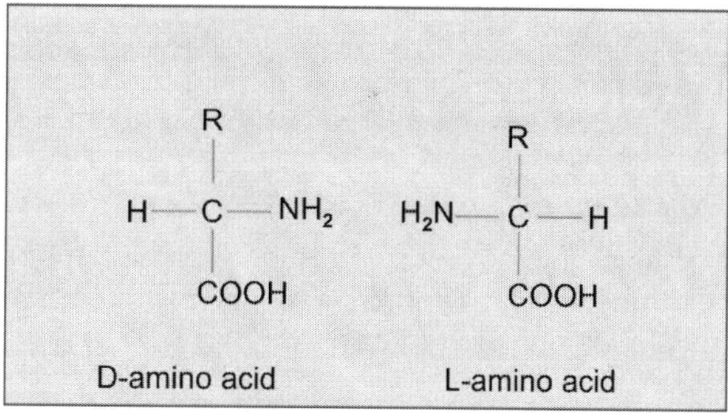

Fig. 3.2 Amino acid stereoisomers

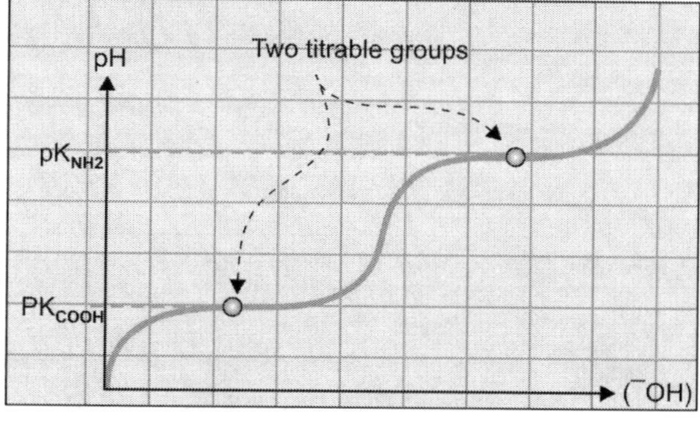

Fig. 3.3 Two titrable/ionizable groups in amino acids

- At isoelectric pH both carboxyl and amino groups are ionized, the molecule as a whole is electrically neutral, and does not move when placed in an electric field. Thus the name isoelectric pH.
- This form of amino acid is known as a *Zwitterion.*
- Isoelectric pH is constant for every amino acid. The solubility and electrical field mobility of an amino acid is the least at its isoelectric pH.

Decarboxylation

Decarboxylation of amino acids gives biogenic amines. Histidine – Histamine, Tyrosine – Tyramine, Tryptophan – Tryptamine, Glutamic acid – GABA.

Transamination and Deamination

- *Transamination*—It involves the transfer of the $-NH_2$ group of an amino acid to an alpha keto acid giving a new amino acid and a new keto acid in the presence of transaminases.
- Alanine + α Ketoglutarate $\xrightleftharpoons{\text{SGOT}}$ Pyruvate + Glutamate
- Here the $-NH_2$ group of alanine (amino acid1) is transferred to alpha ketogluterate (keto acid1) to give pyruvate (keto acid 2) and glutamate (amino acid 2). This reaction plays an important role in catabolism of amino acids and also in synthesis of nonessential amino acids.
- *Deamination*—When the alpha $-NH_2$ group is removed from an amino acid as NH_3 to gives a keto acid, it is termed as deamination. Deamination may be oxidative or nonoxidative. This is important in the pooling of the NH_2 groups of all amino acids into glutamate during NH_3 transport, which finally carries the NH_3 to the liver for urea synthesis.

Reactions of Sulfydryl Groups

- The sulfhydryl group of cysteine can undergo reversible oxidation and reduction, can form disulfide bonds and are essential for the activity of certain enzymes and coenzymes, e.g. Glutathione peroxidase.

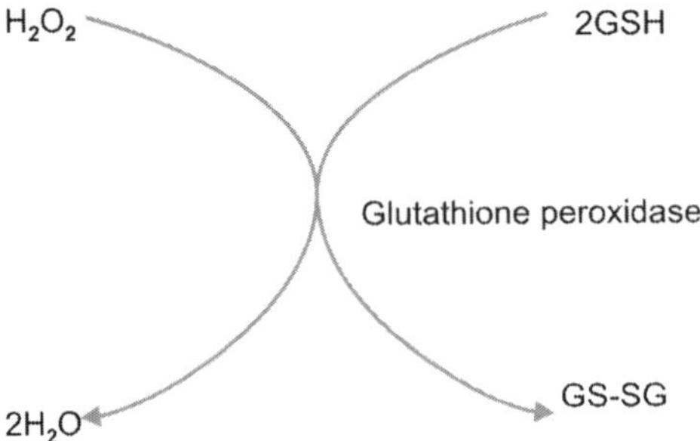

Color Reactions Used for Identification and Quantitation of Individual or Groups of Amino Acids

- Specific chemical reaction can be used to identify individual or group of amino acids, for example, some of the important reactions are:
  - Ninhydrin reaction—for identifying all alpha amino acids.
  - Xanthoproteic reaction—for identifying aromatic amino acids like Phe, Tyr, Trp.

- Millon-Nasse reaction—for identifying tyrosine.
- Aldehyde reaction—for identifying tryptophan.
- Hopkins-Cole reaction—for identifying tryptophan.
- Sakaguchi's reaction—for identifying arginine.
- Lead sulfide reaction—for identifying sulfur releasing amino acids.

Formation of Peptide Bonds

- One of the most important reactions of amino acids is the formation of peptide bonds (Fig. 3.4).
- A dipeptide is formed on polymerization of 2 amino acid residues, tripeptide when 3 amino acid residues polymerize and so on till nonapeptide (with 9 amino acids) more than 10 up to 100 amino acids are termed as polypeptides.
- Peptides with more than 100 amino acid residues are termed as proteins.
- Each peptide and protein has a $-NH_2$terminal end (N terminal end) and a – COOH terminal end (C terminal end).
- During protein synthesis, it is from the N-terminal end that the new protein starts synthesizing. Biologically active peptides are of variable sizes. Some important biologically active peptides are shown in Table 3.1.

$$\underset{\text{Amino acid}}{H_2N-\overset{R_1}{\overset{|}{CH}}-COOH} + \underset{\text{Amino acid}}{H_2N-\overset{R_2}{\overset{|}{CH}}-COOH} \xrightarrow{-H_2O} \underset{\text{Dipeptide}}{H_2N-\overset{R_1}{\overset{|}{CH}}-\overset{O}{\overset{\|}{C}}-\overset{H}{\overset{|}{N}}-\overset{R_2}{\overset{|}{CH}}-COOH}$$

Fig. 3.4 Peptide bond formation

Table 3.1 Biologically important peptides

Glutathione	Tripeptide(γ–glu-cys-gly)	Required for enzymatic activity, for detoxication of peroxides
Angiotensin	Octapeptide	Renin-Angiotensin system plays important role in regulation of blood pressure
Vasopressin (ADH)	Cyclic nonapeptide	Regulates permeability of renal tubules and also increases peripheral vascular resistance
Oxytocin	Nonapeptide	Neuromodulator in brain and acts on breast tissue and uterine tissue.
Thyrotropin-releasing hormone (TRH)	Tripeptide	Stimulates release of TSH from anterior pituitary
Met – enkephalin	Pentapeptide	Relieves pain

Reactions Used for Determination of the Amino Acid Sequence of Peptides and Proteins

- Generally, the N-terminal amino acid is tagged with specific reagent. The tagged amino acid is split off by hydrolysis, and is identified. The reaction is, then, repeated with the new N-terminal amino acid and so on. Reagents used are – *Edman's and Sanger's Reagent. (to be discussed in detail later in the chapter with protein sequencing and separation techniques)*

Classification of Protein

Proteins are large polymers of amino acids having complex structure which perform important functions in all living organisms. They can be classified in a number ways.

Functional Classification of Proteins

Proteins can be classified on the functional basis as:

Structural Proteins

Proteins which make the structural components of the body like – keratin of skin and hair, collagen of cartilages and bones etc.

Catalytic Proteins

All biocatalysts (enzymes) are proteins with exception of 'ribozymes'.

Defensive Proteins

Immunoglobulins are the defence line of our body.

Storage Proteins

Certain proteins have storage function like ferritin is an iron storage protein.

Transport Proteins

Proteins bind to hydrophobic or non - polar molecule for an easy transport in the aqueous medium of plasma/blood, e.g. albumin transports unconjugated bilirubin from RE cells to the liver, or the transport of various lipids as lipoprotein complexes.

Respiratory Proteins

Hb and Mb have the capacity to bind to respiratory gases and exchange them at the tissue level.

Buffering Function

Plasma proteins act as important physiological buffers, preventing the alteration in the pH of plasma from the normal (7.35 – 7.45). Similarly Hb also has the capacity to act as a buffer, owing to the presence of imidazole ring of His.

Fluid Balance

Plasma proteins exert the colloid osmotic pressure and thus help in the retention of fluid in the ECF.

Proteins Classification Based on Their Structure

Proteins can be broadly classified into three classes—*Simple, conjugated and derived.*

Simple Proteins

- These are simply made up of amino acids, e.g. albumin, globulin, etc. Simple proteins can be further classified on the basis of their solubility into:
  - *Albumins:* These are soluble in water and dilute salt solutions. They are heat-coagulable. They are precipitated when their solutions are saturated completely with solid ammonium sulfate, e.g. lactalbumin, ovalbumin.
  - *Globulins:* These are soluble in dilute salt solutions but are insoluble in water. They are heat-coagulable. They are precipitated when their solutions are half saturated with ammonium sulfate, e.g. Ovglobulin, lactglobulin.
  - *Glutelins:* These are soluble in dilute acids and alkalis but are insoluble in water, e.g. Glutenin of wheat and oryzenin of rice.
  - *Prolamines:* These are soluble in 70% ethanol but insoluble in water and absolute ethanol. These are rich in proline, e.g. Gliadin of wheat and zein of corn.
  - *Protamines:* These are soluble in water and ammonium hydroxide, e.g. Salmine and sturine found in the sperms of the fishes, salmon and sturgeon respectively.
  - *Histones:* Histones are soluble in water but are insoluble in ammonium hydroxide. They are rich in arginine, e.g. Histones (H1, H2A, H2B, H3 and H4) are present in nucleus in association with DNA.
  - *Albuminoids:* These are also known as scleroproteins. They are insoluble in most of the solvents. These are structural constituents of tissues, and provide strength to the tissues, e.g. Collagen, keratin, elastin, etc.

Conjugated Proteins

- As the name suggests are made up of a protein part and an additional (conjugated 'or' prosthetic) part called as the apoprotein, e.g.
  - *Glycoprotein:* Contain carbohydrate as prosthetic group. When more than 4% carbohydrate present, it is a mucoprotein and up to 4% carbohydrate, it is a glycoprotein, e.g. Hormones, FSH, LH are glycoproteins and mucin is a mucoprotein.
  - *Metalloprotein:* Metal prosthetic group is present, e.g. Cytochromes, Hb, Mb, carbonic anhydrase, etc.
  - *Phosphoprotein:* Phosphoric acid as the prosthetic group is present, e.g. Casein of milk, vitellin of egg.
  - *Lipoprotein:* Contain lipids as the prosthetic group, e.g. Chylomicron, LDLc, HDLc, VLDL.
  - *Chromoprotein:* Contain a pigment as prosthetic group, e.g. Hb, Mb, cytochromes, etc.
  - *Nucleoproteins:* Contain nucleic acids as their prosthetic group and are present in nucleus in chromosomes.

Derived Proteins

- They are formed from naturally occurring proteins by the action of physical agents, e.g. Heat, ultrasonic waves, etc. or chemical agents, e.g. Acids, alkalis, enzymes, etc.

- *Primary derived proteins:* These are formed by some intramolecular changes in the native proteins not involving hydrolysis of the proteins. These are insoluble and biologically inactive, e.g. Acid metaproteins, denatured proteins and coagulated proteins.
- *Secondary derived proteins:* These are formed by hydrolysis of native proteins. These include primary proteoses, secondary proteoses and peptones in the decreasing order of size.

Structural Organization of Proteins

This section of the chapter deals with the exploration of the 3D structure of proteins, with an emphasis on:

- The sequence of amino acids determining the 3D structure of proteins.
- Stabilization of protein structure due to noncovalent forces.
- Structural and functional relationship of proteins.
- Identification and separation of various types of proteins:
  - Proteins are polymers of amino acids linked up by covalent peptide bonds. The covalent backbone of proteins contains hundreds of peptide bonds.
  - Proteins assume conformations that can be achieved without breaking these covalent bonds.
  - Although the rotation about the peptide bond is restricted, it is possible about the other bonds such that there is minimum entropy and maximum stability.
  - Due to the free rotation about many of these bonds, proteins assume various conformations. (Spatial arrangement of atoms in a protein is called its conformation).
  - The task of understanding the structure of a large macromolecule as protein, the study is done in a hierarchical manner. The proteins are organized at 4 levels of structural organization:
    - Primary
    - Secondary
    - Tertiary
    - Quaternary.

Primary Structural Organization

- This is the most fundamental level of structural organization. It denotes the sequence of amino acids in the polypeptide chain.
- It has an amino terminal end and a carboxyl terminal end. The synthesis of a polypeptide, the numbering and the naming of a polypeptide chain always begins from the amino terminal end (Fig. 3.5).

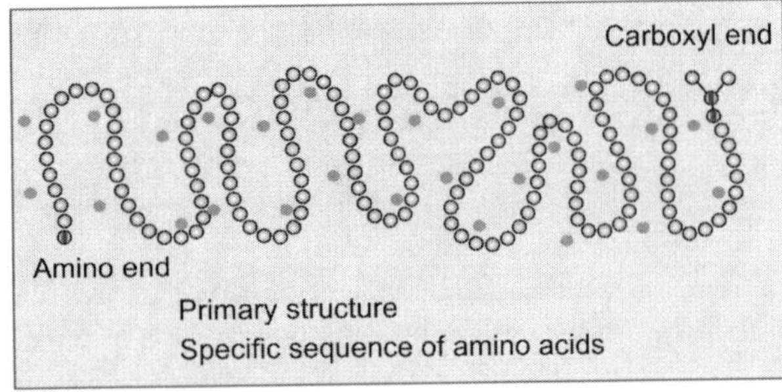

Fig. 3.5 Primary polypeptide chain

- This level of proteins structure is maintained by the peptide bonds between the different amino acids.
- All proteins are made up of 20 amino acids but vary in the sequence and number of amino acids.

- The sequence of amino acids is very important as it determines the further levels of organization, 3 –D structure of the protein and the function of the proteins.
- Any variation in the type of amino acid or the sequence of amino acids may cause loss of normal structure and function of the protein, e.g. HbS has Val instead of Glu at β 6 position. This causes a loss in the functional capacity of the Hb molecule, which converts to HbS.
- The HbS on giving up its O_2 at tissues develops a sticky patch and due to the sticking of several such deoxy HbS molecules it precipitates out forming crystals of deoxy HbS. Such deoxy HbS molecules can now no longer carry new O_2 molecules and the crystals rupture the RBCs *causing sickle cell anemia.*

Secondary Structural Organization

- This is the next higher level of organization. The polypeptide chain is not straight. It becomes specifically twisted, turned and coiled to form various types of regular folding pattern such that amino acids placed 3 – 4 residues apart in straight chain come closer, e.g. α-helix, β-pleated sheet, β-bend, etc. It is maintained by—

Hydrogen Bonds

- These weak bonds are formed between two peptide linkages which may be present in the same polypeptide chain or in two different polypeptide chains.
- In hydrogen bonds, the hydrogen atom of the N–H group participating in a peptide bond is shared between nitrogen of –NH and carbonyl (C=O) oxygen atoms.
- The nitrogen atom involved in this sharing belongs to one peptide bond, and the oxygen atom belongs to another peptide bond.

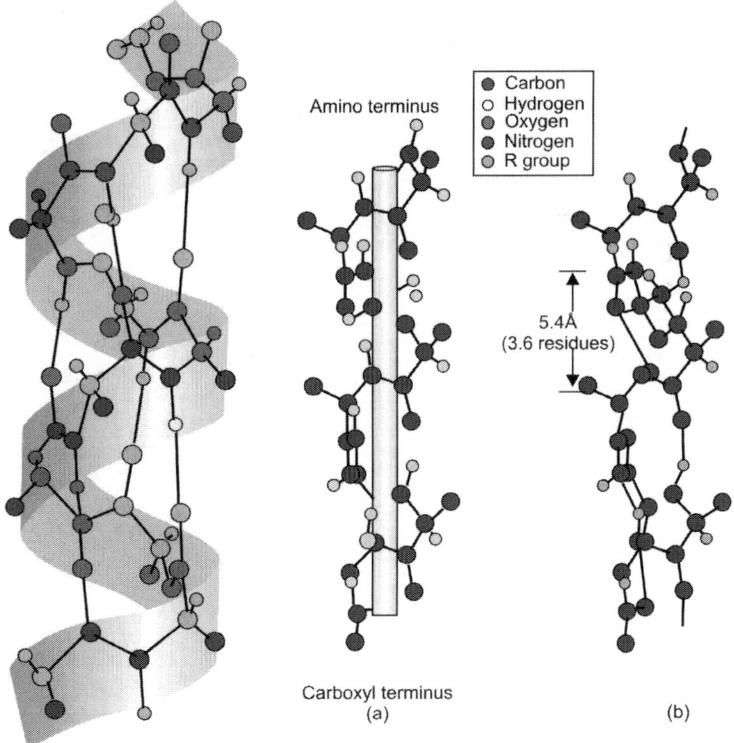

Fig. 3.6 Alpha helix form

Disulfide Bond

- A disulfide bond is formed between two cysteine residues. The sulfhydryl groups of the cysteine residues are linked together.
- Disulfide bond may be formed between two cysteine residues in the same polypeptide chain or in two different polypeptide chains. In the latter case, the two polypeptide chains will be linked together.

Alpha helix

- This is the most commonly encountered secondary structure. In this structure the primary polypeptide chain backbone is tightly wound around an imaginary axis drawn longitudinally through the middle of the helix, with the R groups of the amino acids projecting at right angles to the axis (Fig. 3.6).

Characteristic features of alpha helix

- The α-helix is stabilized by formation of hydrogen bonds between peptide linkages four amino acid residues apart.
- Each peptide linkage in the polypeptide chain participates in hydrogen bonding.
- There are 3.6 amino acid residues in each turn of the helix.
- The pitch of the helix is 5.4 Å i.e. a single turn of the helix extends for 5.4Å.
- The helix may be right-handed or left-handed.
- The right-handed helix is more stable.
- Some amino acid residues, e.g. Proline and hydroxy proline, tend to disrupt the helix, and produce turns or kinks. They are seen in Hb, Mb, Collagen.

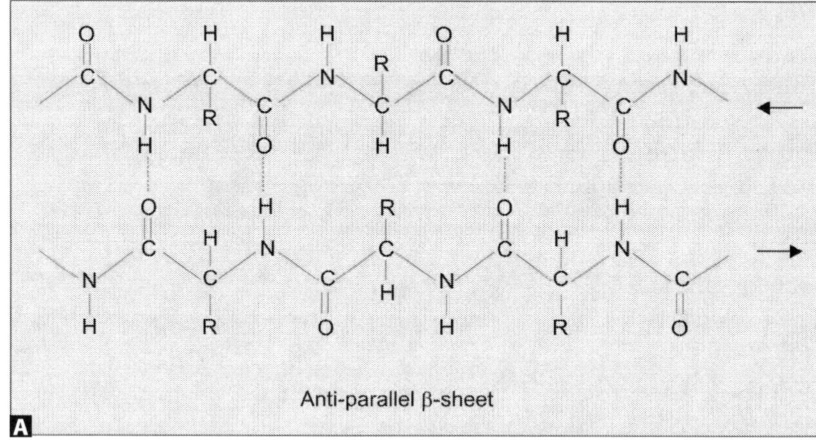

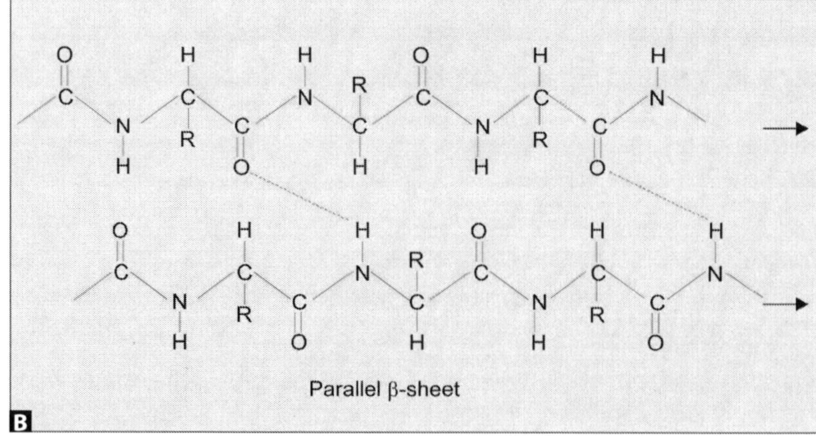

Figs 3.7A and B β-pleated sheet form

β-pleated sheets

- In β-pleated sheets, the polypeptide backbone is extended into zigzag pattern rather than helical structure.
- These when arranged side by side, form a structure resembling series of pleats, thus the name β-pleated sheets.
- The β-pleated sheets may be arranged either parallel or antiparallel sections of same or different polypeptide chain (Figs 3.7A and B).
- They are stabilized by H bonds between 2 parallel or antiparallel sections of β-pleated sheets.
- The R groups of the amino acids of adjacent polypeptide chains (or segments of single polypeptide chain) protrude in the opposite directions.
- When 2 or more β-pleated sheets are layered closely, the R group of the amino acids on touching surfaces must be small like Gly or Ala as can be seen in silk fibroin or β-keratins.

Tertiary Structural Organization

- The overall 3D arrangement of all the atoms in a protein is referred to as the protein's tertiary structure (Fig. 3.8).
- In this arrangement, the secondary structure of the polypeptide chain is folded in such a way that some amino acid residues which are quite distant from each other in the polypeptide chain are brought closer.
- This spatial arrangement of amino acid residues forms a specific three-dimensional conformation—***Native protein*** (tertiary structure).
- Some residues are buried into the interior of the molecule and some are exposed on the surface of the molecule. The hydrophobic amino acid residues usually are buried in the interior of the 3D structure and polar residues occupy the surface of this structure.

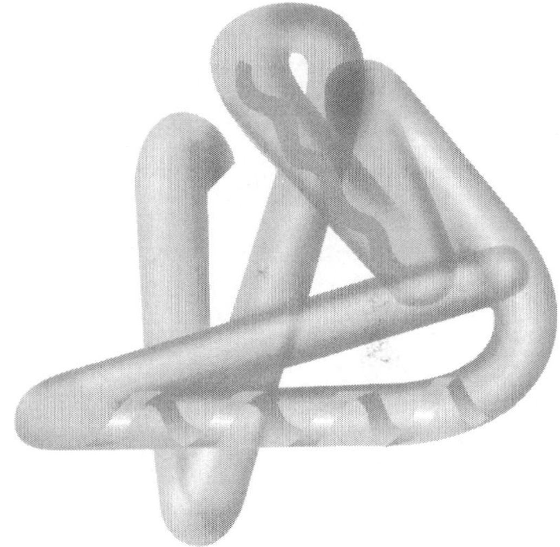

Fig. 3.8 Tertiary structure

The folding occurs due to formation of:

- Disulfide bonds—between 2 cysteine residues.
- H bonds—sharing of H atom between 2 electronegative atoms like N or O.
- Electrostatic bonds—between 2 polar amino acid R groups.
- Hydrophobic interactions—weak interactions between 2 nonpolar amino acid R groups.
- Vander Waals forces—between 2 nonpolar amino acid R groups.

Quaternary Structural Organization

- Many proteins are active functionally at the quaternary level where 2 or more tertiary level protomers assemble together.
- Each chain is known as a protomer or a subunit.

- The subunits may be similar or dissimilar.
- The subunits are combined with each other by noncovalent bonds to form the quaternary structure of the protein (Fig. 3.9).

The various bonds maintaining quaternary structure

- Hydrophobic interactions
- Vander Waals forces
- Some examples of proteins having quaternary structure are—Hemoglobin (tetramer), Lactate dehydrogenase (tetramer), Creatinine kinase (dimer).

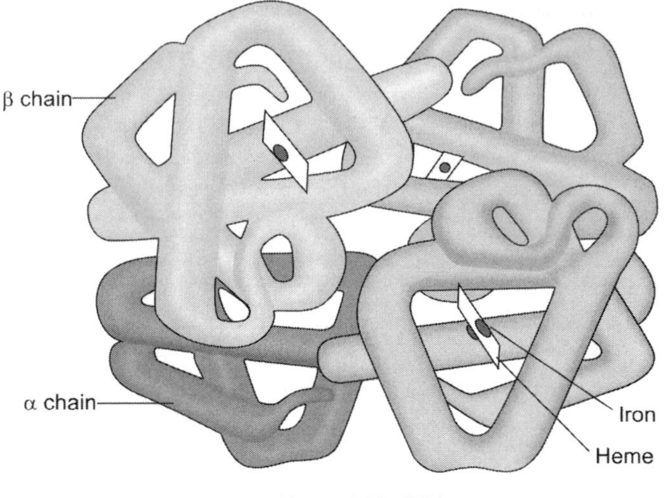

Fig. 3.9 Structure of hemoglobin

Protein Folding and Misfolding

- If a correct primary structure has been formed, the nascent protein will fold spontaneously and attain higher orders of structure and the correct conformation. However, spontaneous folding is a slow process. Rapid and correct folding of the newly-synthesized protein is ensured by some enzymes, protein factors known as chaperone proteins and chaperonins.
- Misfolding can occur due to:
  - Change in primary structure
  - Defects in molecular chaperones
  - Exogenous agents
- A misfolded protein is usually degraded.
- Some misfolded proteins are resistant to degradation, e.g. Amyloid protein and lead to diseases like—Scrapie in sheep, mad cow disease in cattle, Alzheimer's disease and Creutzfeldt – Jacob disease in human beings (Mad cow disease in Humans).

Structural and Functional Relationship

The function of a protein depends upon its structure. Each protein has a unique conformation suited to its biological function. A small change in the primary structure of a protein can alter its conformation resulting in a decrease in or loss of function. Thousands of inherited diseases occur because of synthesis of abnormal proteins, many of which are fatal and many others lead to severe clinical abnormalities.

Catalytic Proteins

- One of the most important functions of proteins is to serve as biological catalysts, i.e. Enzymes. Except for some ribozymes (RNA enzymes), all enzymes are proteins. Biochemical reactions can occur at a significant rate only in the presence of enzymes. Most enzymes have a unique substrate binding site to which only one particular substrate can bind. Certain amino acid residues (or cofactors or coenzymes) are located strategically to catalyze the reaction. *The catalytic site of the enzyme may not be properly formed so that no substrate would bind.*

Structural Proteins

- Quantitatively, the structural proteins constitute the largest functional group of proteins. Structural proteins are present both inside and outside the cells. Inside the cells, they form the cytoskeleton of the cells, e.g. actin, tubulins. Outside the cells, they are present in the connective tissue, e.g. collagen, elastin, keratin, fibronectin, etc.
- Any alteration in the amino acid sequence at the primary structural level would alter the further folding of the polypeptide chain to higher levels of organization, such that the protein may lose its normal functional capacity. *Similarly structural proteins if abnormally synthesized may lead to compromised function of these proteins as is seen in collagen disorders.*

Collagen

- Collagen is the most abundant protein in mammals, constituting about one-fourth of the total protein content.
- There are different types of collagen, type I through type XIX, encoded by different genes. Each type of collagen is a triple helix made up of three polypeptide chains.
- Each polypeptide chain is coiled into a left-handed helix in which three amino acid residues are present in each turn.
- Glycine is the most abundant amino acid in collagen, followed by proline and hydroxy proline.
- Lysine and hydroxy lysine are also present in significant amount.
- Three polypeptide chains are intertwined to form a right-handed triple helix.
- The coiling of three left-handed helices into a right-handed triple helix gives immense tensile strength to collagen.
- The tensile strength is further increased by crosslinks between the three polypeptide chains and between different triple helices running parallel to each other.
- Abnormal collagens may be formed due to mutations or nutritional deficiencies (vitamin – C deficiency).
- Genetic defects leading to the formation of abnormal collagens may involve the genes encoding collagens or the genes encoding enzymes involved in post-translational modifications of procollagens (e.g. different types of Ehlers-Danlos syndrome in which joints are hypermobile, skin is hyperelastic and tissues are fragile).

Denaturation of Proteins

- The normal structure of proteins may be disrupted by physical or chemical agents leading to their denaturation or coagulation. Disruption of structure is associated with loss of function. Thus it is biologically inactive. Exposure to physical agents, e.g. Heat, X-rays, ultraviolet light, high pressure, vigorous shaking, etc. or chemical agents, e.g. Acids, alkalis, heavy metals, organic solvents, etc. may disrupt the secondary, tertiary and quaternary structures of Proteins. The primary structure remains unaffected. The denatured protein is less soluble and is easily precipitated.

Separation of Proteins

- Biological fluids contain a variety of proteins. Levels of these proteins get altered in many pathological conditions. The identification of the proteins would be of great significance in diagnosis and prognosis of these conditions. Many techniques have been developed for the separation and identification of the proteins. Briefly, the methods for fractionation of proteins include:
  - Salt fractionation
  - Alcohol fractionation
  - Centrifugation
  - Electrophoresis
  - Chromatography.

Salt Fractionation

- When a mixture of proteins is treated with varying concentrations of salts, different proteins are precipitated at different salt concentrations.
- This process is known as salting out, and can be used for fractionation of proteins. The salting out of proteins is based upon the fact that proteins form colloidal solutions with water. The colloidal particles are kept in solution by opposing charges on the particles repelling each other and by a shell of hydration around each particle, preventing the coalescence of these particles. However, addition of a neutral salt like ammonium sulfate removes the shell of hydration and neutralizes the charges, causing precipitation of the protein. The amount of salt needed depends upon the particle size of the protein. If the particle's size is small, a greater surface area of protein would need removal of shell of hydration and also the number of charges would also be more. Thus a higher concentration of the salt is needed, to completely saturate the shell of hydration and charges as in full saturation (solid ammonium sulfate). Conversely, if the particle size is large (globulins) the number of charges would be less and surface area would be smaller with a smaller shell of hydration needing lower concentration of neutral salt (ammonium sulfate).
- When a mixture of albumin and globulins is half saturated with ammonium sulfate, globulins are salted out.

Alcohol Fractionation

- Different proteins are precipitated at different concentrations of alcohol.
- Thus, differential alcohol precipitation can also be used for protein fractionation.

Centrifugation

- If a solution containing proteins is centrifuged at a high speed (ultracentrifugation), the proteins are separated into different layers depending upon their relative density.
- This technique is frequently used for the separation of lipoproteins present in plasma.

Electrophoresis

- Electrophoretic separation is based on the movement of charged particles in an electric field.

- If the charged particles, e.g. Proteins, differ in the number and type of charges, they will move at different rates in an electric field and will form different bands after sometime.
- *Discussed in detail in Practical Biochemistry section.*

Chromatography

- Chromatography can be used for the separation of proteins, amino acids, lipids, carbohydrates and several other classes of compounds.
- Basically, a chromatographic system consists of a stationary phase and a mobile phase. Separation occurs on the basis of relative solubilities or affinities towards the two phases.
- *Discussed in detail in Practical Biochemistry section.*

Protein Sequencing

- The modern clinical biochemistry has advanced tremendously over the years, to the extent that today we know the sequence of amino acids in several proteins and are even synthesizing them in laboratories.
  - Before the proteins are to be sequenced, they are first separated and purified using the above-mentioned techniques.
  - Next the amino acid composition is first determined. Peptides are homogenized and the peptide bonds linking them are hydrolyzed using 6N HCl at 110°C in sealed evacuated glass tubes for 24, 48, 72 and 96 hours.
  - The Val –Val, Ile – Ile, Val – Ile, Ile – Val bonds are highly stable. However, there may be some loss of Trp, Cys, Met and Tyr. Gln and Asn get deaminated to Glu and Asp.
  - To overcome these problems, Cys is oxidized to Cysteic oxide which is acid resistant. Trp can be estimated after alkaline hydrolysis. This destroys Cys, Arg, Ser and Thr.
  - Ser and Thr are reported from the hydrolysis mixture at zero hours. Gln and Asn are reported according to their dicarboxylic acid derivatives. Val and Leu are reported from 96 hours sample.
  - Sequencing is then done using 2 reagents—Sanger's and Edman's.

Sanger's Reagent

- More than 5 decades ago, Sanger sequenced the protein hormone Insulin. This was the first protein to be sequenced. He used 1–flouro – 2, 4–dinitrobenzene (Sanger's Reagent).
- He reacted the reagent to the amino terminal end of the peptide chain and then sequentially removed them one at a time. By comparing the amino acid sequences of overlapping peptides, complete sequence of both A and B chains of Insulin were deduced.

Edman's Reagent

- Today automated sequencing of proteins is carried out using the Edman's reagent—phenyl iso-thio-cyanate. In this technique, the amino terminal amino acid is removed as a phenylthiohydantoin derivative, to be identified by high pressure liquid chromatography. The next amino acid in the left-peptide sequence is derivatized and the process is repeated.

A Quick Look at the Proteins and Amino Acids Chemistry

- Proteins are biopolymers of amino acids.
- There are 20 different amino acids—8 essential, 2 semiessential and 10 nonessential.
- Based on chemical structure amino acids can be classified as aliphatic, aromatic, acidic, basic amino acids.
- Amino acids have a chiral carbon atom—show stereoisomerism and optical isomerism.
- Naturally occurring amino acids are L–isomers.
- Proteins are the classified as simple, conjugated and derived.
- Proteins are organized into 4 levels of organization—primary, secondary, tertiary and quaternary.
- The sequence of amino acids determines the structural organization and the functions of the proteins.
- Primary structure is maintained by peptide bonds.
- Secondary structure is maintained by disulfide bonds and H bonds.
- Tertiary structure is maintained by weak noncovalent interactions.
- Quaternary structure is maintained by weak noncovalent interactions.
- Proteins can be separated by various techniques—salt fractionation, alcohol fractionation, centrifugation, chromatography, and electrophoresis.

CHAPTER

4

Chemistry of Nucleic Acids

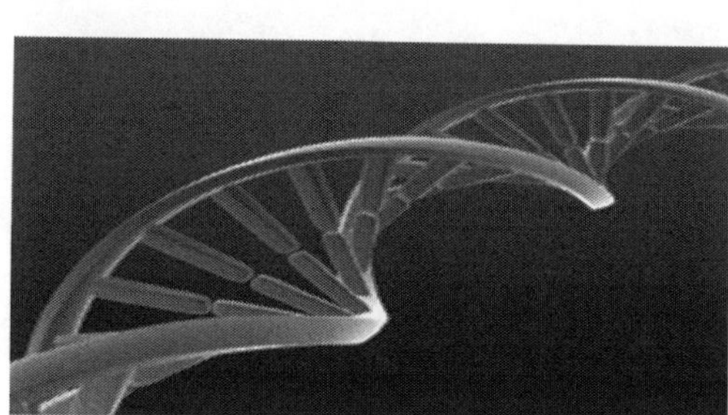

Chapter Framework

- Introduction
- Definition
- Chemistry of Nucleic Acids
- Classification of Amino Acids
- Some Biologically Important Nucleotides
- Structure of Nucleic Acids

Introduction

Nucleic acids are also termed as the 'information macromolecules' since they carry the genetic information of an organism with great accuracy and precision to their progeny. Thus, life perpetuates courtesy these information molecules. They are found in all cells in association with proteins like histones and protamines. Nucleic acids are negatively charged at physiological pH. They determine the properties of a cell, tissue, organ and finally the organism.

Definition

Nucleic acids are the biopolymers of nucleotides, just like proteins are polymers of amino acids and polysaccharides are polymers of monosaccharides. Nucleic acids are of two types—Deoxy - ribonucleic acid (DNA) and ribonucleic acid (RNA).

Chemistry of Nucleic Acids

The nucleic acids are composed of pentose sugars, nitrogen bases and phosphoric acid (Figs 4.1A and B).

There are two types of pentose sugars present in nucleic acids. Depending upon the type of nucleic acid, it may be ribose (in RNA) or deoxyribose (in DNA).

There are 5 types of nitrogenous bases present in nucleic acids—2 purines and 3 pyrimidines.

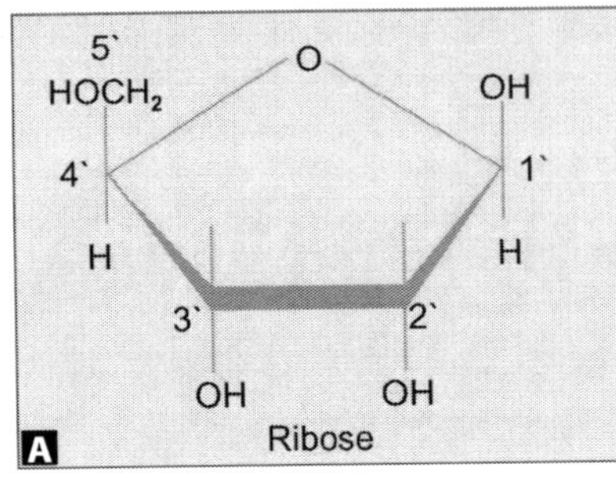

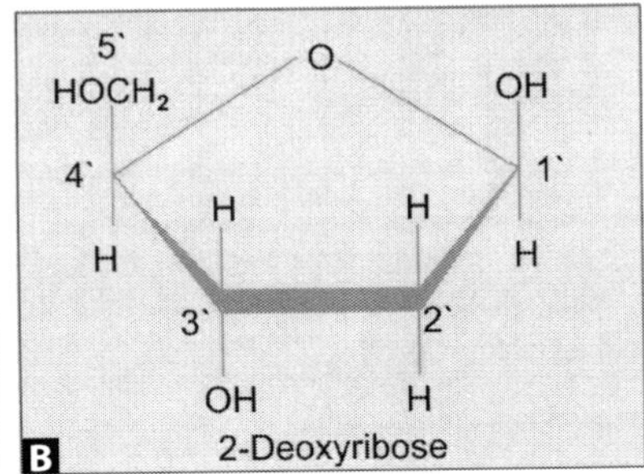

Figs 4.1A and B Pentose sugars

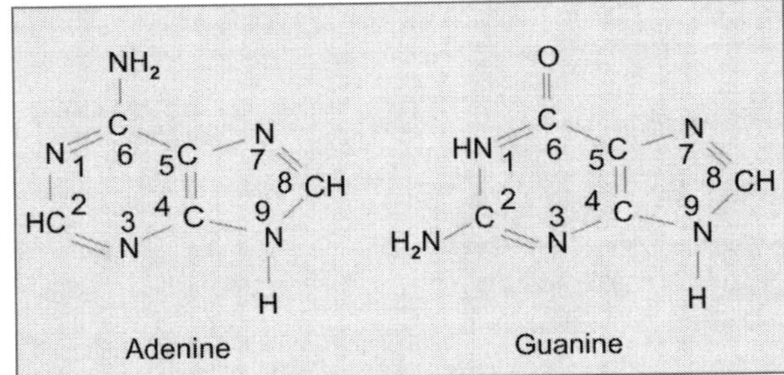

Fig. 4.2 Purines

Purines

The purines are double-ringed compounds (Fig. 4.2). They are:

- Adenine
- Guanine.

Pyrimidines

The pyrimidines are single-ringed compounds. They are:

- Cytosine
- Thymine
- Uracil.

The numbering of these bases occurs in a specific pattern, i.e. the purines are numbered in an anticlockwise manner while pyrimidines are numbered in clockwise manner, as seen in the Figures 4.2 and 4.3.

The fundamental repeating units of nucleic acid are nucleotides. A nucleotide is a phosphorylated form of a nucleoside (i.e. nucleotide = nucleoside + phosphoric acid). Each nucleoside is composed of a nitrogenous base and a pentose sugar linked by an ester linkage of the OH group of the sugar and the NH_2 hydrogen of the nitrogenous bases. Thus, types of nucleosides are:

- Adenosine
- Guanosine
- Cytidine
- Uridine (when ribose).

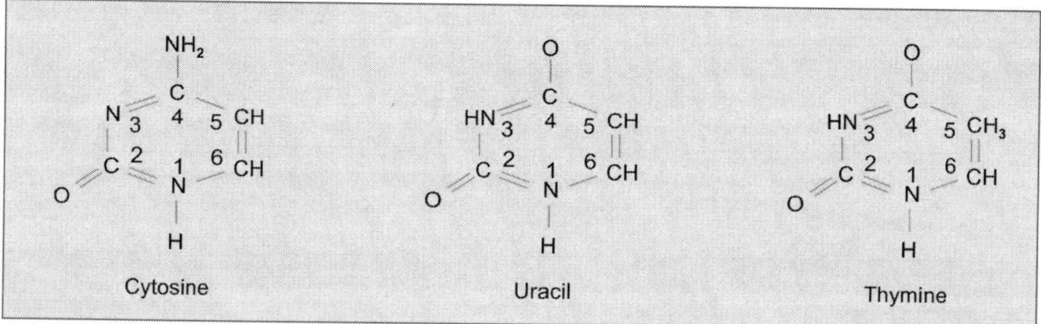

Fig. 4.3 Pyrimidines

- Thymidine (when deoxy ribose)
- Deoxy-adenosine
- Deoxy-guanosine
- Deoxy-cytidine.

The pentose sugar gets phosphorylated at C3' or C5' OH groups during formation of a nucleotide from nucleoside. For example Adenylate, Guanylate, Cytidylate, Uridylate (when ribose) and Thymidylate (when deoxy ribose).

- Deoxy-adenylate (dAMP)
- Deoxy-guanylate (dGMP)
- Deoxy-Cytidylate (dCMP)

The pentose sugar links up with the nitrogenous bases by N–glycosidic linkage.

It is formed between C1' OH group of pentose sugar and N9 of purines and N1 of pyrimidines.

Either of the two OH groups on the pentose sugars at C5' or C3' may be involved in the formation of the phosphodiester linkage (Fig. 4.4).

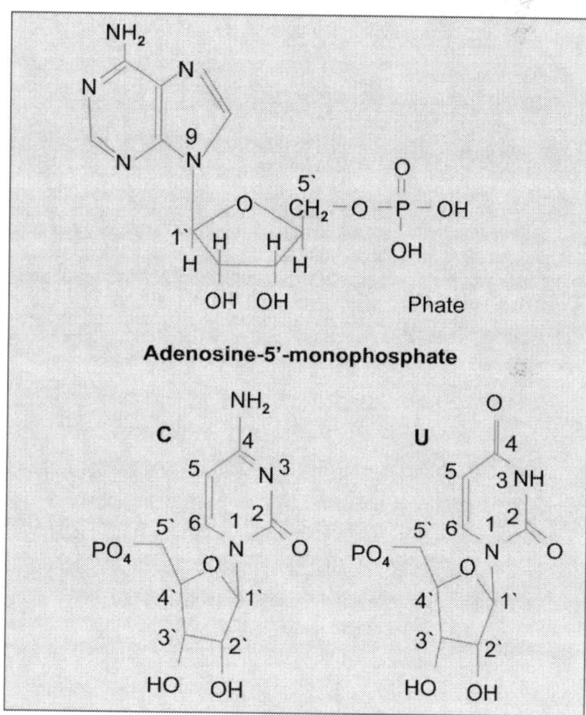

Fig. 4.4 Adenosine nucleotide – AMP and cytosine nucleotide

Some Biologically Important Nucleotides

Certain nucleotides function as **free nucleotides** and play important physiologic or pharmacologic roles:

- Adenine derivatives
- Guanine derivatives
- Hypoxanthine derivatives
- Cytosine derivatives
- Uracil derivatives

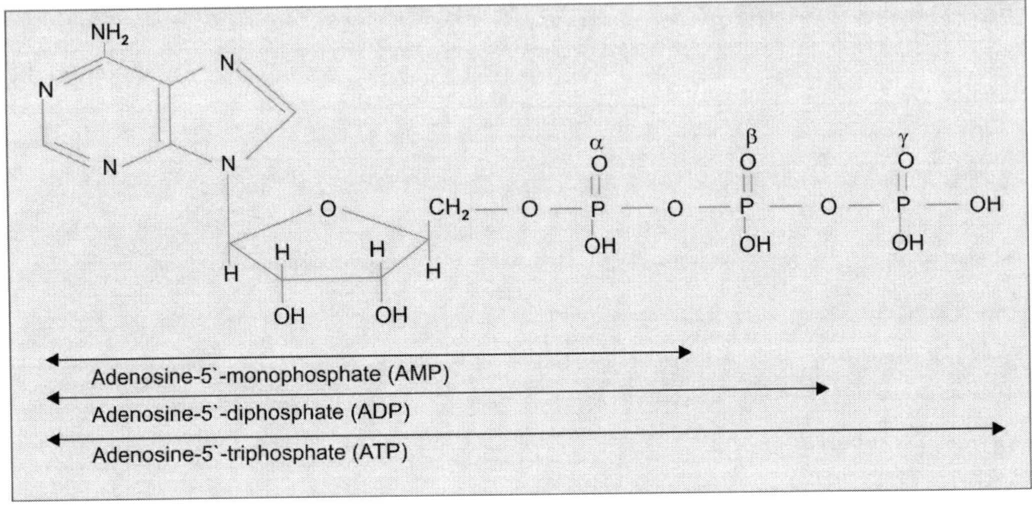

Fig. 4.5 ATP structure

- Coenzymes
- Synthetic derivatives.

Adenine Derivatives

- Important adenine nucleotides are AMP, ADP and ATP (Fig. 4.5).
- ATP and ADP are described as high-energy phosphates. Hydrolytic removal of the terminal phosphate of ADP and the last two phosphates of ATP liberates a large amount of energy.
- Another important adenine nucleotide is c – AMP (cyclic AMP) which acts as a second messenger for various peptide hormones (Fig. 4.6).

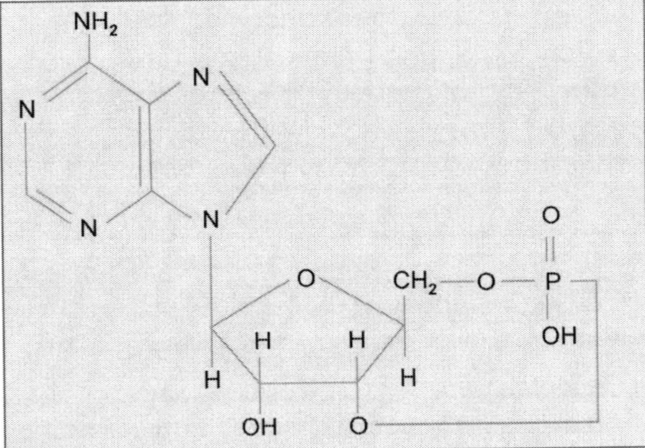

Fig. 4.6 Cyclic AMP

Guanine Derivatives

- Like adenine nucleotides, the guanine-containing nucleotides are GMP, GDP, GTP and cyclic GMP with identical roles.

Hypoxanthine Derivatives

- Hypoxanthine and ribose form a nucleoside, inosine. Inosine monophosphate (IMP) is the nucleotide formed from inosine which is an intermediate in the synthesis of purine nucleotides.

Cytosine Derivatives

- CMP, CDP and CTP are the nucleotides formed from cytosine. CDP and CTP are high-energy phosphates.

Uracil Derivatives

- UMP, UDP and UTP are the uracil-containing nucleotides. UDP and UTP are the high-energy analogs of ADP and ATP respectively.
- Some derivatives of UDP, e.g. UDP-glucose, UDP-galactose and UDP-glucuronic acid, are intermediates in some pathways of carbohydrate metabolism.

Coenzymes

- Most water-soluble vitamins perform their biochemical functions in the form of coenzymes.
- Many of these coenzymes are nucleotides containing adenine, ribose, phosphate and some other groups. For e.g. NAD^+, $NADP^+$ of niacin, FAD, FMN of riboflavin, CoA of pantothenate.

Synthetic Derivatives

- Some synthetic nucleosides and pyrimidine are important pharmacological agents. They function on the basis of the principle that—cell division requires replication of cellular DNA for which a ready supply of nucleotides is essential.
- If substitutions are made in the structures of purine or pyrimidine bases or the sugar portion of the nucleosides, and the substituted bases or nucleosides are given to a subject, they will be incorporated in the nucleic acids.
- DNA containing these abnormal bases or sugars cannot be replicated, and this prevents cell division. For, e.g. 6-Mercaptopurine, 6-Thioguanine, 5-Fluorouracil, Cytosine arabinoside.

Structure of DNA

- Chargaff (1950) studied the base composition of DNA obtained from diverse sources.
- He discovered that the number of adenine residues is always equal to the number of thymine residues, and the number of guanine residues is always equal to that of cytosine residues in a molecule of DNA.
- Maurice Wilkins and Rosalind Franklin carried out extensive X-ray crystallographic studies on DNA, and showed that DNA has a helical structure.
- James Watson and Francis Crick analyzed:
  - The X-ray crystallographic data
  - Chargaff's observations
  - Structures of purine and pyrimidine bases
  - Other facts.
- On the basis of their analysis, Watson and Crick proposed a model of DNA molecule.
- They announced their structure of DNA on Feb 28, 1953.
- Their model was consistent with all the known features of DNA.
- According to Watson and Crick model, DNA is a double-stranded helix, resembling helical ladder. Each strand of DNA is a polymer of mononucleotides.
- The successive nucleotides in a strand are linked by 3′,5′-phosphodiester bonds.
- Four bases—Adenine, guanine, cytosine and thymine are present in these nucleotides.
- The sugar is deoxyribose.
- Each strand possesses a polarity or direction. It has a 3′-end at which the –OH group attached to carbon atom 3 of the sugar is unesterified.

- The other end is the 5′-end at which the –OH group attached to carbon atom 5 of the sugar is esterified with phosphate.
- The two strands are antiparallel, i.e. they are parallel but run in opposite directions.
- The strands are held together by hydrogen bonds between their purine and pyrimidine bases—Adenine is paired with thymine, and guanine with cytosine. This is known as the base-pairing rule.
- Adenine and thymine are linked up by two H bonds and cytosine – guanine by three H bonds.
- The bases are present in the interior of the molecule while the sugar and phosphate groups are present on the outer side. Thus, sugar and phosphate make the side rails of the helical ladder and nitrogen bases the steps of the helical ladder.

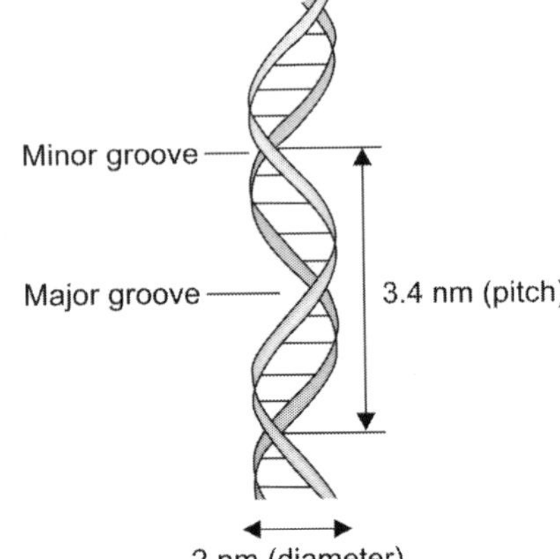

Fig. 4.7 DNA double helix

- The two strands are not straight. They are wound around each other to form a double helix.
- Each turn of the helix contains ten base pairs, and has a pitch of 3.4 nm.
- The diameter of the helix is 2 nm.
- The helix is right-handed.
- Two grooves are seen in the double helix which are termed as the major groove and the minor groove (Fig. 4.7).

Structure of RNA

RNA is also a polymer of mononucleotides. It differs from DNA in the following respects:

- The sugar in RNA is ribose instead of deoxyribose.
- The pyrimidine bases are cytosine and uracil instead of cytosine and thymine of DNA.
- The RNA molecule is single-stranded.
- The numbers of adenine and guanine residues are not necessarily equal to those of uracil and cytosine residues respectively.
- RNA may be folded upon itself and H bonds may be formed between complementary bases on parts of the same strand.
- This may give a double-stranded appearance in certain regions of the molecule.

There are three types of RNA:

- Messenger RNA (mRNA)
- Transfer RNA (tRNA)
- Ribosomal RNA (rRNA).

mRNA

- It acts as a messenger for the genetic information contained in DNA. The RNA molecule is synthesized complimentary to the template DNA strand. The information on the RNA strand guides the sequence of amino acids in a protein.

Table 4.1 Structure and functions of different types of RNA

	Structure	*Function*
mRNA	Single, uncoiled strand	Transmits information from DNA and serves as a template for protein synthesis
tRNA	Single strand, folded back on itself	Brings amino acids to ribosomes for protein synthesis
rRNA	Globular	rRNA and proteins make up ribosomes

- The mRNA of eukaryotes has come unique feature like:
  - At the 5′end, a 7–methyl GTP cap is present that protects against the 5′exonuclease activity.
  - At the 3′ end a poly A tail, i.e. a sequence of about 250 polyadenylate residues is present that protect against the 3′exonuclease activity.
  - The poly A tail also helps in separating the mRNA molecules from a mixture of RNAs by adhering oligo dT to a solid substrate, which polymerizes with the poly A tails of mRNA, isolating them.

tRNA

- This is made up of about 75 nucleotides, and has a molecular weight of about 25,000.
- Its function is to transport amino acids from the cytosol to the ribosomes where proteins are synthesized.
- Proteins are synthesized from 20 amino acids. For each of these amino acids, there is at least one specific tRNA. For some amino acids, there are more than one species of tRNA.
- One species of tRNA transports only one specific amino acid.
- The single strand of tRNA folds upon itself to form a 3D clover leaf structure (Fig. 4.8).
  - The Acceptor arm accepts activated amino acid during the translation process.
  - The Pseudouridine arm helps recognize the correct amino acyl tRNA synthase enzyme.
  - The Dihydrouracil helps bind on to the ribosome.
  - The Anticodon loop has a three nucleotides complimentary to the triplet codon on the DNA coding for specific amino acid.
  - The lump or the extra arm helps in categorising the tRNAs as class I and II. Class – I tRNA have 3–7 nucleotides and class – II tRNAs have 13–21 nucleotides.

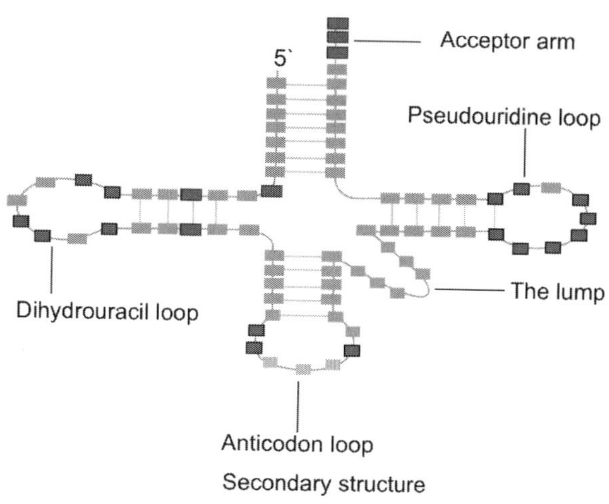

Fig. 4.8 tRNA

Ribosomal RNA

- This is present in the ribosomes. The ribosomes are made up of two subunits known respectively as the 40S subunit and the 60S subunit in eukaryotes.

Features of rRNA

- The 40S subunit is made up of 18S rRNA and about 30 different polypeptides.
- The 60S subunit is made up of three types of rRNA—5S rRNA, 5.8S rRNA and 28S rRNA – and about 50 different polypeptides.
- The 5.8S, 18S and 28S rRNAs are formed from a single 45S precursor
- The 5S rRNA is formed as such.
- The rRNA and polypeptides combine to form globular subunits.
- When proteins are not being synthesized, the two subunits remain separate.
- At the time of protein synthesis, the two subunits combine to form an 80S unit on which mRNA and tRNAs interact to synthesize a protein.
- During protein synthesis, a single mRNA is translated simultaneously by several ribosomal particles, in different regions of the mRNA located at least 80 nucleotides apart. Such a structure is called a Polysome (Fig. 4.9).

Small Nuclear RNAs

- These are made up of about 70–91 nucleotides.
- They help in the processing of heteronuclear RNA.

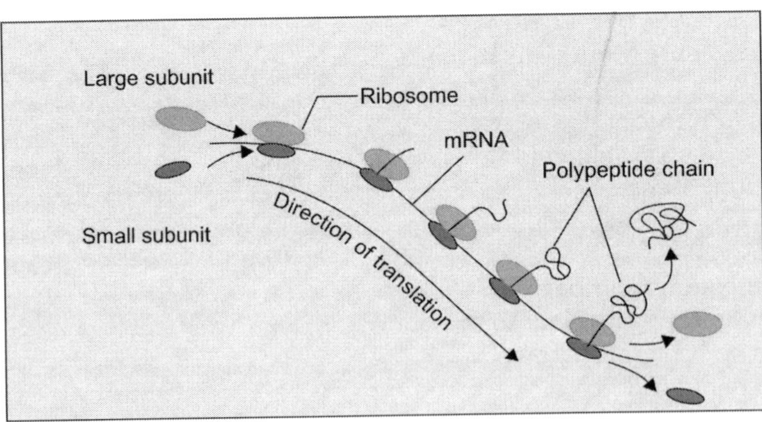

Fig. 4.9 Polysome

A Quick Look at the Chemistry of Nucleic Acids

- Nucleic acids are the polymers of nucleotides.
- Two types of nucleotides are DNA and RNA.
- DNA is the hereditary basis of life.
- DNA has a double helical structure, first described by Watson and Crick.
- DNA differs from RNA in the pentose sugar which is deoxyribose and not ribose , and has pyrimidine thymine instead of uracil.
- Three types of RNAs are known—t-RNA, m-RNA, r-RNA.
- All three participate in translation.
- tRNA carries the amino acids to site of protein synthesis.
- mRNA acts as a template on which new polypeptide chain is synthesized.
- rRNA is the component of ribosomes which the site of translation.
- Small nuclear RNAs help in the RNA processing.

Section – 2

Biocatalysts, Vitamins, Minerals and Nutrition

- Biocatalysts: Enzymes, Enzyme Kinetics and Clinical Enzymology
- Vitamins
- Mineral Metabolism
- Nutrition

CHAPTER

5

Biocatalysts: Enzymes, Enzyme Kinetics and Clinical Enzymology

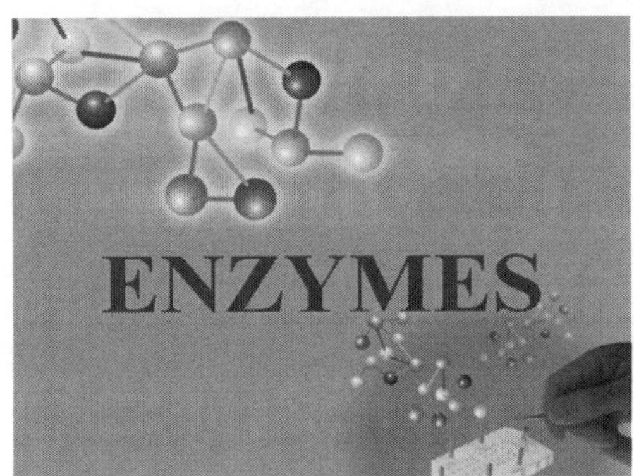

Chapter Framework

- Introduction
- History of Enzymes
- What are Enzymes?
- Nomenclature and Classification of Enzymes
- Coenzymes and Cotactors
- Properties of Enzymes
- Kinetics of Enzymes
- Enzyme Inhibition
- Regulation of Enzyme Activity
- Clinical Enzymology

Introduction

For life to sustain there are two prerequisites:

- The living organism must be able to self-replicate.
- The organism must be able to catalyze chemical reactions efficiently and selectively so as to generate energy necessary for thriving and perpetuating.
    - The biocatalysts, enzymes are highly specialized biomolecules (mostly proteins with exception of ribozymes) that act in a highly organized manner, catalyzing hundreds of stepwise reactions that metabolize nutrient molecules and entrap their chemical energy as utilizable form of energy.

History of Enzymes

- The existence of enzymes has been known for well over a century.
- By the late 1700s and early 1800s, the digestion of meat by stomach secretions and the conversion of starch to sugars by plant extracts and saliva were known. However, the mechanism by which this occurred had not been identified.
- In the 19th century, while studying the fermentation of sugar to alcohol by yeast, **Louis Pasteur** came to the conclusion that this fermentation was catalyzed by a vital force contained within the yeast cells called ferments.
- In **1878** German physiologist **Wilhelm Kühne (1837–1900)** first used the term 'enzyme'.
- *Buchner (1897)* found that the sugar was fermented even when there were no living yeast cells in the mixture. He named the enzyme that brought about the fermentation of sucrose; zymase.

What are Enzymes?

- Enzymes are biocatalysts, i.e. they catalyze and enhance the rates of biochemical reactions without themselves undergoing any change, i.e. they increase the rates of biochemical reactions.
- Most enzymes are Proteins (tertiary and quaternary structures).
- They are not permanently changed in the process.
- Almost all processes in a cell need enzymes in order to occur at significant rates.
- The reactant on which the enzyme acts; is known as the substrate of the enzyme. The enzyme converts the substrate into a product.

Nomenclature and Classification of Enzymes

- The nomenclature of enzymes has undergone many changes over the years.
- Some of the earliest names, e.g. pepsin, ptyalin, zymase, etc. indicate neither the substrates of the enzymes nor the type of reactions catalyzed by them.
- Later, suffix –'ase' was added to the name of the substrate e.g. lipase, protease, ribo-nuclease etc.
- Still the type of reaction catalyzed by the enzyme remained unclear. To make the names of enzymes precise, fully informative and unambiguous, International Union of Biochemistry and Molecular Biology (IUBMB) devised a method of nomenclature and classification of enzymes.

International Union of Biochemistry and Molecular Biology System of Enzyme Nomenclature and Classification

- The enzymes have been divided into six classes (numbered 1 to 6).
- Each class is divided into subclasses.
- Subclasses are divided into sub-subclasses.
- Sub-subclasses are divided into individual enzymes:
  - While naming an enzyme the first part includes the name(s) of the substrate(s) including coenzyme(s) if they act as second substrate(s).
  - The second part includes the type of reaction ending with –ase. If any additional information is to be given, it is put in parenthesis at the end. For example, the enzyme having the trivial name glutamate dehydrogenase.
  - According to IUB system, this enzyme in known as L-Glutamate:NAD(P) oxidoreductase (deaminating).
  - Thus, the name gives complete information about the reaction catalyzed by the enzyme.
  - Furthermore, each enzyme has been given a code number consisting of four digits which, successively, denote the number of the class, subclass, sub-subclass and the individual enzyme.
  - The code number of L-glutamate: NAD(P) oxidoreductase (deaminating) is EC 1.4.1.3 which shows that it is the third enzyme of sub-subclass 1 of subclass 4 of class 1.
  - Thus according to IUB classification, the enzymes are divided into the following six classes:
    1. Oxidoreductases
    2. Transferases
    3. Hydrolases
    4. Lyases
    5. Isomerases
    6. Ligases

Oxidoreductases

These are the enzymes that catalyze oxidation-reduction reactions. Oxidation involves the removal of H from the substrate and simultaneously, the coenzyme is reduced by accepting the H, thus acting like a co-substrate. One of the substrates is oxidized and the other is reduced. There are several subclasses of oxidoreductases, each subclass acting on a particular chemical group. These enzymes use NAD^+, $NADP^+$, FMN and FAD as co-substrates. Examples of oxidoreductases are glutamate dehydrogenase, lactate dehydrogenase, malate dehydrogenase, glycerol-3-phosphate dehydrogenase, etc.

Transferases

These enzymes transfer a group other than hydrogen from one substrate to another. Such groups include methyl group, amino group, phosphate group, acyl group, glycosyl group, etc. Examples include hexokinase, glucokinase, glutamate oxaloacetate transaminase (SGOT), ornithine carbamoyl transferase, etc.

Hydrolases

These are hydrolytic enzymes which hydrolyze bonds such as peptide, ester, glycosidic bonds, etc. These enzymes are commonly found in the digestive secretions and lysosomes. Examples are amylase, lipase, pepsin, ribonuclease, sucrase, lactase and maltase, etc.

Lyases

These enzymes remove chemical groups from substrates by mechanisms other than hydrolysis and may introduce a double bond. The groups removed may be water, amino group, etc. Examples include aldolase, enolase and fumerase, etc.

Isomerases

These enzymes catalyze interconversion of isomers of a compound. Examples include racemase, triose phosphate isomerase, phosphohexose isomerase, ribose-5- phosphate ketoisomerase, etc.

Ligases

These enzymes ligate or bind two compounds together. Since the binding occurs by a covalent bond, a source of energy is required, usually a high energy phosphate. Examples are glutamine synthetase, squalene synthetase and acetyl CoA carboxylase, etc.

Coenzymes and Cofactors

- Some enzymes require the presence of a nonprotein prosthetic substance for their catalytic activity.
- If the nonprotein substance is organic, it is known as a **coenzyme.**
- If it is inorganic, it is known as a **cofactor.**
- The coenzyme or the cofactor may be an integral part of the enzyme molecule or its presence may be required during the reaction.
- The protein portion of an enzyme that requires a coenzyme is called apoenzyme.
- The apoenzyme combines with the coenzyme to form the holoenzyme which is the catalytically active form of the enzyme.

- The apoenzyme provides for the three-dimensional protein structure of the holoenzyme and the coenzyme part acts as a cosubstrate.
- Apoenzyme + Coenzyme = Holoenzyme
- Depending upon the type of group being transferred by the coenzyme, it is of two types:
  - Type – I transferring Hydrogen
    - FAD (Flavin adenine dinucleotide)
    - FMN (Flavin mononucleotide)
    - NAD^+ (Nicotinamide adenine dinucleotide)
    - $NADP^+$ (Nicotinamide adenine dinucleotide phosphate)
      Coenzyme Q
  - Type – II transferring other groups:
    - TPP (Thiamin pyrophosphate) or TDP (Thiamin diphosphate)—Hydroxy ethyl group.
    - CoA (Coenzyme A)—Acyl group.
    - PLP (Pyridoxal phosphate)—Amino group.
    - H4- Folate (Tetrahydrofolate)—1 – C moieties (like formyl, methyl, methylene, etc.)
    - Cobamides (B_{12}- Coenzymes)—Methyl group.
    - Biotin—CO_2.
    - ATP (Adenosine triphosphate)—Phosphate group.

Properties of Enzymes

Enzyme Specificity

- Enzymes are highly specific in their mechanism of action. This is of great significance, because if a single enzyme catalyzes a large number of reactions, it will be impossible to regulate the rates of individual reactions and will cause futile cycling of pathways causing a burning away of essential fuel.
- One of the properties of enzymes that makes them important as diagnostic and research tools is the specificity they exhibit toward the biochemical reactions they catalyze. The degree of specificity may have the following orders:

Group Specificity

Enzymes with group specificity are specific for a chemical group or bond present in the substrate. Such enzymes are usually present in the digestive juices like the lipases, glycosidases, proteolytic enzymes, etc.

Substrate Specificity

Enzymes with substrate specificity are specific for one particular substrate, e.g. Glucokinase, Sucrase, and Fructokinase.

Stereo Specificity

Biomolecules like carbohydrates and amino acids (L – amino acids and sugars are D – sugars) exhibit stereoisomerism. Biochemical reactions of such biomolecules are catalyzed by enzymes specific for a particular stereoisomer.

Structure of Enzyme

- Most enzymes are proteins (with exception of ribozymes). An enzyme has a substrate binding site, active site.
- The active site is a small cleft or a crevice on the enzyme molecule where the various chemical groups are arranged in an order appropriate for substrate binding (Fig. 5.1).

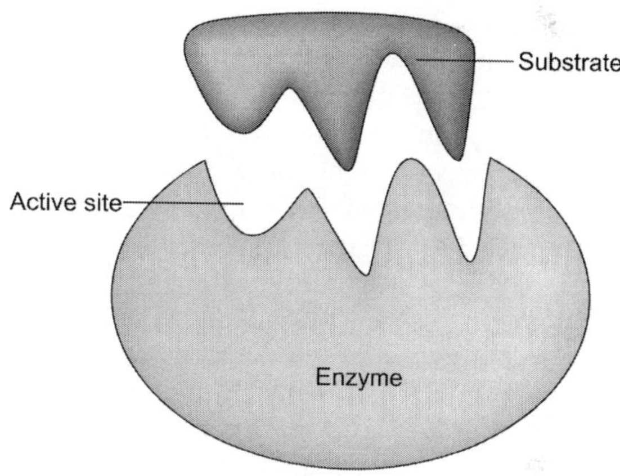

Fig. 5.1 Active site of enzyme

Mechanism of Action of Enzyme

- For the biochemical reactions to go to completion activation energy is needed that raises the substrate to a higher energy level so that the substrate splits into product spontaneously.
- Enzymes catalyze biochemical reactions which otherwise would need a large amount of energy or extremes of temperature and pH for completion.
- In the presence of enzymes, there is reduction in the activation energy required by the substrate molecules for spontaneously breaking down into products. This is like drilling a tunnel in a hill and crossing over without going all around and over the hill (Fig. 5.2A and B).

Enzyme-Substrates Interaction

Enzymes interact with substrates to form enzyme substrate complex (ES). The ES complex then dissociates to give product and free enzyme. The interaction of enzymes with substrates can be explained by two models:

- ***Lock and Key Theory of Emil Fischer:*** According to this theory, the substrate binding site on an enzyme molecule is a rigid 3–dimensional structure having chemical groups arranged

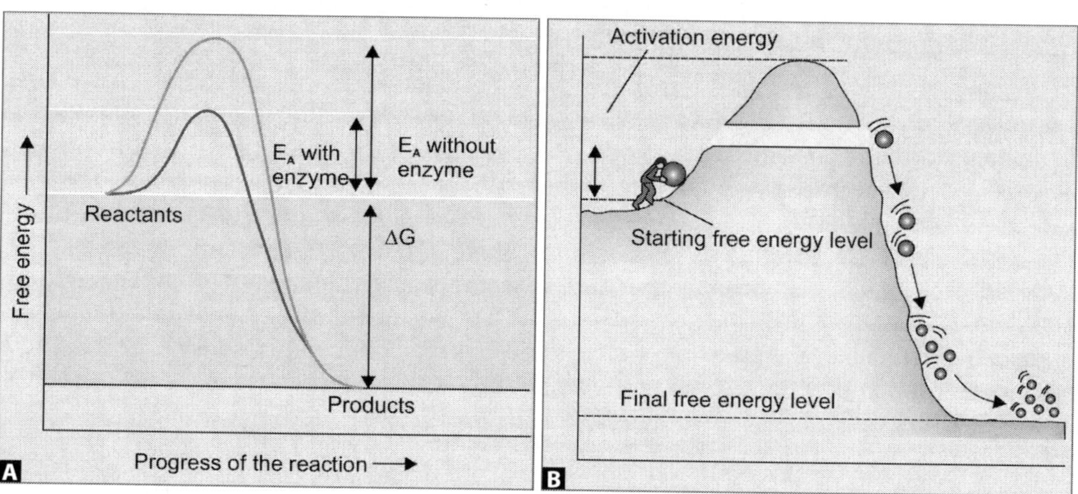

Figs 5.2A and B Reduction in activation energy by enzymes

complimentary to the groups on the substrate. Thus the enzyme fits on like a key fits its specific lock. However, this theory cannot explain the action of single enzyme on multiple substrates and was discarded (Fig. 5.3).

- ***Induced Fit Theory of Koshland:*** According to this theory, the chemical groups on the active site of an enzyme get rearranged when a substrate molecule is approached, according to the chemical groups on the substrate molecule. This realignment helps proper binding of enzyme and substrate. Since the realignment is induced by the close proximity of the substrate, it is termed as induced fit theory (Fig. 5.4).

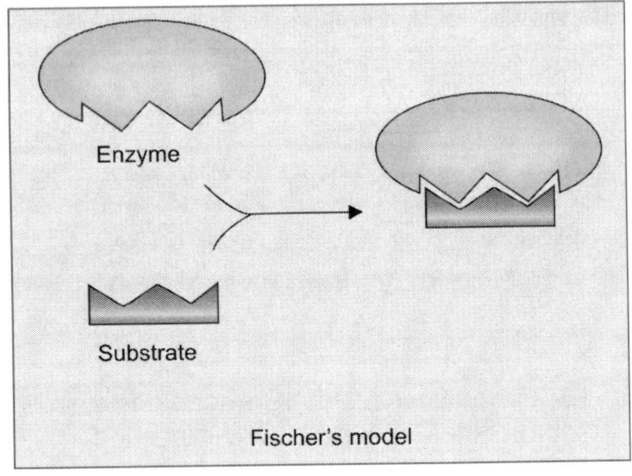

Fig. 5.3 Fischer's model

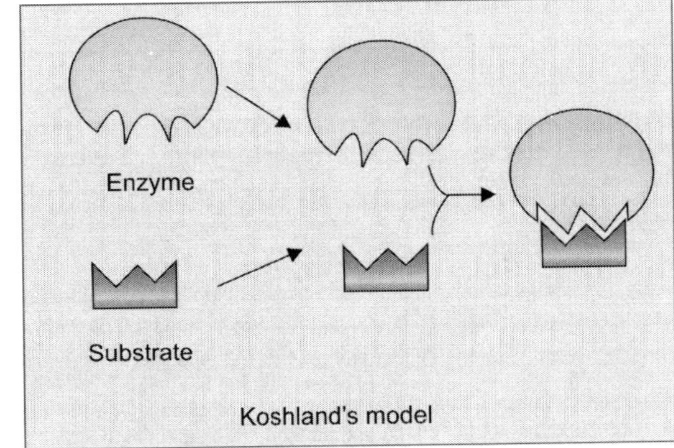

Fig. 5.4 Induced fit theory

Enzyme Kinetics

Factors Affecting Enzyme Activity

The enzyme activity gets affected by the following factors:

- Temperature
- pH
- Enzyme concentration
- Substrate concentration.

Effect of Temperature on Enzyme Activity

During any chemical or biochemical reaction, the molecules react by colliding against each other. The collision occurs due to the inherent kinetic energies of the reacting molecules. A rise in the temperature of the reaction medium would further enhance the kinetic energies of these molecules and the reaction rate. The same holds true for the biochemical systems. However, biologic systems cannot withstand extremes of temperature as the enzymes catalyzing these reactions are proteins and get denatured at extreme of temperatures. Therefore, the rate of an enzymatic reaction increases initially with the rise in temperature, reaches its maximum (at optimum temperature) and then decreases on further increase in temperature due to enzyme protein denaturation. In human, the optimal temperature for enzyme activity is the body temperature, i.e. 37.5°C. There are a few exceptions like the enzymes of a few bacteria of thermal springs.

Effect of pH

Enzymes are highly specific for their optimal pH range, considering the fact that most of the enzymes are proteinaceous in nature. This is because the amino acids are amphoteric in nature and they ionize according to the pH of the medium, and any alteration in the pH of the medium shall cause the ionization of the amino acids groups and radicals. Most human enzymes work optimally at the physiological pH (7.35 – 7.45), however, there are exceptions like the enzymes of gastric juice act at an optimal pH of 1–2; enzymes like alkaline phosphatase (ALP) acts at a pH around 10; acid phosphatase pH range 4–5; pancreatic juice enzymes pH range 8–8.3 etc. Extreme changes in pH, from the optimal range cause the enzyme proteins to denaturate and lose their physiological activity. The enzymes show peak activity at the optimal pH (Fig. 5.5).

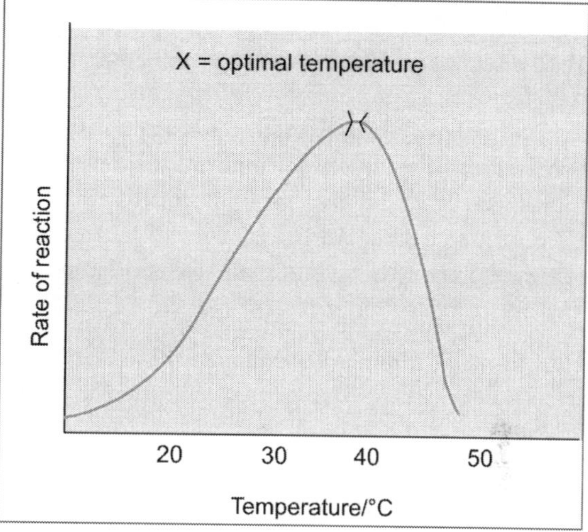

Fig. 5.5 Effect of temperature on enzyme activity

Effect of Concentration of Enzymes

An enzyme binds to a substrate to form the enzyme-substrate complex, which dissociates to form product and enzyme molecule remains unaltered. The rate of a biochemical reaction increases with the increase in the concentration of the enzyme molecules, provided substrate molecules concentration is not a limiting factor (Fig. 5.6).

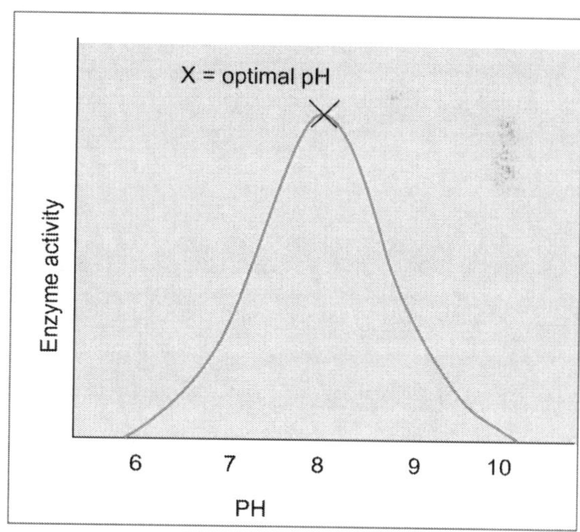

Fig. 5.6 Effect of pH on enzyme activity

Effect of Substrate Concentration

Just as the rate of the reaction is proportional to enzyme concentration, theoretically it should be proportional to substrate concentration also provided that enough enzymes are available to bind the substrate. When the substrate concentration rises, initially there is a proportionate increase in the velocity of the reaction but later the rise in velocity becomes slower until a maximum

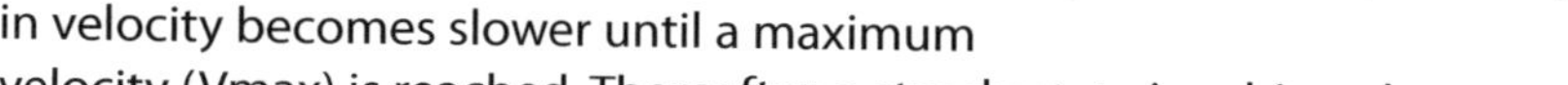

velocity (Vmax) is reached. Thereafter, a steady state is achieved.

At the maximum velocity (Vmax) of the enzyme, all the enzyme active sites are bound to substrate, and the amount of ES complex is the same as the total amount of enzyme. The substrate concentration at half the Vmax is termed as (Km) Michealis constant. The number of substrate molecules handled by one active site per second is given by Kcat or the specificity constant. It is useful for reactions where there are multiple substrates, with multiple rate constants affecting the overall enzyme activity (affinity and catalytic ability). So the efficiency of an enzyme = Kcat/Km

Michealis-Menten Equation

Michealis and Menten proposed a theory to help understand the enzyme kinetics. According to their proposed theory, the enzyme molecules and the substrate molecules react to give an ES complex. This ES complex formation is a reversible step regulated by two rate constants K_1 and K_2. The ES complex dissociates into free E and product (P), the rate of which is depicted by the rate constant $K_{3.}$

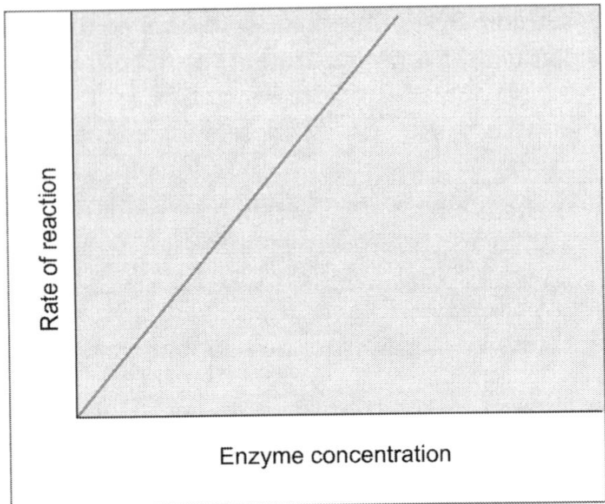

Fig. 5.7 Effect of enzyme concentration

$$E + S \underset{K_2}{\overset{K_1}{\rightleftarrows}} ES \xrightarrow{K_3} E + P$$

$$\frac{V_0 = K_2\,[E]\,[S]}{[S] + [K_3 + K_2]/K_1}$$

$$\frac{K_m = K_3 + K_2}{K_1}$$

$$\frac{V_0 = K_2\,[E]\,[S]}{[S] + K_m}$$

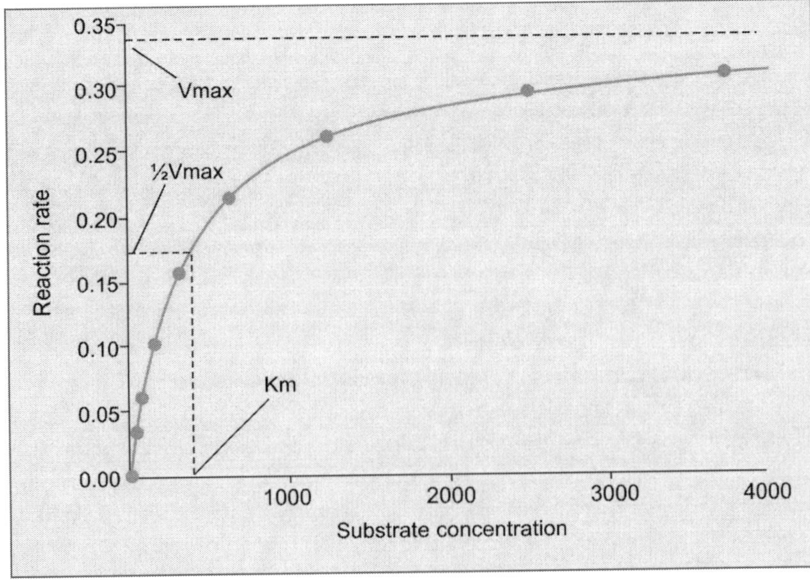

Fig. 5.8 Effect of substrate concentration

According to the Michealis-Menten equation, the rate of the enzyme catalyzed reaction (V_0) varies with substrate concentration according to the equation below:

$$V_0 = \frac{Vmax\,[S]}{Km + [S]}$$

Where, V_0 is initial reaction velocity
Vmax is maximal velocity,
[S] Substrate concentration,
When Km = [S]

$$V_0 = \frac{Vmax}{2}$$

Characteristics of Km

- Every enzyme has got its specific Km, like each individual has a unique finger print.
- Determination of Km is important in the study of enzyme kinetics, assay of enzyme activity and evaluation of enzyme inhibitors.
- Km is inversely proportional to affinity of the enzyme to its substrate, i.e. higher the Km lesser the affinity (high substrate concentration needed to get Vmax/2)
- Low Km high affinity so less substrate concentration needed to get Vmax/2, e.g.
  Glucokinase – Km 5mmol/L
  Hexokinase – Km 0.05 mmol/L
  This suggests that hexokinase will phosphorylate glucose even at low concentrations (0. 05 mmol/L) whereas glucokinase needs high BSL. This is useful too since, the portal vein carries the blood with high blood sugar which induces the secretion of insulin. Insulin then causes the hepatic glucokinase synthesis, which in turn phosphorylates glucose so that more and more glucose is taken up into the hepatocytes down a concentration gradient from blood into the hepatocytes. However, other tissues have hexokinase for phosphorylating and utilizing glucose. Its low Km value assures a high affinity for glucose that enables them to utilize glucose as a source of energy at low concentrations also.

Lineweaver-Burk Plot (Fig. 5.9)

- Sometimes, it is impractical to achieve Vmax as very high [S] are required. Thus, the substrate concentrations are plotted in reciprocals across the reciprocal values of rate of enzymatic reactions.
- This 1/V versus 1/[S] plot is known as Line weaver-Burk plot or double reciprocal plot.

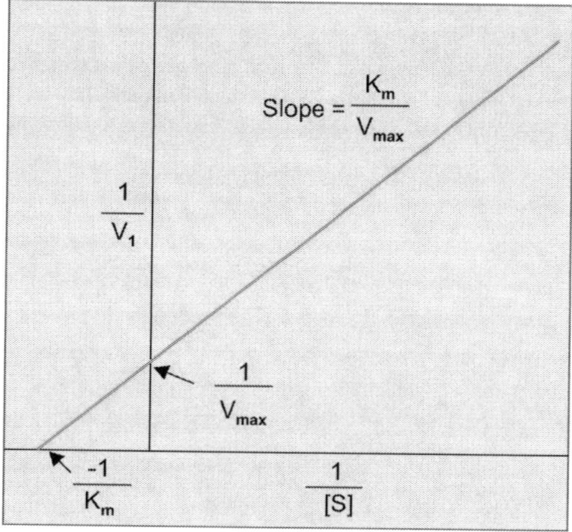

Fig. 5.9 Lineweaver-Burk plot

Enzyme Activation

Some enzymes are secreted in their inactive forms—zymogens. The zymogens are activated when their activity is required, e.g. Proteolytic enzymes—trypsinogen, chymotrypsinogen, and pepsinogen, coagulation factors.

The activation involves splitting of a portion of the peptide chain such that their active site would be exposed to bind the substrate molecules.

Allosteric Enzymes

- Some enzymes are termed as allosteric enzymes. These are multisubunit enzymes with a separate allosteric site in addition to the catalytic/active site.
- Allosteric site is a physically distinct site at which specific modifiers of enzyme activity bind and alter the enzyme activity by causing conformational change in the active site.
- Some allosteric regulators prevent the conformational change required for the binding of the substrate—**Allosteric inhibitors.**
- The enzymes subject to allosteric inhibition are generally present in the beginning of long metabolic pathways.
- If the product is not being utilized and accumulates, it inhibits the allosteric enzyme, and further synthesis of the product is stopped.
- **Allosteric activators** alter the active site conformation such that there is an enhanced binding of the substrate to the active site and thus in turn the rate of catalysis.

Enzyme Inhibition

Enzyme activity is inhibited by a number of inhibitors. Some of the inhibitors act as enzyme poisons and others are used as pharmacologic agents. The different types of inhibitions are:

- Competitive inhibition
- Noncompetitive inhibition
- Suicide inhibition.

Competitive Inhibition (Fig. 5.10)

In this type of inhibition, the inhibitor is a structural analog of the substrate, i.e. it has structural similarities with the substrate. Thus, it competes with the substrate for binding to the active site of the enzyme. In the presence of a competitive inhibitor, the effective concentration of the enzyme molecules is reduced, so there is less availability of enzyme for the substrate. This means a greater substrate concentration is needed to achieve Vmax. Or the affinity of the enzyme for the substrate decreases (Km increases) for achieving same Vmax. When the concentration of substrate is increased, this inhibition may be completely reversed since the substrate molecules would out-number the inhibitor molecules.

■ E + S	⟶	ES	⟶	E + P
■ E + I	⟶	EI	⟶	I + E
■ E + I + S	⟶	EI + ES		
100 100 100		50 50		
■ E + I + S	⟶	ES + EI	⟶	E + P
100 100 900		90 10		90

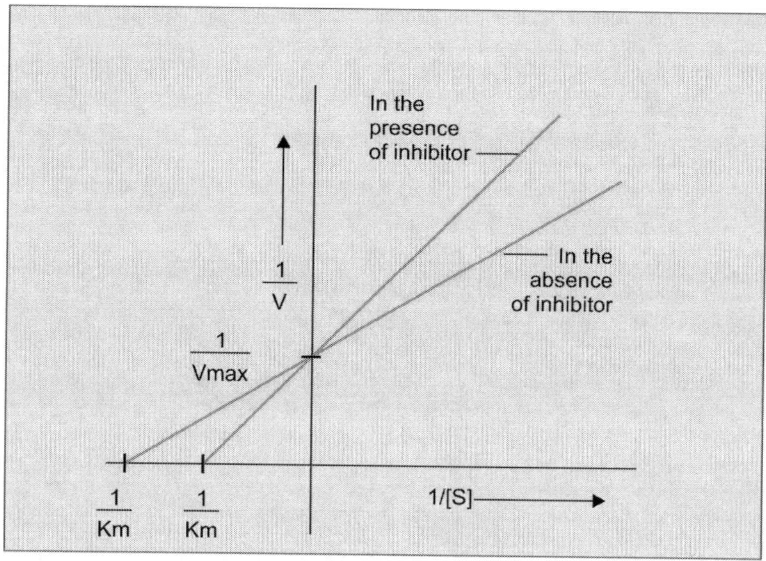

Fig. 5.10 Lineweaver-Burk plot of competitive inhibitor

Pharmacologic Application

- **Sulfa drugs:** Bacteria synthesize folic acid necessary for DNA synthesis, from PABA + Pteroyl glutamic acid. Sulfa drugs are structural analog of PABA. Sulfa drugs compete and prevent formation of folic acid. Thus killing bacteria showing anti-bacterial action.
- **Methotrexate:** It is an anticancer drug. It inhibits enzyme folate reductase competitively and thus inhibits multiplication of cancer cells.
- **Dicoumarol:** Competitively inhibits the Vitamin – K cycle which regenerates reduced vitamin K (quinol form) necessary for activation of clotting factors. Thus it prevents activation of clotting factors and acts like anticoagulant. Dicoumarol poisoning may lead to death due to internal hemorrhages.
- **Allopurinol:** Structural analog of hypoxanthine and inhibits enzyme xanthine oxidase.

  Hypoxanthine —✗→ Xanthine —✗→ Uric acid

  Thus, it is used in treatment of hyperuricemia of gout.

Noncompetitive Inhibition (Fig. 5.11)

- Inhibitor not structural analog of substrate. It binds irreversibly to site other than active site and acts as enzyme poison.
- The Km value is same but Vmax is reduced since the number of functional enzyme molecules is reduced. However those functional have same affinity towards substrate.
- Increasing the substrate concentration does not reverse it.
- For example, **Iodo acetate** poison enzymes with SH group, **CN** poisons Cytochrome oxidase, **Flouride** ions remove Mg^{++} and Mn^{++} ions to inhibit **Enolase** of glycolysis, **British Anti Lewsite (BAL)** used in heavy metal poisoning as it has multiple SH groups and heavy metals bind to them and not to enzymes.

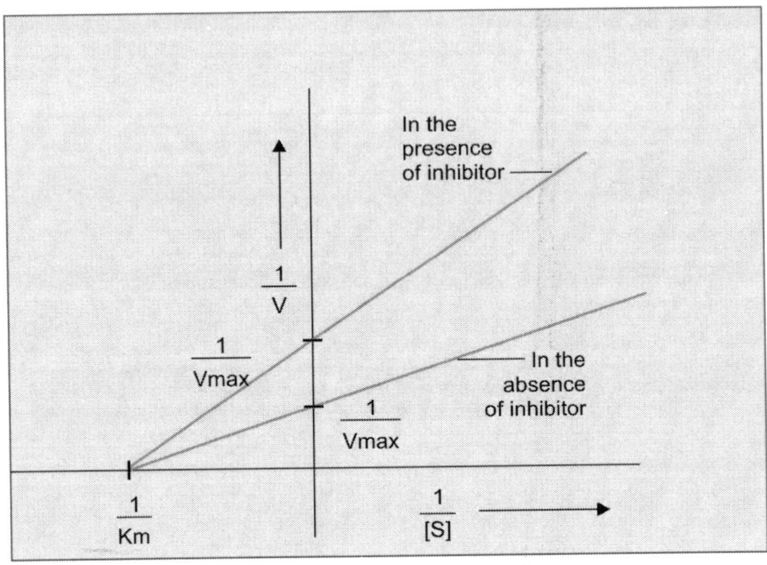

Fig. 5.11 Lineweavers-Burk plot of noncompetitive inhibition

Suicide Inhibition

- It is a type of irreversible competitive inhibition.
- In this, the inhibitor is a structural analog of substrate, which catalyzes a few steps of the enzymatic reaction to be converted into a much stronger inhibitor.
- Thus it inhibits the enzyme which converts it into a stronger inhibitor so it is called suicide inhibition, e.g. **Difluoromethyl ornithine** (DFMO) inhibition of ornithine decarboxylase (ODC) to treat African sleeping sickness caused by Trypanosoma. DFMO reacts with coenzyme of ODC, i.e. Pyridoxal phosphate and becomes active inhibitor to inhibit ODC strongly. Thus, there is no putrescine formed, no polyamines and DNA synthesis, inhibiting multiplication of trypanosoma in the host.
- However, human cells are unaffected since, their rate of turnover of ODC is very high.
- Ornithine —⊖→ Putriscine ——→ Polyamines ——→ DNA
- Aspirin inhibits enzyme cyclo-oxygenase by acetylating the serine residues on active site.

Regulation of Enzyme Activity

Regulation of enzyme activity is a must for the prevention of futile cycling of substrate and to prevent the loss of energy in carrying out unnecessary metabolic reactions.

- **Fine regulation**
  - Covalent modification
  - Allosteric modification.
- **Coarse regulation**
  - Induction
  - Repression

Fine Regulation

- Fine regulation of enzymes activity involves the alteration in the existing enzymes molecules in such a way so as to either increase or decrease their activity as needed. It is achieved by –

Covalent Modification

Addition of or removal of a group that binds to the enzyme covalently like phosphate (phosphorylation), acetyl group (acetylation). This alters the enzyme activity, e.g. Activity of glycogen synthase and phosphorylase during glycogen metabolism.

Allosteric Modification

Positive or negative modifier alters the activity of the enzyme by binding on to the allosteric site of the enzyme.

Coarse Regulation

Coarse regulation alters the concentration of number of enzyme molecules by increasing or decreasing their synthesis at gene level. This is achieved by:

Induction or Repression

- It is induction or repression of specific genes of the enzymes by inducer or repressor molecules, e.g. **Heme** synthesis is reduced by the inhibition of enzyme **ALA synthase** by heme that acts like repressor for ALA synthase gene.
- **Lactose** acts as an inducer for genes of *Lac operon* so that lactose gets metabolized.
- **Glucokinase** gets induced by **insulin**.

Clinical Enzymology

Clinical Significance of Enzymes

Enzymes are of great clinical significance in the modern clinical laboratory. The various areas with significant role for enzymes in clinical laboratory science are:

- Diagnostic
- Therapeutic
- Analytical.

Diagnostic

Enzymes can be used in the clinical biochemistry for diagnosis of various disorders by estimating plasma enzymes. *Enzymes circulating in plasma are of 2 types:*

1. Functional or plasma specific
2. Nonfunctional or plasma nonspecific
   - *Specific enzymes:* These enzymes are purposely secreted into circulation to perform specific catalytic functions and have their substrate in plasma.These are present in high concentration in plasma, e.g. lipoprotein lipase, blood coagulation factors, complement proteins, etc.

- *Nonspecific enzymes:* These are present within cells and are added into plasma on normal wear and tear of cells and tissues. They are present in high concentration within cells but in low concentration in plasma. If the enzyme has a selective tissue distribution or if it is present in far higher concentration in some tissues than elsewhere in the body, it can help identify the site of the disease. Thus, it is the nonfunctional plasma enzymes, having a selective tissue distribution which can provide information of diagnostic importance, e.g. enzymes of secretion (amylase, lipase, ALP, ACP) and enzymes of intermediary metabolism (CPK, LDH, SGOT, SGPT).

Therapeutic use of Enzymes

Some enzymes have therapeutic significance, e.g. Streptokinase and urokinase are used to lyse blood clots in curing myocarclial infarction, pencillinase is used in treating patients allergic to penicillin, bacterial asperginase is used in treating some types of leukemia.

Analytical Use of Enzymes

The modern clinical lab sciences have advanced to a great extent in the evaluation of various biochemical parameters due to the highly specific and sensitive enzymatic reactions forming the basis of these evaluations. Enzymes can be used as reagents and labels.

As reagents they are used for estimation of serum biochemical parameters like sugar, urea, cholesterol, triglycerides, creatinine, etc.

As labels enzymes are used in immunoassays ELISA for determining the serum concentration of hormones like – thyroid, insulin, FSH, LH, etc.

Isoenzymes

Definition

Isoenzymes are physically distinct forms of same enzyme activity. OR Isoenzymes are different molecular forms of same enzyme synthesized by different tissues.

Characteristics of Isoenzymes

- These may be products of different genes located on different chromosomes, e.g. salivary and pancreatic amylase.
- These may be products of different genes on same chromosome like cytoplasmic and mitochondrial Malate dehydrogenase.
- Isoenzymes are made up of multiple sub-units (homo or hetero-multimer), e.g.
  - LDH-4
  - CPK-2
- Isoenzymes may differ in their prosthetic groups e.g. ALP isoenzymes have varying amount of sialic acid groups.
- Isoenzymes can be differentiated by:
  - Agar/PAGE electrophoresis
  - Heat stability
  - Sensitivity to inhibitor (as Km value would alter)

- Tissue localization
- Immunologically by preparing Abs specific for an isoenzyme.

Lactate Dehydrogenase (60 – 250 IU/L)

- There are 5 isoenzymes of LDH. (LDH1, LDH2, LDH3, LDH4, LDH5), each made up of 4 polypeptide chains of 2 types – (H type and M type)
  - LDH 1 – HHHH (Heart)
  - LDH 2 – H3M
  - LDH 3 – H2M2
  - LDH 4 – HM3
  - LDH 5 – M4 (Muscle).

Characteristics of LDH

- Electrophoresis of these causes separation of all 5 in an order LDH 5,4,3,2,1 from cathode to anode.
- LDH5 is the slowest to move as it is least negative and LDH1 is fastest as it is strongly negative.
- Significant elevation of LDH 1 and 2 within 24–48 hours of MI.
- LDH 1 and 2 are elevated in megaloblastic anemia and renal disorders.
- LDH 2 and 3 are elevated in leukemia and various other cancers.
- LDH 4 and 5 are elevated in liver disorders and muscle damage.

Creatine Phosphokinase (Males: 20–80 IU/L and Females: 20 – 50 IU/L)

- CPK has 3 isoenzymes made up of 2 polypeptide chains:
  - CPK 1 – BB (Brain)
  - CPK 2 – MB (Heart)
  - CPK 3 – MM (Muscle).

Characteristics of CPK

- CPK starts increasing within 3 hours of MI and is useful in early diagnosis of MI in cases where ECG changes are not evident.
- CPK has advantage over LDH as it is not altered by the hemolysis.
- CPK is also raised in muscular dystrophies, trauma, crush injuries, fractures.

Table 5.1 Some clinically important enzymes with their specifically associated disease

Enzyme	*Level*	*Increased in*
SGOT	3 IU – 15 IU/L	Viral hepatitis, liver cirrhosis, jaundice, MI.
SGPT	4 IU – 17 IU/L	Viral hepatitis, liver cirrhosis jaundice.
Amylase	80 – 180 Somogyi units	Pancreatitis, parotitis, peptic ulcers.
ALP	3 KÅ – 13 KÅ units	Bone disorders, Rickets , Pagets', Gauchers' disease, obstructive jaundice, etc.
ACP	0.6 KÅ – 3 KÅ units	Prostatic cancer.
γ– GT	10 IU – 47 IU/L	Alcoholic cirrhosis, obstructive jaundice.
LDH	60 IU – 250 IU/L	Megaloblastic anemia, MI, muscular dystrophies, leukemia.

A Quick Look at the Enzymology

- Enzymes are biocatalysts.
- All enzymes with exception of ribozymes are proteins.
- Enzymes are classified into 6 classes by IUBMB (1965) – Oxidoreductases, Transferases, Hydrolases, Lyases, Isomerases, Ligases.
- Some enzymes need coenzymes and cofactors for their optimal activity.
- Enzymes act by reducing the energy of activation needed by the substrate for reaching a transition state and then spontaneously disintegrate into product and enzyme is liberated unaltered.
- Enzyme activity is affected by – concentrations of enzyme, substrate, pH, temperature.
- Michealis constant is (Km) the substrate concentration at half the maximal velocity.
- Inhibitors inhibit the enzyme activity – competitively (reversible) and noncompetitively (irreversible) and suicide inhibition.
- Km is increased and Vmax is unchanged in competitive inhibition. This has pharmacologic use as drugs like sulfa drugs, methotrexate act on the same principle.
- Km is same and Vmax is reduced in noncompetitive inhibition as the affinity of the enzyme molecules not poisoned by inhibitors is not altered.
- Suicide inhibitors are also used as drugs for, e.g. Difluoro methyl ornithine and aspirin.
- Allosteric enzymes are multi subunit enzymes with a separate allostric site that modifies enzyme activity by binding to positive or negative allosteric modifiers, increasing or decreasing enzyme activity respectively.
- Enzyme activity is regulated by—Coarse regulation (induction and repression at gene level) and by Fine regulation (allosteric and covalent modification of existing enzyme molecules).
- Clinically enzymes are useful tools in analytical, diagnostic and therapeutic techniques.
- Isoenzymes are physically, structurally and immunologically distinct forms of the same enzyme activity, e.g. LDH, CPK, ALP, etc.

CHAPTER

6

Vitamins

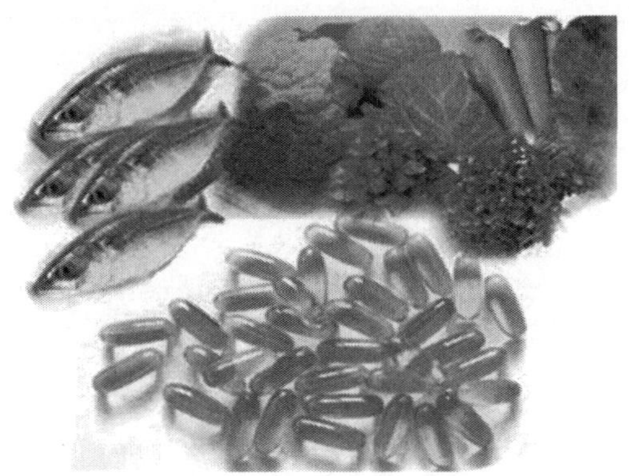

Chapter Framework

- Definition and Classification
- Water-soluble Vitamins
- Chemistry, Biochemical Roles and Deficiency Diseases of B–Complex and Vitamin–C
- Fat-soluble Vitamins
  - Vitamin – A
  - Vitamin – D
  - Vitamin – E
  - Vitamin – K

Definition

Vitamins are heterogeneous group of organic compounds needed in trace amounts for maintenance of good health, homeostasis and reproduction. Most vitamins cannot be synthesized by the human body and needs to be consumed in daily diet (except vitamin of B – complex group like Biotin, Pantothenate, and fat-soluble vitamin like vitamin – K). Vitamins are generally needed in catalytic quantities and do not function as structural elements in the cell.
Vitamins are named so because some of the earlier vitamins discovered were chemically amines and were found to be vital for normal health, vigour and vitality.

Classification

The vitamins are grouped into 2 major groups—Fat-soluble (A, D, E, K) and water-soluble (B – complex and vitamin–C) (Table 6.1).

Table 6.1 Classification of vitamins

Water-soluble	*Fat-soluble*
Soluble in water	Soluble in nonpolar solvents
Absorbed with normal diffusion	Absorbed with dietary fats
Does not need any transport protein (except B_{12} which is transported with transcobalamin)	Transported with lipoproteins and plasma proteins
Not stored in body (except B_{12} at liver) and does not cause toxicity as excess is excreted in urine	Stored at liver (except Vitamin – E at adipose tissue and excess causes toxicity
Act as coenzyme	Do not act as coenzymes
No provitamin forms	Vitamin A and D have provitamin forms

Water-soluble Vitamins

B – Complex Vitamins

The B – complex group of vitamins are water-soluble vitamins, differing structurally as well as functionally. However, they have been grouped together due to the water-soluble nature, the minute quantities they are needed in and the vitality they possess. Most of them act as coenzymes for various metabolic reactions.

B – complex vitamins can be further segregated as:
- Energy releasing—Thiamin, riboflavin, niacin, pantothenate.
- Hematopoietic – Cobalamin, folate, pyridoxine.

Thiamin (B_1)/Antiberiberi Vitamin

Chemical Nature

Chemically B1 comprises of a substituted pyrimidine ring joined by a methylene bridge to a substituted thiazole ring.

RDA and Sources

- 1 – 1.5 mg/day.
- Thiamine is present in the outer layer of rice and whole cereals, on polishing, this layer is lost and in areas where polished rice/cereals are the staple diet deficiency is commonly seen. Requirement increases in hypermetabolic states and increased consumption of carbohydrates.
- Whole cereals (unpolished), legumes, dried yeast, parboiled rice (parboiling causes the aleuron layer to fuse with the seed, preventing the loss associated in refining and polishing of rice).

Active form (Coenzyme form) – Thiamin Pyrophosphate (TPP)

$$\text{Thiamine} \xrightarrow[\text{ATP} \;\rightarrow\; \text{AMP}]{\text{Thiamine diphosphotransferase}} \text{TPP}$$

Biochemical Role

Thiamin is an energy-releasing vitamin that participates in the carbohydrate metabolism and liberates energy from carbohydrate molecules. Its coenzyme form (TPP) is important in the oxidative decarboxylation of α-ketoacids like α-ketoglutarate (of CAC) and pyruvate (of Glycolysis) and in the Transketolase activity of HMP shunt. Both these enzymatic reactions are concerned with carbohydrate metabolism. If carbohydrate-rich diet is taken, more thiamine is required.
- Oxidative decarboxylation of α–keto acids.
  - **Pyruvate dehydrogenase**

$$\text{Pyruvate} \xrightarrow[\text{Lipoic acid, Mg}^{+2}\text{, CoASH}]{\text{Py dh TPP, NAD}^{+}\text{, FAD}} \text{Acetyl CoA}$$

– **α-ketoglutarate dehydrogenase**

$$\xrightarrow[\text{Lipoic acid, Mg}^{+2}\text{, CoASH}]{\alpha\text{-KG, dh, TPP, NAD}^{+}\text{, FAD}} \text{Succinyl CoA}$$

- **Transketolase**

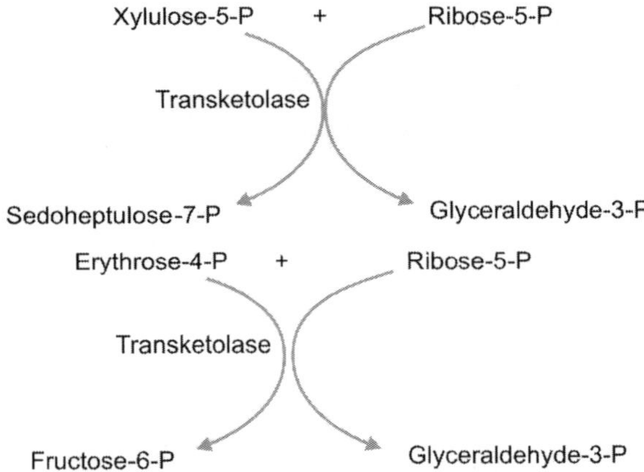

Deficiency Symptoms

In thiamine deficiency, the enzymes requiring TPP as cofactor can no longer execute their biological function and various reactions catalyzed by these enzymes are blocked. This causes accumulation of substrates of these enzymes like—Pyruvate, lactate, pentose sugars**.** Its deficiency mainly affects:

- CNS
- CVS
- GIT
- **Early symptoms** *are anorexia, dyspepsia, and lack of energy so that easily fatigued***.**
- Deficiency of thiamin precipitates as beriberi. It is of 3 types
  - *Dry beriberi*—Predominantly affects the CNS. It is characterized by peripheral neuritis with symptoms of numbness/tingling sensations in extremities, hyperesthesia, ataxia, and person cannot walk and needs support.
  - *Wet beriberi*—Predominantly involves the CVS. The substrates of the enzymes requiring TPP get accumulated and there is edema of legs, face, trunk and serous cavities due to accumulation of various substrates. Palpitation and breathlessness is observed, calf muscles are tender on pressure.
  - *Infantile beriberi*—It occurs in infants (2-5 months) nursing on thiamine deficient mothers. Characteristic features are of tachycardia (>140 beats/min), restlessness, bouts of mimic abdominal pain.
- **Wrenicke's Korsakoff Syndrome**—This is typically seen in chronic alcoholics, since they are nutritionally deprived of the vitamin due to poor eating habits. Besides, the alcohol needs more thiamin for its own metabolism and it also reduces the absorption of dietary thiamin, worsening the situation.

- *Wernicke's encephalopathy* characterized by ataxia, to and fro movement of eyeballs, confusion.
- *Korsakoff's psychosis* characterized by amnesia.

Biochemical Assay for Detecting the Deficiency of Thiamin

- Erythrocyte transketolase activity will be reduced.
- Blood levels of thiamin will be reduced.
- Blood levels of pyruvic acid will be raised.
- Urinary levels of thiamin after a dose are reduced.

Riboflavin (B_2)

Chemical Nature

Chemically riboflavin comprises an isoallaxine ring attached to a ribitol.

RDA and Sources

- 0.6 mg/1000 calories.
- Sources are milk, egg, dried yeast, germinating cereals, liver, kidney, heart (Fig. 6.1).
- Intestinal bacterial flora also synthesizes riboflavin.

Active form (Coenzyme form)

There are two coenzymes of riboflavin—FMN and FAD. The riboflavin molecule is phosphorylated by the intestinal enzyme flavokinase to FMN and later FMN is further phosphor-ribosylated to FAD by FAD synthase.

- Riboflavin + Phosphoric acid = FMN
  FMN + AMP = FAD

Biochemical Roles

- The FMN and FAD are important coenzymes of the oxidoreductases type of enzymatic reactions.
- These two coenzymes can undergo reversible oxidation and reduction, and participate in a number of oxidation-reduction reactions.
- It exists in tissues tightly bound with enzymes.
- The riboflavin portion of FMN and FAD can reversibly combine with two hydrogen atoms.
- Enzymes containing riboflavin coenzymes are called flavoproteins.

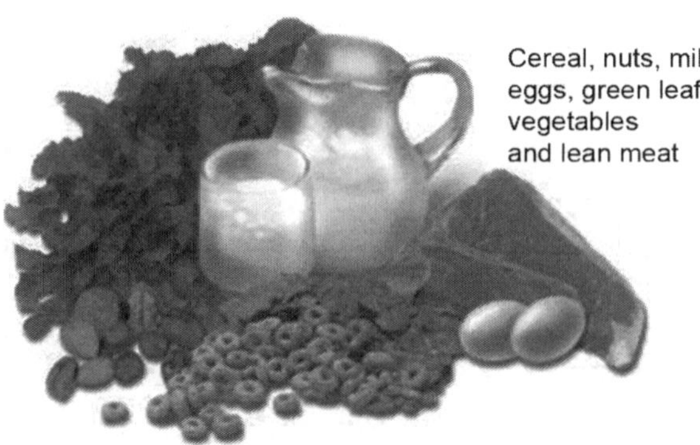

Fig. 6.1 Food sources of riboflavin (vitamin B_2)

- The enzyme complex may contain Mo and Fe.
- During oxidation 2H atoms are accepted from substrate to coenzyme FMN or FAD at N1 and N10 to be reduced to $FMNH_2$/$FADH_2$. Thus the substrate is oxidized and coenzyme is reduced.
- *FMN is a* Coenzyme for L-amino acid oxidase (Fig. 6.2)

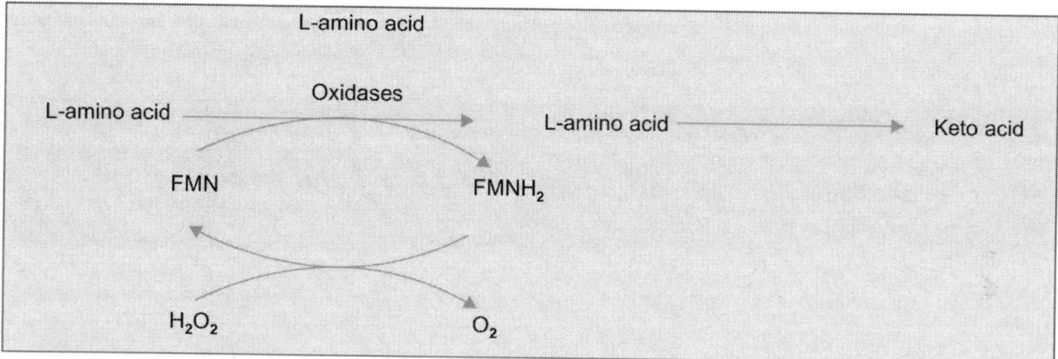

Fig. 6.2 Coenzyme activity of FMN in aminoacid oxidase activity

- **Component of respiratory chain**
  - In respiratory chain, the enzyme NADH dh contain FMN, the electrons are transported from NAD linked dehydrogenases through FMN to CoQ.
    NAD ⟶ FMN ⟶ Co Q
- **FAD acts as a coenzyme in a number of oxidoreductases enzymatic reactions.**
  - *Succinate Dh (CAC)*

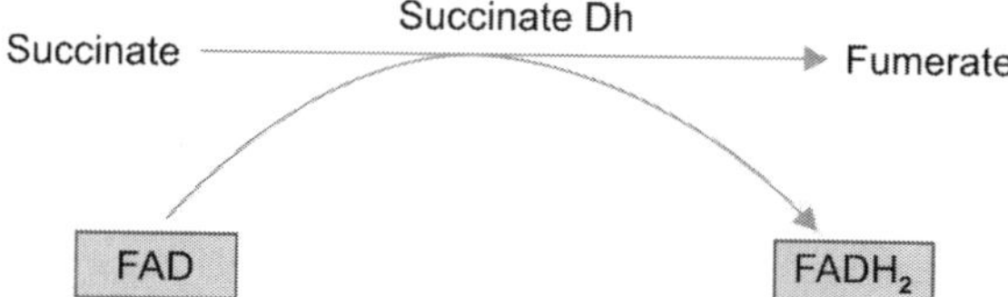

  - *Acyl CoA dehydrogenase (Fatty acid synthesis)*

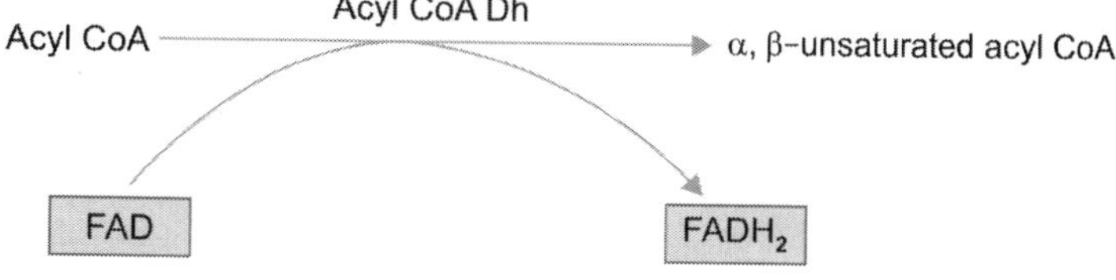

  - *Xanthine oxidase*

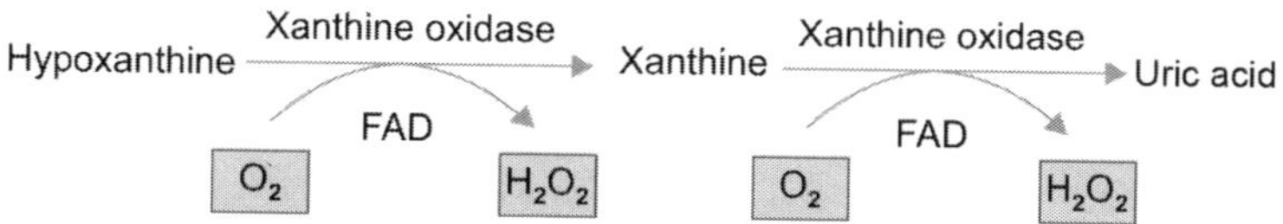

- *Erythrocyte glutathione reductases*

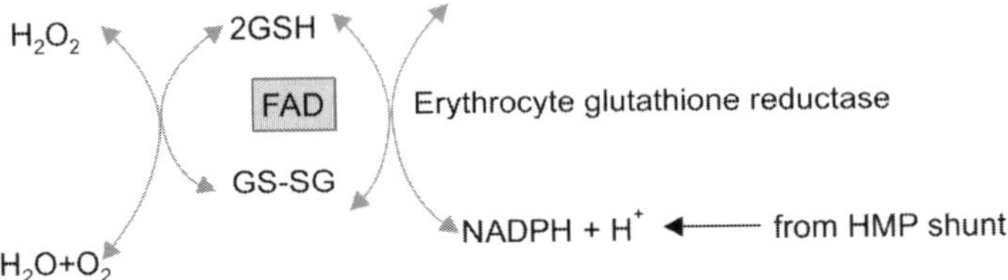

- *Mitochondrial glycerol – 3 – Phosphate dehydrogenase*

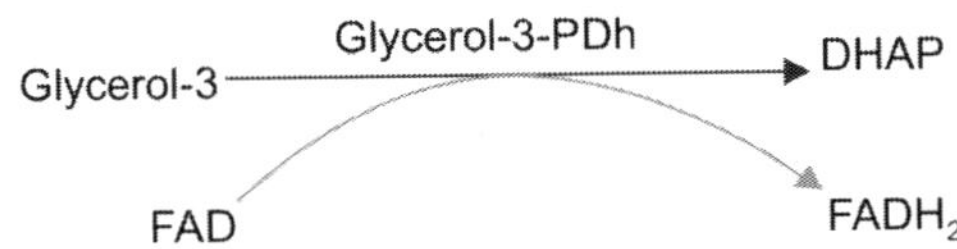

Deficiency

Natural deficiency of riboflavin is **uncommon in humans** because it is synthesized by intestinal bacteria. Its deficiency accompanies other deficiency diseases like—beriberi, pellagra, Kwashiorkor.

It is also seen in infants treated for neonatal jaundice by phototherapy but it is harmless.

Symptoms

Symptoms of riboflavin deficiency include:

- Glossitis—Inflammation of tongue, magenta colored tongue, atrophy of lingual papillae.
- Cheilosis—Fissuring of lips
- Angular stomatitis—Inflammation at corners of mouth
- Seborrheic dermatitis
- Circum-corneal visualization.

Biochemical Assay of Deficiency

- Flourimetric assay of vitamin in blood.
- Erythrocyte glutathione reductases activity in blood.

Niacin (B_3)

Chemical Nature

- Chemically niacin is a pyridine ring with a carboxylic acid group—Nicotinic acid or an amide group—Nicotinamide.
- Both nicotinic acid and nicotinamide have vitamin – B_3 activity.

RDA and Sources

- 20 mg/day.
- Green leafy vegetables, tomatoes, yeast, milk, egg, meat and liver. Niacin is not a vitamin in true sense as it can be synthesized in the body by tryptophan.
- 60 mg of tryptophan gives 1 mg of niacin.

Active form (Coenzyme)

- The coenzyme forms of niacin are NAD^+ and $NADP^+$. They act as co-substrate in the oxido-reductases group of biochemical reactions.
- The niacin gets activated to NAD^+ and $NADP^+$ as follows (Fig. 6.3):
  - During the oxidation–reduction reactions, the reducing equivalents are removed as 2H atoms.
  - The 2H are accepted by the NAD^+ or $NADP^+$ molecule as H^- ion, one H atom is accepted fully and the second atom ionizes to H^+ and e^-. The e^- is accepted by the NAD and H^+ is liberated into the medium.
  - Thus, NAD^+ is reduced to $NADH+H^+$, similarly $NADP^+$ is reduced to $NADPH+H^+$.

Biochemical Role

- These two coenzymes can undergo reversible oxidation and reduction, and can act as coenzymes for several oxidoreductases.
- NAD and NADP act as coenzymes in many metabolic pathways e.g.:
  - Glycolysis
  - Hexose monophosphate shunt
  - Citric acid cycle
  - Synthesis of fatty acids and steroids
  - Oxidation of fatty acids
  - Oxidative deamination of amino acids
  - Generally, NAD acts as coenzyme in catabolic pathways and NADP in anabolic pathways where the $NADPH+H^+$ donate its reducing equivalents for the synthesis of new biomolecules. Thus, the process is termed as *reductive biosynthesis.*
- **NAD requiring enzymes**

  Some examples of enzymes which require NAD as a coenzyme are—
  - Glyceraldehyde-3- phosphate dehydrogenase, (Glycolysis)
  - Lactate dehydrogenase, (Anaerobic glycolysis)
  - Pyruvate dehydrogenase, (CAC)
  - Isocitrate dehydrogenase, (CAC)

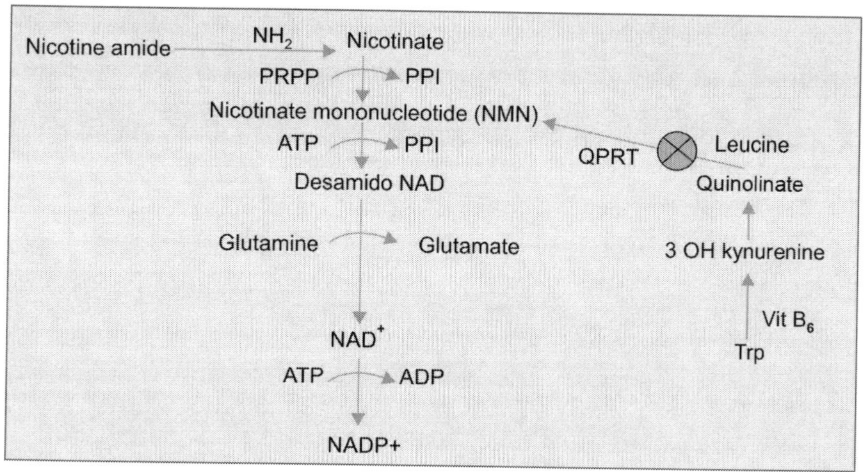

Fig. 6.3 Activation of niacin

- α-ketoglutarate dehydrogenase, (CAC)
- Malate dehydrogenase, (CAC)
- β-hydroxyacyl CoA dehydrogenase (Beta oxidation)
- Glutamate dehydrogenase (NH_3 transport)
- IMP dehydrogenase (Purine biosynthesis).

- **NADPH and NADP requiring enzymes**
  Examples of enzymes requiring NADP as a coenzyme include:
  - Glucose-6-phosphate dehydrogenase (HMP shunt) } NADP+ requiring
  - 6-phosphogluconate dehydrogenase (HMP shunt) } NADP+ requiring
  - β-ketoacyl CoA reductase (FA synthesis)
  - β-hydroxy-β-methyl glutaryl CoA (HMG CoA) reductase (Cholesterol biosynthesis) } NADPH + H^+ requiring
  - Squalene synthetase, (Cholesterol biosynthesis) } NADPH + H^+ requiring
  - Cholesterol 7-α hydroxylase, (Bile acid synthesis). } NADPH + H^+ requiring

Deficiency of Niacin

Causes

- Dietary deficiency of niacin.
- Consumption of maize as a staple diet—Niacin is present bound as niacytin.
- Consumption of sorghum—It has excess of leucine, which inhibits the conversion of dietary Trp to NAD^+.
- Dietary deficiency of tryptophan.
- Hartnup's disease—It is characterized by malabsorption of tryptophan.
- Carcinoid syndrome – In this condition there is a tumor secreting excess of serotonin which is synthesized from tryptophan. Thus less Trp is available for the synthesis of NAD^+.
- Deficiency of Vitamin B_6 – Vitamin B_6 is an important coenzyme required for the conversion of Trp to NAD^+. Deficiency of Vitamin B_6 can lead to added deficiency of vitamin B_3.
  - Deficiency of niacin causes *Pellagra*. The condition is characterized by 4 D's –
    - **D**igestive disorders and diarrhea
    - **D**ermatitis
    - **D**ementia (mental degeneration) and if not cured
    - **D**eath
  - Dermatitis usually affects the parts of the body exposed to direct sunlight like—neck, back of ankles, skin of hands, etc. *Casal necklace* is characteristically seen as dermatitis around neck region.

Pantothenic Acid (Vitamin B_5)

Chemical Nature

It is composed of β alanine + pantoic acid.

RDA and Sources

- Intestinal bacteria can also synthesize it. Therefore, the RDA is less than 10 mg per day.
- It is widely distributed in different food groups—Green leafy vegetables, cereals, yeast, egg, milk, intestinal bacteria.

Active form (Coenzyme)

Pantothenic acid performs its biochemical functions as a constituent of coenzyme A (CoA) and acyl carrier protein (ACP).

Both these compounds contain pantothenic acid in the form of **4′-phosphopantetheine** (Fig. 6.4).

Biochemical Roles of Coenzyme-A

- Coenzyme-A is also represented as CoA-SH.
- Its terminal –SH group binds various compounds.
- This coenzyme participates in a variety of reactions in the metabolism of carbohydrates, lipids and amino acids. Some examples of such reactions are:
  - Oxidative decarboxylation of alpha-keto acids
  - Activation of fatty acids
  - Activation of some amino acids.
- An important role of CoA is to provide **active acetate** (acetyl CoA) for various reactions, e.g.
  - Synthesis of fatty acids
  - Cholesterol
  - Ketone bodies
  - Acetylcholine
  - Acetylation of drugs.
- **Active succinate** (succinyl CoA) is required for hemesynthesis and for gluconeogenesis from some amino acids.

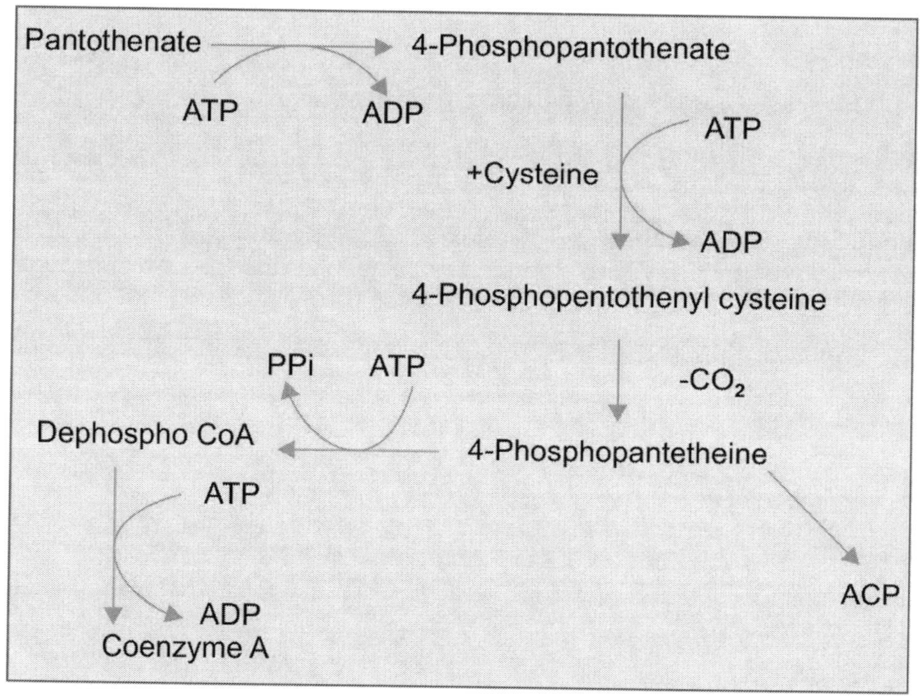

Fig. 6.4 Formation of Coenzyme – A and ACP from Vitamin B_5

Biochemical role of Acyl Carrier Protein (ACP)

- Acyl carrier protein is a constituent of the multienzyme complex, which catalyzes de novo synthesis of fatty acids.

Deficiency of Pantothenate

- Deficiency of pantothenic acid has not been seen in human being normally, since it is synthesized by the intestinal bacterial flora.
- Human deficiency can be produced experimentally, which causes neurological and gastrointestinal disturbances.
- Deficiency in prisoners of war or in famine struck areas was seen with typical symptoms of paraesthesias of lower extremities, fatigue, staggering gait termed as Burning foot syndrome.

Pyridoxal (Vitamin B_6)

Chemical Nature

- Vitamin B_6 consists of three closely related pyridine derivatives, pyridoxine, pyridoxal and pyridoxamine.
- All the three are equally active as vitamins (Fig. 6.5).

Active form (Coenzyme)

- Pyridoxine, pyridoxal and pyridoxamine are phosphorylated by ATP in the presence of pyridoxal kinase to form pyridoxine phosphate, pyridoxal phosphate and pyridoxamine phosphate respectively. Human brain contains pyridoxal kinase in abundance.
- The three form are interconvertible.

Sources and RDA

- Green leafy vegetables, yeast, egg, milk, organ meats like liver, kidney and heart. Daily requirement is 2 mg/day.

Biochemical Roles

- **Role in amino acid metabolism**—Pyridoxal phosphate and pyridoxamine phosphate serve as coenzymes, mainly in the metabolism of amino acids. Pyridoxal phosphate (PLP)

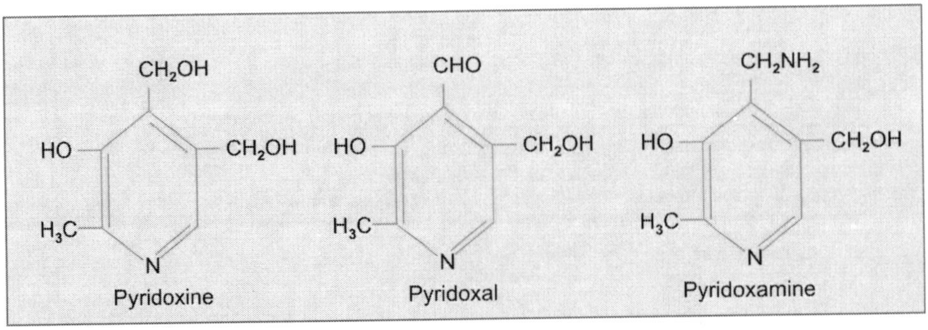

Fig. 6.5 Vitamin B_6

forms a Schiff base with an α-amino acid. The amino acid, thus bound, can undergo various reactions.

- *Transamination*—Transaminases group of enzymes catalyze transamination reactions using PLP as a coenzyme. During transamination NH_2 group of all α -amino acid is first accepted by pyridoxal to form an aldimine. Schiff's base which then transfer the NH_2 group to an α–keto acid to form corresponding 2nd amino acid and 2nd α-keto acid (Fig. 6.6).

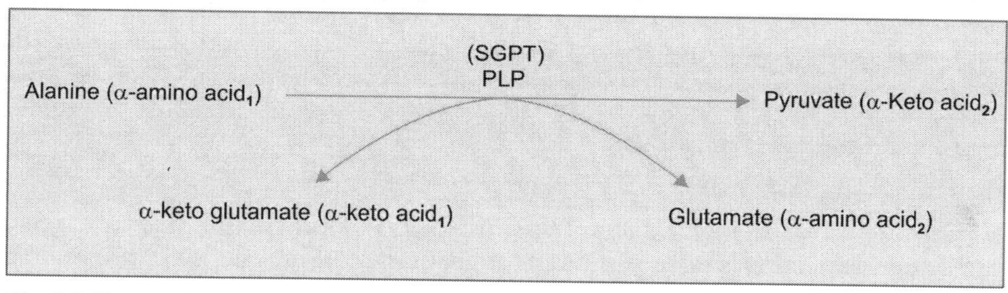

Fig. 6.6 Transamination of α-amino acid by serum glutamate pyruvate

- *Decarboxylation*—Some important biogenic amines are synthesized by the decarboxylation of α-amino acids in the presence of a decarboxylases group of enzymes and PLP as the coenzyme. For example, Histidine gives histamine (vasodilator), glutamate gives gamma amino butyric acid (GABA – inhibitory neuropeptide), tryptophan gives tryptamine that further on methylation gives serotonin etc.
- *Oxidative deamination*—During amino acid catabolism, α-amino acids are deaminated to their keto acid and the amino groups get pooled up as glutamate. The reaction is catalyzed by glutamate dehydrogenase and it needs PLP as a coenzyme.
- *Nonoxidative Deamination*—Nonoxidative deamination of amino acids occur in the presence of pyridoxal phosphate as a coenzyme.

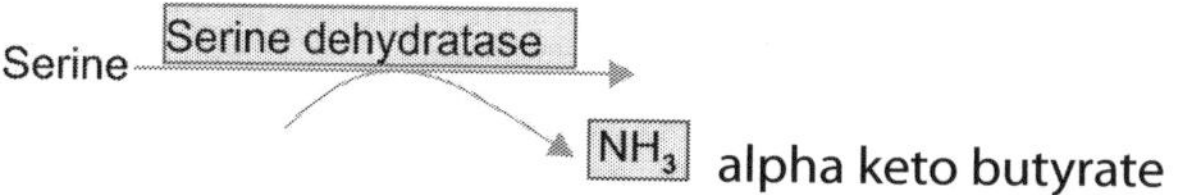

- *Tryptophan metabolism*—PLP is an important coenzyme of Trp catabolism and is part of the reaction sequence that synthesizes niacin coenzyme from Trp.

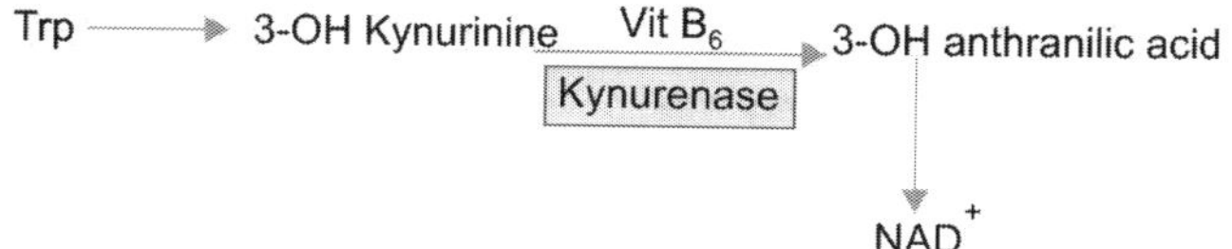

- *Metabolism of Sulfur containing amino acids*—Pyridoxal phosphate is an important coenzyme of the metabolism of S–containing amino acids.

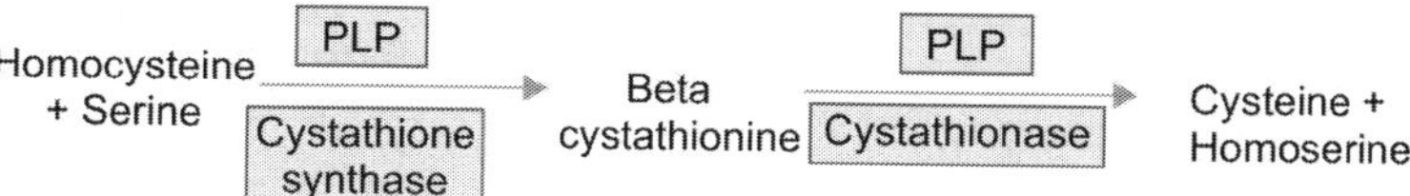

- **Synthesis of heme**—PLP is an important coenzyme of the key enzyme catalyzed reaction of heme synthesis.

$$\text{Glycine + Succinyl CoA} \xrightarrow[\text{PLP}]{\text{ALA synthase}} \text{ALA} \longrightarrow \text{Heme}$$

- **Glycogenolysis**—Key enzyme of glycogenolysis, phosphorylase needs Vitamin B_6 as coenzyme. Almost 60% of the total body pyridoxal is present in the muscles as pyridoxal phosphate bound to the muscle phosphorylase.
- **Sphingomyelin synthesis**—Formation of sphingomyelin requires Vitamin B_6 as coenzyme.

Deficiency Signs and Symptoms

- Neurological symptoms
  - Children with B_6 deficiency show hyperirritability and convulsions due to lack of GABA.
  - Peripheral neuritis is observed due to defect in sphingomyelin synthesis and defective synthesis of niacin from Trp.
- Typical symptoms of pellagra are seen.
- Hypochromic microcytic anemia due to blocked heme synthesis.
- Antitubercular drug isoniazid causes B_6 deficiency because, it forms hydrazones with B_6 and gets eliminated in urine. Also these hydrazones inhibit the pyridoxal kinase enzyme.

Assay for the Deficiency

- Trp load test
  - On giving Trp load in B_6 deficiency there is accumulation of 3 – OH anthranilic acid which gets oxidized to xanthurinic acid and gets excreted in urine.
- Homocystinuria is observed in B_6 deficiency.
- Blood levels of PLP can be assayed.

Biotin

Chemical Nature

- Biotin is a heterocyclic, sulfur-containing, monocarboxylic acid.
- Biotin is also known as **anti-egg white** injury factor. When raw egg white is fed to rats, they develop biotin deficiency. It has been shown that raw egg white contains a protein, **avidin**, which forms a complex with biotin preventing its intestinal absorption. This leads to a deficiency of biotin. Avidin is inactivated by heat, therefore, cooked eggs do not hamper absorption of biotin. Biotin is heat-stable.

Sources and RDA

- Bacterial synthesis in the intestine provides ample amounts of biotin.
- Dietary sources include egg yolk, liver, kidney, yeast, peas, tomatoes, cauliflower, etc.
- Biotin requirement is not known with certainty as the intestinal bacteria meet most of the requirement.

Biochemical Roles

- **Biotin is a coenzyme for carboxylases** and is, therefore, also known as co-carboxylase. The carboxyl group of biotin forms a bond with the epsilon-amino group of a lysine residue of the apoenzyme. Some examples of carboxylation reactions in which biotin is required are:
  - Carboxylation of pyruvate to oxaloacetate **(Pyruvate carboxylase)**
  - Carboxylation of acetyl CoA to malonate **(Acetyl CoA carboxylase)**
  - Carboxylation of propionyl CoA methyl malonyl CoA **(Propionyl CoA carboxylase).**

Deficiency

- Deficiency of biotin is unknown in human beings as sufficient vitamin is provided by intestinal bacteria, and the vitamin is widely distributed in both animal and plant foods.
- Deficiency may occur in animals when they are fed raw egg white.
- It is clinically characterized by **retarded growth, loss of weight, dermatitis, loss of hair, muscular incoordination and paralysis.**

Folic Acid

Chemical Nature

- Chemically folate comprises of a pteridine ring fused with a para-amino benzoic acid which then links up with one or more glutamic acid residues.

Sources and RDA

- Folic acid is obtained from green leafy vegetables, yeast, liver, kidney, meat, fish, milk, etc. Intestinal bacteria also synthesize folic acid.
- Infants and children : 100 μg/day
- Adult men and women : 100 μg/day
- Pregnant women : 300 μg/day
- Lactating women : 150 μg/day.

Digestion, Absorption and Activation of Folate

- Folic acid is found in foodstuffs as pteroyl monoglutamate, pteroyl triglutamate and pteroyl hepta glutamate. The last two are converted into pteroyl monoglutamate in the intestinal mucosa. Absorption of folate occurs at jejunum. Folic acid forms a coenzyme, tetrahydrofolate (5, 6, 7, 8 – H_4 folate) (Figs 6.7A and B).

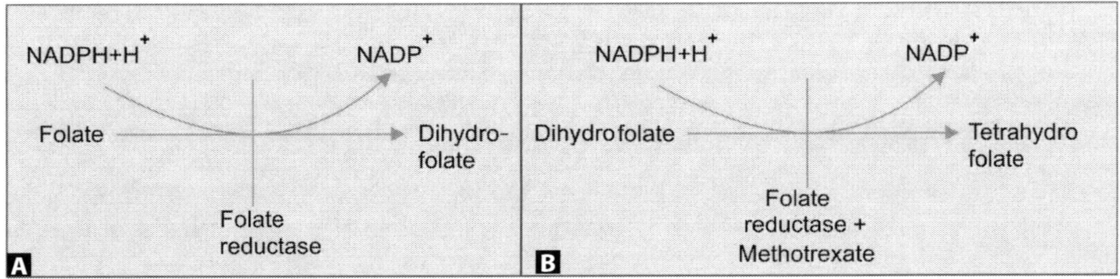

Figs 6.7A and B Reduction of folate and action of methotrexate.

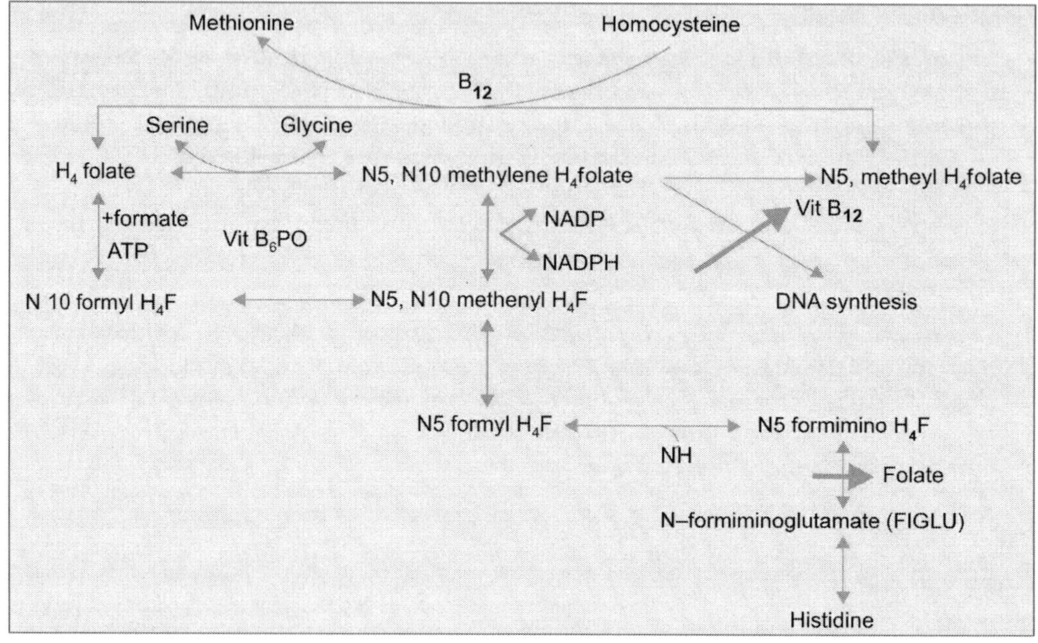

Fig. 6.8 One–carbon metabolism of folate

- H_4 folate is the active coenzyme form of folate. H_4 folate acts as a carrier of activated one-carbon units like methyl, methylene, methenyl, formyl, formino, hydroxy methyl, etc. All these are metabolically interconvertible. These involve N5 and or N10 of the H_4 Folate. N5, N10 methylene H_4F plays a central role in 1-C unit metabolism (Fig. 6.8).

Biochemical Role of Folate

- It is required as a coenzyme in the reaction catalyzed by thymidylate synthase (Figs 6.9A and B).
- N_5- methyl H_4F is required for regeneration of CH_3 cobalamin which is a coenzyme for methionine synthase reaction.
  - In this reaction, homocysteine is methylated to methionine, the methyl group is donated by CH_3 B_{12}.
  - The free cobalamin is again methylated by N_5 - CH_3H_4F.
  - The methionine acts as a donor of CH_3 group in transmethylation reactions like synthesis of choline, creatine etc.
  - The formation of N_5-CH_3H_4F is an irreversible step (Fig. 6.8). The only way of regenerating free H_4F is via this methionine synthases step. In case of B_{12} deficiency folate gets trapped in N_5- CH_3H_4F—Methyl folate trap leading to an associated folate deficiency.

Deficiency of Folate

Causes:

- During pregnancy due to increased demand for the growth and development of the fetal tissues.
- Due to malabsorption or defective absorption as is observed in chronic alcoholism or in sprue and celiac diseases.

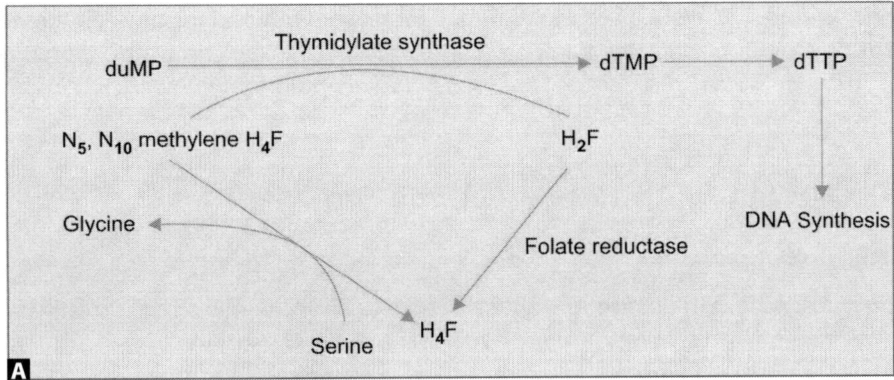

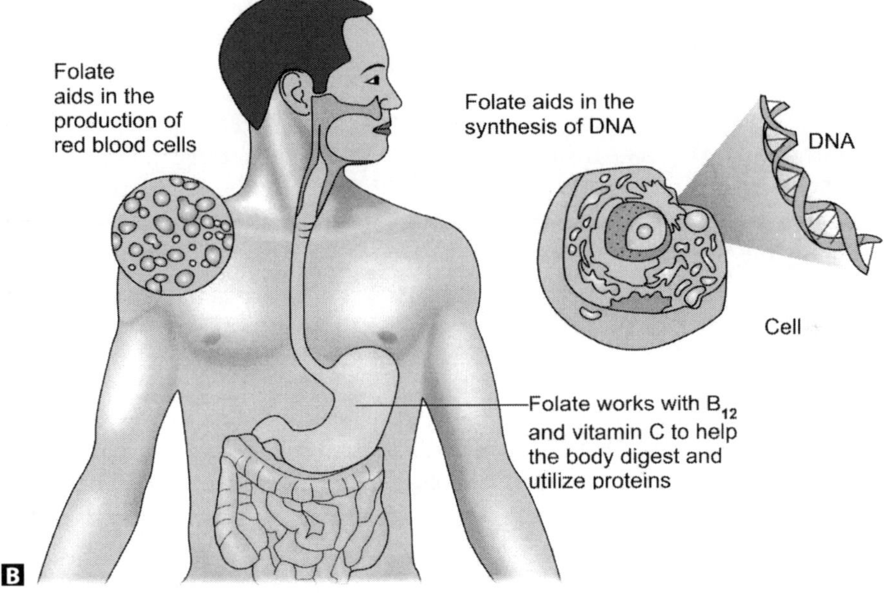

Figs 6.9A and B Role of folate in DNA synthesis

Effects and Symptoms

- The principle manifestation of folate deficiency is **megaloblastic anemia.**
  - This is because the thymidylate synthase does not get the active folate as N_5 N_{10} – methylene tetrahydrofolate and gets blocked, so there is no conversion of d-UMP into d-TMP, and no TTP is available for DNA synthesis causing cell division to be arrested.
  - As a result rapidly dividing cells of bone marrow and intestinal mucosa are badly affected. During erythropoiesis due to folate deficiency, the S-phase of cell cycle gets prolonged and cell division is delayed.
  - In the prolonged S-phase there is more and more synthesis of protein so Hb accumulates in cytoplasm. Thus the cytoplasm is mature but DNA synthesis is delayed.
  - This leads to an asynchrony in maturity of nucleus and cytoplasm, and macrocytic/ megaloblastic RBCs are released in circulation.

- These macrocytic RBCs are abnormal and get rapidly trapped in spleen to be destroyed causing megaloblastic anemia as production of RBCs is slow and destruction is rapid.
- **Neural tube defects (Spina bifida)** are seen in infants born to folate deficient mothers.

Assay of Folate Deficiency:

- **Histidine load test**—FIGLU is excreted in folate deficiency (*see* Fig. 6.8).

Folate Antagonists

- *Sulfonamides:* Sulfonamides are structurally similar to PABA. Humans can use only preformed folate but bacteria can synthesize folate by combining PABA, pteridine ring and glutamate but cannot use preformed folate. Sulfonamides are used as antibacteria drugs. They complete with PABA to combine with pteridine ring and Glu causing folate deficiency. So the thymidylate synthase activity is blocked resulting in inhibition of DNA synthesis so the bacteria are killed. The human cells are not affected as preformed folate is used by them but the bacterial cells are unable to utilize the preformed folate.
- *Methotrexate:* Powerful inhibitor of folate reductase. This acts as an anticancer drug since it inhibits the activation of folate to its active form, depriving the rapidly multiplying cancer cells of the much needed substrate nucleotide – d –TTP.
- *Trimethoprim:* Also inhibits folate reductase but in bacteria and is thus used in combination with sulfonamides as bactericidal drugs.

Cobalamin (Vitamin B_{12})

Chemical Nature

Chemically the structure of B_{12} is similar to that of porphyrins. It has four pyrrole rings with a cobalt atom at the center (corrin ring). This Co has coordination number 6 out of which 4 valencies are satisfied by 4 substituted pyrrole N and 5th valency is linked to a substituted benz imidazole ring. 6th valency of Co is satisfied by either CN– or OH– or CH_3 or adenosyl group depending upon the cobalamin derivative cyanocobalamin or hydroxy cobalamin or methyl cobalamin or ado B_{12} respectively (Fig. 6.10).

Depending upon the substituent group:

- CN—Cyanocobalamin is common oral drug preparation.
- OH—Hydroxycobalamin is injectable preparations.
- Adenosyl - ado B_{12}/adenosyl Cobalamin—It is the major storage form in liver.
- CH_3 - Methyl cobalamin—It is the major form in blood circulation.
- AdoB_{12} and CH_3 B_{12} are functional coenzymes of B_{12}.

RDA and Sources

- Infants and children : 0.3 μg – 0.5 μg/day
- Adult men and women : 1 μg/day
- Pregnant and lactating women: 1.5 μg/day.
- B_{12} is not present in vegetables. It is synthesized by micro-organisms and is stored in liver, making liver a good source. Besides liver, yeast is a good source. Egg and curd also provide B_{12}. Curd is a very good source since lactobacillus of curd can synthesize B_{12} (Fig. 6.11).

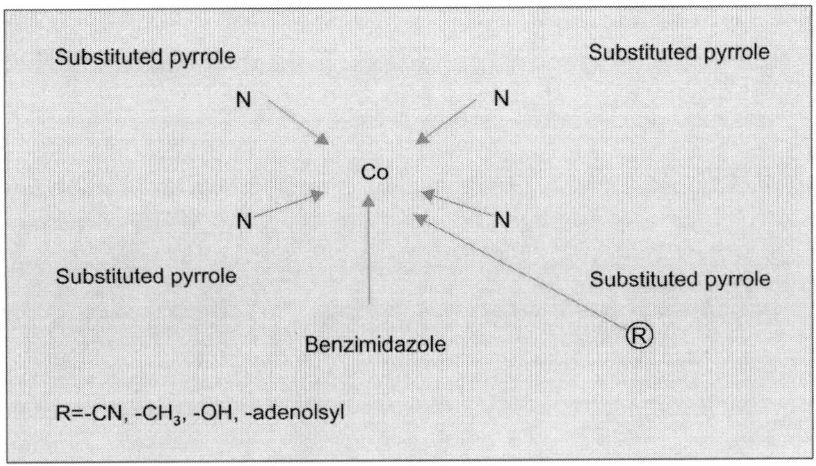

Fig. 6.10 Composition of cobalaonin

Absorption

- Dietary B_{12} is attached to dietary proteins, and the intestinal enzymes release it.
- The free B_{12} now binds to an intrinsic factor of castle (IF) [a glycoprotein secreted by the parietal cells of gastric mucosa] for absorption at ileum therefore, B_{12} is also known as extrinsic factor.
- The IF $-B_{12}$ complex is internalized in the intestinal mucosal cell where IF is hydrolyzed and B_{12} absorbed into blood.
- In the blood B_{12} is transported bound to transcobalamin-II.
- In cytosol of cells, it is present as CH_3 B_{12}. Hydroxy B_{12} is either converted in cytosol to CH_3 B_{12} or it enters mitochondria to be converted to adoB_{12}.

Storage

- It is stored in liver cells as adoB_{12}, bound to transcobalamin-I. Liver stores about 2mg B_{12} sufficient for 2–3 years.

Biochemical Role

- **Methyl malonyl CoA Isomerase (Fig. 6.12)**
  - Ado B_{12} is a coenzyme for the enzyme L – methyl malonyl CoA isomerase.
  - This reaction helps in shuttling the metabolic end product of odd chain fatty acids oxidation into the gluconeogenic pathway, as Succinyl CoA is an intermediate of CAC.

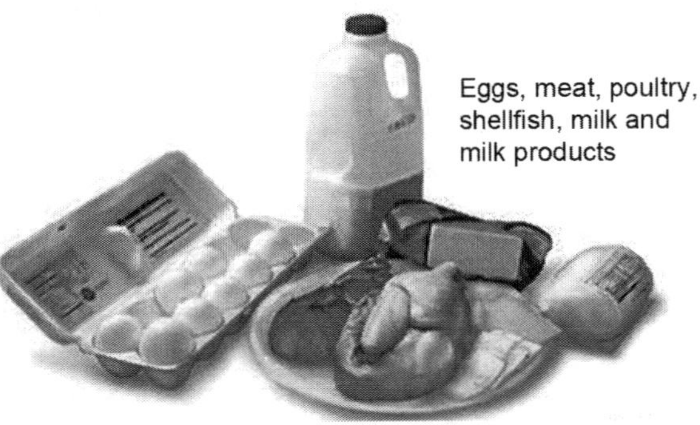

Fig. 6.11 Food sources of Vitamin B_{12}

- **Methionine Synthase (Fig. 6.13)**
  - The synthesis of methionine from homocysteine is a methylation reaction catalyzed by methionine synthase.
  - The enzyme requires methyl B_{12} as a coenzyme.
  - Methionine synthesized acts as a methyl group donor in trans methylation reactions (synthesis of biogenic amines like—choline, epinephrine) as active methionine (SAM).
  - The reaction a junction of interaction of vitamins B_{12} and folate, as the regeneration of methyl B_{12} occurs by the transfer of a methyl group from N_5 methyl H_4F. This releases folate of folate trap.
  - A deficiency of vitamin B_{12} is thus associated with a codeficiency of folate due to **methyl folate trap** and will have the typical symptoms of folate deficiency, i.e. megaloblastic anemia.

Deficiency and Symptoms

Causes

- Dietary deficiency
- Partial or total gastrectomy

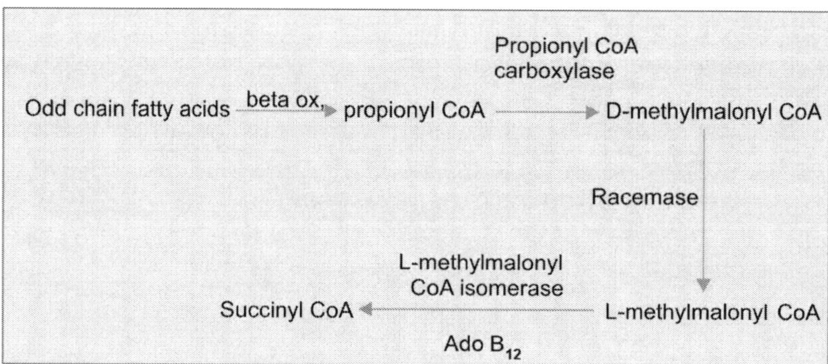

Fig. 6.12 Methylmalonyl CoA isomerase

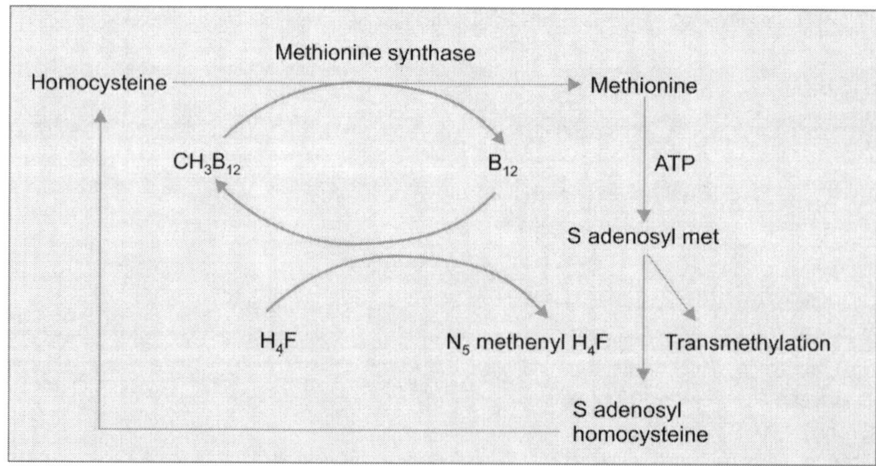

Fig. 6.13 Methinone synthase reaction

- Addisonian pernicious anemia
- Chronic iron deficiency
- Consumption of raw fish (infested with *Diphilobothrium latum*)
- Pure vegetarians (who do not consume even milk and curd as being animal products).

Deficiency Manifestations

- *Megaloblastic anemia*
  - Deficiency of vitamin – B_{12} leads to an associated deficiency of folic acid due to methyl folate trap.
  - The enzymatic reaction catalyzed by thymidylate synthase is blocked due to folate trap, leading to a deficient supply of thymidylate for DNA synthesis.
  - The tissues with rapid turn—over (bone marrow and intestinal) are badly affected, the S-phase is prolonged such that there is a synthesis of cytoplasmic proteins (Hb) but the nucleus is immature.
  - There is release of immature nucleated RBCs called megaloblasts (with mature cytoplasm and immature nucleus) into circulation.
  - The megaloblasts are removed as abnormal cells by the spleen rapidly.
  - More megaloblasts are added into the circulation to keep up with the RBC count.
  - Finally megaloblastic anemia is precipitated.
  - Blood picture shows megaloblasts.
- *Neurological manifestations*
  - The deficiency of vitamin – B_{12} blocks the methionine synthase and L – methyl malonyl CoA isomerase reactions causing their substrates to accumulate.
  - These substrates are the odd chain fatty acid metabolites, Succinyl CoA, homocysteine.
  - The substrates accumulate in the myelin sheath of the nerves causing a defect in the nerve impulse conduction.
  - Besides, the defect in methionine synthase causes a deficiency of methionine and transmethylation reactions requiring active methionine are badly affected.
  - The biogenic amines are not appropriately synthesized, further adding up to the neurological symptoms.

Neurologic Signs and Symptoms

- Paraesthesias of extremities, unsteadiness of gait, later stages loss of memory, confusion.

Assay of B_{12} Deficiency (Fig. 6.14)

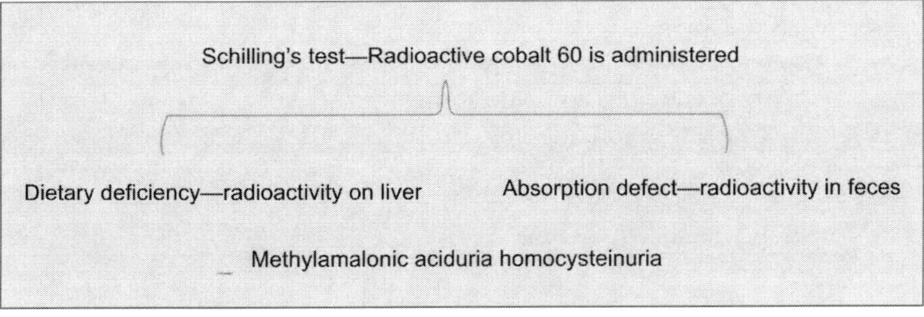

Fig. 6.14 B_{12} deficiency assay

Vitamin – C (Ascorbic acid)

Chemical Nature

- Chemically vitamin-C resembles hexoses, i.e. it is a polyhydric compound with a carbonyl functional group.
- Due to structural similarity with hexoses, vitamin-C also possesses reducing property.

RDA and Sources

- Daily requirement of vitamin-C is 60 mg.
- Richest source of vitamin-C is Indian gooseberry (Amla). Other good sources are citrus fruits like—oranges, lemon, green leafy vegetables, guava, tomato, germinating pulses, etc.
- Vitamin C is synthesized by all plants and animals except guinea pigs and primates, which lack L-gulonolactone oxidase, the enzyme that converts L-gulonolactone into L-ascorbic acid.

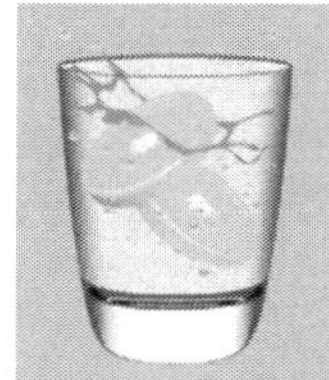

Fig. 6.15 Sources of vitamin-C

Biochemical Roles

- Vitamin C is required for the formation and maintenance of intercellular cement substance.
- Since it can undergo reversible oxidation and reduction, it takes part in some oxidation reduction reactions.
- There is considerable evidence in support of the role of vitamin C in the oxidation of phenylalanine and tyrosine.
- It is required for post-translational hydroxylation of proline and lysine residues, and is, therefore, essential for the conversion of procollagen into collagen which is rich in hydroxyproline and hydroxylysine.
- Through collagen synthesis, it plays a role in the formation of matrix of bones, cartilages, dentine and connective tissue.
- By converting ferric ions into ferrous ions, it helps in the absorption of iron.
- It is required for the formation of bile acids from cholesterol.
- It acts as an anti-oxidant.
- It inhibits the formation of nitrosamines (carcinogens) during digestion.
- Ascorbic acid may play a role in the synthesis of adrenocortical steroid hormones as ascorbic acid content of adrenal gland is found to decrease rapidly in stressful conditions.

Deficiency Signs and Symptoms

- Deficiency of vitamin C produces scurvy
- A full-blown picture of scurvy is rare these days but isolated signs and symptoms of vitamin C deficiency are still seen. The signs and symptoms include:
  - Swollen, spongy and bleeding gums all
  - Loosening of teeth
  - Petechial hemorrhages
  - Hypochromic and microcytic anemia
  - Retardation of skeletal growth.

Table 6.2 Summary of B – complex vitamins

Vitamin	*Sources/RDA*	*Coenzyme form*	*Biochemical reaction*	*Deficiency*	*Assay*
Thaimin (B_1)	Whole cereals, dried yeast, legumes etc. 1– 1.5 mg/day	TPP	Oxidative decarboxylation of alpha-keto acids and transketolase	Beriberi (Dry, wet, infantile), Wernicks's Korsakoff syndrome	RBCs Transketolase activity and Blood levels of pyruvate
Riboflavin (B_2)	Milk, egg, dried yeast, germinating cereals, liver, kidney, heart. 0.6 mg/1000 Cal	FMN, FAD	FMN – L amino acid oxidase, Resp chain, microsomal hydroxylase, FAD – succinate dh, acylCoA dh.	Cheilosis, angular stomatitis, seborrheic dermatitis, corneal vascularization	RBC riboflavin levels, urinary B_2 levels low
Niacin (B_3)	Green leafy vegetables, tomatoes, yeast, milk, egg, meat, liver. 20 mg/day	NAD^+, $NADP^+$	NAD oxidoreductases reactions of carbohydrate and lipid metabolism and NADPH reductive biosynthesis of FAs, Cholesterol bileacids	Pellegra –(4Ds) Digestive disorders and Diarrhea, Dermatitis, Dementia, Death	-
Pantothenic acid (B_5)	Green leafy vegetables, cereals, yeast, egg, milk, intestinal bacteria. <10 mg/day	CoA, ACP	CoA – several derivatives in carbohydrate and lipid metabolism, drug acetylation, ketone body synthesis, cholesterol synthesis. ACP – FA synthesis	Burning foot syndrome	-
Biotin	Egg yolk, liver, kidney, yeast, peas, tomatoes, cauliflower, etc.	Biotin	Propionyl CoA carboxylase, AcetylCoA carboxylase, Pyruvate CoA carboxylase	Not known in humans but in experimental animals retarded growth, loss of weight, dermatitis, loss of hair, muscular in-coordination and paralysis	-
Pyridoxal (B_6)	Milk, egg, dried yeast, germinating cereals, liver, kidney, heart. 2 mg/day	B_6 PO_4	Amino acid metabolism – Transamination, Deamination, Decarboxylation, Heme syn, Glycogenolysis, Sphingomyelin synthesis, etc.	Neurologic symptoms, pellegra like symptoms Hypochromic microcytic anemia	Trp load test Homocysteinuria Blood levels of PLP
Folate	Green leafy vegetables, yeast, liver, kidney, meat, fish, milk, etc. 100 μg/day	H_4 Folate and its 1 C derivatives	Thymidylate synthase Methionine synthase	Megaloblastic anemia, Spina bifida	FIGLU test
Cobalamin (B_{12})	Egg, milk, meat, shell fish, etc but no vegeterain food. 1 μg-day	Ado B_{12}, CH_3 B_{12}, OH B_{12}	Methionine synthase, Methyl malonyl CoA isomerase	Neurologic defects Megaloblastic anemia	Schilling's test, Methyl malonic aciduria Homocysteinuria

- Easy fracturability of bones (Scorbutic bones), as the ground substance of the bones is not Properly laid down.
- Delayed union of fractures all
- Delayed healing of wounds.

- Most of the symptoms of vitamin – C deficiency are due to the defective synthesis of supporting tissue of mesenchymal origin.

Scurvy may be seen in infants feeding on mother's milk, as vitamin – C is lacking in milk and the lack of dietary supplementation may cause infantile scurvy – *Barlow's disease*.

Fat-soluble Vitamins

- Fat-soluble vitamins are hydrophobic, nonpolar molecules, which cannot be synthesized by the body in adequate amounts and therefore must be supplied in the diet.
- These are absorbed along with dietary lipids.
- Once absorbed they are transported in lipoproteins or with specific binding proteins.
- There are four fat-soluble vitamins—A, D, E and K.

Vitamin – A

Chemical Nature

- Chemically vitamin A comprises of a cyclo – hexenyl ring (beta – ionone ring) and an isoprenoid side chain with an "R" group that may be either alcohol (retinol), aldehyde (retinal/retinine) or a carboxylic acid group (retinoic acid).
- β-carotene is chemically made up of 2 molecules of retinal joined at aldehyde end.
- One molecule of β carotene splits to give two moles of retinal.

RDA and Sources

- Males—1000 μg/day
- Females—800 μg/day
- Preformed vitamin-A is present in animal foods like—egg, fish liver oil, milk, butter, cream, cheese, etc (Fig. 6.16).
- Provitamin form—β carotene is present in colored fruits and vegetables like—papaya, mangoes, carrots, tomatoes, spinach, beet root, plums, etc.

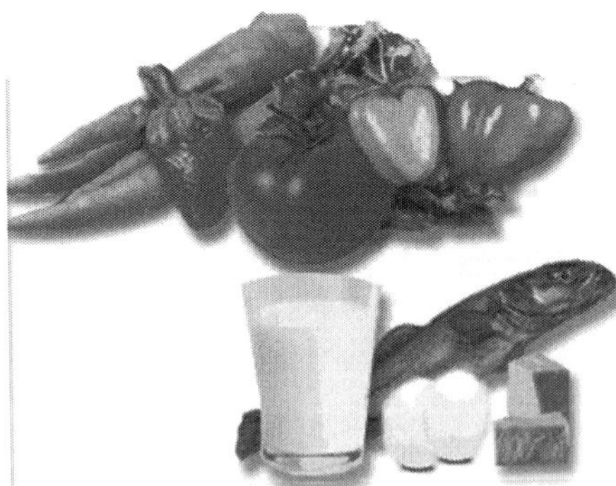

Fig. 6.16 Sources of vitamin A

> Provitamin—Provitamins are organic compounds which do not possess vitamin activity but are converted to vitamin when taken in the body.

Active Form

- Retinoid is the term used to include retinol and its related derivatives retinal and retinoic acid.
- All the 3 retinoids, i.e. retinol, retinal and retinoic acid in the body carry out the Vitamin A activity.
- Retinoids exist in *Cis* and *Trans* forms. [for e.g. 11 – cis retinal and All trans retinal]

Absorption, Storage and Transport of Vitamin – A

- Dietary fat contains retinyl esters dissolved in it.
- These dietary retinyl esters are dispersed by bile salts and hydrolyzed in the intestinal lumen by pancreatic lipase, followed by absorption directly into the intestinal epithelium.
- Dietary β-carotenes are oxidatively cleaved by β –carotene dioxygenase to produce two molecules of retinaldehyde in the intestinal lumen.
- The reaction is facilitated by bile salts and molecular oxygen.
- The retinal is then absorbed into the intestinal mucosal cells.
- Further, within the intestinal mucosal cell, retinal is reduced to retinol utilizing NADPH dependent *retinaldehyde reductase.*
- A small fraction of retinal is oxidized to retinoic acid irreversibly.
- Most of the retinol in the intestinal mucosal cells is esterified with saturated fatty acids and incorporated into chylomicrons.
- The chylomicrons enter the blood stream, where these are converted to chylomicron remnants, as they lose their fat content at different tissues, while still retaining their retinyl ester content.
- Retinyl esters are picked by the hepatocytes along with the chylomicron remnants and stored as retinyl palmitate forming a lipoglycoprotein complex in the hepatocytes.
- The retinyl palmitate is stored within the hepatocytes bound to cellular apo – retinol binding protein (apo –RBP) to form a holo RBP.
- When needed, the retinyl esters are hydrolyzed and released from the hepatocytes to be transported in the blood bound to a RBP and carried to different target tissues.

Biochemical Roles of Vitamin – A

- Role in vision (retinal)
- Role as a steroid hormone (retinol and retinoic acid)
- Role in maintenance of epithelial surfaces (retinoic acid)
- Role as an antioxidant (beta carotene).

Role in Vision

- The retinal cells rods and cones have two visual pigments—Rhodopsin and conopsin for vision in dim light and bright light respectively.
- Vitamin – A is an important component of both these pigments.

Vision in dim light – Wald's visual cycle

- In a dimly lit area, the rhodopsin of the rod cells helps in vision.
- Rhodopsin is photo–isomerized (bleached) sequentially from lumi to batho to meta – I to meta –II rhodopsin and finally into all – trans retinal and protein opsin.
- All – trans retinal is isomerized to 11–cis retinal in the retina cells by the **retinine isomerase** enzyme to again combine with opsin and regenerate rhodopsin.
- Some of the all – trans retinol is carried with blood to the liver.
- At the liver alcohol dehydrogenase reduces all trans retinal to all trans retinol.
- All – trans retinol esterifies with palmitate to be stored at the liver as retinyl palmitate.
- Once the liver stores are furnished, the all trans retinol then is isomerized to 11 – cis retinol at the liver.

- 11 – cis retinol finally is oxidized to 11–cis retinal that binds to opsin and regenerates rhodopsin.
- This complete cycle of bleaching of rhodopsin by light photons and the regeneration of rhodopsin is termed as the Wald's visual cycle (Fig. 6.17).
- When a person suddenly moves from brightly lit area to a dimly lit area, all the rhodopsin is completely bleached and it takes some time to regenerate rhodopsin, which would help in vision in dim lit area.
- This time taken for the regeneration of rhodopsin for vision in dim lit area is called the **dark adaptation time.**

Mechanism of generation of visual impulse by transducin protein

- The photoisomerization of rhodopsin is associated with generation of a nerve impulse (to visual cortex) via a trans-membrane protein – **transducin** present in close vicinity to rhodopsin.
- The transducin is a G–protein made up of 3 subunits—α, β and γ. Its α–subunit normally remains bound to GDP and is inactive.
- During photoisomerization, the GDP is displaced by GTP causing the dissociation of α subunit from β and γ and activation of α – subunit.
- Activated α–sub unit activates the c–GMP phosphodiesterase, which in–turn reduces the concentration of c–GMP within the rod cells, causing the hyperpolarization of rod cell membrane by closure of the cation specific channels.
- This hyperpolarization generates a nerve impulse which is sent to the visual cortex and vision is perceived.
- The α–subunit has an innate GTPase activity and hydrolyses the GTP to GDP and re- association of α-subunit occurs with the β and γ-subunits.

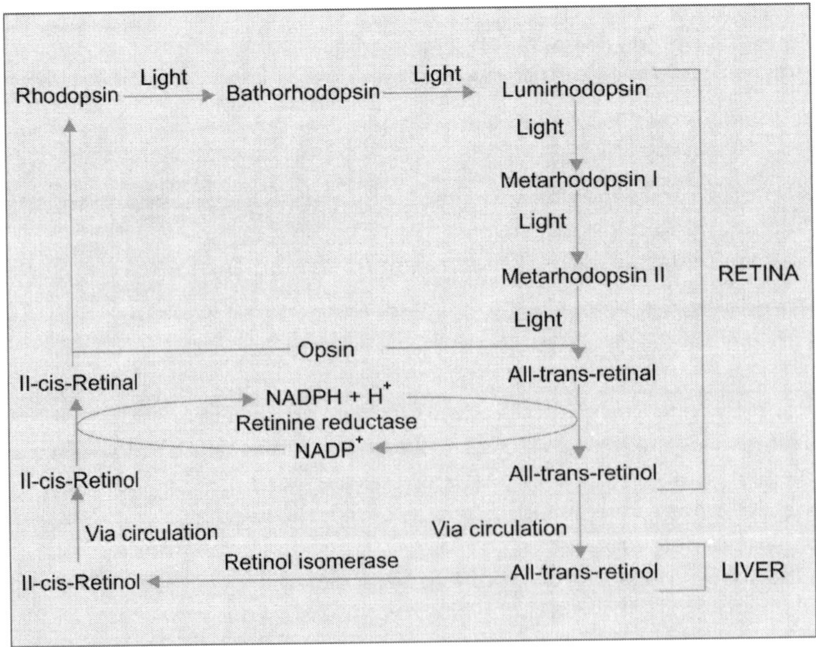

Fig. 6.17 Wald's visual cycle

Role as a Steroid Hormone

- Retinol and retinoic act as steroid hormone. Their whole mechanism is similar to the mechanism of action of steroid hormones.
- Retinol and retinoic acid being fat-soluble easily pass through biological membranes.
- Once inside the target cell, they bind to a cellular retinol/retinoic acid binding protein (CRBP).
- Bound to CRBP, they are transported to nucleus. At the nucleus retinol or retinoic acid enter the nucleus and bind to specific genetic sequences and cause gene expression.
- Binding to specific DNA sequences, they cause gene expression and protein synthesis. Role of retinol for normal reproduction is probably based on this.

Role in Maintenance of Epithelial Surfaces

- Retinoic acid is involved in glycoprotein synthesis.
- It has been experimentally proved that retinoyl phosphate acts as a carrier of oligosaccharide units across cell membranes by cis-trans isomerization.
- This is responsible for glycoprotein synthesis and synthesis and secretion of MPS.
- Therefore, retinoic acid helps in the growth and differentiation of tissues, various epithelial and embryonic tissue differentiation.
- It also helps in the maintenance of various epithelial surfaces by secretion of mucin which is mucoprotein composed of MPS and protein moiety.
- Mucin keeps the various epithelial surfaces moist, soft, supple and infection free for, e.g. epithelia of GIT, GUT, respiratory tract, urinary tract, etc.
- Thus retinoic acid helps maintain various epithelial surfaces.
- It also helps in overall growth including the skeletal growth.

Role of Beta Carotene as an Antioxidant

- β - carotene acts an antioxidant at low partial pressure of oxygen.
- It does so due to its ability to stabilize the peroxy free radical within its conjugated alkyl in chain structure.
- Since, at acts at low O_2 partial pressure, it complements the antioxidant properties of vitamin E which acts as high O_2 tension.

Deficiency of Vitamin – A

Deficiency of vitamin-A leads to:

- Eye manifestations
- Skin and epithelial manifestations
- Risk of cancer
- Overall growth retardation.

Eye Manifestations

- Deficiency of vitamin-A causes the dark adaptation time to increase. Typical symptoms of night blindness are seen, where vision in dim lit area or after night fall is badly impaired. The person finds it difficult to read, work or drive in night. Night blindness is seen in prolonged deficiency and is one of the early symptoms of vitamin – A deficiency, when the blood circulating levels are reduced and the liver stores too are depleted. Further deficiency causes typical eye manifestations, which if not cured therapeutically may progress to complete blindness.

Typical eye symptoms include

- **Xerophthalmia**—The conjunctiva becomes dry, wrinkled, lustreless, hazy and pigmented. The tear glands stop secreting tears which normally keeps the eye moist, washing away, bacteria and other foreign matter—resulting in dry, inflamed eyelids and loss of the glistening transparent appearance of the eye.
- **Bitot's spot**—Xerophthalmia is at times associated with Bitot's spots which are well-demarcated foamy-white or grayish irregular areas found on the temporal side of the cornea.
- **Keratomalacia**—When xerophthalmia persists for a long time, the dryness spreads to the cornea. The cornea becomes soft, ulcerated, infected and perforated and may progress to complete blindness.

Eye manifestations till bitot's spot are completely reversible by supplementing vitamin – A in diet. However, once there is keratomalacia, reversal is not possible.

Skin and Epithelial Manifestations

- The deficiency of vitamin–A leads to a defect in the synthesis and secretion of MPS and glycoprotein.
- The skin becomes dry, wrinkled and there is perifollicular hyper-keratosis.
- Epithelial surfaces become dry, keratinized and are prone to repeated infections, especially the epithelia of respiratory tract, urinary tract, GIT, etc.

Risk of Cancer

- There is an enhanced rate of cancers reported in populations with low consumption of beta carotene. Many human cancers arise in the epithelial tissues that depend on retinoids for normal cellular differentiation.

Overall Growth Retardation

- There is an overall retardation of growth in vitamin–A deficiency due to defective MPS synthesis, that is the needed for good skeletal growth.

Hypervitaminosis–A

- Excessive intake of Vitamin–A causes hypervitaminosis–A due to the raised unbound retinol as retinol levels exceed the binding capacity of RBP.
- The signs and symptoms include pruritic skin, chapping of skin about mouth, headache, etc.

Vitamin – D (Antirachitic Factor)

Chemical Nature

- Chemically vitamin – D has a steroid nucleus similar to cholesterol.
- There are two provitamin forms 7–Dehydrocholesterol (derived from cholesterol biosynthesis in skin) and ergosterol (from ergot fungus).

- Both ergosterol and 7–Dehydrocholesterol are converted to ergocalciferol and cholecalciferol respectively on exposure to UV rays of sunlight.
- Calciferol is then activated to active vitamin – D, i.e. Calcitriol.

RDA and Sources

- Infants, children and pregnancy—400 IU
- Adults – 200 IU
- Plant foods are poor sources of vitamin – D. However, some important plant sources include green leafy vegetables.
- Ergocalciferol may be present in some plant food infected with fungus ergot, but the intestinal absorption is poor.
- Rich sources of vitamin–D are fish, fish liver oil, butter, cheese, egg yolk, etc.

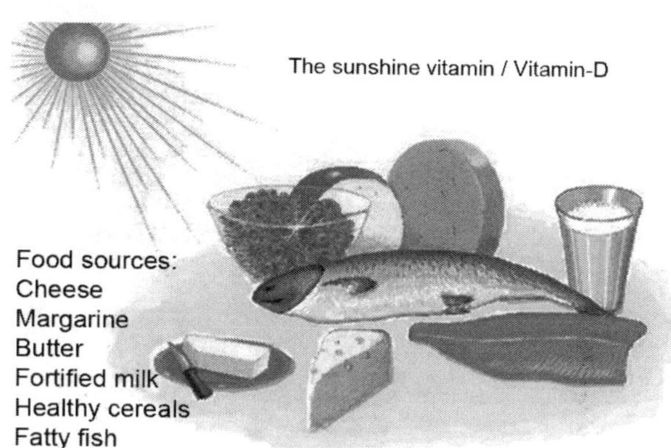

Fig. 6.18 Sources of vitamin – D

Absorption, Transport, Storage and Activation

- Absorption of vitamin – D occurs with dietary fats, assisted by the bile salts.
- Cholecalciferol is most efficiently absorbed.
- Once absorbed the cholecalciferol is transported in the chylomicrons.
- The chylomicrons unload their lipid content at various tissues to finally reach the liver as chylomicron remnant with the cholecalciferol content.
- At the endoplasmic reticulum of the hepatocytes, the cholecalciferol is hydroxylated at 25th position by the enzyme 25–hydroxylase.
- Cholecalciferol is converted to 25–hydroxy cholecalciferol (25–HCC).
- It is the storage form of vitamin–D.
- 25–hydroxylase requires coenzymes and cofactors—
  - $NADPH^+ + H^+$
  - Molecular oxygen
  - Cyt P450
  - Mg^{+2}
- Some of the cholecalciferol is also hydroxylated at 24th position, to form 24–HCC which is the inactive form of vitamin–D.
- 25–HCC is then transported in blood bound to plasma protein albumin (1 albumin + 2 moles 25–HCC) to the proximal convoluted tubules (PCT) of kidneys.
- At the PCT mitochondria, there occurs the second hydroxylation reaction at position1 of cholecalciferol to produce 1, 25–di-hydroxy cholecalciferol (1, 25–DHCC) in the presence of rate limiting enzyme 1α – hydroxylase.
- 1 α–hydroxylase requires following as coenzymes and cofactors
  - $NADPH^+ + H^+$
  - Ferrodoxin
  - Renal Ferrodoxin reductase

 - Molecular oxygen
 - Cyt P 450
 - Mg^{+2}

- 1, 25–DHCC is also termed as *Calcitriol* since it has 3 OH groups.
- Calcitriol acts like a steroid hormone, thus cholecalciferol is also termed as prohormone. Calcitriol is the active vitamin–D.
- Calcitriol can also be synthesized by the UV rays activation of 7–Dehydrocholesterol of malphigian layer of skin into cholecalciferol. This cholecalciferol then follows the same route of hepatic and renal hydroxylation till formation of calcitriol. Thus vitamin – D is also called the **sunshine vitamin. Biochemical role of Calcitriol**
- Calcitriol has three major target tissues—Bones, intestines and renal tubules (Fig. 6.19).
- Calcitriol acts like a steroid hormone, crossover the cell membranes of the target tissues, reaches the nucleus of target tissues bound to a cellular binding protein and enters the nucleus.
- At the nucleus, calcitriol causes gene expression of specific DNA sequences.
- At the intestines and the DCT of renal tubules, it causes the synthesis of calcium binding protein—**Calbindin.**
- One calbindin can bind 2 molecules of calcium.
- At the intestine, calbindin increases the absorption of dietary calcium and phosphorous. Thus increasing serum calcium.
- At the renal tubules, calbindin increases the reabsorption of filtered calcium and decreases the reabsorption of filtered phosphorous. Thus, increasing serum calcium and decreasing serum phosphorous.
- At the bones, calcitriol increases the osteoblastic activity and enhances the secretion of alkaline phosphatase by the osteoblasts. Thus the organic phosphorous converts to inorganic phosphorous and when ionic product of Ca^{+2} and P is greater than 40, bone gets deposited (mineralization of bone).

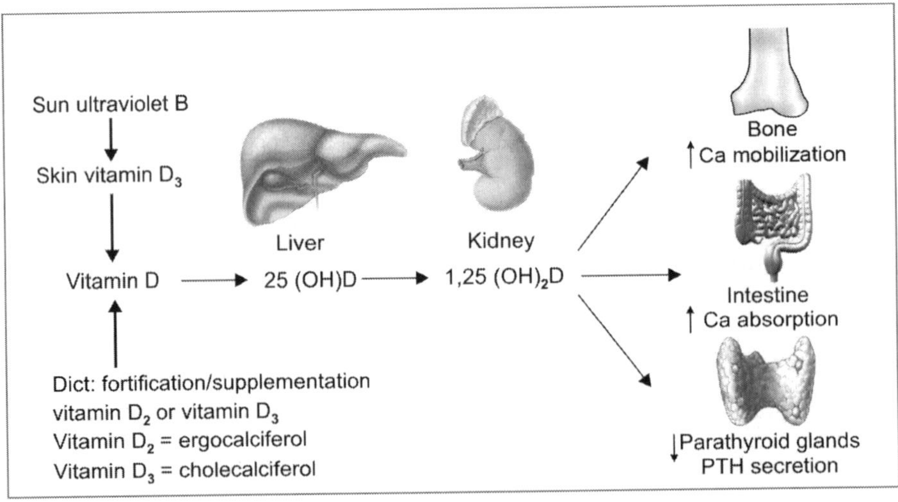

Fig. 6.19 Absorption, transport, activation of dietary vitamin – D and its target tissues

Regulation of Calcitriol Synthesis

Regulation of calcitriol synthesis occurs at three levels:

- Feedback inhibition of its own synthesis by inhibiting 1–α hydroxylase is the strongest regulatory pathway.
- Serum PTH levels.
- Serum levels of Ca and P.
  The 2nd and 3rd are interrelated.

Ca homeostasis by Calcitriol, PTH and Calcitonin – A Coordinated System

- Parathyroid hormone is secreted by the parathyroid gland in response to the serum calcium levels.
- It maintains serum Ca level by increasing bone resorption (increased osteoclastic activity), renal tubular reabsorption of Ca and increased 1 – α hydroxylase activity.
- It decreases serum phosphorous level by decreasing renal tubular reabsorption of P.
- Calcitonin is secreted by the c–cells of thyroid and works antagonistically to PTH and Vitamin–D.

Hypocalcemia

- PTH is secreted by the parathyroid gland so as to maintain the serum Ca levels.
- PTH increases serum calcium level by:
  - Increasing bone resorption/dissolution.
  - Increasing synthesis of calcitriol.
  - Increase renal tubular reabsorption of Ca.
- Simultaneously, it reduces serum P level by increasing its excretion thus preventing the ionic product of Ca and P to cross the saturation level.
- Calcitonin is reduced under these circumstances.

Hypercalcemia

- Reduced PTH secretion.
- Reduced reabsorption of Ca from renal tubules.
- Reduced dietary Ca absorption.
- Reduced bone osteoclastic activity and more of osteoblastic activity (bone deposition).
- Calcitonin levels rise and increase excretion of Ca.
  - Thus Calcitriol, PTH and Calcitonin act as a coordinated system to maintain a normal serum-calcium level.

Deficiency of Vitamin - D

Causes

- Dietary deficiency.
- Obstructive jaundice and fat malabsorption.
- Multiparous women with dietary deficiency.
- Women residing in purdah in certain communities along with dietary deficiency.
  - Deficiency of vitamin – D in children causes **Rickets** and in adults causes **Osteomalacia.**

Rickets

- Rickets is the vitamin – D deficiency disease of children.

Causes

- Dietary deficiency
- Genetic defect –Hypophosphatemic rickets (X – linked) and Vitamin – D receptor involving rickets (truly vitamin – D resistant).

Symptoms and Biochemical Defect

- It is mostly seen during periods of active growth, i.e. in infants and during puberty.
- Deficiency of vitamin – D during the active growth periods causes a defective mineralization of the new bone matrix, making the bones soft and pliable.
- The defectively mineralized bones are deformed and bone deformities are seen (Figs 6.20A to F):
  - Craniotabes
  - Bossing of frontal bones of skull
  - Delayed closure of fontanels
  - Undue prominence of sternum—Pigeon chest
  - Enlargement of costochondral junctions—Rickety rosary
  - Bending of the soft weight bearing bones—Bow legs
  - Knock knees *(genu valgum)*
  - Vertebral column maybe bent laterally (scoliosis), forwards (kyphosis) or backwards (lordiosis)
  - Enlarged wrists and knees due to overgrowth of epiphyseal ends:
    - Besides these skeletal deformities, there is overall skeletal growth retardation.
    - Biochemically, the plasma levels of vitamin – D, Ca and P are reduced.
    - Serum alkaline phosphatase is increased.

Osteomalacia

- It is a vitamin – D deficiency disease of adults (Figs 6.21A and B).

Causes

- Dietary deficiency.
- Purdah system in some communities in women.
- Multiparous women with dietary deficiency (as each pregnancy draws on the mothers skeletal system for deposition of fetal skeleton).
- Post-menopausal women (as the levels of estrogen are reduced, which reduces the bone deposition and increases bone resorption).
- Ageing (risk of osteomalcia in females : males is 2:1).

Symptoms and Biochemical Defect

- The vitamin – D levels are reduced so dietary Ca and P are not absorbed.
- Serum Ca and P are reduced.
- PTH is secreted in response to hypocalcemia and reduced vitamin –D levels.

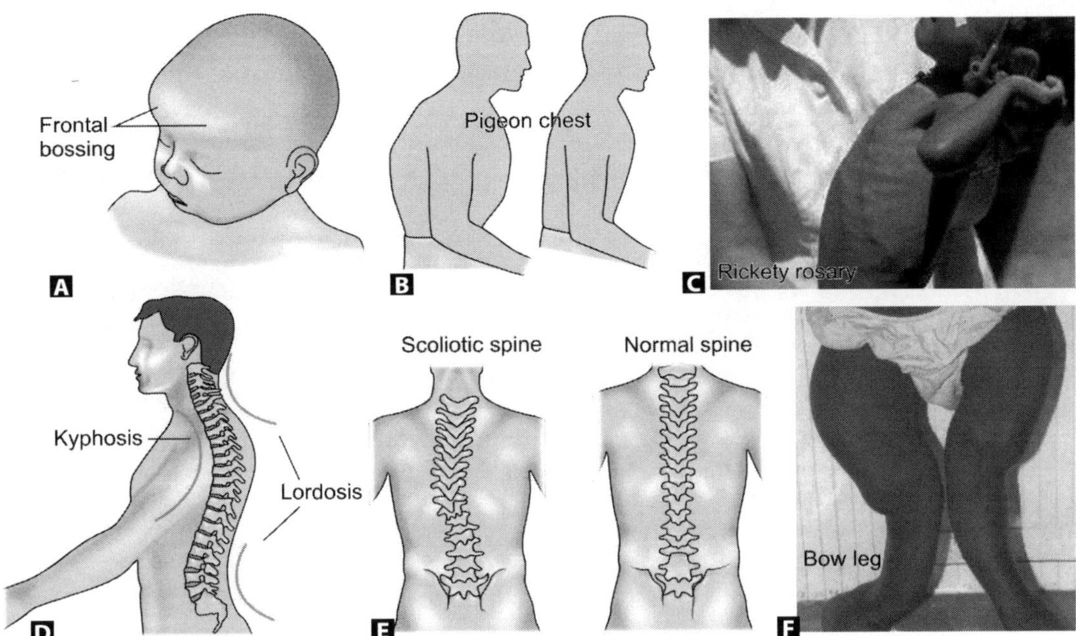

Figs 6.20A to F Skeletal deformities in rickets

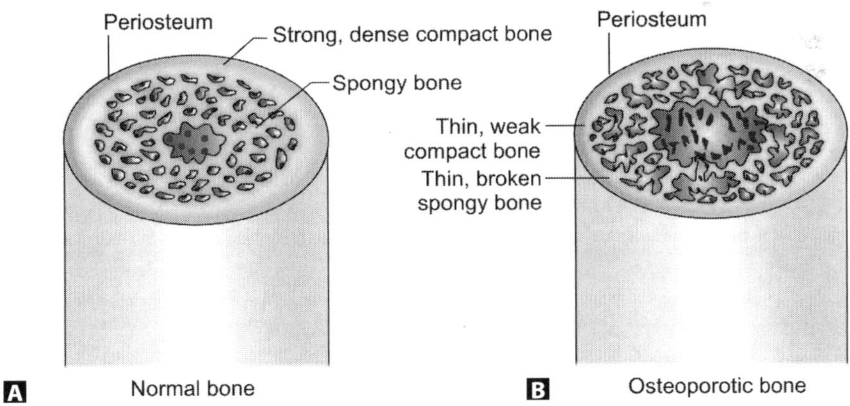

Figs 6.21A and B Normal and osteoporotic bone

- There is demineralization of the mature bones (bone resorption) for maintenance of serum Ca and P levels.
- Such bone becomes spongy due to demineralization.
- Demineralization of the mature bones makes the bones brittle, which fracture easily.
- Typical symptoms of bone aches and pains.

Hypervitaminosis – D

- Prolonged intake of large doses of vitamin-D in pharmacological form may cause hypervitaminosis-D
  - Serum calcium is raised.
  - Hypercalcemia may cause loss of appetite, polydipsia, polyuria, constipation, muscular weakness, etc.
  - Calcification may occur in soft tissues, e.g. arteries, bronchi, muscles, kidneys, etc.
  - Stones may be formed in the kidneys.

Vitamin – E (Tocopherol)

Chemical Nature

- Chemically tocopherols are isoprenoid substituted 6- hydroxychromanes.
- There are several naturally occurring tocopherols like α-tocopherol, β-tocopherol,γ-tocopherol and δ-tocopherol.
- α-tocopherol is the most abundant and with maximum vitamin activity.

RDA and Sources

- Vegetable oils, e.g. wheat germ oil, rice bran oil, corn oil, soya bean oil, cottonseed oil, etc. are very rich in vitamin E.
- Other good sources are green leafy vegetables, nuts, legumes, milk, eggs and meat.
- Adult men—15 IU/day.
- Adult women—12 IU/day.
- Pregnant and lactating women—15 IU/day.

Absorption and Transport

- Digestion and absorption of dietary vitamin – E occurs along with dietary fat.
- Furthermore, it is transported by the chylomicrons to the liver and exported from liver in VLDL.
- It is stored in the adipose tissue.

Biochemical Role

Antioxidant Nature of Vitamin-E

- Vitamin – E acts as an antioxidant at high partial pressure of O_2. Vitamin – E is concentrated at the cellular and subcellular membrane phospholipids of mitochondria, ER, Plasma membranes and RBC membranes.
- Tocopherols act as antioxidants due to their ability to transfer phenolic hydrogen to a peroxy free-radical of a PUFA. Thus scavenging it and simultaneously itself is converted to a phenolic free-radical. This phenoxy radical can follow 2 paths:
  - Either it reacts with vitamin- C and regenerates tocopherol
  - Or it reacts with another peroxy radical so that the chromane ring and side chain are oxidized to a nonfree radical product. This nonfree radical product then conjugates with glucuronic acid and is excreted from the body causing a net loss of the vitamin.

- Vitamin- E reduces the risk of myocardial infarction by reducing the oxidation of LDLc.
- It prevents peroxidation of unsaturated fatty acids, and protects the tissues against the harmful effects of lipid peroxides.
- It protects the RBC membrane from oxidants, and makes the RBCs resistant to hemolysis.
- It protects the pulmonary tissue from atmospheric oxidants.

Synergistic Activity of Vitamin-E and Selenium (Se)

- Vitamin-E and Se act synergistically against the peroxidation of PUFA by free radical, i.e. they reinforce each others' action.
- Se is a cofactor of enzyme glutathione peroxidase, which provides the 2nd line of defense against the hydroperoxides damage on the biological membranes.
- Vitamin-E reduces Se requirement by preventing its loss from the body.
- Conversely Se is necessary for the normal pancreatic function, which is necessary for digestion and absorption of the dietary lipids.

Ageing and Vitamin-E

- Owing to its antioxidant activity, vitamin-E has been shown to fight ageing.

Deficiency of Vitamin-E

- Deficiency of vitamin-E is uncommon due to its widespread distribution in foods.
- Moreover, the foods which are rich in PUFA, e.g. vegetable oils, are also rich in vitamin-E.
- Deficiency may occur in severely undernourished children and in premature infants fed on artificial milk not containing vitamin-E.
- The clinical manifestations of deficiency are edema, hemolytic anemia and thrombocytosis.

Vitamin – K (Koagulation Vitamin)

Chemical Nature

- Chemically vitamin – K activity is seen in isoprenoid substituted naphthoquinones.
- There are 3 major types of vitamin–K compounds:
  - Phylloquinone (derived from plant sources like alfalfa, spinach, etc.)
  - Menaquinone (derived from putrid fish meal)
  - Menadione (synthetic derivative).

RDA and Sources

- Green leafy vegetables (alfalfa, spinach, cabbage, etc.) are rich in vitamin-K.
- Cauliflower and peas are also good sources.
- Liver is a fair source. Small amounts are present in milk and eggs also. A very important source is bacterial synthesis in the intestine. The intestinal bacteria synthesize a good deal of vitamin-K which is available to the host.
- Since bacterial synthesis supplies enough vitamin–K. RDA is not known precisely and less than 0.1 mg per day is needed.

Biochemical Roles

Role in Maturation of Clotting Factors

- Vitamin K is essential for normal coagulation of blood. Concentrations of several coagulation factors in plasma are decreased in vitamin K deficiency. These include Prothrombin **(Factor II),** Proconvertin **(Factor VII),** Christmas factor **(Factor IX)** and Stuart-Prower Factor **(Factor X)**.
- The clotting factors are synthesized at the liver in zymogenic form. They are activated by a post-translational modification. Post-translational modification involves the gamma- carboxylation of their glutamic acid residues by a vitamin- K dependent carboxylase (Fig. 6.22).
- At physiological pH, the carboxyl groups attached to the γ-carbon of carboxy glutamate residues are ionized.
- The two negatively charged carboxyl groups act as a Ca^{++} binding site. Thus, the function of vitamin-K is to create Ca^{++} binding sites on the prothrombin molecules as a result of which they become biologically active. Similar Ca^{++} binding sites are probably created by vitamin-K on Factors VII, IX and X also thus helping in blood coagulation.

Therapeutic Role of Vitamin – K

- Another important function of vitamin–K is its therapeutic use as an **antidote to poisoning** by dicoumarol type drugs.
- The administration of vitamin-K would by-pass the epoxide-reductase step.

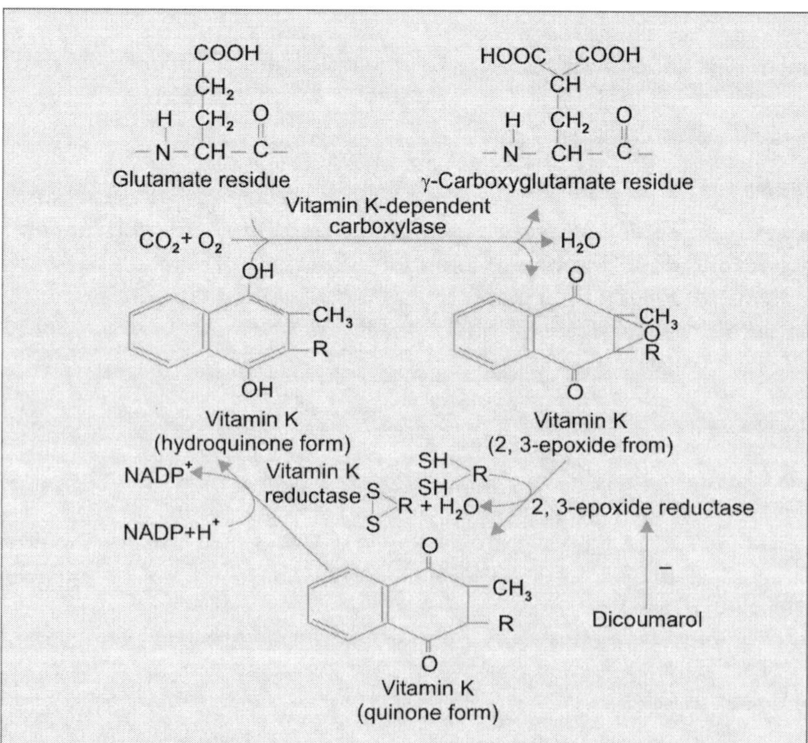

Fig. 6.22 Vitamin K cycle

Deficiency of Vitamin – K

- Deficiency of vitamin-K leads to a disturbance in the normal mechanism of coagulation of blood. Even a slight injury causes prolonged bleeding in a subject deficient in vitamin K.
- Diagnosis can be made by measuring prothrombin time, which is prolonged in vitamin K deficiency.
- Prothrombin time may also be prolonged in patients with liver damage due to inability of the liver to synthesize prothrombin. However, these two conditions can be distinguished by parenteral administration of vitamin-K. Prothrombin time returns to normal in subjects' deficient in vitamin-K but not in patients with liver damage.

A Quick Look at the Enzymology

- Vitamins are classified as water-soluble (B – complex and Vitamin – C) and fat-soluble vitamins (A, D, E, K).
- Most B – complex group of vitamins are present in dries yeast, green leafy vegetables, cereals and egg.
- B – complex vitamins are not stored in body , with an exception of vitamin – B_{12} , which is stored at liver.
- B – complex vitamins act as coenzymes.
- B – complex group of vitamins are important in metabolic reactions of carbohydrates, lipids and amino acids (thiamin, riboflavin, niacin, pyridoxal, Pantothenate, biotin) and in synthesis of DNA (B_{12} and folate).
- Vitamin –C cannot be synthesized by humans and higher primates due to lack of an oxidase enzyme that converts L – gulonate into ascorbic acid.
- Vitamin – C maintains connective tissue of mesenchymal origin, osteoid, dentine, ground cementing substance of capillaries, helps in wound healing, iron absorption, metabolism of tyrosine amino acid.
- Vitamin – C is an antioxidant water-soluble vitamin.
- Fat-soluble vitamins are digested and absorbed with dietary fats.
- Vitamin – A has importance in maintaining vision in dim light, epithelial tissues, tissue differentiation.
- Vitamin – D is responsible for the maintenance of calcium homeostasis along with PTH.
- Vitamin –D helps in bone deposition.
- Vitamin – E is the first line of defense against lipid peroxidation by free radicals.
- Vitamin – K acts as a coenzyme for the maturation of clotting factors II, VII, IX and X at liver by gamma carboxylation of glutamic acid residues of these factors.
- Beta carotene and tocopherols are fat-soluble antioxidants.
- Beta carotene acts as an antioxidant at low partial pressure of oxygen and tocopherols at high partial pressure of oxygen.
- All fat-soluble vitamins are stored at liver, with exception of vitamin –E (at adipose tissue).
- Deficiency of vitamin –A causes nyctolopia, vitamin – D causes rickets (in children), osteomalacia (in adults), vitamin – E causes hemolytic disease of new born and vitamin –K causes hemorrhagic tendencies.

CHAPTER

7

Mineral Metabolism

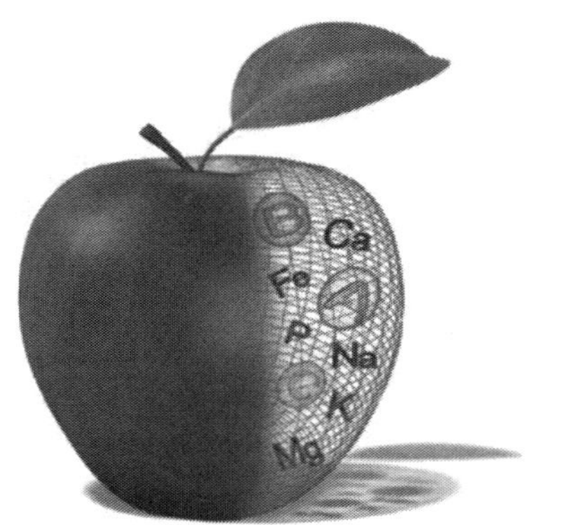

Chapter Framework

- Introduction
- Macrominerals
  - Calcium
  - Phosphorus
  - Sodium
  - Potassium
- Microminerals
  - Iron
  - Copper
  - Zinc
  - Selenium
  - Magnesium
  - Fluoride

Introduction

Dietary minerals are inorganic substances that our body needs in adequate amounts for vital body processes and body developments. Although minerals may be required in small quantities, they are still very important for our general health and well-being. Dietary minerals we consume can be broadly classified into:

- Macro minerals – required in amounts greater than 100 mg/day, e.g. Ca, P, Na, K, Mg, Cl, etc.
- Micro minerals – required in amounts lesser than 100 mg/day, e.g. Fe, Cu, Se, Zn, Cr, F, Co, I, etc.

Macrominerals

Calcium (Ca)

Total Body Ca

- Calcium is the most abundant mineral of human body, measuring a whopping 1 kg in an adult.
- Most of the calcium (99%) is present in the bones and teeth as hydroxy apatite crystals [$Ca_{10}(PO_4)_6(OH)_2$].

- However, calcium is also present in the circulation as ionized calcium, bound calcium (bound to plasma protein albumin) and complexed calcium (complexed with organic acids).

RDA and Sources

- Daily requirement of Ca is 800 mg/day for adults.
- More than 1500 mg/day for pregnant and lactating women.
- 1200 mg/day for growing children.
- Milk and milk products, cheese, cereals, legumes, nuts and vegetables like cabbage, cauliflower, green leafy vegetables, etc. are good sources of Ca.

Absorption of Ca

- Absorption of dietary Ca is carried out by a calcium binding protein—*Calbindin,* which is synthesized and secreted by the intestinal cells.
- The intestinal cells synthesize and secrete calbindin under the potent effect of Vitamin–D (Calcitriol) *[see Chapter 6].*

Factors Enhancing Absorption of Ca

- Acidic pH
- Amino acids Arg, Lys, Met, Isoleu, Trp
- PTH
- Vitamin–D
- Ideal Ca: P ratio of 1:1, absorption can occur across a ratio of 1:2 to 2:1.

Factors Reducing Ca Absorption

- Alkaline pH
- Phytates and oxalates of vegetables, as they form insoluble complexes with Ca.
- Obstruction of bile duct leading to fat malabsorption, which causes Vitamin–D deficiency and a defective absorption of Ca.
- Chronic renal failure, as Vitamin–D activation to calcitriol gets impaired.
  - Excretion of Ca occurs partly through the kidneys, but predominantly in the feces. Small amount is also lost through sweat.

Functions of Ca

Formation of Bones and Teeth

- Calcium phosphate is first deposited in an amorphous form, which is later converted into crystalline form.
- The crystalline form is known as hydroxyapatite, and its rough composition is $Ca_{10}(PO_4)_6(OH)_2$.
- There is a continuous exchange of calcium between bones and extracellular fluid.

Excitability and Conductivity of Nerves

- Ca can influence the excitability of sensory neurons.
- It serves as a charge carrier through voltage gated Ca channels, leading to depolarization of membrane and generation of action potential.

Neuromuscular Transmission

- In a classic synapse, calcium's main role is to trigger the release of chemicals (called neurotransmitters) from the presynaptic neuron.
- How calcium does, this is well-established and is achieved through voltage-gated calcium channels located on the membrane of the presynaptic terminal.
- These channels open in response to membrane depolarization, the type of signal carried by an action potential.

Excitability and Contractility of Myocardium

- The cardiac muscle depends upon the extracellular Ca level for its contraction.
- Systole is prolonged in hypercalcemia.

Coagulation of Blood

- Blood coagulation occurring by intrinsic or extrinsic pathway requires the Ca^{++} for the formation of active prothrombin activator.

Role in Hormone Action

- Ca acts as second messenger for hormones like—Glucagon, Oxytocin, etc.
- It also helps in the release of certain hormones from their storage granules, e.g. Insulin.

Role in Enzyme Action

- Ca helps in action of certain enzymes by activating a calmodulin mediated phosphorylating cascade.

Serum Ca Level and its Homeostasis (Fig. 7.1)

- The normal serum Ca level is 9–11 mg/dL.
- Serum Ca is present in three forms:
  - Ionized – 50% it is the functional calcium
  - Bound – 40% bound to plasma protein albumin
  - Complexed – 10% with organic acids like—citrate, oxalate, etc.
- Maintenance of a normal serum Ca is of prime importance and is achieved by a coordinated action of:
  - Vitamin–D
  - PTH
  - Calcitonin

Role of Vitamin–D in Serum Ca Maintenance

- Calcitriol acts like a steroid hormone and increases the synthesis of Calbindin at the:
  - Intestines—Increasing absorption of dietary Ca and P.
  - Kidneys—Increasing reabsorption of Ca filtered at the glomerulus.
- Thus, Vitamin–D increases the serum Ca level.

Role of PTH in Maintenance of Serum Ca

- During hypercalcemia secretion of PTH is inhibited.

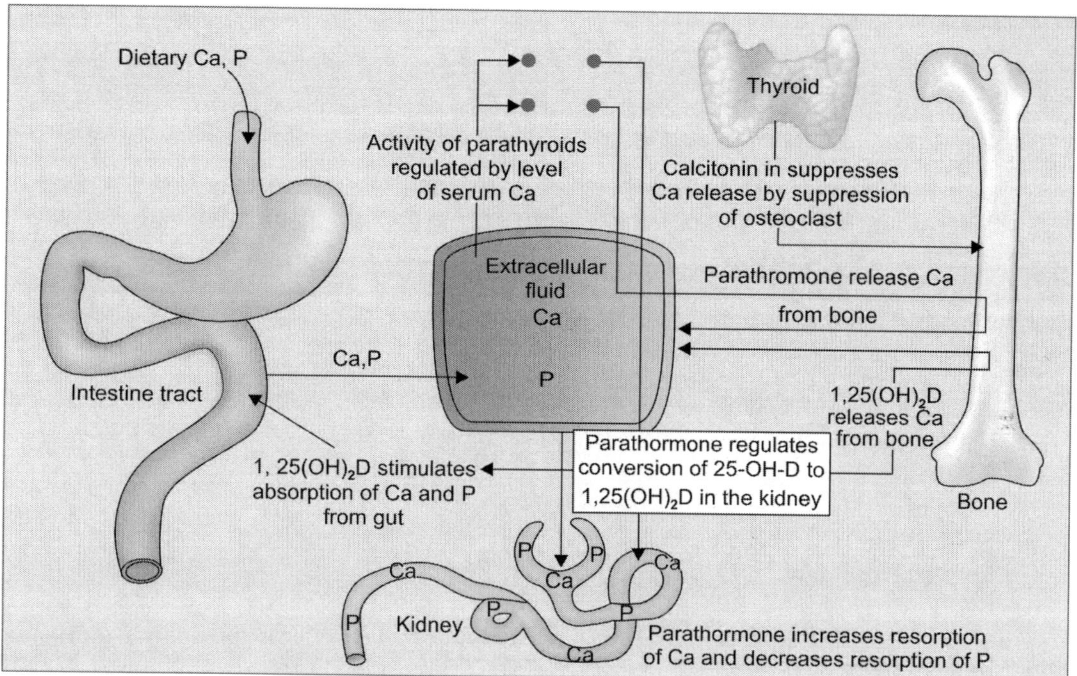

Fig. 7.1 Maintenance Ca homeostasis by a concerted action of vitamin-D, PTH and calcitonin

- Reduced PTH reduces bone resorption by inhibiting its osteoclastic activity at bones.
- Reduced PTH reduces the activity of 1-α hydroxylase on 25-HCC, so calcitriol is not synthesized. Thus, reducing absorption of dietary Ca and reabsorption of filtered Ca at renal tubules.
- Reduced PTH directly reduces reabsorption of Ca at renal tubules. Thus, maintaining serum Ca.
- During hypocalcemia secretion of PTH is enhanced, which has the following influences:
  - Increased osteoclastic activity at bones.
  - Increased activation of 25–HCC to 1, 25–DHCC (Calcitriol).
  - Increased reabsorption of Ca at renal tubules (DCT).

Role of Calcitonin in Maintenance of Serum Ca

- Calcitonin acts antagonistic to PTH, i.e. it increases the excretion of Ca by reducing renal tubular reabsorption of Ca.

Hypercalcemia

Causes

- A rise in serum calcium level (hypercalcemia) occurs in:
  - Hyperparathyroidism
  - Hypervitaminosis D
  - Bone cancer

- Multiple myeloma
- Leukemia
- Polycythemia
- Milk-alkali syndrome
- Sarcoidosis
- Idiopathic infantile hypercalcemia, etc.

- If serum calcium level remains elevated over a long period, calcium may get deposited in soft tissues, such as kidneys, liver, arteries, etc.

Hypocalcemia

Causes

- A decrease in serum calcium level (hypocalcemia) is seen in:
  - Hypoparathyroidism
  - Rickets
  - Osteomalacia
  - Steatorrhea
  - Chronic renal failure
  - Nephrotic syndrome, etc.
- A drop in serum calcium below 8.6 mg/dL is hypocalcemia. Tetany is seen below 8.6 mg/dL.
- A sudden decrease in serum calcium may cause tetany—involuntary contraction of skeletal muscles. Typical symptoms include *carpopedal spasm, laryngospasm (can be fatal) and Chvostek's sign.*
- Levels below 8.1 are fatal.

Phosphorus (P)

Total Body Distribution

- The total phosphorus in human body is 700 gs, with 85% in the skeletal system, 15% in the soft tissues and less than 1% in circulation.
- In the skeletal system, it is a component of the hydroxy apatite crystals.
- Among the soft tissues, it is abundantly present in the muscles and nerves as compared with other tissues.

RDA and Sources

- Children—800 mg/day
- Adolescents—1200 mg/day
- Adults—800 mg/day
- Pregnant and lactating women—1200 mg/day
- Milk, cheese, eggs, meat, nuts and beans are particularly good sources of phosphorus.

Digestion and Absorption

- Phosphorus is absorbed from the small intestine along with calcium.
- If calcium absorption is normal, so will be that of phosphorus.

Serum Phosphorus

- Phosphorus is mainly an intracellular mineral.
- Serum inorganic phosphorus level is 2.5 mg – 4.0 mg/dL in adults and 4 mg – 7 mg/dL in children.
- The product of serum calcium concentration (mg/dL) and serum inorganic phosphorus concentration (mg/dL) remains nearly constant.
- Adults –
  - [Serum calcium] × [serum inorganic phosphorus] =40
- Children –
  - [Serum calcium] × [serum inorganic phosphorus] =50.

Functions of Phosphorus

Formation of Bones and Teeth

Phosphorus along with Ca forms the hydroxyapatite crystals of bones and teeth. 85% of P is present as these crystals.

Formation of High-energy Compounds

Phosphorus is an important component of the energy currency of the cell, i.e. ATP and on hydrolysis of the ATP to ADP there is release of utilizable form of energy for the cell. Similarly, P is an important component of many other high energy compounds, where it helps to store the utilizable energy in the form of chemical bond, e.g. GTP, TTP, CTP, phosphoenol pyruvate, creatine phosphate, etc.

Role in Metabolism

Phosphorus, being an important component of the energy currency of the cell, it plays important role in energy metabolism. Besides, the phosphorylation and dephosphorylation of enzymes of metabolic pathways activates or deactivates them.

Formation of Nucleic Acids

Phosphorus is an important component of both the nucleic acids, DNA and RNA in the form of phosphoric acid.

As a Component of Compound Lipids and Conjugated Proteins

Phosphorus is an important component of phospholipids (lecithin, sphingomyelin etc.) and phosphor – proteins (like Casein, vitellin).

Formation of Membranes

Phosphorus is an important component of biologic membranes, as these membranes comprise of phospholipids (having phosphoric acid as its components).

Formation of Nervous Tissue

The nervous tissue is abundant in P, since sphingophospholipids are important components of the myelin sheath.

Maintenance of pH

The maintenance of a normal pH of blood is achieved by a concerted action of various plasma buffers like—bicarbonate, phosphorous and ammonia buffer systems. The phosphorus buffer system at the renal tubules and is responsible for the acidification of the urine along with the ammonia buffer system (*see Chapter 31*).

Hypophosphatemia

Causes

- *Hyperparathyroidism*—Due to increased osteoclastic activity and reduced renal tubular reabsorption of P under the influence of PTH.
- *Malabsorption*—Due to reduced absorption of dietary P.
- *Steatorrhea*—Due to malabsorption of dietary fat and fat-soluble vitamins leading to deficiency of vitamin –D.
- *Starvation*—Due to reduced dietary intake of P.
- *Vitamin – D deficiency*—Rickets and osteomalacia.
- *Chronic renal failure*—Due to defective activation of 25 – HCC to 1, 25 –DHCC.
- *Symptoms include*—Ectopic calcification.

Hyperphosphatemia

Causes

- *Hypoparathyroidism*—The low PTH levels cause reduced renal tubular reabsorption of P.
- *Bone cancer*—Due to increased turnover of bones.
- *Hypervitaminosis-D*—Due to increased absorption of dietary vitamin – D and reabsorption at renal tubules.
- *Diabetes mellitus*—Due to defect in carbohydrate metabolism.

Symptoms Include

Muscle weakness, dysfunction, reduced cardiac output, confusion, delirium, WBC dysfunction susceptibility to infection, large pulp cavities in teeth, hemolytic anemia.

Sodium (Na)

Total Body Na

- Total body Na is 60 gs of which about 20 gs is present in the muscles and rest in various tissues.
- It is the principle extra cellular cation, with a concentration of 135 mMol – 140 mMol/L.
- It is found associated with chloride ions as NaCl and with bicarbonate ions as $NaHCO_3$.
- The intracellular concentration of Na is less (10 mMol/L).

RDA and Sources

- The daily requirement of Na is 4.0–6.0 (i.e. approximately 10–16 of common salt).
- However, the requirement of Na may vary depending upon the daily losses of Na via sweating or in hypertensive individuals where the intake has to be reduced.
- Sodium is widely distributed among different food groups.
- Meat, fish, fowl, eggs, milk, cheese and cereals are rich in sodium. Carrot, radish, cauliflower, spinach, turnip, legumes and nuts are also good sources of sodium. Besides, the common salt used as a flavouring agent is one of the most significant sources of Na in daily diet.

Absorption of Na

- Absorption of dietary Na takes place along the whole of the intestinal lumen, i.e. both small and large intestines.
- The absorption occurs down a concentration gradient from the intestinal lumen into the intestinal mucosal cell, since the intracellular concentration of Na is low.
- The low intracellular concentration is maintained by the action of a membrane located $Na^+ - K^+$ ATPase pump, which pumps Na absorbed into the circulating blood with the expenditure of a high energy phosphate.

Functions of Na

Role in the Maintenance of the Osmolarity and Fluid Balance

Osmotic pressure is exerted by the solute particles across a membrane. Sodium being abundant extracellularly exerts the maximum osmotic pressure and is responsible for the maintenance of the fluid balance.

Role in the Resting Action Potential and Membrane Potential

Sodium concentration within the cell is low and plasma membrane is as such impermeable to Na. However, during the nerve and muscle excitation, this distribution of Na is disturbed as the Na moves in due to the generation of an action potential. The maintenance of the normal resting membrane potential is important for the next action potential. This is achieved by the $Na^+ - K^+$ ATPase pump, which pumps 3 Na^+ out of the nerve/muscle cell for an inflow of 2 K^+. Thus the normal resting membrane potential (– 70 to – 95 mV) is maintained across the membrane. Such a membrane is said to be polarized membrane.

Maintenance of the Blood pH

Sodium is an important cation of the plasma buffers. It is present as $NaHCO_3$ in the bicarbonate buffer, as Na_2HPO_4/NaH_2PO_4 in phosphate buffer. It is reabsorbed at the renal tubules in exchange for the secretion of H^+ that help in acidification of the urine and also maintain the blood pH (For detail mechanism, *See* Chapter 31).

Maintenance of the Viscosity of Blood

Sodium helps in hydration of the plasma proteins thus contribute towards maintaining the viscosity of blood.

Active Transport of Biomolecules

The active transport of glucose, galactose and amino acids is achieved by the $Na^+ - K^+$ ATPase pump (*See* in Chapter 10)

Hypernatremia

Hypernatremia is generally not caused by an excess of sodium, but rather by a relative deficit of free water in the body. For this reason, hypernatremia is often synonymous with the less precise term, dehydration.

Water is lost from the body in a variety of ways, including perspiration, insensible losses from breathing, and in the feces and urine. If the amount of water ingested consistently falls below the amount of water lost, the serum sodium level will begin to rise, leading to hypernatremia.

Causes

- It can occur due to excessive loss of water with inadequate rehydration causing hemoconcentration as in excessive sweating or diarrhea, inadequate intake of water, typically in elderly or otherwise disabled patients who are unable to take in water as their thirst dictates, excessive losses of water from the urinary tract, which may be caused by glycosuria, or other osmotic diuretics.
- Excessive excretion of water from the kidneys caused by diabetes insipidus, which involves either inadequate production of the hormone vasopressin, from the pituitary gland or impaired responsiveness of the kidneys to vasopressin making the renal tubules impermeable to water and no reabsorption of water occurs and excessive water is lost in urine (diuresis) causing hypernatremia.
- Intake of a hypertonic fluid (a fluid with a higher concentration of solutes than the remainder of the body), e.g. excessive use of saline in children or during management of acidosis by excessive use of $NaHCO_3$ or ingesting seawater also causes hypernatremia because seawater is hypertonic.
- Mineralocorticoid excess due to a disease state such as Conn's syndrome or Cushing's disease—any rise of these hormones would lead to retention of Na and excretion of K. Or in prolonged steroid therapy.

Symptoms of hypernatremia include—Lethargy, muscle weakness, edema, irritability, neuromuscular excitability, seizures and coma.

Hyponatremia

Hyponatremia is an electrolyte disturbance in which the sodium concentration in the serum is lower than normal.

Causes

- Hyponatremia is observed in cirrhosis, congestive heart failure, nephrotic syndrome, and massive edema of any cause when both water and Na content increase but the water content is greater than Na.
- Total body water increases, but the body's sodium content stays the same hypothyroidism, glucocorticoid deficiency.
- Water and sodium are both lost from body, but the sodium loss is greater.
  - Any cause of hypovolemia such as prolonged vomiting, decreased oral intake, severe diarrhea.
  - Diuretic use (due to the diuretic causing a volume depleted state and thence ADH release, and not a direct result of diuretic-induced urine sodium loss).

Symptoms include—Nausea and vomiting, headache, confusion, lethargy, fatigue, appetite loss, restlessness and irritability, muscle weakness, spasms or cramps, seizures, and decreased consciousness or coma.

Potassium (K)

Total body Potassium (K)

- Total amount of potassium in an average adult is about 140 gram.
- Potassium is the chief cation of the intracellular compartment, and is present in all cells.

RDA and Sources of K

- Approximately 4 gs of K intake daily is sufficient.
- Potassium is very widely distributed in foodstuffs. Meat, fish, fowl, cereals, vegetables, apricots, peaches, oranges, bananas and pineapples are rich in potassium.

Absorption of K

- Absorption of potassium occurs in the intestine along concentration gradient.
- Serum potassium level is 3.5 mEq – 5 mEq/L.

Functions of K in the Body

Maintenance of Intracellular Osmotic Pressure

Potassium maintains the intracellular osmotic pressure just as Na maintains the extra cellular osmotic pressure.

Component of Intracellular Buffers

Just as sodium is a part of bicarbonate and phosphate buffer in the extra cellular compartment, K is a component of bicarbonate and phosphate buffer in the intracellular compartment.

Nerve Excitability and Conduction

- Potassium maintains the normal excitability of nerves.
- It also maintains the contractility of muscles, especially the cardiac muscles.

Cofactor of Enzymes

For for example in Pyruvate Kinase.

Active Transport

It is a part of the $Na^+ – K^+$ ATPase pump and thus helps in the active transport of glucose, galactose and amino acids.

Hypokalemia

Causes

- Inadequate intake (rare)
  - Hypokalemia may occur due to inadequate intake or starvation.
- GI losses:
  - A more common cause of hypokalemia is flushing losses of GI fluids as in diarrhea or after surgical procedures. Sometimes, it is also observed in vomiting. However, K losses in

vomitus are not very significant but postemetic urinary losses of K are significant so as to compensate for alkalosis associated with vomiting.

- Urinary losses:
  - Conn's tumor (causing primary hyperaldosteronism) leads to urinary losses of K. Cushing's syndrome (hyperaldosteronism) hypokalemia is a rule. Thiazide diuretics also increase urinary losses of K.
- Other causes of hypokalemia: Renal tubular acidosis:
  - In the heart, hypokalemia causes hyperpolarization in the myocytes' resting membrane potential. The more negative membrane potentials in the atrium may cause arrhythmias.

Hyperkalemia

Causes

- Increased intake:
  - Hyperkalemia due to increased intake is rare but can be seen if there is increased intravenous infusion of K.
- Anuria:
  - Anuria is the condition where there is a complete shut down of kidney function. Under these circumstances, there is a rise of serum K, which may be severe if the intra cellular K is added up by some other tissue.
- Tissue damage:
  - Crush injuries with excessive damage of muscle mass adds up to the serum K levels.
- *Addison's disease*
  - Reduced secretion of aldosterone reduces the losses of K (hyperkalemia) and increases the loss of Na.
- Diabetic ketoacidosis:
  - The acidosis of diabetes mellitus causes initially a rise of serum K. Due to the increased activity of $Na^+ - K^+$ ATPase.

Symptoms include—palpitation, cardiac arrhythmias, sudden heart failure, metabolic acidosis, muscle weakness, etc.

Magnesium (Mg)

Total Body Mg

- The total magnesium in an average adult is about 20 g.
- Of the total Mg 89% is in the bones and muscles, with bones having 60% of the total body content.
- Most of the remaining Mg is distributed equally between muscles and nonmuscular soft tissues.
- Approximately, 1% of the total body content of Mg is extracellular.
- Serum magnesium level is 2 mg – 3 mg/dL.
- Concentration of magnesium in the intracellular compartment is higher than that in the extracellular compartment.

- Of the extracellular Mg, one-third is bound nonspecifically to plasma proteins.
- The rest of the extracellular Mg is diffusible or ionized and is the biologically active component. The ratio of bound to unbound Mg remains constant.

RDA and Sources

- Children—150 mg – 25mg/day
- Adult men—350 mg/day
- Adult women—300 mg/day
- Pregnant and lactating women—450 mg/day
- Nuts, beans, wheat, milk, eggs, orange and spinach are good sources of Mg.
- Almond is particularly rich in magnesium.

Absorption, Secretion and Excretion of Mg

- Absorption of dietary Mg occurs at jejunum and duodenum, assisted by vitamin–D.
- About 12% – 40% of Mg is absorbed.
- There is secretion of Mg in the intestinal secretions, so much so that hypomagnesemia is observed in patients with large losses of Mg in intestinal fluids and less reabsorption.
- Most of the Mg which is absorbed into the body is excreted by the kidneys.
- Aldosterone plays a role in the renal regulation.
- A high aldosterone level decreases the tubular reabsorption of magnesium.
- Fecal excretion largely accounts for the unabsorbed fraction.

Functions of Mg

- Magnesium is involved in excitability of nerves.
- A low magnesium level increases the excitability, and a high magnesium level decreases the excitability.
- Magnesium is a cofactor for some enzymes.
- Magnesium is a cofactor for all the enzymes requiring ATP as a second substrate as ATP participates in biochemical reactions as Mg^{++}-ATP complex, e.g. Hexokinase.
- Phosphofructokinase, pyruvate kinase, thiokinase, mevalonate kinase, squalene synthetase, glutamine synthetase, carbamoyl phosphate synthetase, PRPP synthetase, etc.

Hypomagnesemia

- Serum magnesium level is decreased (hypomagnesemia) in chronic alcoholism, chronic diarrhoea, hyperparathyroidism and aldosteronism.

Hypermagnesemia

- A high serum magnesium level (hypermagnesemia) is commonly seen in renal failure.

Microminerals

Iron (Fe)

Total Body Iron Distribution

- Total body iron is 3.5 – 4.5 g.
- Iron is stored bound to ferritin and hemosiderin.
- Iron is transported bound to transferrin.
- 60% – 70% is in Hb
- 5% – 10% is in Mb
- 10% – 15% is in the form of storage iron (Ferritin and Hemosiderin)
- 5% is in transport protein transferrin
- <1% in iron requiring enzymes and cytochromes.

RDA and Sources

- *Males* – 10 mg/day
- *Females* – 18 mg/day
- *Pregnancy and lactation* – 40 mg/day
- *Sources* – Organ meats, green leafy vegetables, pulses, cereals, jaggery, apples.
- Dietary iron is present in two forms:
  - Heme iron present in the nonvegetarian foods as Hb or Mb. This is easily absorbed as it has iron in the Fe^{++} form.
  - Nonheme iron present in the vegetarian foods, which is in the Fe^{+++} form and has to be reduced to Fe^{++} form for absorption.

Absorption and Transport

- Iron is absorbed at the duodenum. Of the total iron consumed in diet, only 10% is absorbed into the gut, rest is excreted unabsorbed.

Factors Which Increase Absorption of Iron

1. *Vitamin–C*—It converts in vegetarian foods ferric form to ferrous form for easy absorption.
2. *Acidity*—Optimal pH for absorption of iron is acidic.

Factors Which Decrease Absorption of Iron

1. *Phytates*
2. *Oxalates*
3. *Phosphates*

- All these organic ions are present along with the nonheme iron of vegetarian food and they reduce the absorption of iron by complexing with it preventing its absorption.
- The ferrous form of dietary iron is absorbed across the duodenal mucosa into the mucosal cell.
- Within the mucosal cell, ferrous form is oxidized to ferric form by a copper dependent ferroxidase – I (having Ceruloplasmin activity).
- The ferric form of iron now combines with the apo–ferritin to form ferritin that is stored in the mucosal cell.

- *Mucosal block theory*:
  - Iron absorption is regulated at the level of the intestinal mucosal cell.
  - The mucosal cell stores iron in the form of ferritin.
  - One ferritin can bind 4500 Fe^{+++}.
  - When the iron stores of the body are replete (sufficient), this mucosal layer blocks further absorption of iron across this layer into plasma by storing it as ferritin.
  - When the iron stores of the body are depleted the iron is drawn from the stored iron of the mucosal cell thus the mucosal block is removed.
- Once the mucosal block is removed, now the ferro-reductase of mucosal layer reduces Fe^{+++} to Fe^{++} which can now crossover into the general circulation.
- In the circulating blood, Fe^{++} is reoxidized to Fe^{+++} in the presence of a copper-dependent ferroxidase – II.
- The Fe^{+++} now combines with the apo–transferrin to form the transport protein transferrin.
- One transferrin can bind 2 Fe^{+++}.
- Normally transferrin remains 30% – 35% saturated with iron.
- Its main function is to carry iron to the various target tissues to be either utilized or stored.
- Iron is a one-way element.
- Iron once absorbed into the plasma cycles within the body between tissues. It cannot be excreted from the body.
- The only loss of iron is through the desquamation of the mucosal cells storing iron as ferritin and trace amounts by occasional RBCs in urine.
- Iron requirement is increased in pregnancy to form the foetal blood and for sequestering (storing) iron in foetal liver.
- Iron requirement is also high in active growth period like puberty.
- Once the demand is satisfied, in adults the total body iron is recycled and very little is lost (1 mg – 2 mg/day).
- This is mainly due to the renewal of the mucosal layer by desquamation (Fig. 7.2).

Iron Overload

- Hemosiderin is iron overload protein.
- Hemosiderin is ferritin with its protein shell removed a little bit to incorporate more ferric ions. It is present in liver, spleen, RE cells.

Hemosiderosis

- Iron overload may occur in thalassemia patients due to repeated blood transfusion (as the mucosal block is bypassed) (Fig. 7.3).
- Hemosiderosis is a harmless condition where the iron deposits in body tissues but does not damage them.

Bantu Siderosis

It is seen in African tribe – *Bantu*—as they cook meals (corn staple diet) in iron pots.

- Corn is low in phosphate so more iron available for absorption.
- There is some defect in their mucosal block leading to excess absorption.

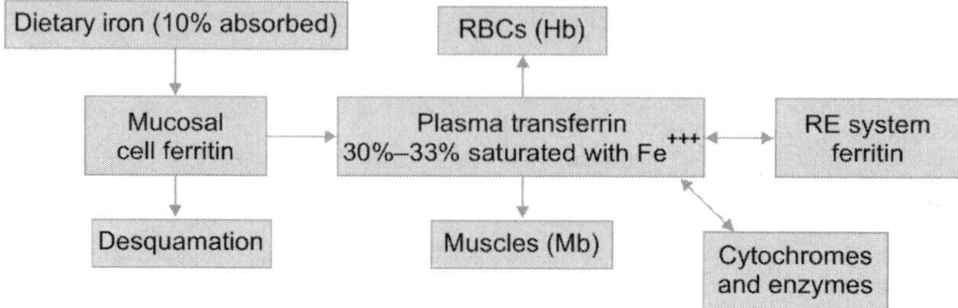

Fig. 7.2 Iron as one-way element

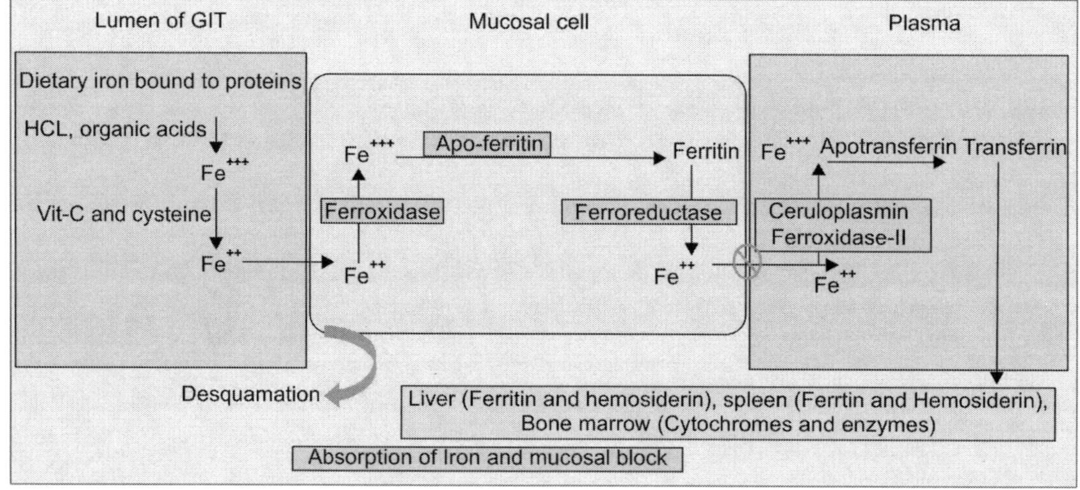

Fig. 7.3 Absorption of iron and mucosal block theory

Hemochromatosis—Rare genetic disorder. Iron damages the tissues where it deposits.

- It is characterized by the accumulation of iron in liver (cirrhosis), pancreas (diabetes), skin (bronze coloration) – Bronze diabetes.

Iron Deficiency

- Iron deficiency—30% worldwide and 70% in Indian population.
- More in Indians because we are mainly vegetarian.

Causes of Fe Deficiency

- Hookworm infection
- Achlorhydria

- Chronic bleeding as in peptic ulcers and piles
- Sudden accidental blood loss
- Pregnancy, lactation, growing children—dietary deficiency.

Blood Picture

- Hypochromic microcytic.

Symptoms

- Apathy, anorexia, weakness, fatigue, palpitation, pale skin—Metabolic processes are sluggish so lack of energy.

Copper (Cu)

Total Body Copper

- Total body copper—100 mg – 150 mg
- Distributed in RBCs, bones, muscles, brain and liver.
  - In RBCs—erythrocuperin
  - In Liver—hepatocuperin
  - In Brain—cerebrocuperin.

RDA and Sources

- Adults—2.5 mg/day.
- Children—0.05mg/kg body weight/day.
- *Sources* – Cereals, legumes, nuts, meat, shell fish.
- Milk and dairy products are poor sources.

Absorption of Dietary Copper

- Absorption of dietary copper occurs at the duodenum.

Absorption Inhibited by

- Cd, Mo, Zn, Ag, Hg and Phytates and high amount of Vit–C.
- An unidentified factor secreted in saliva and gastric juice complexes with the insoluble dietary Cu^{++} and helps to solubilize it for easy absorption.
- Absorbed into intestinal mucosal cells, Cu combines with metallothionin.
- Cu then is secreted into plasma where it combines with histidine and albumin.
- Liver removes the absorbed Cu from blood in less than one hour.

Fate of Copper at Liver:

- Some of the absorbed copper is secreted in the bile and finally excreted in feces. This is the principle means that maintains copper homeostasis.
- Liver synthesizes glycoprotein apo–ceruloplasmin that incorporates copper to form ceruloplasmin.
- 1 ceruloplasmin binds to 6 – 8 copper ions—half as Cu^{++} and half as Cu^{+}.

Serum Copper

Copper is present in two forms in serum:

- Direct reacting—4% present in this form and is loosely bound to albumin.
- Bound form—96% is present in this form and is bound to apo–ceruloplasmin.
- *Excretion*—85% – 99% is via feces and 1% – 15% is via urine.

Functions of Copper

Role in Enzymatic Activity

- Copper is integral part of enzymes like—Cytochrome oxidase, mono–amine oxidase (MAO), lysyl oxidase, super oxide dismutase (SOD), tyrosinase.
- Cytochrome oxidase—Final acceptor of respiratory chain.
- Lysyl oxidase—Maturation of pro-elastin to elastin.
- MAO—Metabolism of epinephrine and norepinephrine.
- SOD—Endogenous antioxidant
- $O^{2-} + O^{2-} + 2H^{+} \longrightarrow H_2O_2$
  - SOD has two forms—Cytosolic containing Cu^{++} and Zn^{++}
  - Mitochondrial containing Mn^{++}.
- Tyrosinase—Melanin synthesis.

Role in Iron Metabolism

- Fe^{++} is oxidized to Fe^{+++} by the ferroxidase activity of copper containing protein ceruloplasmin.

Role in Maturation of Pro-elastin

- Copper containing enzyme lysyl oxidase oxidizes the Lys side chains of pro-elastin to –CHO and helps cross-linking the soluble pro-elastin fibers into mature insoluble elastin fibers.

Role in Bone and Myelin Sheath Formation

- Copper has been reported to help maintain bones and myelin sheath.

Deficiency of Copper

- Weight loss.
- Anemia (Hypochromic microcytic).
- Bone disorder—Deficient trabeculae, thin cortices and wide epiphysis.
- Graying of hair.
- Myocardium atrophy.

Inherited Disorders of Copper Metabolism

Wilson's Disease (Autosomal recessive)/Hepatolenticular Degeneration

- Metabolic defect in incorporation of Cu in ceruloplasmin and impaired ability of liver to secrete Cu – Copper toxicity.

- Total body copper retention especially in brain, liver, kidney, cornea –Hepatolenticular degeneration.
- Liver cirrhosis.
- Dysfunction of lenticular region, necrosis and sclerosis.
- Aminoaciduria.
- Copper deposition around cornea in Deschmet's membrane – Kyserfleischer ring (greenish ring around cornea)

Menke's Disease (Kinky hair disease)

- *Metabolic defect* – Defect in copper absorption.
- Ist and IInd phase of absorption are normal.
- IIIrd phase of absorption is abnormal.

Clinical Feature

Mental retardation, abnormal bone formation, kinky hair that are graying, lusterless and brittle.

Zinc (Zn)

Total Body Zn

- The total amount of zinc in an average adult is 1.4 g – 2.3 g.
- Its tissue distribution is very wide.
- Prostate, liver, kidneys, muscles, heart, skin, bones and teeth are particularly rich in zinc.
- Blood cells, erythrocytes and leukocytes, have a higher concentration of zinc than plasma.

RDA and Sources

- Children—10 mg/day.
- Adult men—15 mg/day.
- Adult women—12 mg/day.
- Pregnant women—15 mg/day.
- Lactating women—20 mg/day.
- Zinc is widely distributed in foodstuffs.
- Liver, kidney, meat, fish, eggs, milk, yeast and whole grain cereals are good sources of zinc.

Absorption of Dietary Zn

- Zinc is absorbed from the small intestine (duodenum). Copper, cadmium and calcium interfere with the absorption of zinc. Phytates also retard zinc absorption by forming an insoluble complex with zinc.
- Zinc absorbed may be either retained in the intestinal cells bound to metallothionins until needed in the body or it may be transported to different tissues. Some reaches the pancreas and is secreted with pancreatic juices during digestion. Zinc secreted in the small intestine is reabsorbed to be transported back to the pancreas—enterohepatic circulation of Zn. Thus, absorption of Zn is similar in some respects to that of iron.

Functions of Zn

- Zinc is essential for normal growth and sexual development.
- It is required for the synthesis of nucleic acids, which is essential for cell division and growth.
- In the form of zinc fingers, it is a constituent of some proteins which regulate transcription.
- Many enzymes require zinc for their catalytic activity. These include carbonic anhydrase, carboxy peptidase, lactate dehydrogenase, malate dehydrogenase, glutamate dehydrogenase, alcohol dehydrogenase, alkaline phosphatase, super oxide dismutase, DNA polymerase, etc.
- Zinc is present in the β-cells of the islets of Langerhans. It is required for the storage and release of insulin.
- Zn accumulates in and around tissues during their healing. Thus is important in wound healing.
- It helps in vitamin–A activity as it is present in retinine isomerase of Wald's visual cycle. It also helps in release of vitamin–A from liver into blood.

Deficiency of Zn

Causes

- A dietary deficiency of zinc may occur in vegetarians taking refined wheat flour as their staple diet.
- It can also occur in *acrodermatitis enteropathica*. It is an inherited disorder of Zn malabsorption. It leads to—dermatological, ophthalmological, gastrointestinal and neuropsychiatric features.

Deficiency manifestations

- It causes retardation of growth, dwarfism, delayed puberty and hypogonadism.
- A milder deficiency may cause poor wound healing and impaired perception of taste.

Selenium (Se)

Total Body Selenium

- Selenium is present in human body in minute amounts. About 6 mg of selenium is present in the body of an average adult.
- It is widely distributed in the body.
- Renal cortices, liver, muscles, pancreas, pituitary, nails and skin contain selenium in relatively large amounts.

RDA and Sources

- The daily requirement for selenium is about 70 µg in adult man and 55 µg in adult women.
- Good sources include mainly cereals, fruits. Dairy products are poor sources.
- Biologic forms are selenocysteine and selenomethionine.

Absorption of Dietary Selenium

- Absorption of selenium occurs at the duodenum.

Functions of Selenium

The role of selenium in the nutrition of animals has been known for some time now. A few functions of importance are discussed below:

- It is involved in normal growth, reproductive functions and prevention of hepatic necrosis and muscle dystrophy in several animal species.
- Its exact role in human beings is still being investigated. It may be involved in the *synthesis of coenzyme Q.*
- It is also believed to play a role *in immune reactions.*
- It is a component of some proteins in the form of *selenocysteine.*
- The most definitive role of selenium, discovered so far, is in the prevention of peroxidation of lipids and other compounds.
  - Hydrogen peroxide, formed in the tissues by the action of aerobic dehydrogenases and superoxide dismutase, is a toxic compound.
  - It is detoxified by reduced glutathione.
  - The reaction is catalyzed by glutathione peroxidase.
    $2G - SH + H_2O_2 \longrightarrow GS - SG + 2H_2O$
  - Selenium is a constituent of glutathione peroxidase.

Deficiency of Selenium

Causes

- It may be seen in total parenteral nutrition, kwashiorkor.
- Some cases of endemic selenium deficiency have been seen in regions deficient in selenium in soil.
- *Keshan's disease:* It is seen in Keshan province of N-E China. It manifests as cardiomyopathy with clinical symptoms of:
  - Acute/chronic cardiac enlargement.
  - Arrythmias.
  - ECG changes.
- It is endemic as the dietary intake in the region is very low—7µg – 11µg/day.
- *Kaschinbeck's disease:* It is seen in several parts of eastern Asia and manifests as osteoarthritis. It is particularly seen in children 5–13 years of age. Their fingers and long bones are shortened with severe enlargement of joints resulting in growth retardation.

Selenium Toxicity

- Toxicity to Se is seen in industrial exposure as in glass, paint or electronic industry.
- Early manifestation is a garlicky breath due to dimethyl selenide.
- Later there occurs dermatitis, hair loss and nails become brittle.

Fluoride (Fig. 7.4)

Total Body Fluoride

- About 2.6 g of fluorine is normally present in the human body.
- More than 95% of it is present in bones and teeth.

RDA and Sources

- Fluorine is ingested in the form of fluorides.
- A fluoride content of 0.5 – 1 parts per million (ppm) in water will provide sufficient fluoride.
- Fluoride is present in the drinking water, beverages made by fluoridated water like—tea, coffee, beer, wine, etc. Food cooked in fluoridated water like—rice, pasta, etc. and fluoridated toothpaste.

Metabolism of Fluorine in Human body

- Fluoride is readily absorbed from the gut and enters the extracellular fluids.
- The absorbed fluoride is distributed in bones, teeth and soft tissues by the circulating blood (Fig. 7.4).
- Excretion of fluoride occurs via urine (50% – 70%) and sweat.

Functions of Fluoride

- Fluoride's high chemical reactivity and small radius allow it to either displace the larger hydroxyl (–OH) ion in the hydroxyapatite crystal, forming fluoroapatite, or to increase crystal density by entering spaces within the hydroxyapatite crystal. Fluoroapatite hardens tooth enamel and stabilizes bone mineral.
  - It makes the teeth resistant to dental caries. At the teeth, fluoride combines with hydroxy apatite crystals to form the fluoroapatite crystals. These fluoroapatite crystals then form

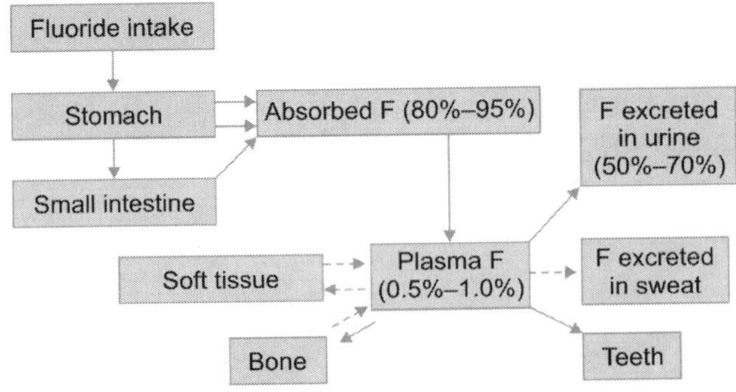

Fig. 7.4 Absorption, transport and metabolism of fluoride

a layer of CaF on the enamel, making it hard and resistant to action of bacteria. Thus, it prevents dental caries. Certain bacteria, which are normal inhabitants of the oral cavity, act upon dietary carbohydrates and convert them into lactic acid. Lactic acid corrodes the enamel of the teeth and produces cavities (dental caries). Fluoride hardens the enamel of the teeth and makes it resistant to attack by lactic acid.

- It helps to retain Ca and P in bones, making the bones stronger. Thus, fluoride makes the bones resistant to osteoporosis in later life.

Fluoride Toxicity—Fluorosis

- Fluoride is potentially toxic.

Acute Fluoride Intoxication

- The acute effects of the ingestion of massive doses of fluoride are first those of an irritant poison with an early involvement of the alimentary, cardiovascular, respiratory and central nervous systems, with corresponding symptoms, is a characteristic feature and such cases commonly have a fatal outcome in two to three days.
- After ingestion of fluorine compounds in high doses, there is diffuse abdominal pain, diarrhoea and vomiting. There is excessive salivation, with thirst, perspiration and painful spasms in the limbs.

Lethal Dose

The acute lethal dose of fluoride for man is probably about 5 gram as NaF.

Chronic Fluoride Ingestion

Toxic Effects on Human Beings

- Fluorosis is the chronic ingestion of high doses of fluoride over duration of time. Fluorosis may cause—skeletal fluorosis, dental fluorosis, Nonskeletal manifestations, or any combination of the above and in final stages it causes premature aging.
- If the fluoride content of drinking water exceeds 1.2 ppm (or the daily fluoride intake exceeds 3 mg), it may cause fluorosis.
- Fluoride >2 ppm drinking water—Gastrointestinal disturbances. Fluoride is known to combine with hydrochloric acid of the stomach and is converted to hydrofluoric acid (F+HCL = HF + Cl). Hydrofluoric acid is highly corrosive and hence the stomach and intestinal lining (mucosa) is destroyed with loss of microvilli.
- Fluoride > 5 ppm drinking water—Teeth affected and skeletal fluorosis is seen (Figs 7.5 and 7.6).

Dental fluorosis
Faint yellow
Brown stain
Pitting. Chipped off
White opacities
Black discoloration
Delayed eruption
Enamel hypoplasia

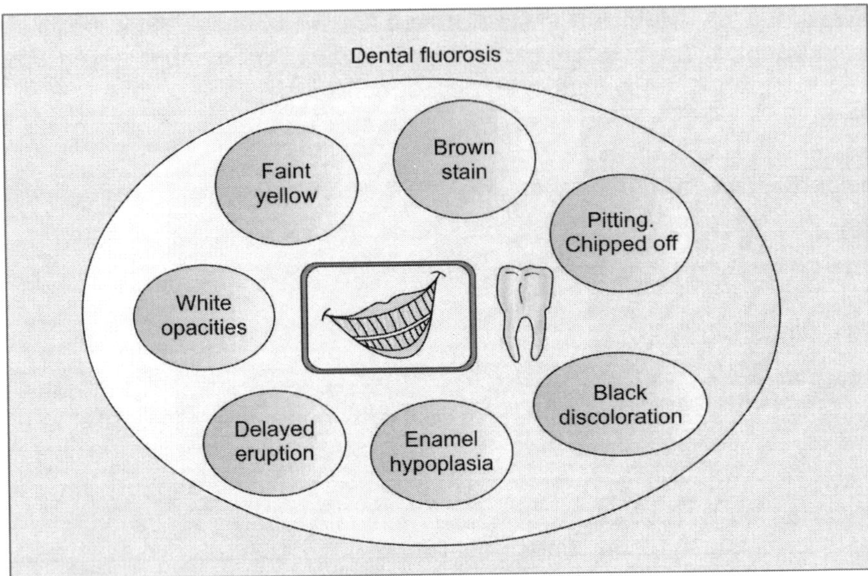

Fig. 7.5 Dental fluorosis

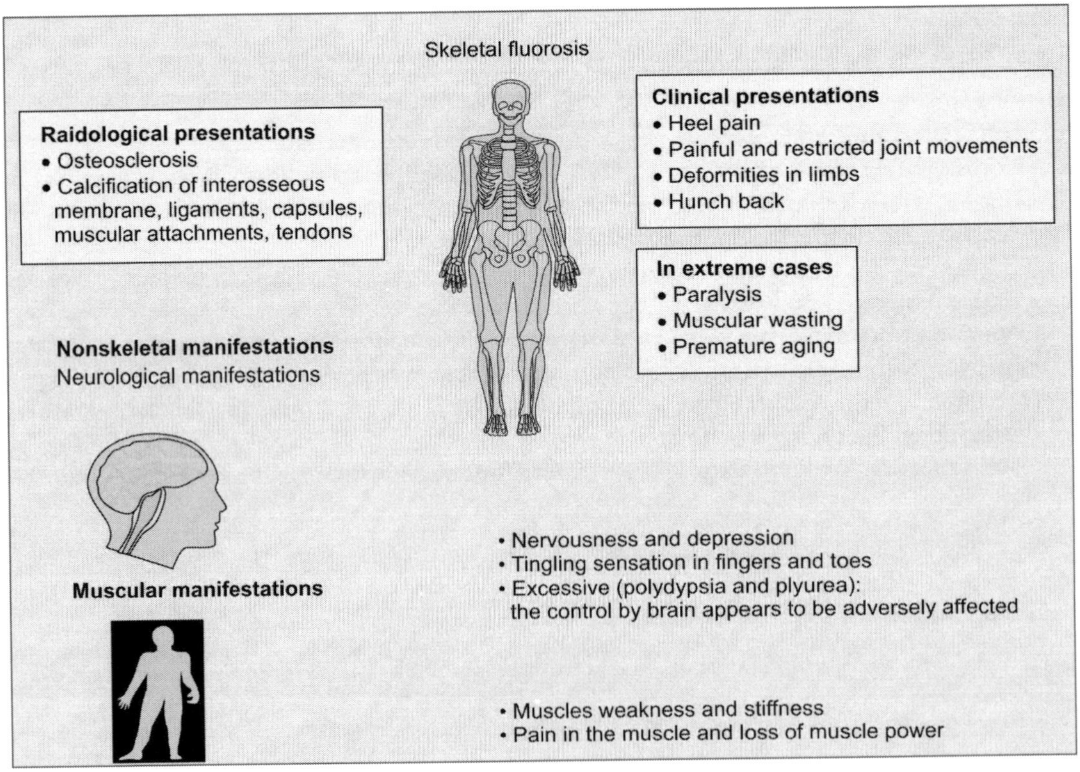

Skeletal fluorosis
Raidological presentations
• Osteosclerosis
• Calcification of interosseous membrane, ligaments, capsules, muscular attachments, tendons
Clinical presentations
• Heel pain
• Painful and restricted joint movements
• Deformities in limbs
• Hunch back
In extreme cases
• Paralysis
• Muscular wasting
• Premature aging
Nonskeletal manifestations
Neurological manifestations
• Nervousness and depression
• Tingling sensation in fingers and toes
• Excessive (polydypsia and plyurea): the control by brain appears to be adversely affected
Muscular manifestations
• Muscles weakness and stiffness
• Pain in the muscle and loss of muscle power

Fig. 7.6 Skeletal and nonskeletal fluorosis

A Quick Look at the Mineral Metabolism

- Minerals though needed in small amounts are important for maintenance of normal health and well-being.
- Macro – minerals are needed in amounts greater than 100 mg/day, e.g. Na, K, Mg, Cl, Ca, P.
- Micro – minerals are needed in trace amounts, i.e. less than 100 mg/day, e.g. Fe, Cu, Zn, F, Se, Cr, etc.
- Na is important in maintenance of normal fluid balance, pH of blood, action potential.
- K is important for nerve muscle excitability, contractility of heart.
- Mg is important for the activity of various enzymes of carbohydrate, lipid and amino acid metabolism.
- Ca is present in bones and teeth, acts as second messenger for hormones action, important for muscle contractility, neuromuscular transmission, blood coagulation and hormones storage and secretion.
- P is present in bones and teeth, is important for enzyme activity in metabolism, high energy compounds, compound lipids, conjugated proteins, membranes, nerves and maintenance of blood pH.
- Fe is important component of Hb, Mb, cytochromes, enzymes like—aconitase, catalse, etc.
- Fe absorption occurs as Fe ++ form and is regulated by mucosal block theory.
- Fe deficiency causes hypochromic microcytic anemia and toxicity causes hemosiderosis and hemochromatosis.
- Cu is required for normal growth, maintenance of bones, nerves myelin sheath, Fe absorption and maturation of elastin.
- Zn is required for normal growth, reproduction, wound healing and action of various enzymes like SOD, carbonic anhydrase, DNA polymerase, retinine isomerase, etc.
- Se acts as an antioxidant as a part of glutathione peroxidase.
- Fluoride is present in bones and teeth, and helps retain Ca and P in bones and teeth.
- F toxicity causes fluorosis.

CHAPTER

8

Nutrition

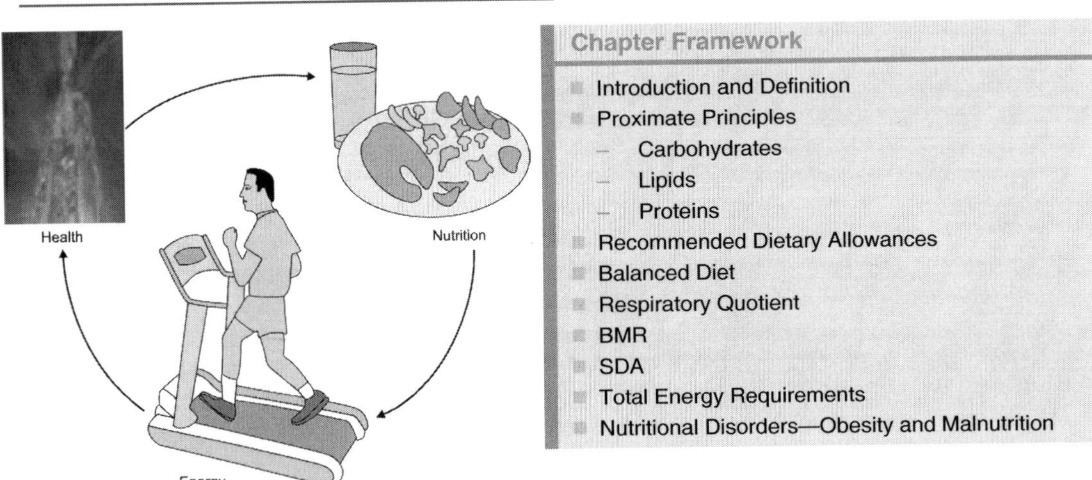

Chapter Framework

- Introduction and Definition
- Proximate Principles
  - Carbohydrates
  - Lipids
  - Proteins
- Recommended Dietary Allowances
- Balanced Diet
- Respiratory Quotient
- BMR
- SDA
- Total Energy Requirements
- Nutritional Disorders—Obesity and Malnutrition

Introduction

We need a wide range of nutrients to lead a healthy and active life. The various components of diet provide the energy essential for survival. The human body needs energy constantly throughout life for:

- Maintenance of body temperature.
- Supporting the physical activity and growth.
- Various physiological activities like digestion, absorption, circulation of blood, respiration, excretion, etc.
- Maintaining and regulating the metabolic activities of cells to release energy from nutrients and to store extra supplies for use in periods of dearth.

Definition

The study of food and nutrients, both qualitatively and quantitatively, necessary for the maintenance of an optimum health, is known as the science of nutrition.

The food we eat is made up of several nutrients, which can be divided into two major categories:

- *Proximate principles:* These liberate the energy necessary for survival by various metabolic processes. They include—dietary carbohydrates, lipids and proteins.

- *Regulatory principles:* These regulate the process of metabolism by participating as coenzymes and cofactors. Thus, they are important for the enzymatic activities of metabolic pathways. For example Vitamins and minerals. These regulatory principles are required in trace amounts and many of them cannot be synthesized in the body. Therefore, an inadequate intake of one or more of these nutrients adversely affects the human health, leading to various deficiency disorders like—beriberi (Vitamin B_1), pellagra (Niacin), megaloblastic anemia (Folate and B_{12}), hypochromic microcytic anemia (Iron deficiency), etc.

Proximate Principles

Dietary Carbohydrates

- Carbohydrates are the chief source of energy supplying approximately 60%–70% of the total energy requirement. However, Indians being predominantly vegetarians, procure almost 80%–90% of their daily caloric supply from carbohydrates. This makes the Indian diet vegetarian unbalanced.
- The major dietary carbohydrate sources are—Cereals, legumes vegetables and fruits.
- The calorific value of the carbohydrates is 4.1kcal/g, i.e. 1 gram of a carbohydrate can release 4.1 kcal of energy.
- Types of dietary carbohydrates:
  - *Available/digestible*
    These are the dietary carbohydrates that can be easily digested in the gut of humans. For example Starch, glycogen, disaccharides and monosaccharides.
  - *Unavailable/indigestible (Dietary fibers)*
    The dietary carbohydrates, which cannot be digested in the gut due to the lack of enzyme catalyzing their hydrolysis are included in this group. For example, Cellulose, lignin, pectin, hemicellulose, gums and mucilages, etc.

Functions of Dietary Carbohydrates

Major Source of Energy

Dietary carbohydrates are the most important source of energy, since they are mainly absorbed as glucose—the principle sugar of the blood.

Brain, CNS and RBCs utilize Glucose as an Exclusive Fuel Source

Normal functioning of the brain, CNS and RBCs is achieved due to the supply of glucose by dietary carbohydrates.

Protein Sparing Action

Since carbohydrates are used as the principal fuel source, therefore, the dietary proteins are spared oxidation. Instead, the dietary proteins are used for tissue protein synthesis for new tissue formation, differentiation, repair of old tissues and regeneration of damaged tissues.

Help in Oxidation of Lipids

Glucose during oxidation by glycolysis gives pyruvate. This pyruvate on carboxylation gives rise to oxaloacetate (OAA). Minor concentrations of OAA help maintain the CAC, which is the final common pathway of oxidation of all the three proximate principles including the dietary lipids. *Thus, lipids are oxidized in fuel of carbohydrates.*

Provide Energy for Muscle Contraction

Dietary carbohydrates are the principle energy source for all body cells. However, in skeletal muscles during intense muscular activity, there is limited supply of oxygen, even to the extent that anaerobic conditions may prevail. Under these anaerobic circumstances, it is the anaerobic glycolysis that generates ATP to help sustain the muscle activity.

Pentoses are Present in Nucleic Acids

Ribose is a component of RNA and deoxyribose of DNA.

Synthesis of Nonessential Amino Acids

The intermediates of the citric acid cycle provide the carbon skeletons for the synthesis of nonessential amino acids.

Excess Carbohydrates Stored as Lipids

The excess of dietary carbohydrates are stored in the adipose tissue as triglycerides, which serve as a source of energy during periods of leanness.

Importance of Dietary Fibers

- Dietary fibers are the unavailable carbohydrates, which do not supply energy. They are present in the plant cell wall. These are categorized as:
  - *Soluble dietary fibers:* Gums, pectins and mucilages.
    - *Improves glucose tolerance:* The soluble dietary fibers improve the glucose tolerance, since they reduce the gastric emptying rate. This prevents the sudden large surge in the blood glucose level which might occur if there is increased gastric emptying due to large amount of absorbable carbohydrate reaching the intestines in shorter duration. Thus, these can help manage the blood glucose levels in diabetic patients.
  - *Insoluble dietary fibers:* Cellulose, hemicellulose and lignin.
    - *Roughage:* The insoluble dietary fibers form the bulk of the diet, i.e. roughage.
    - *Satiety:* Since the dietary fibers form the bulk of the diet, therefore they give a feeling of stomach fullness without consumption of excess calories.
    - *Prevent constipation:* The insoluble dietary fibers are hygroscopic and thus imbibe water. This helps in proper bowl motility and the feces become soft, prevent constipation.
    - *Lower serum cholesterol:* The insoluble dietary fibers bind to the dietary cholesterol and prevents its absorption. Besides, these dietary fibers also bind to the bile salts secreted into the gut lumen and prevent their enterohepatic circulation. This causes the loss

of bile salts in the feces and the pool of bile acids at the gall bladder gets depleted. However, a constant pool has to be maintained for the bile acids. Thus the liver draws on serum cholesterol and oxidizes it to bile acids. This reduces the serum cholesterol level. Therefore, the patients with hypercholesterolemia and coronary heart disease are advised to consume higher amounts of raw vegetables as salads to help regulate their serum cholesterol.

- *Adsorb carcinogens, neutral sterols, bile acids, bacterial toxins:* The dietary fibers have the tendency to adsorb onto the harmful chemical carcinogens and bacterial toxins. Thus protect against their harmful effects. Also they can adsorb bile acids and neutral sterols leading to their excretion in feces.
- *Prevents colon cancer, diverticulosis, piles, coronary heart disease, and diabetes mellitus.*

Adverse effects of dietary fibers

- *Trace element deficiencies*—Dietary fibers can bind trace elements like iron, copper, selenium, etc. prevent their absorption and lead to their deficiencies.
- *Bacterial fermentation of dietary fibers causes discomfort and flatulence* – Excess of dietary fibers when consumed can cause discomfort due to bacterial fermentation and flatulence.

– *Dietary Lipids*
  - Dietary lipids should supply 15%–20% of total caloric supply.
  - The calorific value of dietary lipids is 9 kcal/g.
  - These are the most important cooking medium and provide taste and palatability to the food.
  - Important sources of dietary fats are vegetable seeds, butter, ghee, milk, milk products, egg yolk.
  - The major dietary fats are saturated (butter, ghee, cheese, etc.), monounsaturated (olive oil), polyunsaturated (vegetable oils) and trans fats. Out of these the saturated fats (especially lauric, myristic and palmitic acid) and trans fats tend to raise the serum cholesterol levels.
  - The MUFA and PUFA tend to reduce the serum cholesterol levels (MUFA : PUFA = 1:1) Thus, patients with hypercholesterolemia and those with coronary heart disease are advised a diet low in saturated and trans fats, with appropriate consumption of PUFA and MUFA.

Functions of Dietary Fats

Cooking Medium

Fats are the major cooking medium of the Indian cuisine. Dietary cooking fats are the prime visible fats that provide taste and palatability to the food.

Provide Energy

The calorific value of dietary fats is the highest amongst the proximate principles (9 kcal/gm). Thus fats supply energy in a highly condensed and concentrated form.

Protein Sparing Action

Like the dietary carbohydrates, the dietary fats too have a protein sparing action as they are the preferred fuel source over the dietary proteins; which are spared to be utilized for the synthesis of structural components of the body and in tissue repair/regeneration.

Provide Fat Soluble Vitamins

The dietary fats like—vegetable oils, butter, ghee, cheese, fish liver oil, etc. provide the fat- soluble vitamins (A, D, E, K).

Provide Essential Fatty Acids

Essential fatty acids linolenic and arachidonic acid are supplied by the vegetable oils used as cooking medium. These essential fatty acids are of great significance (*see* Chapter 1) in the maintenance of serum cholesterol levels, synthesis of potent local hormones like—prostaglandins, leukotriene, thromboxane.

Docosa-hexenoic Acid (DHA)

A polyunsaturated fatty acid (PUFA), DHA is provided by dietary fats. This is important in the early development of brain of the children and also for good vision as it maintains the retinal membrane.

Dietary Proteins

- Proteins are the building blocks of the body. A human being needs a constant supply of excellent quality proteins throughout life, since proteins are not stored in the body like—carbohydrates (as glycogen) or lipids (as triglycerides). Rather proteins are the dynamic proximate principle of the body, they are either utilized by the body or if in excess of the requirement will be completely catabolized to urea and excreted.
- This dynamic nature of the proteins necessitates a continuous supply of protein that contains all the essential amino acids in abundance.
- However, all the dietary proteins do not contain appropriate amount of essential amino acids. Depending upon their essential amino acid content, the dietary proteins can be classified as:
  - *Excellent quality (Ist class proteins):* These are mainly the nonvegetarian proteins and contain all the essential amino acids in abundance. For example organ meats and egg.
  - *Good quality proteins:* These are the poultry, milk and milk products. They contain all the essential amino, acids, however not in abundance or surplus, rather in just appropriate amount.
  - *Fair quality proteins:* These comprise predominantly the vegetarian proteins. Such proteins do not have all the essential amino acids rather they lack at-least one essential amino acids. However, for strict vegetarians, the dietary supply of essential amino acids can be achieved by consumption of the fair quality proteins in combination, such that deficiency of one protein is fulfilled by the other one. Such proteins when consumed in combination are termed as the *Complimentary proteins.* For, e.g. Cereals lack lysine but contain methionine and pulses lack methionine but contain lysine. On consuming cereals and pulses in combination a complete good quality protein is supplied, like eating dal – chaval (pulses

– rice) or dal – chappati (pulses – wheat).
- Dietary proteins should provide for 10%–15 % of the total caloric requirement.

RDA of Dietary Proteins

Infants
2.4 g/kg body weight.

Children Up to 10 Years
Boys 1.75 g/kg body weight and girls 1.6 g/kg body weight.

Adults
Men and women 1 g/kg body weight.
- Pregnancy 2 g/kg body weight.
- Lactation 2.5 g/kg body weight.

Functions of Dietary Proteins

Importance of dietary proteins is in:
- *Maintain a state of nitrogen balance:* Dietary proteins are the important source of nitrogen and sulfur in our body. In a healthy adult the amount of nitrogen consumed as protein is equal to amount of nitrogen lost in urine, feces and skin added together.
  - *Positive nitrogen balance:* It is seen when amount of nitrogen excreted is less than consumed as in conditions of active growth as in infants, growing children, adolescence, pregnant and lactating mothers, convalescence from sickness, under influence of anabolic hormones like growth hormone, insulin, etc.
  - *Negative nitrogen balance:* It is seen when the amount of nitrogen lost is more than consumed as in chronic illnesses, cancer, old age, burns, malnutrition, under influence of excess of hormones like—Thyroxine, stress hormones.

Supply Essential Amino Acids

Essential amino acids cannot be synthesized in our body, therefore, dietary proteins of good quality supply sufficient amounts of these.

Building Blocks of Body

Proteins are the building block of our body synthesizing and repairing tissues. The dietary proteins are used for the purpose of building new tissue proteins and repair of the worn out ones since proteins cannot be stored and should be consumed daily.

Source of Energy

Proteins are spared oxidation for energy production as dietary carbohydrates and lipids are used preferentially over them. This is because the oxidation of proteins requires a larger amount of energy to be spent than carbohydrates and lipids. Thus dietary proteins are the last to be oxidized as a fuel source.

Assessing the Quality of Dietary Proteins

A number of indices help assess the quality of dietary proteins. These are based upon the digestibility of dietary proteins and their essential amino acid content (Table 8.1).

Biologic Value of Protein

Biologic value of protein $= \dfrac{N_2 \text{ retained} \times 100}{N_2 \text{ absorbed}}$

For, e.g. Ingested protein = 127 mg
Excreted N_2 in feces (unabsorbed) = 4 mg
Absorbed N_2 = 127 – 4 = 123 mg
Excreted N_2 in urine = 24 mg
N_2 retained = Absorbed N_2 – Excretion in urine, i.e. 123 – 24 = 99 mg

BV $= \text{BV} = \dfrac{99}{123} \times 100 = 81\%$

However, biologic value of proteins is often a misguiding value, as it does not take into consideration the protein loss during digestion. For e.g., If 5 mg of dietary protein is consumed, 1 mg is absorbed and 0.8 mg of it retained as nitrogen, then the BV would be 0.8/1 × 100 = 80%. However, only 1 mg is absorbed out of 5 mg of dietary protein.

Net Protein Utilization

- It is the ratio of nitrogen retained to nitrogen consumed as dietary protein:

$$\text{NPU} = \frac{N_2 \text{ retained} \times 100}{N_2 \text{ intake}}$$

Protein intake = 127 mg
Retained N_2 = 99 mg

$$\text{NPU} = \frac{99}{127} \times 100 = 78\%$$

Thus, it gives better picture of the nutritional importance of proteins. Considering that out of 5 mg of dietary proteins only 1 mg is absorbed and 0.8 mg retained, the NPU would be

$$\frac{0.8}{5} \times 100 = 16\%$$

Table 8.1 Comparing some important dietary vegetarian and nonvegetarian proteins quality indices

	BV	*NPU*	*PER*	*Chemical score*
Egg	90	91	4.5	100
Milk	84	75	3	65
Meat	80	76	2.8	70
Fish	85	72	3	60
Wheat	58	47	1.7	42

Comparing with the biologic value of this protein, which was 80%, the NPU gives a true picture of the quality of the dietary proteins.

Some other indices are also used like the *protein efficiency ratio (PER)* and the *Chemical score of a protein.*

- *PER* is the weight gain by an experimental animal per gram of protein consumed.
- *Chemical score* (amino acid score).

$$= \frac{\text{mg of amino acid per gram of test protein}}{\text{mg of amino acid per gram of reference protein}}$$

- Egg protein is taken as reference protein since it contains all the essential amino acids in abundance. Its chemical score is taken as 100.

Calorific Value of Nutrients

- Calorific value is the amount of energy contained in each gram of a nutrient.
- It is calculated using a *Bomb calorimeter.*
- Calculation of the calorific value of a nutrient is done by combusting the desired nutrient in the bomb calorimeter (Fig. 8.1).
- The heat liberated on combustion is absorbed by the water surrounding the sample cup.
- The calorific value is taken as the rise in temperature by one degree per gs of the nutrient burnt.

Energy Requirements of a Person

- Direct calorimetry the subject is kept in an insulated chamber surrounded by water.
- The rise in temperature of water is measured over a period of some hours and from this, the energy produced per hour or per minute can be calculated.
- In indirect calorimetry, the energy production is measured from the volume of oxygen consumed and carbon dioxide eliminated by a person over fixed period.

Respiratory Quotient (RQ)

- The ratio of CO_2 produced to O_2 consumed on combustion of nutrient in oxygen with entrapment of ATP is termed as RQ.
- Carbohydrates RQ = 1
  $C_6H_{12}O_6 + 6O_2 \longrightarrow 6\,CO_2 + 6H_2O$
- Lipids have an RQ less than that of carbohydrates as the number of oxygen atoms contained per molecule of a lipid is less. Thus, greater oxygen is consumed for the combustion of fats. Lipids RQ = 0.7.
- RQ of the dietary proteins is also low, since there isn't any general structural formula for the proteins and different proteins vary in their composition of amino acids with varying number of carbon and oxygen atoms. However, the value has been generalized to be 0.8.
- Mixed diet RQ is 0.82 – 0.85 since all the three proximate principles are included in it in varying amounts.

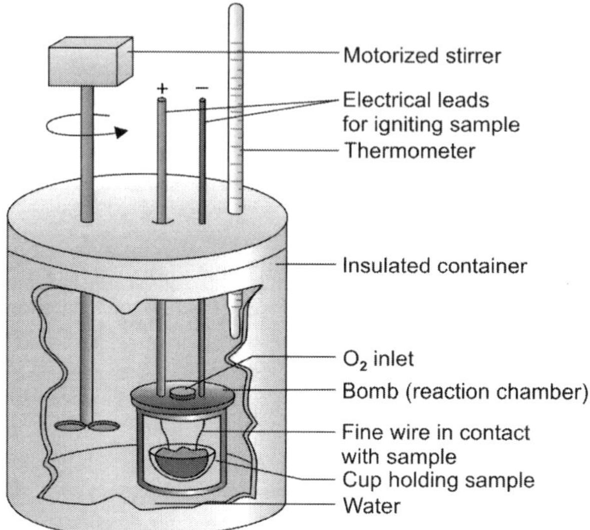

Fig. 8.1 Bomb calorimeter

Significance of Respiratory Quotient

- Measurement of RQ gives an idea about the type of fuel getting metabolized.
- RQ is increased when carbohydrates are deposited as lipids. This is for the reason that an oxygen-rich substance like glucose is being converted into substance which is poor in oxygen. Hence, the volume of expired carbon dioxide may be greater than the volume of inspired oxygen.
- RQ decreases during alkalosis owing to the suppression of the respiratory centers causing retention of CO_2 to maintain the blood pH (respiratory compensation).
- RQ increases in acidosis owing to the stimulation of respiratory centers for hyperventilation flushing out excess of CO_2 and regaining normal blood pH (respiratory compensation).
- RQ is reduced in starvation and ketosis as the principle fuel utilized in this condition is the stored fat of adipose tissue.

Factors which have to be Considered while Calculating Energy Requirement

- Basal metabolic rate (BMR)
- Specific dynamic action (SDA) of food
- Physical activity.

Basal Metabolic Rate (BMR)

It is defined as the amount of energy required by an awake individual at complete physical and mental rest to sustain life. It is measured as kcal/m^2/hour.

Normal Values

- Adult males—35—40 kcal/m²/hour
- Adult females—32—37 kcal/m²/hour
- It can be measured by:
  - Open circuit method—Tissot's and Douglas bag method
  - Closed circuit method—Benedict Roth's method

Conditions for Measuring BMR

- Person should be awake.
- Person should be resting—Physical and mental.
- Person should be in postabsorptive state.
- Environmental conditions should be pleasant.
- Person should be reclining.

Benedict-Roth's Method (Fig. 8.2)

- *Apparatus:* The apparatus used in the procedure comprises of a cylinder kept inverted on a soda lime tower and floating on a water jacket of outer up – right cylinder. The inverted cylinder is connected by means of a pipe to an airway outlet. This airway outlet is guarded by a two-way valve such that the expired air is breathed into the pipe leading to the soda lime tower. The inverted cylinder is joined to a pulley that connects a spirometer to the cylinder, such that any movement of the cylinder will get recorded on the spirometer as volumes of the air displaced from this cylinder.

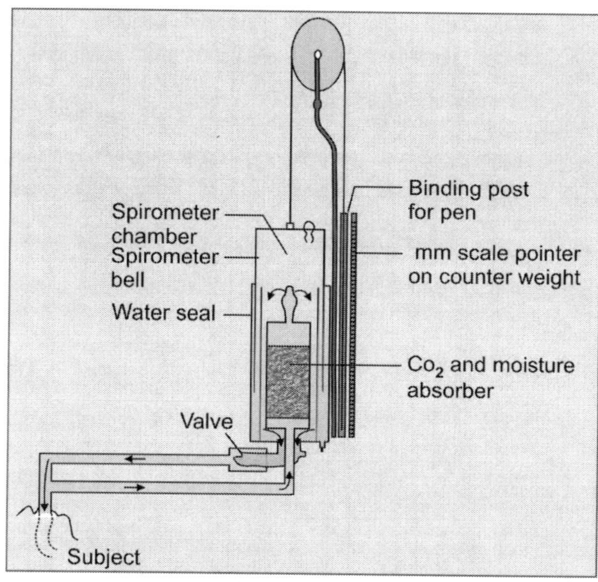

Fig. 8.2 Benedict-Roth apparatus

- *Procedure:* The person is asked to come after an over-night fast. The person is then asked to recline on a comfortable bed in a pleasant environment (normal temperature, pressure and humidity). Now the person is asked to breathe-in through mouth with nose clipped for about 6 minutes. This will cause the volume of oxygen to be utilized in the inverted cylinder. The volume of air inspired would be recorded at the spirometer due to the movements of the cylinder on the water jacket. The CO_2 expired will enter the soda lime tower due to the two-way valve. This would prevent the mixing of the expired air with the air utilized in inspiration.

Calculations

- Average of three sets of readings is taken.
- O_2 consumed for 6 minutes duration multiplied with 10 to convert to per hours.
- The volume of O_2 consumed per hour is then multiplied with 4.825 to convert into kcal.
- The volume of O_2 consumed in kcal / hour is divided by surface area to get values as per square meter.
- Surface area is calculated by a formula Dubois-dubois formula
- Surface area (m) = $W^{0.425}$ (kg) × $H^{0.725}$ (m) × 71.84×10^{-4}.

Factors Affecting BMR

- *Age:* BMR of infants is low and it increases till the age of 5 years. The BMR of the adults starts waning with age. It starts decreasing after the age of 30 years. Thus BMR is lower in old age.
- *Gender:* BMR of males is higher than the female counterparts owing to the greater muscle mass.
- *Surface area:* BMR of lean persons is higher than that of obese persons. This is because the surface of lean persons is more than obese persons.
- *Climate:* The tropical climatic conditions favour a drop in BMR, whereas it is raised in the cold climatic conditions. This is due to the reduced enzymatic activities during hot climates.
- *Race:* The BMR of the Caucasians is higher than that of the Orientals. Furthermore, the Eskimos have a BMR 33% higher.
- *Lifestyle:* The BMR is lower in people with sedentary lifestyle and rose in people with more active lifestyle. So the BMR of a laborer or an athlete would be more than that of an office clerk.
- *Dietary habits:* The vegetarians have a lower BMR as compared to the nonvegetarians.
- *Hormones:* Various hormones affect the BMR. Hormones of adrenal cortex, growth hormone, thyroid hormone enhance the BMR.
- *Pregnancy:* During the third trimester of pregnancy, the BMR of the females is raised owing to the sum total of their own BMR and the growing fetus's BMR.
- *Stress:* BMR is raised during stress due to the secretion of stress hormones—epinephrine and norepinephrine.
- *Drugs:* Certain drugs like nicotine raise the BMR.
- *Sleep:* BMR is lowered during sound sleep and raised during disturbed sleep.

- *Pathologic states:* BMR gets altered during various pathologic states. During fever, polycythemia, hyperthyroidism, Cushing's syndrome, hyperpituitarism, the BMR is raised. Conversely, during anemia, hypothyroidism, Addison's disease, hypopituitarism the BMR is lowered.
  - Accurate measurement of BMR is not possible, therefore an allowance of 24 kcal/kg body weight is taken as a standard.

Specific Dynamic Action (SDA)/Thermogenic Effect of Food

- Consumption of food increases the energy production in the body, even in the basal state. This is due to SDA or thermogenic effect of food.
- After consumption of food, some energy is spent by the body for digestion, absorption, transport, metabolism and interconversion of carbohydrates, lipids and proteins and for their storage.
- The energy spent by the body to metabolize food is known as the SDA of the food.

SDA of Proteins

Proteins have the highest SDA. When 25 gram protein is ingested, about 30 kcal are spent in metabolizing it. The energy value of 25 gm of protein is 100 kcal but 30 kcal have to be spent to gain this energy. So, the net gain of energy from 25 gram of protein will be 70 kcal only. Thus, the SDA of proteins is about 30%.

SDA of Lipids

SDA of lipids is about 13% and SDA of carbohydrates about 5%. When different foodstuffs are taken together, the SDA is less than the sums of SDA of individual foodstuffs. Carbohydrates and lipids have lower the SDA. Lipids cause a greater lowering of SDA than carbohydrates since the storage of lipids needs lesser expenditure of ATP and also lipids have a higher total calorific value, thus producing greater energy per gram. A mixed diet containing proteins, lipids and carbohydrates has an SDA of about 10%.This means that if a mixed diet having a calculated energy value of 3,000 kcal is taken in a day, the net energy gain would be 2,700 kcal only because 300 kcal would be spent on account of SDA to metabolise the foodstuffs. Therefore, an additional provision of 10 % has to be made for SDA while calculating the energy requirement of a person.

Calculating Energy Requirements of an Individual

- *Energy requirement = BMR + Physical activity + SDA*
- In general, physical activity can be divided into three types depending upon one's occupation:
  - Sedentary workers (clerks, teachers, etc.)—30%–40% of BMR
  - Moderate workers (students, housewives)—40%–50% of BMR
  - Heavy workers (laborers, athletes)—50%–60% of BMR
  - *Numerical*, e.g. Student with body weight 55 kg. Calculate the energy requirement.

Ans. BMR of the student = 55 × 24 = 1,320 kcal/h/m^2

Energy required for physical activity = 50% of energy required for BMR = 660 kcal

$$1320+660 = 1980 \text{ kcal}$$

Energy required for SDA = 10% of total energy (BMR + PA) = 1980 + 198 = 2178 kcal

Round off to the nearest whole number = 2200 kcal.

Recommended Dietary Allowance

It is defined as the quantity of nutrients to be provided daily in the diet for maintaining good health and physical efficiency along with an extra provision to prevent the development of deficiencies.

Factors Affecting RDA

- *Gender*—Men have 20% higher RDA (except for iron).
- *Age*—Nutrient requirements are higher in growing age and in old age.

Table 8.2 RDA of an Adult Man

Carbohydrates	400 g
Fats	70 g
Proteins	56 g
EFA	4 g
Vit A	1000 μg
Vit E	10 mg
Vit C	60 mg
Vit B_1	1.5 mg
Vit B_2	2 mg
Vit B_3	20 mg
Vit B_6	2 mg
Folate	100 μg
Vit B_{12}	1 μg
Ca	800 mg
P	800 mg
Fe	10 mg

Balanced Diet

Balanced diet is defined as the diet which contains different types of foods, possessing the nutrients—carbohydrates, lipids, proteins, vitamins and minerals in a proper proportion so as to meet the requirements of the body, to maintain good health, with an extra provision for withstanding short periods of leanness.

- The Composition of Balanced diet
  - Varies with countries
  - Ethnicities
  - Age
  - Gender
  - Local availability
  - Socioeconomic status of the population concerned
  - Palatability.
- The Indian balanced diet comprises of:
  - *Cereals:* Contains carbohydrate as starch, some protein and little lipids.
  - *Pulses:* Pulses are a major source of proteins for Vegetarians.
  - *Green leafy vegetables, roots and tubers, fruits:* Contain vitamins, minerals, add roughage to diet.
  - *Milk and Milk products:* Contains high quality protein with all essential amino acids, has vitamins except Vit – C, has Ca and P, no iron.
  - *Fats and Oils:* Cooking medium, provide fat-soluble vitamins, essential fatty acids.
  - *Sugar:* Source of energy, jaggery provides iron.
  - *Meat, fish and egg in nonvegetarian diet:* Source of high quality protein.
  - *Meat* also provides readily absorbable form of iron. Organ meats like liver provide with fat-soluble vitamins.
  - *Fish* provides with essential fatty acid linoleic acid, iodine and good quality protein.
  - *Egg* is in itself a complete protein with all essential amino acids in abundance. Also provides fat-soluble vitamins, cholesterol and saturated fatty acids.
    - Half of the requirement for pulses can be replaced by one egg (or 30 gram of meat or fish) and 5 gram of oil and fat.

Adjustment in Pregnancy

The additional allowances in pregnancy are:

- Cereals—35 g to provide for the extra energy, protein, iron and Ca requirements.
- Pulses—15 g to provide for the extra proteins requirement.
- Milk—100 mL to provide for the good quality proteins with all essential amino acids in appropriate amounts.

Table 8.3 Adult male and female (vegetarian) balanced diet

	Male	*Female*
Cereals (g/day)	460	410
Pulses (g/day)	40	40
Roots and tubers (g/day)	50	50
Leafy vegetables (g/day)	40	100
Milk (mL/day)	150	100
Oil and fats (g/day)	40	20
Sugar and Jaggery (g/day)	30	20
Other vegetables	60	40

- Sugar and jaggery—10 gram to provide for the extra requirement of iron, especially in the vegetarian females.

Adjustments During Lactation

The additional allowances in lactation are:

- Cereals—60 gm to provide for the extra protein and carbohydrate supply needed for milk synthesis.
- Pulses—30 gm to provide for the extra protein needed for the milk protein synthesis.
- Milk—100 ml to provide for the good quality protein with all.
- Sugar and jaggery – 10 gm to provide for the iron.
- Oil and fat—10 gm to provide for the milk lipids.

Nutritional Disorders

Diseases resulting from inadequate or excessive intake of nutrients are known as nutritional disorders.

Some Important Nutritional Disorders

- *Protein energy malnutrition* is a common condition associated with the deficiency of regulatory principles as well as a lack of dietary excellent quality proteins.
- *Cachexia:* In chronic debilitating disorders, when the person is on total parenteral nutrition, there is under nutrition and wasting of the body tissues. This is termed as **Cachexia.**
- *Obesity:* An excessive deposition of body fat due to a prolonged state of positive energy balance is termed as obesity.
- *Over Nutrition:* An excessive accumulation of a nutrient in the body which becomes toxic to the tissues as in case of hypervitaminosis of fat-soluble vitamin or in iron overload condition – hemochromatosis.

Obesity

Obesity may be defined as accumulation of excess fat in the body:

- Hereditary factors or hormonal disorders.
- *Excessive calorie intake:* When energy intake exceeds the energy expenditure, the extra calories are converted into fat, and are deposited in fat depots. Obesity predisposes the individual to many diseases, e.g. dyspnea on exertion, hypertension, diabetes mellitus, coronary artery disease, cerebral thrombosis, gall bladder stones, arthritis of weight-bearing joints, etc.

Measuring Obesity

- One-way to assess obesity is by measuring *skinfold thickness with calipers.* Skinfold thickness is increased in obesity. A simpler alternative is the calculation of *body mass index (BMI)*
- BMI = Wt (kg)/Ht (m^2)
- The normal BMI is 20–25 kg/m^2 in males and 19–24 kg/m^2 in females. A BMI above the upper limit of normal signifies obesity.

Normal wt	Grade – 1	Grade – 2	Grade – 3
BMI 19–24.9	BMI 25–29.9	BMI 30–39.9	BMI 40 and more

Treating Obesity

- The basic principle of treatment is to decrease energy intake and to increase energy expenditure. Energy expenditure is increased by increasing physical activity. Walking at moderate speed increases the energy expenditure to 300 kcal/hour. The energy expenditure during brisk walking, running, swimming and heavy exercise is 500 to 600 kcal/h. The energy intake should be reduced to 1000 kcal/day, until the ideal body weight or BMI is achieved. Protein intake should be maintained at 1 g/kg of body weight. Fats should provide about 10% energy, and should be in the form of vegetable oils rich in essential fatty acids. The remaining calories should be provided by carbohydrates.
- Intake of sugar and jaggery should be restricted to 15 g/day or less.
- Potatoes and sweet potatoes should be excluded from the diet.
- Other vegetables, raw, boiled or steamed, may be taken as desired.
- 200–250 gram of fruits and 400 mL of skimmed milk should be included in the daily diet.
- Vitamin supplements may be given in the form of one multivitamin tablet daily.

Protein Malnutrition

- Protein malnutrition is defined as a dietary deficiency of good quality protein leading to a state of negative nitrogen balance.
- Protein malnutrition may be associated with a simultaneous lack of energy, the condition observed in protein-energy malnutrition (Kwashiorkor) or purely protein malnutrition (Marasmus) (Table 8.3).
- These are disorders of the poor economic strata world over.
- These are frequently seen in children of poor economic strata.
- Kwashiorkor and Marasmus are the two common protein malnutrition disorders seen in children.
- Most of the Third World countries like the South African countries of Somalia, Nigeria, Latin American countries, and Indian subcontinent have a widespread prevalence of these disorders.

Table 8.4 Comparison of Kwashiorkor and Marasmus

	Kwashiorkor	Marasmus
Prevalence	Children up to age 5 years	Infants less than 1 year
Cause	Due to early weaning, disease the 1st child gets due to early birth of 2nd child	Premature infants, malnourished mother, developmental defects of mouth and palate so problem in feeding, no dietary supplementation
Precipitation of the disease	By infections like mumps, measles or respiratory disorders	–
Biochemical defects	Starchy diet is fed, so there is enough energy supply but the dietary protein is deficient in quantity and quality—*Protein Malnutrition*	Feeds exclusively on breast milk, but mother malnourished so both energy and quantity of protein is deficient—*Protein Calorie Malnutrition*

Contd...

Contd...

	Kwashiorkor	*Marasmus*
Plasma proteins	Hypoproteinemia, A:G ratio reversed	Hypoproteinemia, A:G ratio maintained
Serum lipids	Hypertriglyceridemia and fatty liver	No fatty liver and serum lipids deranged
Electrolytes	Depletion of Na+ and K+	Depletion of Na^+ and K^+
Clinical Symptoms *1. Anemia*	Severe to moderate	Mild anemia
2. Appearance	Pitting Edemadue to hypoproteinemia 1st affecting legs and then spreading upwards. Appears blown up	No edema, child is emaciated grossly
3. Overall growth	Retarded growth	Growth retarded, Subcutaneous fat and muscles are wasted
4. Behavior	Apathy, anorexia, less lively, refuses to eat	Child is hungry, and cries continuously
5. Skin	Skin lesions, hyperpigmentation, exfoliation, ulceration at skin of legs, buttocks, and perineum	Skin thin attached to bony prominences, wrinkled
6. Hair	Hair dry, thin, hypopigmented – flag sign – alternate pigmented and hypopigmented areas of hair	Hair thin lusterless.
7. Diarrhea/vomiting	Vomiting, diarrhea sometimes seen, if there are secondary infections	Vomiting, diarrhea seen
8. BMR	BMR low	BMR low
Prognosis	Bad, mortality rate is high (10%–20%)	Good unless there are severe infections

A Quick Look at the Nutrition

- Nutrition is the science of nutrients necessary to sustain life and health.
- Nutrients comprise of proximate principles and regulatory principles.
- Proximate principles (carbohydrates, lipids and proteins) predominantly are substrates that supply energy and are structural components of the body.
- Regulatory principles (vitamins and minerals) act as cofactors and coenzymes in biochemical reactions.
- Dietary carbohydrates are the principle source of energy.
- Dietary lipids are the cooking medium, provide taste and palatability, supply fat-soluble vitamins, EFAs and are important source of energy.
- Dietary proteins supply essential amino acids.
- Proteins are principally structural components.
- Energy requirements of an individual depend upon physical activity, BMR and SDA.
- BMR is the energy required by an awake individual at complete physical, mental, emotional and digestive rest to sustain energy per square meters of body surface area per hour.
- SDA is the thermogenic effect of food, i.e. the heat generated over and above the calorific value of a nutrient or the energy spent for the digestion, absorption, assimilation of a nutrient.
- The balanced diet composed all the nutrients—proximate principles and regulatory principles in appropriate amounts, just enough to maintain good health and face a period of leanness is important.
- Obesity is a nutritional disorder due to consumption of excess calories, more than can be burnt.
- Protein malnutrition is seen as kwashiorkor and marasmus.

Section – 3

Biological Oxidation and Energy Metabolism

- Biological Oxidation and Respiratory Chain
- Carbohydrate Metabolism
- Lipid Metabolism
- Amino Acid Metabolism
- Purine and Pyrimidine Metabolism

CHAPTER

9

Biological Oxidation and Respiratory Chain

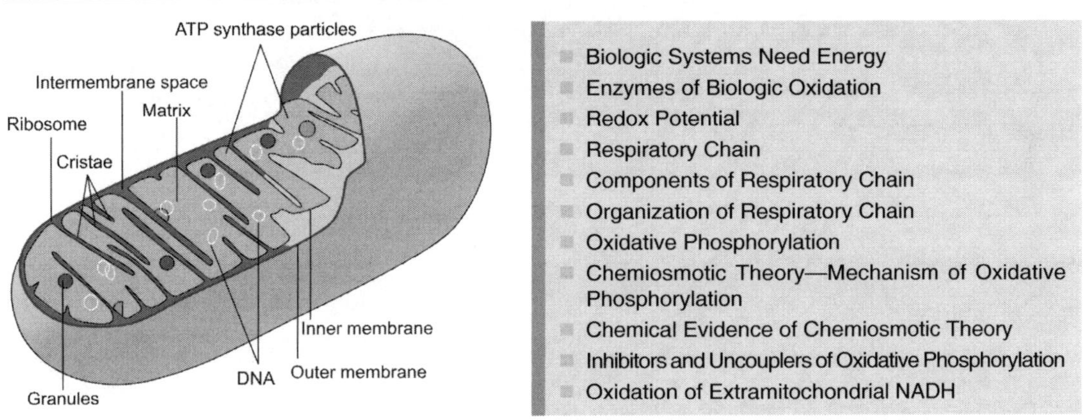

- Biologic Systems Need Energy
- Enzymes of Biologic Oxidation
- Redox Potential
- Respiratory Chain
- Components of Respiratory Chain
- Organization of Respiratory Chain
- Oxidative Phosphorylation
- Chemiosmotic Theory—Mechanism of Oxidative Phosphorylation
- Chemical Evidence of Chemiosmotic Theory
- Inhibitors and Uncouplers of Oxidative Phosphorylation
- Oxidation of Extramitochondrial NADH

Biologic Systems Need Energy

Life on earth is sustained by harnessing energy from the surroundings, entrapping it into utilizable forms (metabolites) and utilizing it for various processes like—growth, locomotion and propagation. Existence of every organism is thus associated with a colossal number of chemical reactions involving generation or utilization of energy (Fig. 9.1).

- Humans obtain energy for survival by oxidizing nutrients collected from food by respiration, and synthesize body constituents using these nutrients. This mechanism also applies to individual cells.
- We require energy for various activities, e.g. muscle contraction, nerve conduction, synthetic reactions, active transport, etc. The ultimate source of energy is the food that we consume. Carbohydrates, lipids and proteins present in food provide us energy.

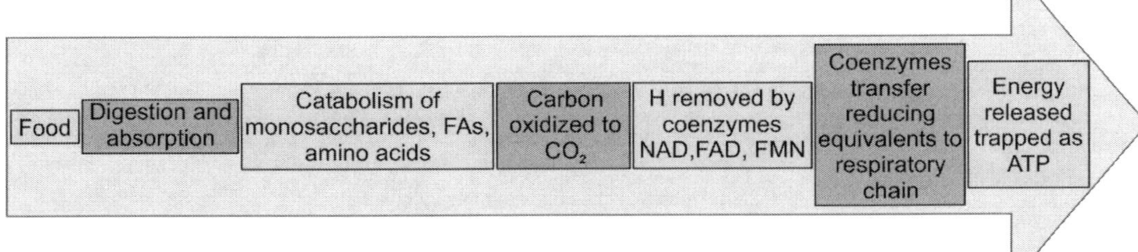

Fig. 9.1 Energy transformation from food to utilizable from ATP

- In cellular activities, thermal, mechanical, electrical and other types of energy are used, and these are generally exchanged using a material called ATP. ATP is readily and widely utilized as the source of energy in numerous biochemical reactions.
- Thus every organism, be it a simple prokaryote or highly complex mammal, has evolved efficient mechanisms of ATP generation and consumption. Therefore, in a way, ATP can be considered as the sole energy currency for the biological world.
- Generation of ATP in humans occurs by the substrate level phosphorylation and oxidative phosphorylation.
- Substrate level phosphorylation occurs when the free energy change between the substrate and product is high, e.g. formation of ATP in the glycolytic step of pyruvate kinase.
- Oxidation is removal of electrons and reduction is addition of electrons. Oxidation coupled with phosphorylation of ADP at the respiratory chain is known as oxidative phosphorylation.
- *Oxidative phosphorylation*, thus, is the mechanism by which the energy present in various nutrients is captured in an easily utilizable form. This utilizable form of energy is the free energy of a system.

High-energy Phosphates

- The energy released during catabolism is captured in the form of a group of compounds known as high-energy phosphates. The most important high-energy phosphate is ATP (Fig. 9.2 and Table 9.1).
- Hydrolysis of ATP into ADP and Pi liberates 7.3 kcal of energy per mol. Similarly, hydrolysis of ADP into AMP and Pi also releases nearly the same amount of energy.
- However, hydrolysis of AMP into adenosine and Pi liberates much less energy (3.4 kcal/mol).

Biological systems have two types of reactions:
Endergonic reactions—These reactions require free energy ATP for completion, e.g. synthetic reactions where a biomolecule is getting synthesized like protein synthesis or fatty acid synthesis, etc.
Exergonic reactions—These reactions liberate energy that free energy that is trapped as ATP, e.g. oxidative reactions like citric acid cycle, glycolysis, fatty acid oxidation, etc.

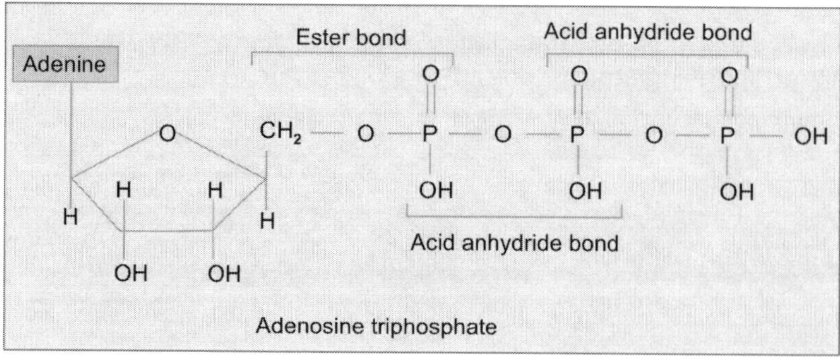

Fig. 9.2 Structure of ATP

Table 9.1 Some important high and low energy compounds

Compound	ΔG_0	*Compound*	ΔG_0
Phosphoenol pyruvate	– 14.8	AMP (→ Adenosine + Pi)	– 3.4
Carbamoyl phosphate	– 12.3	Glucose-1-phosphate	– 5.0
1.3-Biphosphoglycerate	– 11.8	Fructose-6-phosphate	– 3.8
Creatine phosphate	– 10.3	Glucose-6-phosphate	– 3.3
ATP (→ ADP + Pi)	– 7.3	Glycerol-3-phosphate	– 2.2

The compounds having ΔG_0 above that of ATP can transfer their phosphate group to ADP forming ATP

Enzymes of Biological Oxidation

- Material changes in cells are all catalyzed by enzymes. Specifically, all chemical reactions in the living body are rigorously regulated by the synthesis, degradation and activity modulation of enzymes, which are normally made of proteins but may also contain prosthetic groups.
- The various enzymes catalyzing biological oxidation reactions are the enzymes of oxidoreductases class. They can be subdivided into—
  - Oxidases, Dehydrogenases, Hydroperoxidases and Oxygenases.

Oxidases

- These enzymes remove hydrogen from a substrate and transfer it to oxygen forming water or hydrogen peroxide. The enzymes forming water are metalloenzymes that usually contain copper, e.g. cytochrome oxidase and tyrosinase.
  The general reaction catalyzed by these enzymes is:
  $$AH_2 + \frac{1}{2} O_2 \longrightarrow A + H_2O$$
- The enzymes forming hydrogen peroxide are flavoproteins containing FMN or FAD, e.g. L- amino acid oxidase (containing FMN) and xanthine oxidase (containing FAD).
- These enzymes catalyze the general reaction:
  $$AH_2 + O_2 \longrightarrow A + H_2O_2$$

Dehydrogenases

- These are conjugated proteins containing nicotinamide nucleotides or flavin nucleotides or iron-porphyrin as the prosthetic group. They remove hydrogen from a substrate,and transfer it to another substrate.
- The prosthetic group acts as carrier of hydrogen atoms.
- *Those containing NAD:* Lactate dehydrogenase, malate dehydrogenase etc.
- *Those containing NADP:* Glucose-6-phosphate dehydrogenase, 6-phosphogluconate dehydrogenase, etc.
- *Those containing flavin nucleotides:* Succinate dehydrogenase, acyl CoA dehydrogenase, etc.
- *Those containing iron-porphyrin:* Cytochrome b, cytochrome c, cytochrome c_1.

Hydroperoxidases

- These enzymes convert hydrogen peroxide into Water, and protect the tissues against the toxic effects of hydrogen peroxide.

- These include:
  - *Peroxidase*—It catalyzes the reaction

$$H_2O_2 + AH_2 \longrightarrow A + 2H_2O$$

  - Catalase—It catalyzes the reaction

$$2\,H_2O_2 \longrightarrow O_2 + 2H_2O$$

Oxygenases

- These enzymes incorporate oxygen into a substrate. They can be subdivided into:
  - Di-oxygenases
  - Mono-oxygenases.

Di-oxygenases

- These enzymes catalyze the incorporation of both the atoms of oxygen molecule into the substrate.

$$A + O_2 \longrightarrow AO_2$$

  Examples include *homogentisate oxidase and tryptophan pyrrolase.*

Mono-oxygenases

- These enzymes incorporate one atom of the oxygen molecule into the substrate as OH group, i.e. carry out hydroxylation.
- The other atom of oxygen oxidizes another reduced substrate to water
- $AH + O_2 + BH_2 \longrightarrow A\text{–}OH + B + H_2O$
- These enzymes are also known as *hydroxylases or mixed function oxidases.*
- They are used to metabolise xenobiotics (foreign compounds), e.g. drugs *like morphine, phenobarbitone, rifampicin, etc.*
- They also catalyze hydroxylation of endogenous substrates, e.g. *phenylalanine, tryptophan, steroids, cholecalciferol, etc.*
- Two slightly different hydroxylase systems are present in the cells :
  - Microsomal hydroxylase system—hydroxylation of steroids and drugs.
    Containts—NADPH – Cyt P450 and Cyt P450
  - *Mitochondrial hydroxylase system—hydroxylation of steroid hormones.*
    Containts—Adrenodoxin – Cyt P450 and Cyt P 450.

Redox Potential

Reducing equivalents (H^+ or e^-) are generated during the oxidation of major foodstuffs, which are transferred to the respiratory chain.

- The reducing equivalents are not directly transferred to the molecular oxygen, rather is sequentially transferred through a series of carriers (cytochromes, flavoproteins, FeS proteins)
- The enzymes and coenzymes concerned with the removal of reducing equivalents from the substrates and their transfer to oxygen are present in the inner mitochondrial membrane in an ordered sequence.
- This sequence of carriers of reducing equivalents is arranged according to the redox potential of the various components of the Electron transport chain, in an increasing order of *redox potential* [*Table 9.2*].

Table 9.2 Redox potential of various components of respiratory chain

Component	*Redox potential*	*Component*	*Redox potential*
$2H^+ - H$	– 0.42 eV	Cyt c_1 (Fe^{+++}) – Cyt c_1 (Fe^{++})	+ 0.22 eV
$NAD^+ - NADH + H^+$	– 0.32 eV	Cyt c (Fe^{+++}) – Cyt c (Fe^{++})	+ 0.25 eV
$FAD - FADH_2$	+ 0.03 eV	Cyt a (Fe^{+++}) – Cyt a (Fe^{++})	+ 0.29 eV
Cyt b (Fe^{+++}) – Cytb (Fe^{++})	+ 0.08 eV	Cyt a_3 (Fe^{+++}) – Cyt a_3 (Fe^{++})	+ 0. 38 eV
$CoQ - CoQH_2$	+ 0.04 eV	½ $O_2 - H_2O$	+ 0.82 eV

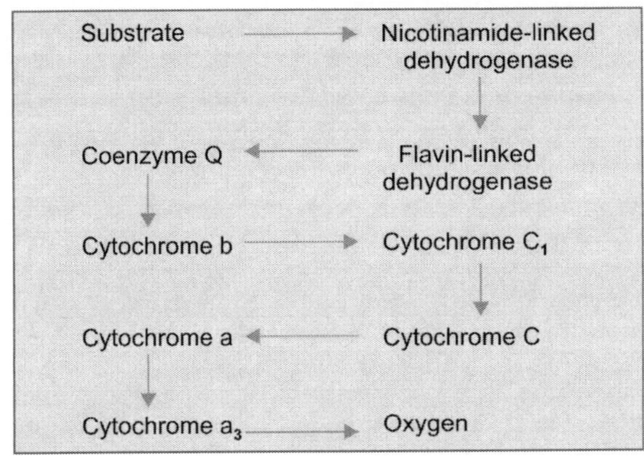

Fig. 9.3 Flow of electrons in respiratory chain

- Redox potential is the tendency of a substrate to donate electron. It is always denoted in eVolts.
- Higher the redox potential lesser the tendency to donate e^- and vice versa.
- The electrons move from a relatively electronegative component to a relatively electropositive component [Fig. 9.3].
- So the electrons move in the ETC from more electronegative NAD-linked dehydrogenases (– 0.32 eV) to more electro positive O_2 (+ 0.82 eV). The redox span of respiratory chain is + 1.1 eV.

Respiratory Chain

- Energy-rich nutrients like—Glucose, fatty acids and amino acids are oxidized stepwise by a series of reactions in various metabolic pathways.
- In many oxidation reactions, reducing equivalents are removed as H^+, from the substrates and are taken up by coenzymes like—NAD^+ and FAD.
- The reduced coenzymes transfer the reducing equivalents to respiratory chain.
- Oxidation of the reducing equivalents in the respiratory chain is coupled with the phosphorylation of ADP to ATP.
- This is the most important mechanism for capturing the energy present in various nutrients.
- As the respiratory chain is located in the mitochondria, the mitochondria have been described as the power house of the cells (Fig. 9.4).

Components of Respiratory Chain

- The respiratory chain is present on the inner mitochondrial membrane.
- Mitochondrial constituents are encapsulated by two highly specialized membranes with a narrow intermembrane space. While the outer mitochondrial membrane act like a sieve that restricts free flow of molecules from the cytoplasm; the inner membrane is further selective in nature and play a critical role in electron transport and ATP generation.
- The inner mitochondrial membrane contains all the proteins involved in electron transport, ATP generation and transport of metabolites (both in and out of mitochondria).
- Under electron microscope, the inner mitochondrial membrane appears to be wrinkled (folded) and organized in layers called cristae (Fig. 9.4).
- Formation of cristae significantly increases the total surface area of the inner membrane.
- The number of mitochondria present in a cell depends upon its metabolic activities and may range from a single large mitochondrion to thousands of mitochondria of various sizes.
- The various proteins of the electron transport chain are—
  - *Cytochromes*—Cytochromes are heme proteins with iron oscillating in Fe^{++} and Fe^{+++} forms during the transfer of the reducing equivalents through them.
  - *FeS* proteins—These are proteins with iron sulfur centers and they too interchange alternatively as Fe^{++} and Fe^{+++} state during electron transport.
  - *Flavoproteins*—These are FAD linked coenzymes.
  - *Ubiquinone*—This is the soluble component of respiratory chain that can move in the respiratory chain and collect reducing equivalents. It is structurally similar to vitamin – E.
  - *Molecular oxygen*—It is the terminal acceptor of respiratory chain.
    - The mitochondrial electron transport chain catalyzes a reaction that can be represented as follows:

$$2\,H^+ + 2\,e^- + \tfrac{1}{2}O_2 \longrightarrow H_2O + \text{energy}$$

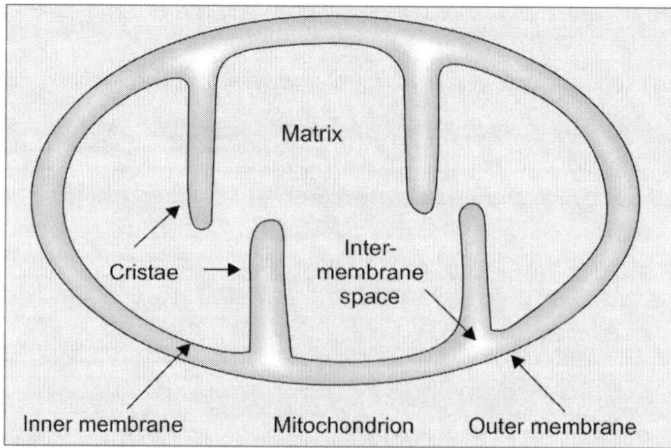

Fig. 9.4 Mitochondria—the power house of cell

Organization of Respiratory Chain

- The respiratory chain is organized as four complexes. Each complex is arranged on the inner mitochondrial membrane in an increasing order of the redox potential of its component proteins and coenzymes [Fig. 9.5].
- Complex I acts as *NADH: Ubiquinone oxidoreductase and* transfers reducing equivalents from NADH to CoQ.
- Complex II acts as *succinate: Ubiquinone oxidoreductase, and* transfers reducing equivalents from succinate to CoQ. It is located at right angles to the rest of the complexes.
- Complex III acts as *ubiquinol: Ferricytochrome C oxidoreductase* and transfers reducing equivalents from reduced CoQ to cytochrome C.
- Complex IV acts as *Ferro cytochrome C: Oxygen oxidoreductase, and* transfers reducing equivalents from reduced cytochrome C to oxygen.
- The redox potential of each protein collectively constitutes the redox potential of each complex and place them in a hierarchical order dictating who will be the oxidant and who will be the reductant when together. Reducing equivalents are accepted by a carrier having a redox potential just above that of the substrate.
- As the reducing equivalents are transferred across the respiratory chain, there is liberation of free energy, which gets entrapped as the chemical form ATP at specific sites.
- The quantum of energy released at any site is proportional to the difference in the redox potentials of the component donating the reducing equivalents and the component accepting the reducing equivalents.
- Thus, different quanta of energy are released at different sites.

Oxidative Phosphorylation

- At the respiratory chain, the quantum of energy released exceeds 10 kcal/mol on the sites where difference between the redox potentials of the donor and the acceptor of reducing equivalents is 0.3 eVolts or more. ADP is phosphorylated to ATP at these sites.
- There are three such sites in the respiratory chain:
  - Site I is between NAD and CoQ
  - Site II is between CoQ and cytochrome C
  - Site III is between cytochrome C and oxygen

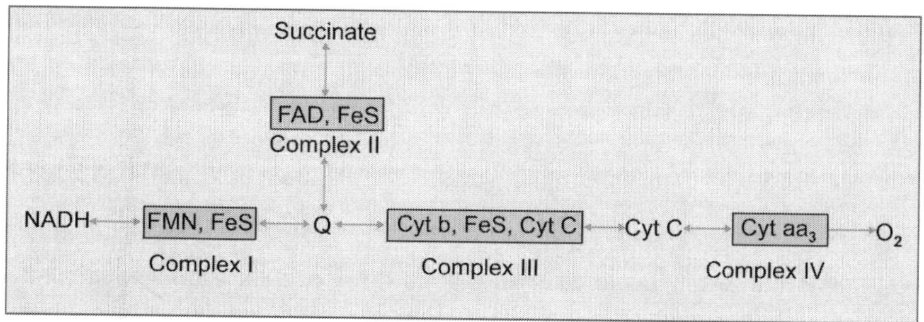

Fig. 9.5 Organization of respiratory chain

- These sites correspond to complexes I, III and IV respectively in the respiratory chain.
  - The various enzymes of metabolic pathways of carbohydrates, lipids and amino acids transfer their reducing equivalents to the different complexes of respiratory chain, guided by their redox potentials.
- The substrates that transfer reducing equivalents to Complex-I, i.e. NAD-linked dehydrogenases, e.g. isocitrate, malate, glutamate, etc. can phosphorylate three molecules of ADP to 3 ATP.
- The substrates that transfer reducing equivalents to Complex–II, i.e. FAD linked dehydrogenases phosphorylate only two molecules of ADP to 2 ATP as site I is bypassed, e.g. succinate, glycerol-3-phosphate, acyl CoA, etc.
- The FAD-linked dehydrogenases are at a higher redox potential than NAD-linked dehydrogenases, thus the first site of ATP synthesis is bypassed and $FADH_2$ releases 2 ATP on transfer of reducing equivalents through the respiratory chain, whereas NADH gives 3 ATP molecules.
- The ratio of ADP molecules phosphorylated to the number of oxygen atoms reduced is known as P: O ratio.
- The P: O ratio is three when the reducing equivalents are accepted by NAD, and is two when the reducing equivalents are accepted by FAD.

Control of Respiratory Chain

- Biological oxidation on respiratory chain is tightly coupled to phosphorylation, i.e. one cannot proceed without the other thus rate of respiration of mitochondria can be controlled by concentration of ADP.
- When a cell is in resting state, ATP stores are fulfilled, no ADP is available, and thus no biological oxidation can occur. Conversely when work is performed ADP concentration is high and rate of biological oxidation increases.
- Besides this other factors controlling rate of biological oxidation are:
  - Availability of ADP
  - Availability of substrate
  - Availability of coenzymes and carriers of respiratory chain
  - Availability of O_2.

Chemiosmotic Theory—Mechanism of Oxidative Phosphorylation

- The reducing equivalents are transferred across the electron transport chain (ETC) as H^+ and e^-.
- The reducing equivalents are transferred to complex – I (from NAD-linked dehydrogenases) FMN and FeS protein. The redox potential difference is large enough to entrap a high energy bond as ATP (ADP $\rightarrow$ ATP).
- In case of FAD-linked dehydrogenases, the reducing equivalents are transferred to complex – II FeS proteins.
- There is then the transfer of reducing equivalents from both complexes (I and II) to ubiquinone (CoQ).
- Ubiquinone, being the mobile carrier, collect these reducing equivalents from both the complex – I and II and transfer to the first cytochrome (of a series on the respiratory chain), i.e. cytochrome – b, reducing the Fe^{+++} to Fe^{++} form.

- The reducing equivalents are then sequentially transferred through cytochrome – C_1, C and AA_3 causing alternately reduction and oxidation of Fe^{+++} to Fe^{++}.
- There is entrapment of a high-energy phosphate when the reducing equivalents are transferred from cytochrome – b to C_1 and from cytochrome – C to AA_3, converting ADP to ATP.
- Thus, 3 ATP are formed when reducing equivalents transfer from NAD-linked dehydrogenases and 2 ATP when they are transferred through FAD-linked dehydrogenases (the 1st site of phosphorylation being bypassed).
- This process of entrapment of a high-energy phosphate coupled with oxidation on the respiratory chain is termed as *oxidative phosphorylation.*
- The high-energy phosphates are trapped at 3 sites only on the ETC, since the free energy change suitable for the process is achieved at three sites only.
- The mechanism responsible for oxidative phosphorylation has been explained by the *Chemiosmotic theory* by *Peter Mitchell.*
- According to this theory, the energy released during the transport of electrons in the respiratory chain is used to actively eject the hydrogen ions (H^+) or protons from the matrix through the innermitochondrial membrane, which is otherwise impermeable to hydrogen ions.
- This ejection establishes an electrochemical gradient across the inner mitochondrial membrane.
- The concentration of hydrogen ions on the outer side of the inner mitochondrial membrane becomes higher as compared to the inner side, making it more electropositive as compared to the inner side.
- This electrochemical gradient increases upto a certain limit.
- When this limit is reached, the hydrogen ions re-enter the matrix releasing energy. However, this re-entry is possible at three sites on the ETC, i.e. at complex – I, complex – III and complex – IV.
- The energy released during influx of protons is used to activate a membrane-bound enzyme, vectorial ATP synthetase which converts ADP and Pi into ATP.
- It has been shown by electron microscopy that vectorial ATP synthetase is made up of F_0 and F_1 components (Fig. 9.6).

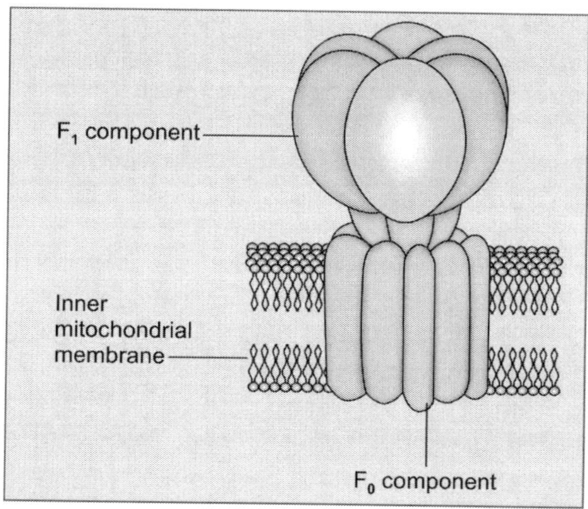

Fig. 9.6 F_0F_1 particle

- F_0 component is embedded in the inner mitochondrial membrane while the F_1 component projects into the matrix.
- F_0 acts as a channel for the passage of hydrogen ions F_1 component possesses ATP synthetase activity, which is switched on when the hydrogen ions pass through the F_0 component.
- According to the mechanism of phosphorylation proposed in the chemiosmotic hypothesis, when hydrogen ions flow back into the matrix, two hydrogen ions combine with two electrons and one oxygen atom of inorganic phosphate forming water and converting inorganic phosphate into a highly reactive form which readily combines with ADP by a high-energy bond.

Chemical Evidence for Chemiosmotic Theory

There is strong experimental evidence in support of chemiosmotic hypothesis. Building up of H^+ gradient is the basic premise of the hypothesis.

- It has been shown experimentally that if H^+ gradient is created artificially by bathing intact mitochondria in a fluid having a relatively high H^+ concentration as compared to the mitochondrial matrix, phosphorylation occurs even in the absence of oxidation.
- The electrochemical gradient one generated across the coupling membrane does not allow further translocation of protons until it is discharge by a vectorial membrane located ATP synthase.
- It has been shown that disruption of the mitochondrial membrane leads to loss of ATP synthetase activity.
- Chemiosmotic theory explains the tight coupling of oxidation with phosphorylation and one cannot proceed without the other. When ADP stores are saturated rate of respiration also falls.

Inhibitors and Uncouplers of Oxidative Phosphorylation

- Certain agents are known to inhibit oxidative phosphorylation at specific sites in the respiratory chain.
- *Amobarbitone, Rotenone and Piericidin A*, which inhibit oxidative phosphorylation at site I have been shown to inhibit the oxidoreductase activity of *complex I.*
- *Malonate and TTFA* inhibit *complex II.*
- *Dimercaprol and antimycin* inhibit the oxidoreductase activity of *complex III.*
- *Hydrogen sulfide, carbon monoxide and cyanide* inhibit the oxidoreductase activity of *complex IV.*
- When oxidation is inhibited, phosphorylation also cannot occur.
- *Oligomycin* inhibits oxidative phosphorylation at all the sites by binding to and inhibiting F_o component of ATP synthetase.
- In fact, the subscript 'o' derives from the tendency of this component to bind oligomycin.
- *Uncouplers* cause the uncoupling of oxidation and phosphorylation, i.e. in presence of uncouplers of respiratory chain, there is no phosphorylation but oxidation occurs.
- It has been shown that they make the innermitochondrial membrane freely permeable to hydrogen ions. This does not allow the electrochemical gradient to build up and, therefore, ATP cannot be synthesized even though oxidation is going on, *e.g. dinitrophenol, dinitrocresol and dicoumarol.*

Physiological Uncouplers

- *Thermogenin,* a protein present in brown adipose tissue, also uncouples oxidation and phosphorylation by acting as a channel for re-entry of hydrogen ions so that the hydrogen ions gradient cannot build up.
- Brown adipose tissue is rich in mitochondria.
- Oxidation occurring in brown adipose tissue without generation of ATP results in production of heat.
- Brown adipose tissue is present in significant amount in infancy and decreases with age.

Oxidation of Extramitochondrial NADH

The respiratory chain receives reducing equivalents from a range of metabolic pathways both mitochondrial (CAC, Beta–oxidation etc.) and extramitochondrial (Glycolysis). The reducing equivalents generated in the cytoplasmic pathways have to be transported into the mitochondria, as the mitochondrial membrane is not permeable to extramitochondrial NADH. This is achieved by some shuttle pathways:

1. Glycerol shuttle
2. Malate shuttle

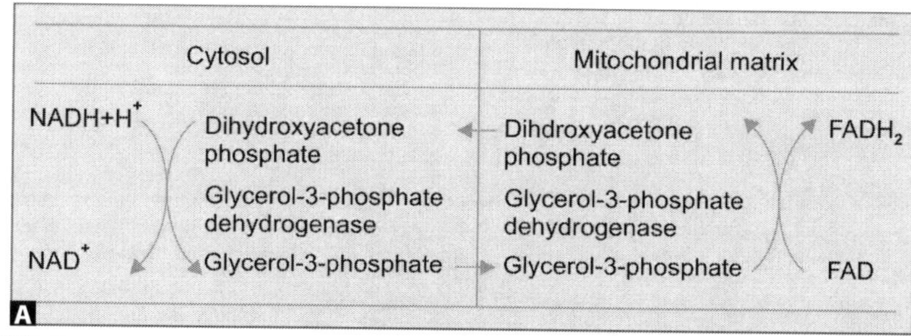

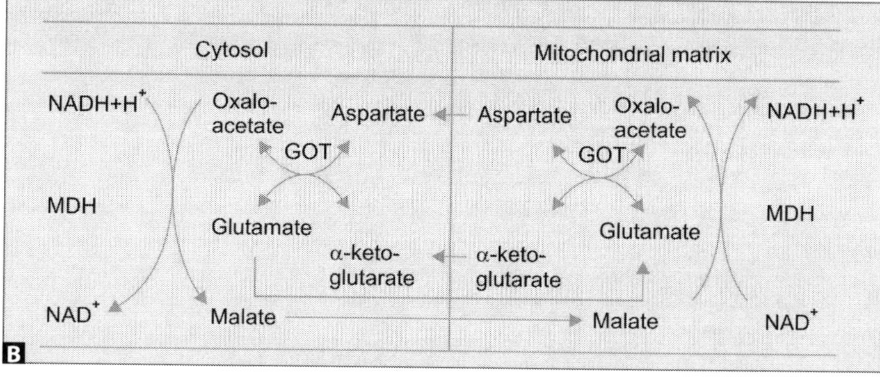

Figs 9.7A and B Oxidation of extramitochondrial NADH

A Quick Look at the Biological Oxidation and Oxidative Phosphorylation

- Human beings sustain life by harnessing energy from the food they consume.
- The food consumed is digested, absorbed and oxidized to produce energy.
- ATP is the energy currency of a cell.
- ATP is generated by the substrate level phosphorylation and by oxidative phosphorylation.
- Substrate level phosphorylation occurs when free energy change in an exergonic reaction is very high.
- Oxidative phosphorylation occurs at the mitochondria and on the respiratory chain.
- Respiratory chain comprises of a series of coenzymes arranged in an increasing order of their redox potential.
- Reducing equivalents generated in various biologic oxidation reactions are transferred to the ETC.
- Energy of oxidation is trapped as high energy phosphate ATP when the free energy change is more than 37 kJoules or the redox potential difference is more than -2eV on the respiratory chain.
- Oxidative phosphorylation generates 3 ATP when NAD-linked dehydrogenases and 2 ATP when FAD-linked dehydrogenases transfer their reducing equivalents.
- Mechanism of oxidative phosphorylation is explained by Chemiosmotic theory of Peter Mitchell.
- Chemiosmotic theory states that the inner mitochondrial membrane is impermeable to H+ and thus a electrochemical gradient is generated across it due to oxidation. This is discharged by a membrane located ATP synthase (Fo) to trap a high-energy phosphate as ATP.
- Uncouplers of oxidative phosphorylation make the inner mitochondrial membrane permeable to H+ thus there is no electrochemical gradient but oxidation occurs without phosphorylation.

CHAPTER

10

Carbohydrate Metabolism

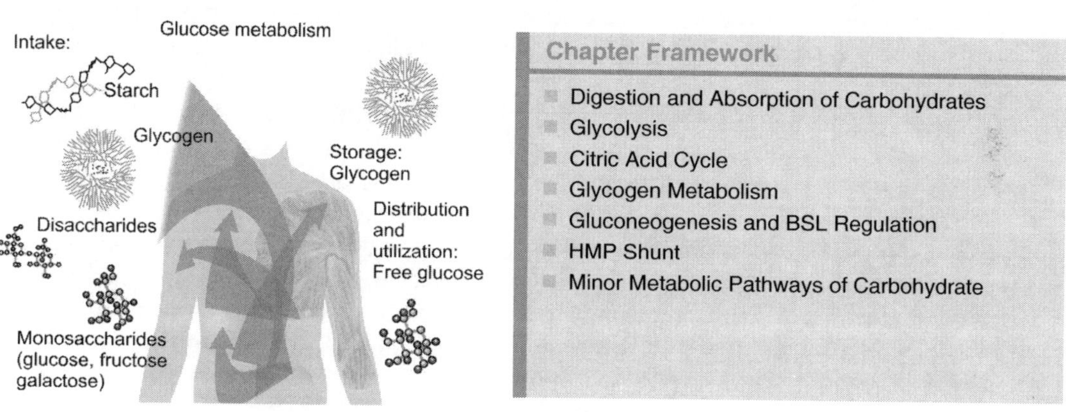

Chapter Framework

- Digestion and Absorption of Carbohydrates
- Glycolysis
- Citric Acid Cycle
- Glycogen Metabolism
- Gluconeogenesis and BSL Regulation
- HMP Shunt
- Minor Metabolic Pathways of Carbohydrate

Introduction

Carbohydrate metabolism includes all the metabolic pathways that help in uptake, utilization and storage of carbohydrates. The dietary carbohydrates are the principle source of energy for humans and form the bulk of our diet. Most of these dietary carbohydrates are complex carbohydrates that are digested into simpler forms—monosaccharides, that are eventually the absorbable forms. Most important monosaccharide is glucose. Other monosaccharides convert to glucose at liver. Once absorbed, the monosaccharides are utilized via energy releasing pathways like glycolysis, CAC to liberate their inherent energy. Some of the excess carbs are stored as glycogen at liver and muscles to be utilized in periods of dearth.

Separate pathways are there for the oxidation of different monosaccharides like galactose or fructose.

Digestion and Absorption of Carbohydrates

Dietary Carbohydrates

- Dietary carbohydrates are the prime source of energy for humans, supplying approximately 60%–70% of the caloric needs. As discussed earlier, the dietary carbohydrates can be classified as 'available' and 'unavailable' carbohydrates. The available carbohydrates are named so since these are acted upon by the enzymes of the gut and add up to the blood sugar level. Thus, these carbohydrates are also the 'glycemic carbohydrates', e.g. monosaccharides (glucose,

fructose from fruits, vegetables, sweets, etc.), disaccharides (lactose, maltose, sucrose) and polysaccharide starch.
- However, the unavailable carbohydrates are not digested by the human gut enzymes and do not add up to the BSL. These primarily form the dietary fibers (soluble and insoluble).

Digestion of Carbohydrates

- The cellular use of carbohydrates depends on their absorption from the gastrointestinal tract into the bloodstream, a process normally restricted to monosaccharides. Polysaccharides and disaccharides therefore must be hydrolyzed to their constituent monosaccharide units.
- The hydrolytic enzymes involved are collectively called glycosidases or, alternatively, carbohydrases.
- The process of digestion of carbohydrates commences from the oral cavity, with the hydrolysis of dietary starch (boiled) by the salivary amylase. Salivary amylase mixes with the starchy products during the chewing of the food. It hydrolyses the α-1 – 4 glycosidic linkage of the boiled starch to generate smaller units dextrin, limit dextrin and maltose.
- Before being swallowed, this phase of digestion produces few monosaccharides. However, the salivary amylase action continues in the stomach until the gastric acid penetrates the food bolus and lowers the pH sufficiently to inactivate the enzyme. By this point, the starches have been partially hydrolyzed, with the major products being dextrins, which are short-chain polysaccharides and maltose.
- Further digestion of the dextrins is continued in the small intestine by the α-amylase of pancreatic origin, which is secreted into the duodenal contents. The presence of pancreatic bicarbonate in the duodenum elevates the pH to a level favourable for enzymatic function.
- If the dietary starch form is amylose, which is unbranched, the products of α-amylase hydrolysis are maltose and the trisaccahride maltotriose, which undergoes slower hydrolysis to maltose and glucose.
- The hydrolytic action of α-amylase on amylopectin (branched starch) produces glucose and maltose, as it does with amylose. However, α-1-6 bonds linking the glucose residues at the branch points of the molecule cannot be hydrolyzed by α-amylase. Consequently, disaccharide units called isomaltose, possessing α-1-6 glycosidic bonds, are released.
- The disaccharides are then further hydrolyzed to their component monosaccharides by the action of disaccahridases on the brush border of the intestine, namely—Sucrase, lactase, maltase, isomaltase for sucrose, lactose, maltose and isomaltose respectively.

Absorption of Dietary Carbohydrates

- The monosaccharides glucose, galactose, fructose are absorbed at the brush border of the small intestine.
- The absorption of glucose and galactose occurs with the cotransport of Na by a sodium-dependent glucose transporter protein (SGLT1) present on the luminal surface of small intestine by secondary active transport. This process is powered by the $Na^+ – K^+$ ATPase.
- SGLT1 is specific for sugars having the specific orientation at C_2 and C_5 similar to that of glucose. Thus galactose is also transported by this transport protein.
- Fructose is absorbed via facilitated transport by the membrane spanning GLUT5 transport protein.

- All the three monosaccharides are finally transported into the portal circulation by a facilitated transport carried out by GLUT2 transporter on the basolateral membrane surface (Fig. 10.1).
- All three main sugars absorbed from the gut (glucose, galactose, and fructose) are transported via the portal vein to the liver (glucose concentrations in the portal vein after a meal can rise to almost 10 mM), but only glucose appears in significant concentrations in the peripheral circulation. Most of the galactose and fructose is removed during first pass through the liver via specific receptors on hepatocytes, so that the blood concentration of these sugars rarely exceeds 1 mM. Within the hepatocytes, galactose is converted to glucose enzymatically and fructose is glycolyzed.
- The principal sugar thus circulating is glucose which then is utilized by glycolysis and CAC (supplying ATP) or is stored as glycogen (liver and muscle) and as triglyceride at adipose tissue.
- Different tissues take up glucose via glucose transporters. There are 6 different types of glucose transporters (Table 10.1).

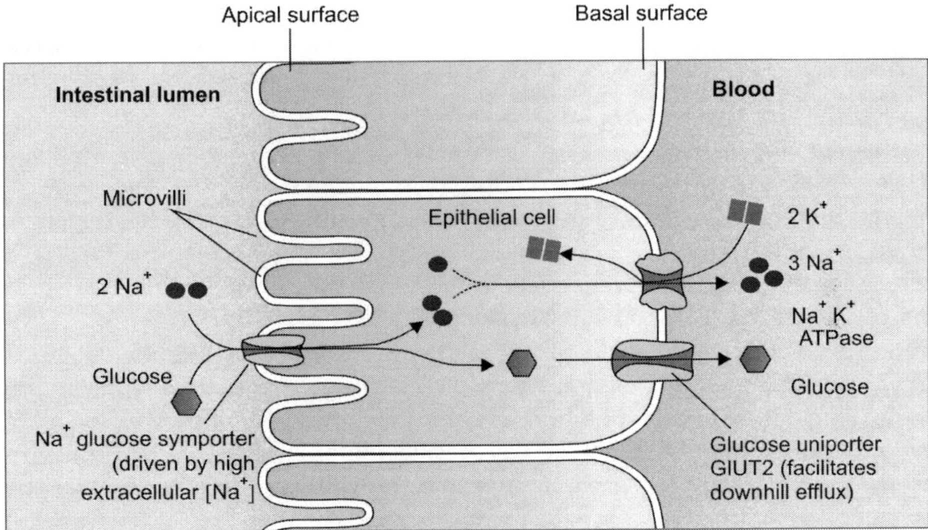

Fig. 10.1 Absorption of monosaccharides

Table 10.1 Types of glucose transporters

Glucose transporter	*Tissue*
SGLT 1 transporting Glucose and Galactose	Luminal side of enterocytes and renal tubular cells
GLUT 1 transporting Glucose	RBCs
GLUT 2 transporting Glucose, Galactose and Fructose	Contraluminal side of enterocytes, liver and fructose renal tubular cells
GLUT 3 transporting Glucose	Brain
GLUT 4 transport Glucose	Adipose tissue, skeletal muscles and myocardium
GLUT 5 transport Fructose	Luminal side of enterocytes and liver

Dietary Carbohydrates and Dental Caries

The resident bacteria in the mouth ferment carbohydrates and yield acidic end-products (mainly lactic acid but also some formic, acetic, and propionic acids), which result in a drop in dental plaque pH.

When the pH falls below 5.5, the dental enamel dissolves in the plaque fluid and repeated exposure to periods of very low pH can lead to caries.

Not all carbohydrates are equally cariogenic. The sugars found commonly in human foods, e.g. sucrose, fructose, glucose, and maltose, are all readily fermented by bacteria in the mouth and are strong cariogenic.

Lactose, galactose, and starches are less cariogenic, while sugar alcohols such as xylitol (used as a sweetener in some confectionery and chewing gums) are not cariogenic.

Eating sugars with meals reduces the risk of caries, as does the consumption of cheese, which provides phosphates to prevent demineralization.

Glycolysis (Embeden Meyerhof Pathway)

Most carbohydrate enters the bloodstream as glucose for transport to the tissues, where it has three possible metabolic fates—it can be used for energy, stored as glycogen in the liver and muscles, or converted to fat.

Importance of Glycolysis

- Glycolysis, the first step in glucose metabolism, is a fundamental pathway by which virtually all cells can produce energy.
- Glucose is oxidized to pyruvate in aerobic glycolysis and to lactate in anaerobic glycolysis.
- It is a cytosolic metabolic pathway that occurs in all the cells of our body. RBCs generate energy by glycolysis exclusively.
- Other tissues that are largely dependent on glycolysis for providing energy are brain, CNS, retina, renal medulla, skin and white skeletal muscle fibers.
- Glycolysis is unique because it can occur in both aerobic and anaerobic conditions. This is of particular significance during strenuous muscular activity when the blood supply to the muscle becomes limiting and anoxic conditions prevail. Under these circumstances, the muscle cells derive energy for sustained contraction by the anaerobic glycolysis.
- Similarly, the RBCs lack mitochondria and thus derive their energy supply by anaerobic glycolysis.
- Glycolytic pathway generates the intermediates of other metabolic pathways like—Hexose monophosphate pathway:
  - Glycogen synthesis:
  - Pyruvate dehydrogenase
  - Fatty acid synthesis
  - Krebs' Cycle
  - Glycerol-phosphate.

Tissue specific functions of glycolysis

- RBC's—Rely exclusively for energy
- Skeletal muscle—Source of energy during exercise, particularly high intensity exercise (anaerobic glycolysis)
- Adipose tissue—Source of glycerol-P for TG synthesis and source of acetyl-CoA for FA synthesis
- Liver—Source of acetyl-CoA for FA synthesis and source of glycerol-P for TG synthesis

Glycolysis Pathway

- The glycolytic pathway is the oxidative pathway of glucose. The complete pathway can be divided into two phases (Fig. 10.2):
  - Preparatory phase
  - Pay-off phase.

Preparatory Phase—ATP is Consumed to Activate Substrate

- During the preparatory phase the substrate glucose is charged to a high-energy intermediate such that in the following pay off phase there is liberation of the free energy contained in glucose as the energy currency of the cells (ATP) and as reducing equivalents ($NADH+H^+$) generated by the oxidation.
- The preparatory phase begins with the phosphorylation of glucose to glucose – 6 – phosphate by hexokinase (all tissues except liver where it is done by glucokinase) (Table 10.2).
  - Glucose – 6 – phosphate is isomerized to fructose – 6 – phosphate by phosphohexose isomerase.
  - Fructose – 6 – phosphate is further phosphorylated to fructose 1, 6-bisphosphate by phosphofructokinase – 1 (PFK-I).
  - Next, the 6 C compound is split into 2 three C compounds by aldolase. Aldolase splits fructose – 1, 6 –bisphosphate into 2 molecules of 3 C sugars – glyceraldehyde – 3 –P and dihydroxy acetone phosphate(DHAP). However, triose phosphate isomerase isomerizes DHAP to Glyceraldehyde – 3- P.

Pay-off Phase-activated Substrate is Oxidized to Liberate Reducing Equivalents and ATP

- During the pay-off phase, the 3 C compound is oxidized and the free energy of oxidation is trapped by substrate level phosphorylation and by oxidative phosphorylation.
- It begins with oxidation of Glyceraldehyde – 3 –P (2 mols) by Glyceraldehyde – 3 – phosphate dehydrogenase using NAD^+ as coenzyme to 1, 3 - bisphosphoglycerate.

Table 10.2 Difference between glucokinase and hexokinase

	Glucokinase	Hexokinase
Kinetic parameters		
K_m	High (10 mM)	Low (< 100 μM)
Vmax	High	Low
Tissue distribution	Liver Pancreatic beta cells	Most tissues
Regulation		
Short-term	Activity responds to changes in glucose concentration	Inhibited by glucose-6-phosphate
Long-term	Synthesis induced by insulin	Constitutive

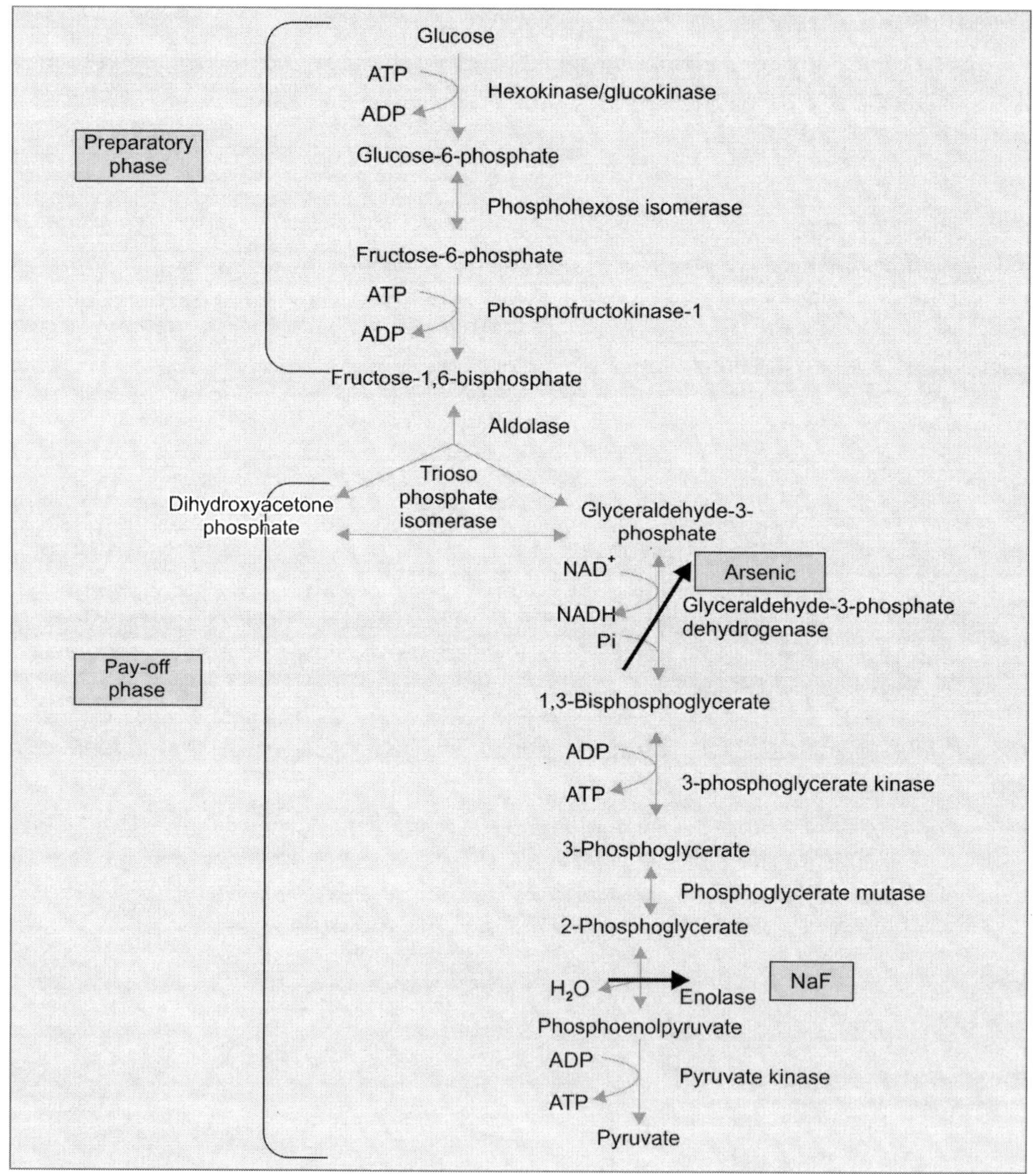

Fig. 10.2 Glycolysis pathway

- This enzyme is unique. It has 4 polypeptide chains with 4 SH groups on each. One of the SH group is present on active site and binds to the substrate by a high-energy thioacetal linkage.
- During oxidation, there is removal of reducing equivalents, which are accepted by NAD^+ to be reduced to $NADH+H^+$.
- The $NADH+H^+$ is only weakly attached to this enzyme and is readily replaced by new NAD^+ molecule.

- And the energy of the high-energy thioacetal linkage is entrapped as a high-energy P bond at C1 giving 1, 3–bisphosphoglycerate.
- 1, 3 BPG (2 mols) is converted to 3–PGA (2 mols) with capture of 2 ATP.
- 3–PGA (2 mols) in presence of phospho-glucomutase converts to 2–PGA (2 mols).
- 2–PGA (2 mols) is dehydrated to 2- Phospho-enolpyruvate (2 mols).
- Finally 2–PEP in presence of pyruvate kinase entraps 2 mols of ATP and converts into 2 mols of pyruvate.
- In RBCs, a shunt pathway works out a way to discharge excess of energy as heat without trapping ATP–Leubring Rappoport Shunt (Fig. 10.3).

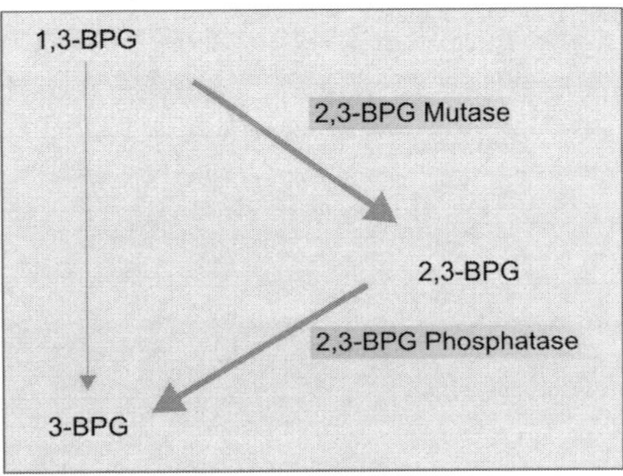

Fig. 10.3 Leubering – Rapport Shunt

Advantages of 2,3–BPG Shunt

- This is advantageous to the economy of the RBC as it dissipates an inorganic PO_4 without trapping it as ATP and so glycolysis can proceed even when need for ATP is minimal.
- Besides 2,3–BPG is a strong anion that has affinity for the beta-chains of deoxy Hb and it decreases the affinity of Hb for O_2 causing unloading of O_2.
- So, when 2, 3–BPG increases in concentration. There is more unloading of O_2 and ODC shifts to right.
- 2, 3–BPG has low affinity for gamma-chains present in HbF, this permits HbF to take up O_2 even at low partial pressure of O_2 found in placental blood.

Anaerobic Glycolysis

- It is particularly seen in RBCs as they lack mitochondria and in skeletal muscles, which contract for some time even in aerobic conditions.
- There is no difference in the step of glycolysis when there is lack of oxygen.
- The only difference is that the end product is lactate.
- This is so because under anaerobic conditions, the reducing equivalents removed as NADH $+H^+$ at glyceraldehyde dehydrogenase step cannot enter the resp. chain. Therefore, for glycolysis to proceed the NAD^+ is regenerated by the reduction of pyruvate to lactate.

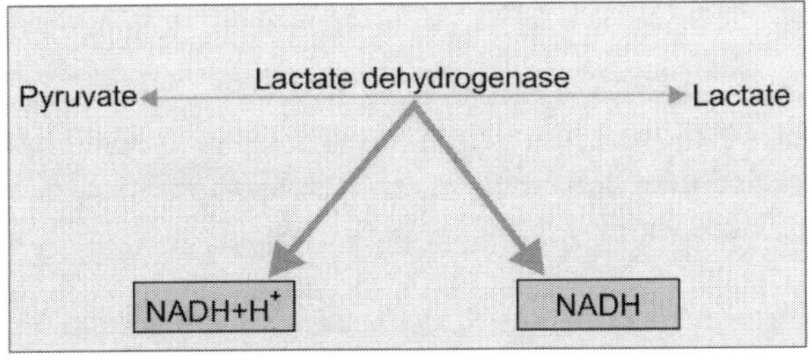

Energetics of Glycolysis

➤ Preparatory Phase-	
1. Hexokinase	– 1 ATP
2. Phosphofructokinase	– 1 ATP
➤ Pay-off Phase	
1. Glyceraldehyde dh	+ 2NADH + H^+ = 6 ATP
2. PGA kinase	+ 2ATP
3. Pyruvate kinase	+ 2 ATP
	Total 8 ATP (aerobic glycolysis)

Regulation of Glycolysis

- Regulation occurs at 3 irreversible steps.
- Hexokinase commits the cell for glucose utilization.
- PFK-1 is rate limiting enzyme and primary site of regulation.
- PFK -1 is the key regulatory enzyme. It reciprocally regulates glycolysis and gluconeogenesis, such that there is no futile cycling of substrates. (*see* regulation of gluconeogenesis and glycolysis in Figure 10.15)

Pyruvate kinase Deficiency
RBC dependent on glycolysis for energy
- Sodium/potassium ion pumps require ATP.
- Abnormal RBC shape a result of inadequate ion pumping.
- Excessive RBC destruction in spleen
  - Hemolysis
  - Jaundice (elevated bilirubin, fecal urobilinogens)
  - Increased reticulocyte count

Fate of Pyruvate

- The metabolic fate of pyruvate generated by glycolysis depends upon the availability of oxygen; if anaerobic conditions exist—pyruvate is reduced to lactate via lactate dehydrogenase activity as in anaerobic glycolysis.
- Under aerobic conditions, the pyruvate is oxidatively decarboxylated to acetyl CoA via pyruvate dehydrogenase activity.
- Pyruvate dh is a multienzyme complex that links glycolysis and citric acid cycle.
- This multienzyme complex has three enzyme activities encrusted into one enzyme molecule, namely:
  - E1: pyruvate dehydrogenase—
    Oxidative decarboxylation of pyruvate
  - E2: dihydrolipoyl transacetylase—
    Transfers acetyl group from TPP to lipoic acid
  - E3: dihydrolipoyl dehydrogenase—
    Transfers acetyl group to CoA, transfers electrons from reduced lipoic acid to produce NADH

- Oxidative decarboxylation of pyruvate by E1 generates a 2 carbon moiety acetyl group that links up with the coenzyme thiamin pyrophosphate.
- E2 transfers the acetyl group from TPP to next coenzyme lipoic acid, such that it converts to acetyl lipoate.
- Finally, acetyl group is transferred to CoA to form acetyl CoA with the oxidation of lipoate and generation of $FADH_2$. Reduced lipoate is regenerated and $FADH_2$ transfers the reducing equivalents to NAD^+ to produce NADH. All this is achieved by the E3 enzyme activity.
- Thus oxidative decarboxylation of pyruvate generates acetyl CoA and $NADH+H^+$.
- Acetyl CoA then has differing fates depending upon the metabolic state of the tissue, i.e. the acetyl CoA may enter the citric acid cycle (low-energy charge to generate more ATP) or may be used for de–novo fatty acid synthesis (when enough substrate and energy available—in anabolic state).
- Regulation of Pyruvate dehydrogenase (PDH) complex
- The enzyme complex PDH is both allosterically and covalently regulated as shown in Figure 10.4.
- Covalently, it is modified by phosphorylation and dephosphorylation, with the phosphorylated form being inactive and dephosphorylated form being active.
- Negative allosteric regulators are acetyl CoA, NADH, ATP and positive are CoA, NAD and ADP

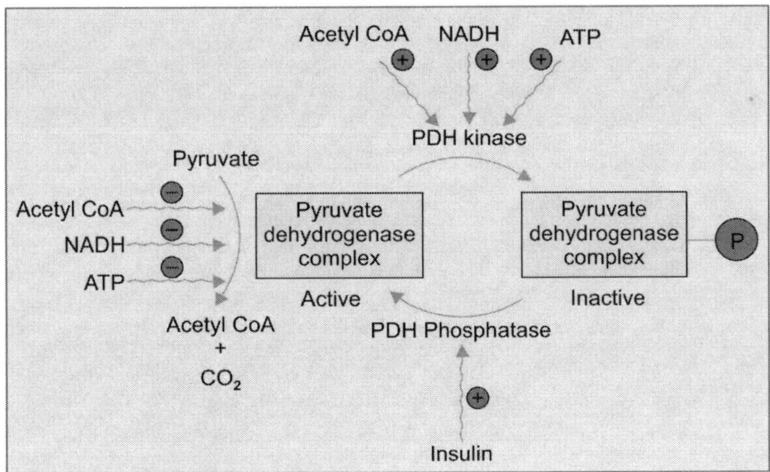

Fig. 10.4 Regulation of pyruvate dehydrogenase

Tissue specific regulation of pyruvate dehydrogenase

- **At muscles**

  When in resting state:

  Energy charge is high, high NADH, Acetyl CoA, ATP will inhibit PDH by accelerating its phosphorylation.

  When exercising:

  ATP used so ADP concentration is high, NADH and acetyl CoA will be reduced activating PDH, such that more and more ATP is generated.

Contd...

Contd...

> ***At liver***
>
> In fed state:
>
> Increased availability of substrate (glucose) and high insulin PDH active so anabolism occurs enhance the availability of acetyl CoA for FA synthesis occurs.
>
> In starved state:
>
> No insulin so PDH inactive.

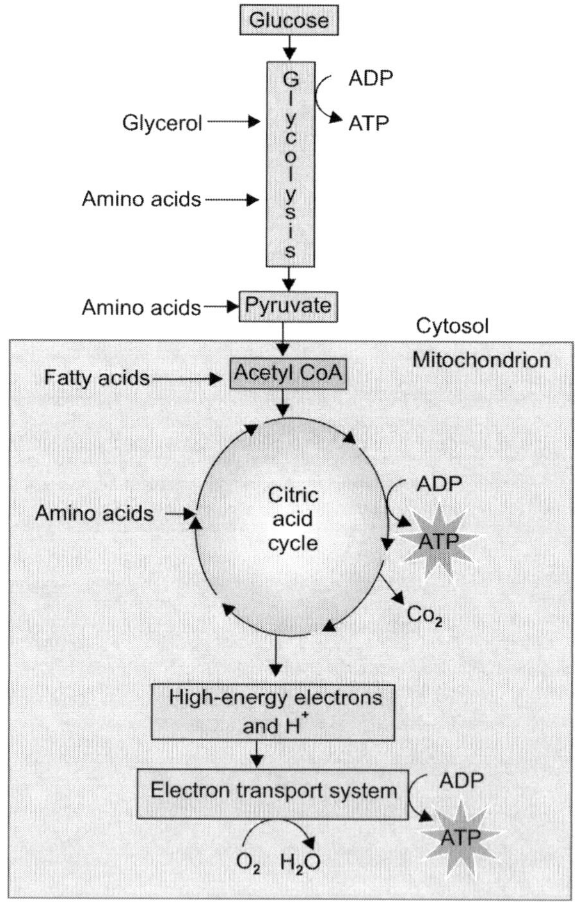

Fig. 10.5 Link of glycolysis and CAC

Tricarboxylic Acid Cycle (TCA)/Citric Acid Cycle (CAC)/Krebs Cycle

Site

The citric acid cycle occurs in the mitochondrial matrix:

- The Krebs cycle is a series of enzymatic reactions that catalyzes the aerobic metabolism of fuel molecules to carbon dioxide and water, thereby generating energy for the production of adenosine triphosphate (ATP) molecules. The Krebs cycle is so named because much of its elucidation was the work of the British biochemist Hans Krebs.

- It is named as citric acid cycle since it begins with citric acid that is further oxidized. Similarly, the other synonym is tricarboxylic acid cycle because the cycle has tricarboxylic acid intermediates.
- This is the final common pathway for oxidation of carbohydrates, lipids and proteins since all these 3 fuel source are converted to acetyl CoA at some stage of metabolism.
- In eukaryotic cells, all but one of the enzymes catalyzing the reactions of the Krebs cycle are found in the mitochondrial matrixes. Succinate dehydrogenase is bound to mitochondrial membrane.
- This pathway brings about the oxidation of acetyl CoA residues, liberating reducing equivalents which are easily transferred to the respiratory chain present on inner mitochondrial membrane and capturing free energy ATP by phosphorylation.

Significance of CAC

Amphibolic Nature of CAC

- CAC is *amphibolic in nature,* i.e. it is both catabolic and anabolic in nature.
- The anabolic nature of CAC is explained by
  - Synthesis of nonessential amino acids
  - Synthesis of glucose by gluconeogenesis
  - Synthesis of fatty acids.
- Intermediates of CAC can give rise to nonessential amino acids by transamination.
- C skeletons of many amino acids form intermediate of CAC after deamination or transamination and indirectly contribute to gluconeogenesis.
- Intermediates of CAC take part in gluconeogenesis and produces glucose from non-carbohydrate precursors, this occurs only in liver and kidney (since all the enzymes for gluconeogenesis are present in these tissues), depending on the BSL.
- Citrate of CAC participates in lipogenesis. Lipogenesis occur in cytosol from acetyl CoA (Fig. 10.6).

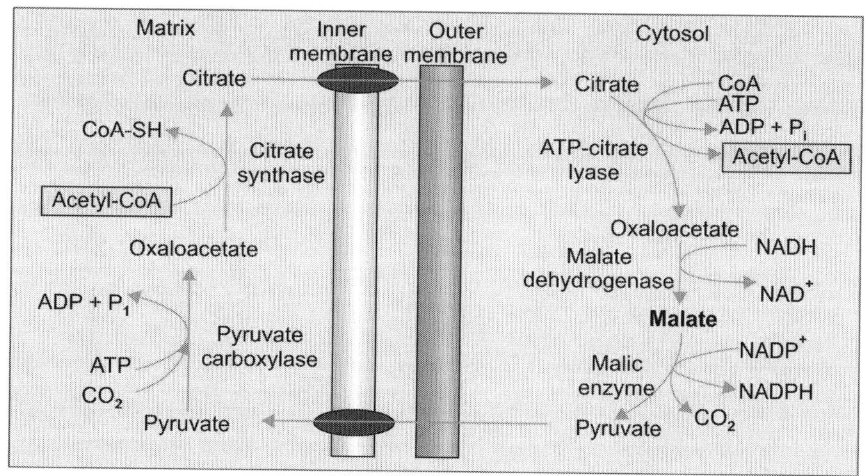

Fig. 10.6 ATP citrate lyase activity and Krebs cycle

- Citrate carries the acetyl unit out of mitochondria into cytosol by a citrate transporter.
- In cytosol citrate breaks down into acetyl CoA and OAA in the presence of ATP citrate lyase acetyl CoA is then used in lipogenesis.

Pathway of Citric Acid Cycle

- CAC begins with the condensation of 2 – C acetyl CoA and 4 – C oxalo acetic acid (OAA), in the presence of condensing enzyme citrate synthase. Oxaloacetate is both the first reactant and the final product of the metabolic pathway. Catalytic amounts of OAA are required during the CAC (Fig. 10.7).
- The product of acetyl CoA and OAA is 6 – C citric acid. After the synthesis of citric acid, the cycle machinery continues through seven distinct enzyme-catalyzed reactions that produce, in order, iso citrate, α –keto glutarate, succinyl coenzyme A, succinate, fumerate, malate, and oxaloacetate.
- The citrate is first dehydrated and then a water molecule added again in the presence of aconitase to form the iso citrate (6 – C).
- Isocitrate is then oxidized to alpha-keto gluterate (5 – C) using NAD^+ as a coenzyme in the presence of isocitrate dehydrogenase. Along with there is also a removal of CO_2 molecule reducing the number of carbon atoms from 6 – 5.

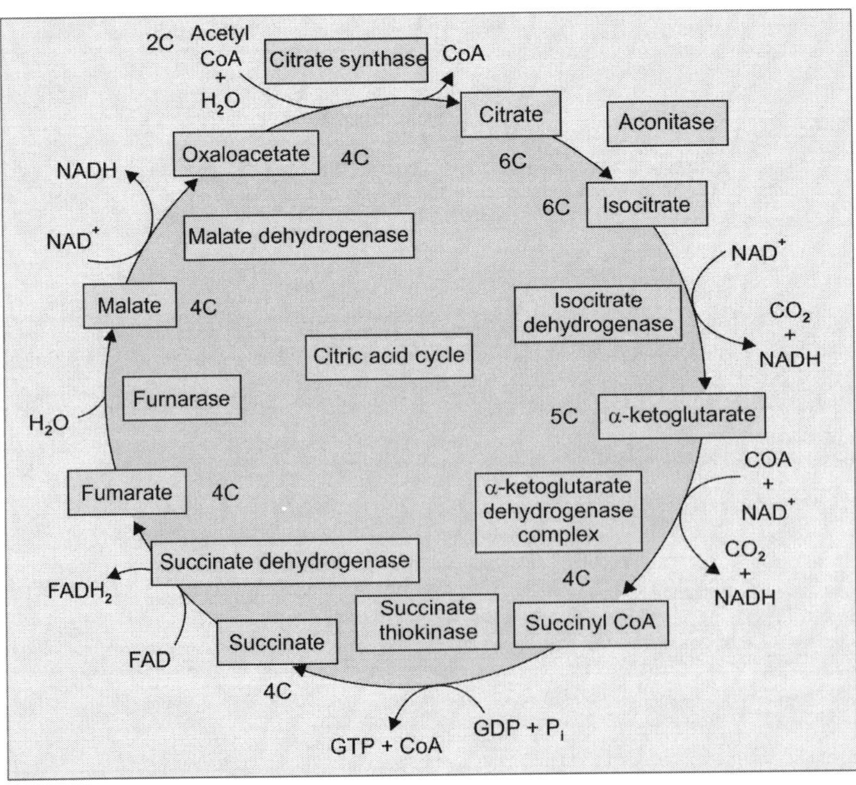

Fig. 10.7 Pathway of citric acid cycle

- The alpha-keto gluterate is then oxidatively decarboxylated to succinyl CoA (4 – C) in the presence of alpha-keto gluterate dehydrogenase enzyme complex. This enzyme complex is similar to PDH in activity and coenzymes requirement. The regulation of the enzyme activity is also carried out in the manner similar to PDH.
- Succinyl CoA in the next step helps trap the free energy of the CoASH at substrate level as ATP from ADP. The enzyme is a kinase succinate thiokinase. In this reaction the succinyl CoA is converted into succinate (4 – C).
- Further succinate is oxidized to fumerate (4 – C) by a membrane bound enzyme succinate dh using FAD as a coenzyme.
- Fumerate is then oxidized to malate in presence of fumerase. Fumerate and malate are geometric isomers.
- Malate is finally oxidized in presence of malate dh and NAD^+ to regenerate OAA.
- Thus OAA is regenerated just as a catalyst is liberated unaltered after a biochemical reaction.

Energetics of CAC

- CAC is closely associated with the oxidative phosphorylation occurring in the mitochondria.
- The proximate presence of the CAC and the respiratory chain serves great as the reducing equivalents are transferred from the CAC to the respiratory chain.
- 3 ATP are generated by each NADH transferred to the respiratory chain and 2 ATP per $FADH_2$.
- Since there are 3 enzymes using NAD^+, thus overall 9 ATP are generated by the NAD^+ using enzymes.
- 2 ATP are generated by succinate dh via $FADH_2$.
- 1ATP is produced by substrate level phosphorylation at the succinate thiokinase step.
- Thus total 12 ATP are produced from each acetyl CoA oxidation in CAC.

1.	Isocitrate dh	NADH+ H^+ = 3 ATP
2.	α-KGdh	NADH + H^+ =3 ATP
3.	Succinate dh	$FADH_2$ = 2 ATP
4.	Malate dh	NADH + H^+= 3 ATP
5.	Succinate thiokinase 1 ATP at substrate level	

– 12 ATP from 1 acetyl CoA

Net ATP from oxidation of 1 glucose molecule aerobically:

- 1 glucose gives 2 pyruvate which is oxidatively decarboxylated to 2 acetyl CoA (24 ATP) + Pyruvate dh gives 6 ATP = 30ATP
- Glycolysis = 8 ATP
- 30 + 8 = 38 ATP

Regulation of CAC

Regulation at the Level of Respiratory Chain

Citric acid cycle is regulated by the energy level of the tissue since it is tightly coupled with the respiratory chain. There is a tight coupling of oxidation with phosphorylation and one cannot proceed without the other. Thus when there is increased rate of work done, ATP is consumed and concentration of ADP is high, thus substrate for phosphorylation is available and oxidative phosphorylation will occur at a high rate enhancing the rate of CAC too. Conversely when the energy charge is saturated as in resting state, concentration of ATP is high and oxidative phosphorylation cannot take place. Thus the availability of the oxidized coenzymes for CAC will not be there reducing the rate of CAC.

Regulation at the Level of Enzymes

The key regulatory enzymes of CAC are citrate synthase, pyruvate dh and alpha-keto gluterate. These enzymes are allosterically and covalently modified enzymes (as seen with PDH especially for alpha KG dh).

Glycogen Metabolism

Introduction

Glycogen is the storage carbohydrate of animals. Hence it is also termed as 'animal starch'. Humans store the excess carbohydrate in the form of glycogen at liver and muscles. The excess carbohydrate is particularly stored as glycogen in humans since it is highly branched yet a compact molecule in structure. Thus it stores greater units of glucose per mol than starch which is the storage polysaccharide of plants. This stored carbohydrate has great significance in the maintenance of the normal blood sugar level (BSL), which in turn is of paramount importance in humans. However, it is the liver glycogen that helps maintains the normal BSL whereas the role of muscle glycogen is as the fuel source for muscle contraction. This stored glycogen is split to add up to blood sugar at liver and at muscles it splits and burns down to produce ATP for muscle contraction.

The synthesis of glycogen is carried out by *glycogenesis* that means genesis (synthesis) of glycogen. The splitting or breakdown of glycogen is carried out by glycogenolysis that means lysis (breakdown) of glycogen.

Glycogenesis

- Glycogenesis occurs in cytosol of almost all the tissues in our body, but the predominant sites for storage of glycogen are liver and muscles.
- Liver stores up to 5% glycogen by wet tissue weight and muscles store up to 1% glycogen by wet tissue weight. What limits the production beyond these levels is till date unknown. Thus, the healthy well-fed adult of 70 kg has approximately 72 g of glycogen stored at liver and about 400 g of glycogen is present as the wet weight of muscle mass.
- Glycogen is a branched homopolysaccahride of repeating glucose units linked up in α-1- 4 glycosidic linkage in the straight chain part and has α-1-6 glycosidic linkage at the branch point.
- The synthesis of glycogen begins on a protein backbone—glycogenin. Glycogenin is a short polypeptide with glycosylated tyrosine residues.
- Glycogenin acts as a priming polypeptide on which the glucose residues polymerise sequentially one after the other.
- The process of glycogenesis begins with the activation of glucose.
- For this the key reaction of glucose phosphorylation initiates the synthesis of Glucose – 6 – P which then converts to Glucose – 1 – P in the presence of phosphoglucomutase.

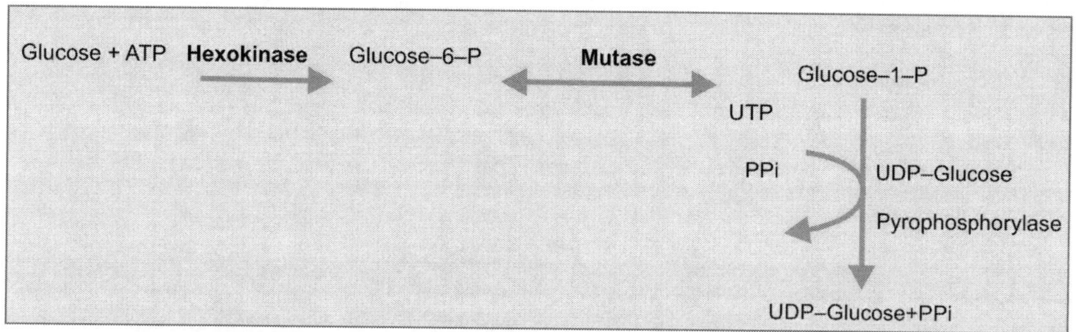

- Finally the enzyme UDP – Glucose Pyrophosphorylase catalyzes the synthesis of Glucose–1–P to UDP – Glucose with a large change in free energy making the reaction irreversible. The hydrolysis of pyrophosphate to PPi is responsible for the large change in free energy.
- UDPG reacts with glycogen primer.
- UDP is released and glucose is added to the glycogen primer.
- Thus, if the glycogen primer had n glucose units before the reaction, it would have n+1 glucose units after the reaction.
- C1 of the new glucose unit forms a glycosidic bond with C4 of the last glucose unit on the nonreducing end of the glycogen primer.
- The reaction is catalyzed by glycogen synthetase.
- This process of addition of glucose units to the glycogen primer continues until the chain contains about eleven glucose units.
- Then, amylo–1,4 α1,6–trans glucosidase (branching enzyme) detaches a fragment of 6–7 glucose units from the growing end, and reattaches it to the chain by an α – 1,6 – glycosidic bond to form a branched structure (Fig. 10.8).
- The two branches start growing again by addition of glucose units by α – 1, 4 – glycosidic bonds catalyzed by glycogen synthetase.
- When the branches contain about 11 glucose units, branching enzyme acts again and create more branches.
- This process of lengthening and branching continues until a large and highly branched glycogen molecule is formed.
- Two branch points are separated by 8–12 glucose units.

Regulation of Glycogenesis

- The process of glycogenesis is regulated by means of covalent modification of the key enzyme glycogen synthetase (Fig. 10.9).
- The regulation occurs in a highly complex yet stringent manner, in-sync with the major BSL regulating hormones—Insulin, glucagon and epinephrine.
- The major sites of glycogen storage—Liver and muscles have similar regulation.

The regulatory hormones insulin and glucagon are peptide hormones and cannot permeate the target cell membranes. Thus they execute their physiological role via the second messenger cAMP and protein kinase.

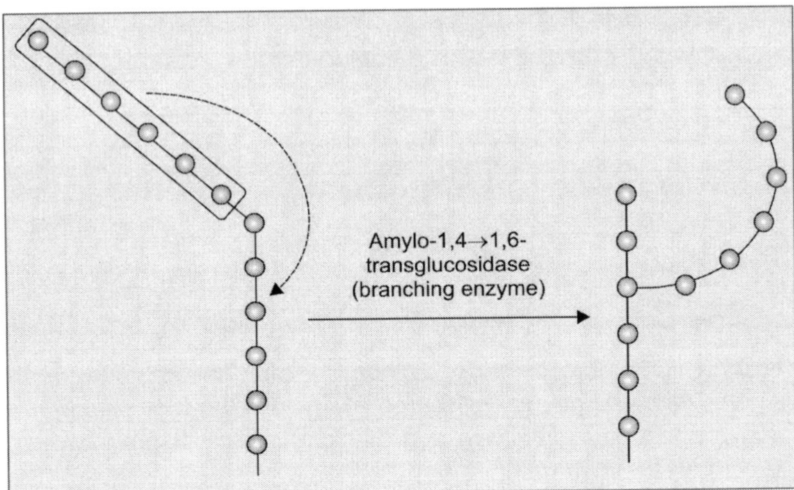

Fig. 10.8 Branching of glycogen

- Protein kinase is a tetramer made up of 2 catalytic and 2 regulatory units. In the inactive form, all 4 subunits are fused together and in active form the catalytic units dissociate from regulatory units due to binding of cAMP.
- The hormones glucagon and epinephrine get released in response to a low BSL. These hormones (epinephrine at muscles and glucagon at liver) enhance the activity of the adenylate cyclase enzyme, thus increasing the concentration of cAMP.
- The cAMP in – turn activates the protein kinase.
- Activated protein kinase phosphorylates the enzyme glycogen synthase making it inactive and preventing the storage of the limiting amount of glucose as glycogen. Thus making it available to the tissues.
- Dual inactivation of glycogen synthase is exerted by the activation of an inhibitor protein that gets phosphorylated in the presence cAMP. Active inhibitor protein inhibits activity of a protein phosphatase enzyme thus reducing the dephosphorylation of glycogen synthase – doubly activating glycogen synthase.
- Thus the inhibitor protein acts as a fulcrum that keeps a balance between phosphorylation and dephosphorylation.
- Conversely when the BSL is high, the hormone secreted in response is Insulin. Insulin enhances the activity of the enzyme phosphodiesterase which hydrolyze the cAMP to 5′ – AMP. The reduced concentration of cAMP is unable to activate the protein kinase and thus there is no phosphorylation of glycogen synthase.
- Simultaneously, the reduced active protein kinase also decreases the concentration of the active inhibitor protein. This leads to a reduced inhibition of protein phosphatase and a dual activation of glycogen synthase since the inactive inhibitor protein can no longer inhibit phosphatase causing a dephosphorylation and activation of glycogen synthase doubly after the initial activation by reduced active protein kinase.
- Thus, the regulation of glycogenesis is a cascading reaction where the activation of a preceding substrate amplifies the activation of the next substrate in the reaction sequence.

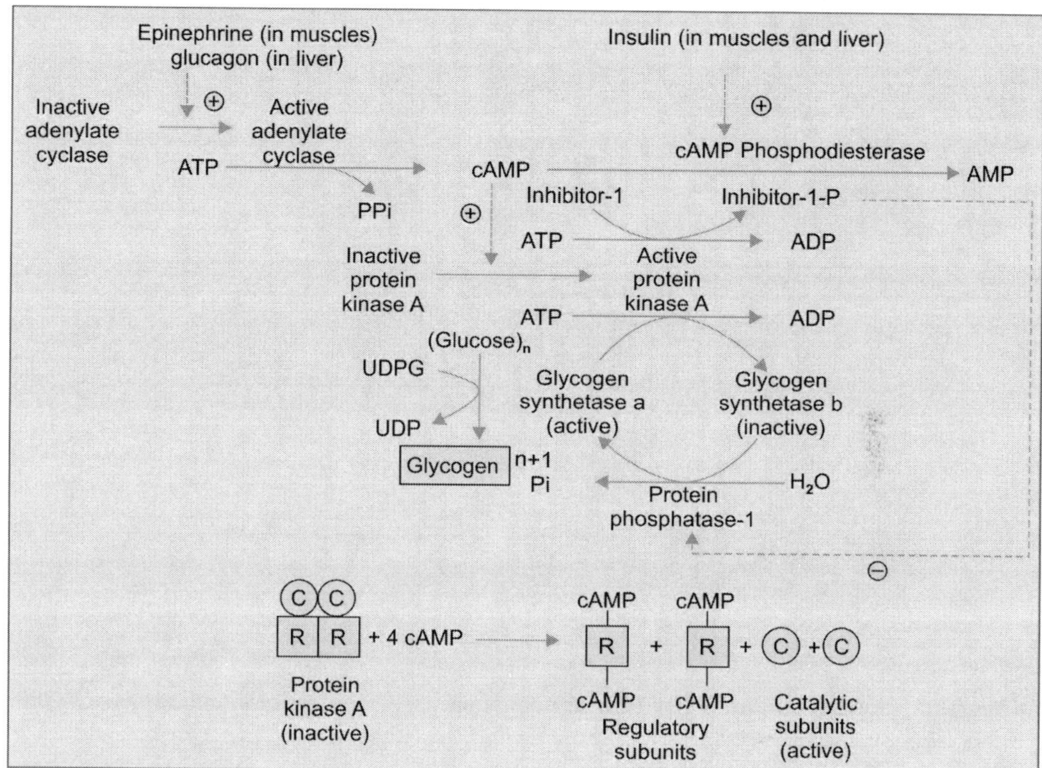

Fig. 10.9 Regulation of glycogenesis

Glycogenolysis

- The process of stepwise breakdown of glycogen into glucose–1–P is termed as glycogenolysis. This process is catalyzed by phosphorylase, in association with glucan transferase and debranching enzymes.
- The key enzyme of glycogenolysis is phosphorylase.
- The key enzyme of glycogenolysis is phosphorylase (glycogen phosphorylase) which catalyzes the phosphorolytic removal of glucose from glycogen as glucose–1–phosphate.
- This enzyme hydrolyses the terminal α–1, 4–glycosidic bonds at the nonreducing ends of the glycogen molecule.
- Presence of a large number of branches in the glycogen molecule facilitates rapid glycogenolysis as the terminal glucose units on all the branches can be split off simultaneously.
- The energy present in the glycosidic bond is conserved by incorporating a phosphate group into the liberated glucose molecule, i.e. as glucose–1–P.
- The process of stepwise removal of glucose units from each branch continues until only *four glucose units* are left distal to the branch points. The molecule so formed is a *limit dextrin.*

After the formation of limit dextrin, *(α–1,4 α–1,4)–glucan transferase* transfers a trisaccahride from one branch to another.

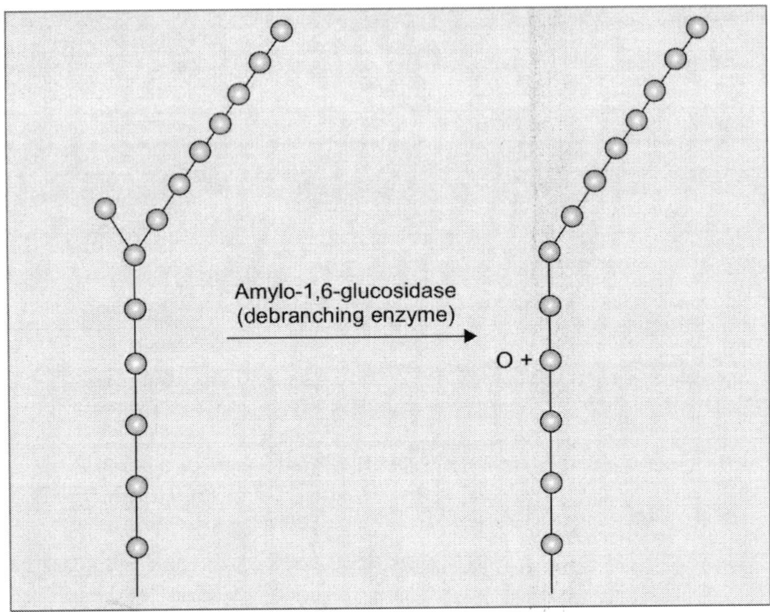

Fig. 10.10 Debranching action at α–1 – 6 branch point

- The single glucose unit attached to the main chain by 1, 6–glycosidic linkage is split off by *amylo–1,6–glucosidase (debranching enzyme)* (Fig. 10.10).
- This is not a phosphorolytic breakdown.
- The glucose unit is liberated as free glucose.

Regulation of Glycogenolysis

- Glycogenolysis is regulated by the covalent modification of the key enzyme phosphorylase.
- Regulation occurs in reciprocal to the regulation of glycogenesis.
- The key enzyme phosphorylase activity is regulated by the cellular concentration of cAMP but in reciprocal to glycogen synthase.
- cAMP levels are in turn regulated by the hormones—Insulin, epinephrine (at muscles) and insulin, glucagon (at liver).
- Key enzyme phosphorylase (glycogen phosphorylase) is active (phosphorylase a) in phosphorylated form and inactive in dephosphorylated form (phosphorylase b).

Muscle Phosphorylase

- Muscle phosphorylase differs from liver phosphorylase.
- It is a *dimer.* Each unit has a *Pyridoxal molecule* and also a *serine residue* which is phosphorylated during activation.
- Phosphorylation is carried out by *Phosphorylase kinase,* which is made up of 4 subunits – α, β, γ, δ.
- α, β *have serine residues,* get phosphorylated by protein kinase A and cause partial activation of phosphorylase kinase.

- *γ has catalytic site.*
- *δ has binding sites for Ca^{++}.*
- During muscle contraction, the Ca^{++} released binds to δ causing complete activation of phosphorylase kinase.
- Further this phosphorylase kinase phosphorylates muscle phosphorylase and activates glycogenolysis in muscles with increase in muscle contraction—*Amplification of glycogenolysis by muscle contraction* (Fig. 10.11).
- Furthermore, this phosphorylase kinase also phosphorylates inhibitor protein to inhibitor protein – 1 – P.
- This then inhibits the phosphatase enzyme, reducing the dephosphorylation of phosphorylase a to phosphorylase b—so glycogenolysis continues.
- Simultaneously, same inhibitor –1–P inhibits the dephosphorylation of glycogen synthase b to glycogen synthase, i.e. inhibiting glycogenesis.
- Muscle glycogenolysis does not add up glucose to blood as muscles lack enzyme *glucose – 6 – phosphatase.*

Liver Phosphorylase

The liver phosphorylase gets activated on phosphorylation by the phosphorylase kinase similar to muscle phosphorylase.

However, the phosphorylase kinase does not have the binding site for Ca unlike the muscle phosphorylase kinase.

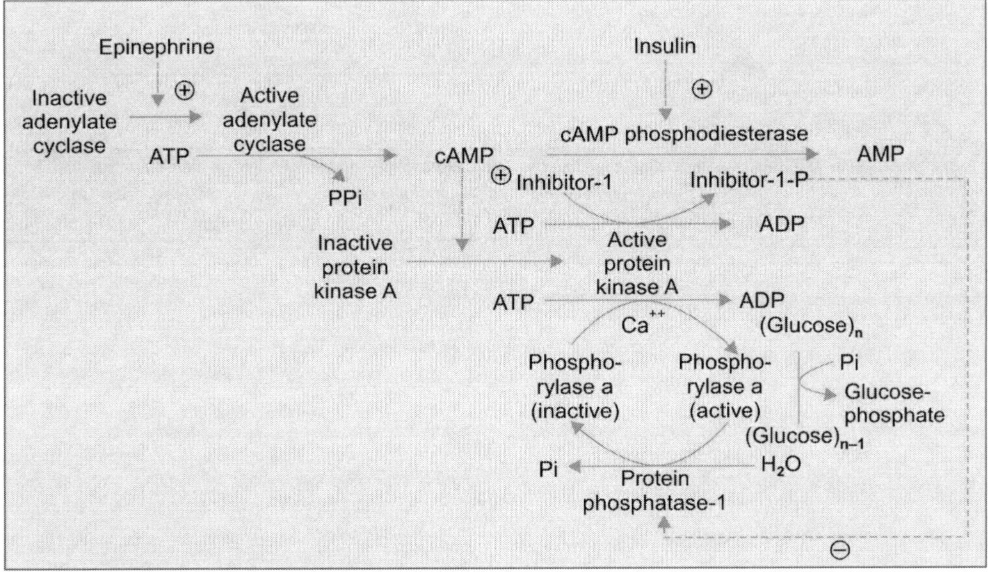

Fig. 10.11 Regulation of glycogenolysis at muscles

Reciprocal Regulation of Glycogen Metabolism during Fed State

- During fed state, when the BSL is high, insulin secreted in response to raised BSL inhibits glycogenolysis by reducing the concentration of cAMP (stimulating phosphodiesterase).
- Reduced cAMP reduces active protein kinase.
- This causes increased concentration of dephosphorylated glycogen synthase (a) and phosphorylase (b).
- Thus, there is more storage of glucose as glycogen during fed state.

Reciprocal Regulation of Glycogen Metabolism during Fasting State

- During fasting state, counter-regulatory hormones of insulin are secreted, i.e. epinephrine and glucagon.
- At liver, the glucagon binds to specific receptors, activates adenylate cyclase.
- This raises cAMP concentration and activates protein kinase A.
- Protein kinase A phosphorylates –
  - Glycogen synthase a—inactivating it.
  - Phosphorylase kinase—activating it.
  - Inhibitor protein—activating it.
- Phosphorylase kinase phosphorylates and activates phosphorylase leading to glycogenolysis —breaking glycogen to glucose –1–P which eventually adds up to BSL.
- Inhibitor –1–P inhibits phosphatase, reducing concentration of dephosphorylated phosphorylase (inactive), i.e. further adding up to glycogenolysis.
- Inhibitor – 1– P also causes a reduced concentration of dephosphorylated glycogen synthase (active) – inhibiting glycogenesis simultaneously and doubly (direct and indirect).

Glycogen Storage Diseases

Table 10.3 Glycogen storage diseases

Disease	*Enzyme defect*	*Biochemical defect and symptoms*
Von Girke's	Glucose – 6 – Phosphatase	Hepatocytes and renal cells loaded with glycogen, hypoglycemia, ketosis, lacticacidemia, hyperlipemia
Pompe's	Lysosomal α – 1–4 and α – 1 –6 glucosidase	Fatal, accumulation of glycogen in lysosomes, heart failure
Limit dextrinosis	Debranching enzyme	Accumulation of characteristic branched polysaccharide
Amylopectinosis	Branching enzyme	Accumulation of polysaccharide with less branching. Death due to cardiac or liver failure
McArdle's	Muscle/Myophosphorylase	Diminished exercise tolerance, muscles have 2.5 – 4% glycogen stored
Her's	Liver phosphorylase	High glycogen in liver, hypoglycemic tendency
Tarui's	PFK in muscles and RBCs	Similar to McArdle's disease but also may have hemolytic anemia
Type VIII	Liver phosphorylase kinase	Same as Her's disease.

Gluconeogenesis and Blood Sugar Level Regulation

Introduction

- The normal fasting blood sugar level is 70 mg – 110 mg/dL. This basal level of blood sugar has to be maintained since the brain, CNS and RBCs can utilize only glucose as a fuel source. The basal BSL is maintained by hepatic glycogenolysis and gluconeogenesis.
- Gluconeogenesis is the 'neo' or new synthesis of glucose from noncarbohydrate sources like lactate, pyruvate, glycerol, odd chain fatty acids or amino acids like alanine and other glucogenic amino acids.

Site of Gluconeogenesis

- Gluconeogenesis occurs in liver and kidneys as these are the tissues that possess the key enzymes of gluconeogenesis.
- The liver accounts for 90% of gluconeogenesis in the body, the kidney's produce the other 10%.

Significance of Gluconeogenesis

- It helps maintain the BSL during prolonged fasting, since a minimal level of glucose is necessary for the optimal functioning of brain and RBCs.
- It helps scavenge the end-products of metabolism of tissues, e.g. lactate produced during muscle contraction, fatty acids and glycerol during lipolysis.
- Adipose tissue needs glucose for the supply of glycerol – 3 P, thus needs gluconeogenesis.
- It provides for the glucose necessary for the synthesis of lactose by the lactating mammary gland.
- Muscles need a constant supply of glucose during anaerobic conditions (persistent, prolonged contraction), lactate converts by gluconeogenesis into glucose.

Principle Gluconeogenic Substrates

The principle substrates for gluconeogenesis are lactate, pyruvate, glycerol, odd chain fatty acids, amino acids with exception of purely ketogenic amino acid – leucine.

Lactate and Pyruvate

At muscles and RBCs the anaerobic glycolysis produces lactate by LDH. With the help of Cori Cycle, the lactate of muscles and RBCs converts to glucose (Fig. 10.12).

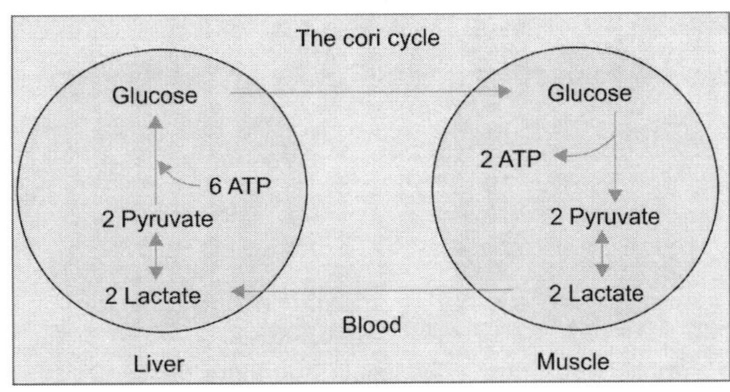

Fig. 10.12 Cori's Cycle

Amino Acids

Glucogenic amino acids like—alanine, glycine, valine, tyrosine, tryptophan, etc. i.e. which can

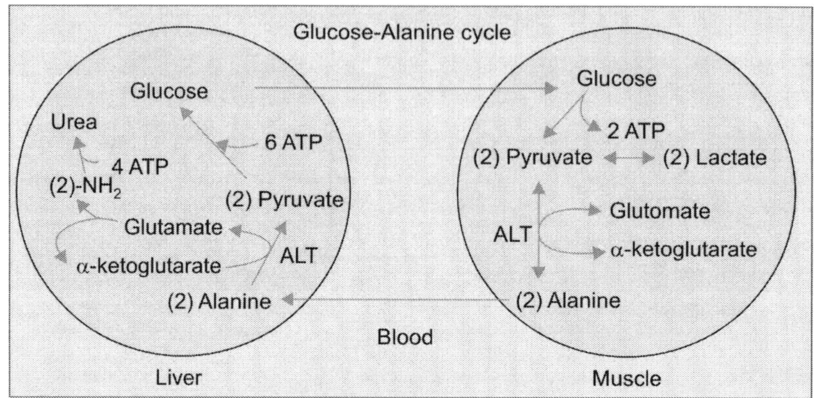

Fig. 10.13 Glucose – Alanine Cycle

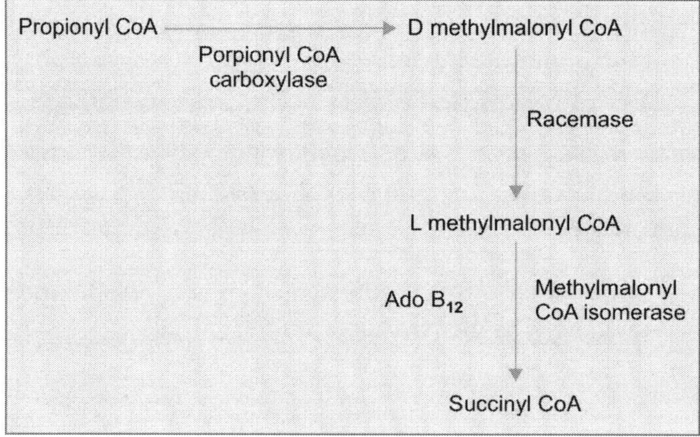

Fig. 10.14 Propionyl CoA conversion to Succinyl CoA

convert into intermediates of CAC can synthesize glucose via gluconeogenesis, e.g. Glucose – Alanine cycle (Fig. 10.13).

Odd Chain Fatty Acids

At the adipose tissue, during oxidation of odd chain fatty acids propionyl CoA is the end product. Propionyl CoA converts into an intermediate of CAC – Succinyl CoA in a stepwise manner that eventually forms glucose via gluconeogenesis (Fig. 10.14).

Process of Gluconeogenesis

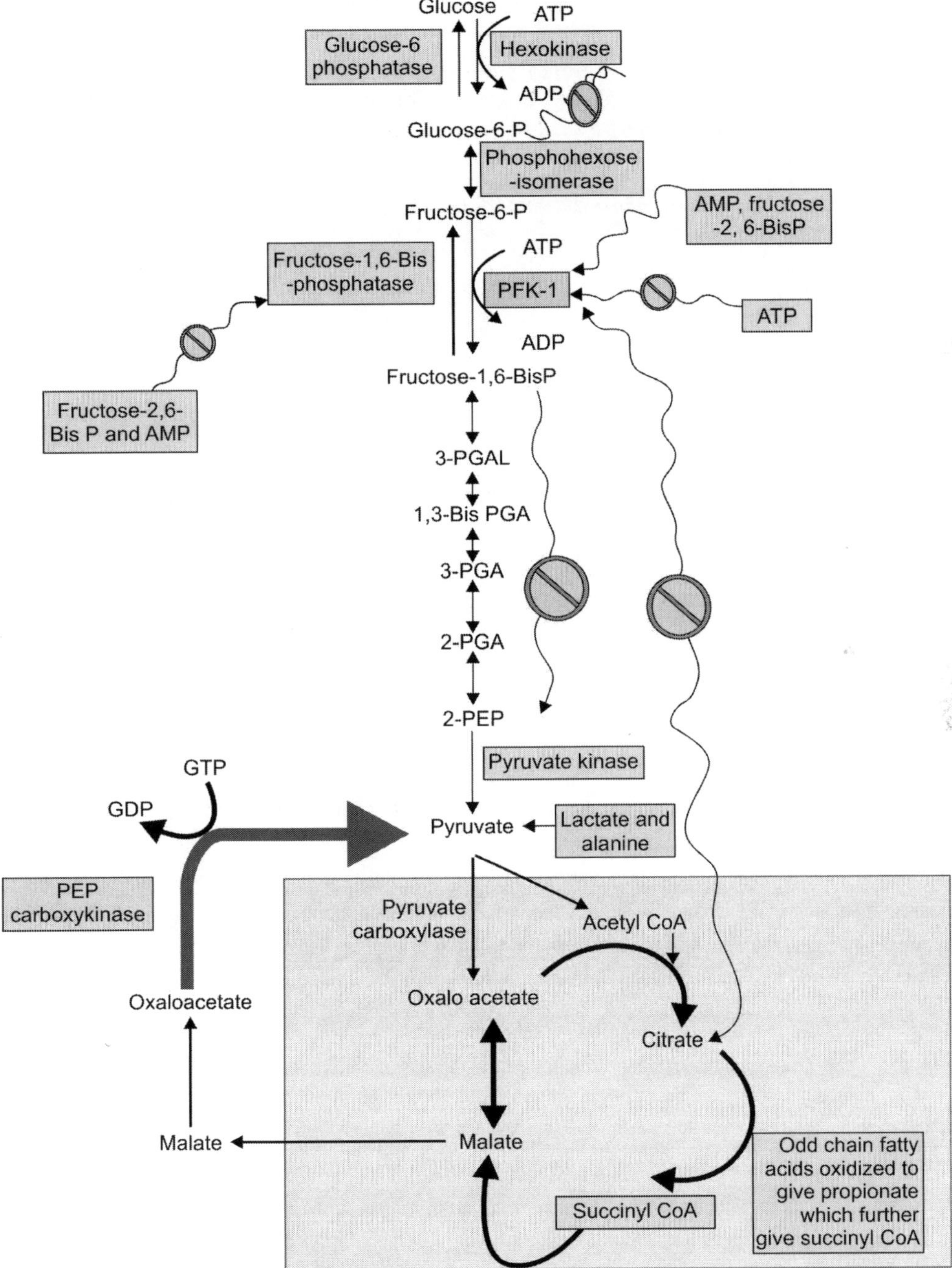

Fig. 10.15 Steps of gluconeogenesis

Key Enzymes of Gluconeogenesis

- Gluconeogenesis involves both the Glycolysis and CAC pathways. It is not the simple reversal of glycolysis because that would be highly endergonic. Rather the gluconeogenic organs have 2 key enzymes that help bypass the irreversible reactions of glycolysis. Besides the conversion of pyruvate back into PEP requires 2 key enzymes. Thus together 4 key gluconeogenic enzymes help circumvent the steps with high free energy change (Fig. 10.15).
- The four key gluconeogenic enzymes:
  - Phosphoenol pyruvate carboxykinase (PEP Carboxykinase)
  - Pyruvate carboxylase
  - Fructose 1, 6 – Bis phosphatase
  - Glucose – 6 Phosphatase

Pyruvate to PEP Conversion

- Two steps are required to convert pyruvate back into PEP.
  - The first step is the carboxylation of pyruvate to form oxaloacetate. This reaction is catalyzed by *pyruvate carboxylase* and requires ATP and Biotin.
  - In the second step oxaloacetate is decarboxylated and phosphorylated to produce phosphoenolpyruvate in presence of *phospho-enol pyruvate carboxykinase.*
- The CO_2 added in the pyruvate carboxylase step comes off in the PEP carboxykinase step. The decarboxylation reaction is very exergonic and helps to drive the otherwise highly endergonic reaction of PEP synthesis.
- Pyruvate carboxylase is found only in the matrix of the mitochondria. The next enzyme involved in gluconeogenesis is PEP carboxykinase which is found in both the mitochondria or in the cytosol or both depending on the organism and the tissue.
- In human livers, PEP carboxykinase is found in both the mitochondria and the cytosol. Pyruvate is transported into the mitochondria where it is either converted into acetyl-CoA by pyruvate dehydrogenase and enters the citric acid cycle, or it is converted into oxaloacetate by pyruvate carboxylase and used for gluconeogenesis.
- In tissues where PEP carboxykinase is found only in the cytosol, oxaloacetate must be reduced to malate so that it can be transported across the mitochondrial membrane to the cytosol where the malate is re-oxidized into oxaloacetate and goes on through gluconeogenesis.

Conversion of Fructose – 1,6 – Bisphosphate to Fructose – 6 – Phosphate

- Since all of the reactions between phosphofructokinase and pyruvate kinase are reversible and near equilibrium, the same enzymes can function in both glycolysis and gluconeogenesis.
- The next irreversible step that must be overcome is to generate fructose-6-phosphate from fructose-1,6-bisphosphate. The enzyme that catalyzes this reaction is *Fructose 1,6-bisphosphatase.*

Conversion of Glucose – 6 – Phosphate to Glucose

- The interconversion of fructose – 6 P and glucose – 6 P is a reversible reaction catalyzed by a hexose isomerase.
- The isomerization of glucose-6-phosphate into glucose is another irreversible reaction with high free energy change and requires circumvention by key gluconeogenic enzyme *Glucose – 6 – phosphatase.*
- The last irreversible step to overcome is the phosphorylation reaction catalyzed by hexokinase. The enzyme that reverses this step, converting glucose-6-phosphate into glucose is glucose-6-phosphatase. This enzyme is a membrane bound protein found in the lumen of the endoplasmic reticulum. This enzyme is not present in the muscles or the brain and hence glucose cannot be produced by these organs.

Regulation of Gluconeogenesis

- Regulation of gluconeogenesis occurs:
  - By allosteric modification of key enzymes.
  - By hormones insulin and glucagon
  - By covalent modification of key enzymes.

Allosteric Regulation

The key enzymes of gluconeogenesis that are regulated allosterically include:

Pyruvate Carboxylase

Regulated by positive allosteric modifiers – Acyl CoA and ATP which indicate that cell has high-energy and enough substrate to convert into glucose so gluconeogenesis occurs and pyruvate converts to OAA. Conversely, if acyl CoA and ATP are low, then the cell is depleted of energy and so CAC occurs for ATP synthesis and pyruvate is oxidatively decarboxylated to acetyl CoA.

Allosteric Reciprocal Regulation of Gluconeogenesis and Glycolysis

- *PFK – 1* – It catalyzes the first committed step of glycolysis. It is allosterically inhibited by ATP and citrate indicating a high energy level and availability of substrate for gluconeogenesis. Thus reciprocally inhibiting glycolysis and simultaneously enhancing gluconeogenesis. It is allosterically activated by fructose – 2,6 – bisP (which is produced by PFK – 2 – a covalently modified enzyme by insulin and glucagon). Thus, fructose 2,6 – bisP enhances glycolysis and inhibits gluconeogenesis.
- *Fructose 1,6 – bis phosphatase*—The enzyme is allosterically inhibited by AMP and fructose – 2,6 – bisP, i.e. when the energy level of the cell is low AMP levels shall be high inhibiting gluconeogenesis and stimulating glycolysis for more ATP production.
- *Pyruvate Kinase*—The enzyme is allosterically activated by fructose 1,6 – bisP. Thus the substrate fructose 1, 6 – bisP makes a provision for its complete catabolism by enhancing the rate of glycolysis.

Hormonal Regulation and Covalent Modification

- Hormones insulin and glucagon regulate the gluconeogenic pathway in reciprocal with glycolytic pathway.
- The regulation is such that there is no futile cycling of the substrates and at a time only one cycle proceeds—glycolysis of gluconeogenesis.
- The hormones insulin and glucagon are responsible for the covalent modification of the enzyme PFK -2.
- Gluconeogenesis is regulated by the covalent modification of key enzyme PFK – 2. The enzyme PFK – 2 has dual enzyme activity – kinase (in dephosphorylated state) and phosphatase (in phosphorylated state). This helps in the reciprocal regulation of glycolysis and gluconeogenesis. (Fig. 10.16)

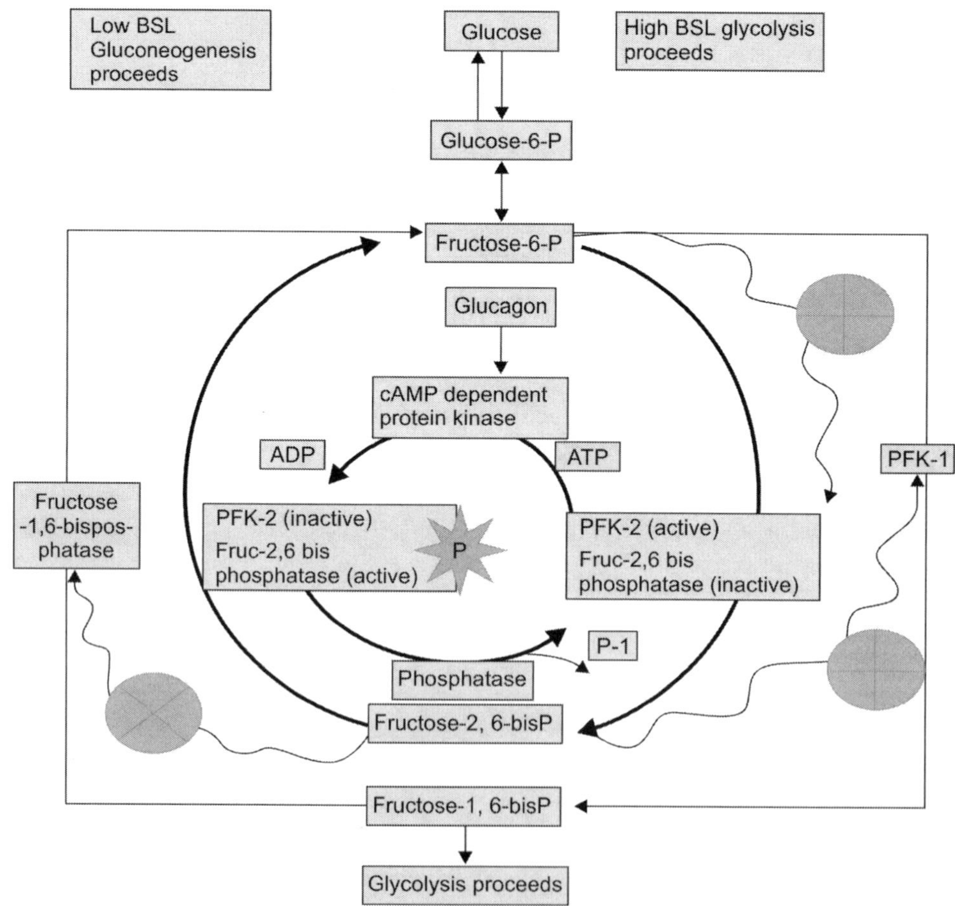

Fig. 10.16 Hormonal and covalent modification of PFK -2 for reciprocal regulation of glycolysis and gluconeogenesis

Regulation of Gluconeogenesis when BSL is High

- Insulin secreted in response.
- Enzymes of glycolysis increased in activity (PFK–1).
- PFK–2 (dual enzyme activity protein) is dephosphorylated so it acts like kinase and concentration of fructose 2,6 – bisP increased.
- Fruct -2,6 – bisP increases activity of PFK –1 and inhibits fructose –1,6 – bis phosphatase.
- Thus inhibition of gluconeogenesis and stimulation of glycolysis.

Regulation of Gluconeogenesis when BSL is Low

- Counter regulatory hormones secreted—Glucagon.
- Glucagon increases concentration of cAMP.
- cAMP dependent protein kinase phosphorylates PFK –2 so that it is inactivated but the 2nd enzyme activity fructose 2,6 – bis phosphatase is activated.
- This reduces concentration of fructose 2,6 – bis P.
- So reduced inhibition of gluconeogenic enzyme fructose 1,6 – bis phosphtase.
- Reduced activation of PFK – 1 so glycolysis stopped.
- Gluconeogenesis proceeds to maintain BSL.

Blood Sugar Regulation

- Glucose is the principal sugar of blood. A normal fasting blood sugar level is 70–110 mg/dL. After meals the blood sugar level rises, however will never exceed the renal threshold (180 mg/dL). The level drops back to the fasting level within 2 hours (post prandial). This maintenance of a normal BSL is a highly regulated homeostatic mechanism (Fig. 10.17). It is primarily achieved by the feedback effect of hormones—Insulin, glucagon, epinephrine, glucocorticoids and growth hormones. Equilibrium in these hormones, i.e. insulin and its counter-regulatory hormones help keep a balance in BSL.
- The factors that add up to BSL are:
  - Dietary
  - Hepatic glycogenolysis
  - Hepatic and renal gluconeogenesis
  - Hepatic conversion of other monosaccharides to glucose.
- The factors that utilize BSL are:
  - Glycogenesis (10%)
  - Glycolysis (50%)

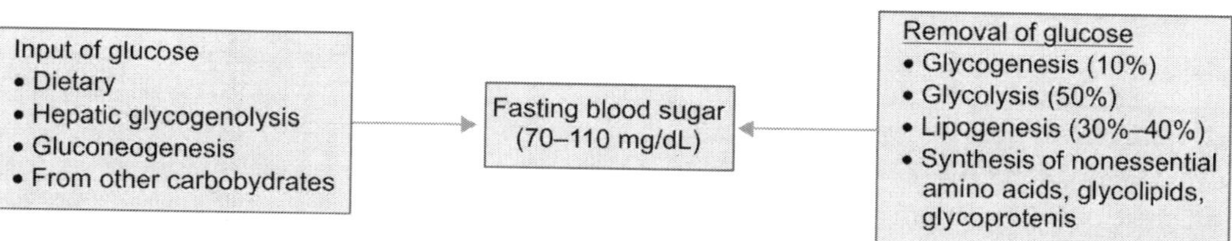

Fig. 10.17 Balance in factors adding to BSL and factors utilizing BSL

- Lipogenesis (30% – 40%)
- Synthesis of nonessential amino acids, glycolipids, glycoproteins
- Kidneys (>180 mg/dL)

- A balance in these two is kept for a proper glucose homeostasis, achieved by hormones.

Regulation of BSL is Mainly under Hormonal Influences

Role of Insulin

- It has hypoglycemic effects.
- Increases glucose uptake.
- Increases glucose utilization.
- Increases hepatic glycogenesis.
- Increases glycolysis.
- Increases lipogenesis.

Role of Counter

- *Regulatory hormones* like—hormones of adrenal cortex, growth hormone, and glucagon. They tend to increase the BSL.
- Increase hepatic glycogenolysis.
- Increase protein catabolism at peripheral tissues (amino acids available as gluconeogenic substrate).
- Increase hepatic uptake of amino acids.
- Increase hepatic gluconeogenesis.

Regulation in Fed Condition (Postprandial)

- Just after meals, the BSL rises (all monosaccharides convert to glucose at liver).
- Pancreatic cells freely permeable to glucose.
- Beta cells secrete insulin.
- Insulin carries out the *hypoglycemic action.*
  - Increase the uptake of glucose at tissues like muscles and adipose tissue via GLUT – 4 transporters.
  - Induces the hepatic glucokinase.
  - Glucokinase phosphorylates glucose to glucose – 6 –P.
  - A concentration gradient pulls more and more glucose into the liver cells to be stored as glycogen.
  - Induces other key enzymes of glycolysis (PFK -1 and pyruvate kinase).
  - Increases hepatic glycogenesis and lipogenesis (storing excess of glucose as glycogen at liver and TG at adipose tissue).
  - Initiates synthesis of nonessential amino acids.
  - Insulin initiates lipogenesis as –
    - It activates the enzymes of HMP shunt which supplies NADPH for fatty acid synthesis.
    - It induces key enzyme of fatty acid synthesis—acetyl CoA carboxylase.
    - It provides glycerol for TG synthesis.

- Muscles rapidly increase its glucose uptake which is critical for dealing with sudden increases in plasma glucose (storing excess glucose as glycogen in fed state).
- Counter – regulatory hormones are reduced during this period.

Regulation in Fasting Condition

- During 12–14 hours fasting, the levels of insulin are reduced and that of the counter – regulatory hormones are raised for maintaining the BSL between 70 – 110mg/dl.
- BSL is maintained by hepatic glycogenolysis for 8 – 10 hrs.
- Counter-regulatory hormones activate key enzymes of gluconeogenesis—
  - PFK – 2,
  - Pyruvate carboxylase,
  - PEP carboxykinase,
  - Glucose – 6 – phosphatase,
  - Fructose – 1, 6 – bis phosphatase
- Adipose tissue TGs are lipolyzed under the influence of adrenal cortical hormones, hormone sensitive lipase, glucagon, GH.
- Glycerol is picked up by hepatocytes as a precursor of gluconeogenesis.
- Fatty acids are taken up by liver to be oxidized as a fuel source of energy.
- Muscles add up to BSL via Cori cycle. The muscle cannot release glucose into circulation (as it lacks glucose – 6 – phosphatase). However, in fasting and prolonged fasting skeletal muscle has an additional role in maintaining plasma glucose levels: it releases free amino acids into circulation to serve as substrates for liver gluconeogenesis.

Regulation in Prolonged Fasting

- Kidneys also become gluconeogenesis site.
- Counter-regulatory hormones cause protein catabolism at peripheral tissues to liberate amino acids.
- Amino acids picked up by liver as precursors of gluconeogenesis. (Glucose – alanine cycle)
- Muscles also add up sugar indirectly via Cori cycle.

Hexose Monophosphate Shunt (HMP) and Minor Metabolic Pathways of Carbohydrate Metabolism

Introduction

- Glucose is at the center of carbohydrate metabolism. It is activated to glucose-6-P which then is either glycolyzed or stored as glycogen at liver and muscle or enters HMP shunt. The pathway is named as hexose monophosphate shunt since it begins with hexose mono-phosphate glucose–6–P. Another name commonly used is pentose phosphate pathway, since the intermediates of the pathway are pentoses like ribose–5–P, ribulose–5–P, xylulose–5–P.
- HMP shunt along with glycolysis is a major glucose oxidative pathway, where glucose–6–phosphate is oxidized via pentose intermediates, using $NADP^+$ as a coenzyme and generates CO_2, Glyceraldehyde–3–P and NADPH + H^+.
- No energy is generated rather; it uses NADP as a coenzyme that on reduction gives rise to the reducing power (NADPH+H^+) for biosynthesis of important biomolecules.

- This pathway is split into oxidative-irreversible and nonoxidative-reversible phases.
- The complete pathway occurs in the cytosol of cells and the overall reaction is:

$$3\ \text{Glucose–6–P} + 3\text{NADP}^+ \longrightarrow 3\ CO_2 + 2\ \text{Glyceraldehyde–3–P} + 3\ \text{NADPH} + H^+ +$$

Tissue Specific Site of HMP Shunt

- HMP shunt occurs in tissues that are rapidly dividing like—
  - Bone marrow
  - Skin
  - Intestinal mucosa.
- In tissues involved in rapid biosynthesis of fatty acids, cholesterol and other steroids like—
  - Adipose tissue
  - Liver
  - Adrenal gland
  - Lactating mammary gland.

  Erythrocytes and lens of eye too possess active enzymatic machinery for HMP shunt.

Significance of HMP Shunt

Each tissue possessing the HMP shunt renders a unique significance to this pathway.

Actively Multiplying Tissues

Such tissues have a high demand for pentose – ribose and deoxy ribose for the rapid rate of cell division and HMP shunt provides for these pentoses.

Reductive Biosynthesis

Tissues involved in the biosynthesis of fatty acids, sterols, steroid hormones, cholesterol, etc. need the reducing power as NADPH derived from HMP shunt. Thus HMP shunt is of significance to these tissues.

Maintenance of Membrane Integrity of Erythrocytes

HMP shunt is very active in RBCs. Nearly 10% of total glucose utilized is oxidized by HMP shunt. The cell membrane of erythrocytes is constantly exposed to O_2, thus there is enhanced risk of free radical damage. However, the RBCs maintain their cell membrane integrity by the enzyme glutathione peroxidase. This enzyme scavenges the peroxides like H_2O_2 and prevents the peroxidation of the PUFA of cell membrane of RBCs. HMP shunt supplies the NADPH+H+ for the maintenance of reduced glutathione as shown in Figure 10.18.

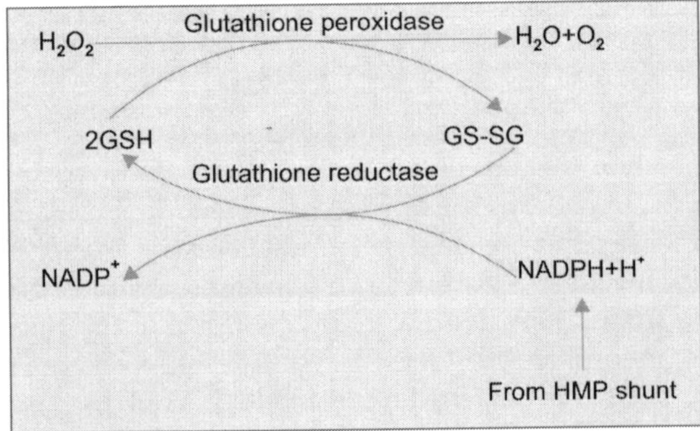

Fig. 10.18 Role of HMP shunt in maintenance of glutathione

Transparency of Lens of Eye

Just as in the RBCs, the HMP shunt generated NADPH+H^+ helps in the maintenance of the transparency of the lens of eye, which too is under a constant attack of free radicals/reactive oxygen species. This helps maintain the transparency of the lens of eye.

The NADPH +H^+ of HMP Shunt

It maintains the glutathione buffers of all cells and helps in proper enzymatic activity of enzymes dependent on these buffers. Thus they can prevent or undo oxidative damage to proteins, lipids, and other sensitive molecules.

Pathway of HMP Shunt

- Although the hexose monophosphate pathway has fewer enzymes than glycolysis, it is somewhat more complicated. It is a multicyclic pathway.
- The complete pathway of HMP shunt is divided into the oxidative reversible and non- oxidative irreversible sections.

Oxidative Phase of HMP Shunt

- The oxidative pathway involves the oxidation of glucose – 6 – phosphate by two enzymes—Glucose – 6 – phosphate dehydrogenase and 6 – Phosphogluconate dehydrogenase using NADP$^+$ as the coenzyme.
- It is shown as in Figure 10.19
- During the oxidative phase the glucose – 6 – P is oxidized sequentially to ribulose – 5 – P and NADPH+H^+. At a time 3 mols of glucose – 6 – P are oxidized so 3 CO_2, 3 NADPH and 3 ribulose – 5 – P are formed.
- The first reaction of the pentose phosphate pathway is the oxidation of glucose 6-phosphate by glucose 6-phosphate dehydrogenase (G6PD) to form 6-phosphoglucono-lactone and NADP$^+$ acts like an electron acceptor.
- The lactone is hydrolyzed to the free acid 6–phosphogluconate by a specific lactonase, then 6–phosphogluconate undergoes oxidation and decarboxylation by 6–phosphogluconate dehydrogenase to form the ketopentose ribulose 5-phosphate. Thus, the second molecule of NADPH is produced.
- Total 6 NADPH and 6 ribulose–5–P are produced from 3 mols of glucose participating in one cycle of HMP shunt.

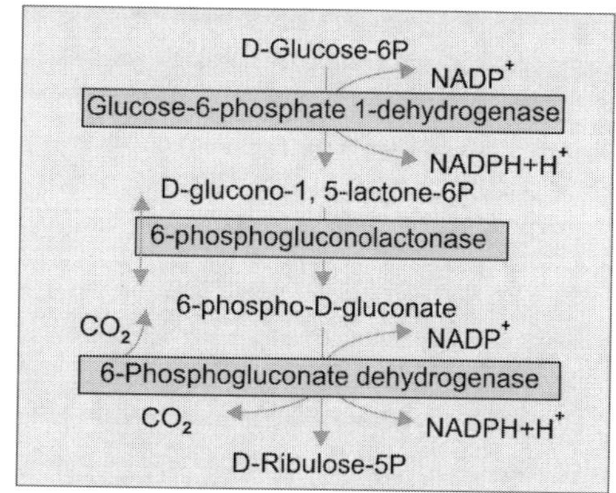

Fig. 10.19 Oxidative phase of HMP shunt

Nonoxidative Phase of HMP Shunt

- In this nonoxidative phase, out of the 3 molecules of ribulose 2 are epimerized to xylulose – 5 – P and one isomerized to ribose – 5 – P. Ribose – 5 – P is used up directly in purine and pyrimidine biosynthesis and ribulose participates further down the nonoxidative phase (Fig. 10.20).

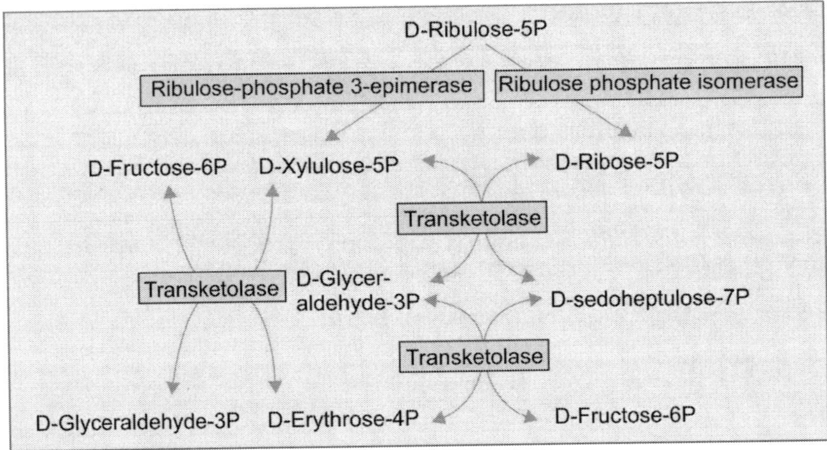

Fig. 10.20 Nonoxidative phase of HMP shunt

- All steps of this phase are reversible, thus tissues not requiring NADPH but only pentoses like ribose, e.g. brain, polymorphonuclear cells, etc. may simply reverse this phase for the synthesis of ribose, to be used in cell division.
- Two enzymes are unique to this phase of HMP shunt—**Transketolase and Transaldolase**. These two enzymes are involved in the rearrangement of the pentose phosphates.
- Transketolase uses TPP as a coenzyme. It catalyzes the transfer of a two-carbon fragments from a ketose donor to an aldose acceptor. In its first appearance in the pentose phosphate pathway, transketolase transfers C–1 and C–2 of xylulose 5–phosphate to ribose 5–phosphate, forming the seven-carbon product sedoheptulose–7–phosphate and a 3–C fragment of glyceraldehyde–3–P is left.
- Next, transaldolase catalyzes a reaction similar to the aldolase reaction of glycolysis: A three-carbon fragment is removed from sedoheptulose 7–phosphate and condensed with glyceraldehyde 3–phosphate, forming fructose 6–phosphate and the tetrose erythrose 4–phosphate.
- Transketolase acts again, forming fructose 6–phosphate and glyceraldehyde 3–phosphate from erythrose 4–phosphate and xylulose 5–phosphate.
- Two molecules of glyceraldehyde 3–phosphate formed by two iterations of these reactions can be converted to a molecule of fructose 1,6–bisphosphate as in gluconeogenesis.
- Finally FBPase–1 and phosphohexose isomerase convert fructose 1, 6–bisphosphate to glucose 6–phosphate.
- In tissues that require primarily NADPH, the pentose phosphates produced in the oxidative phase of the pathway are recycled into glucose 6–phosphate.

Clinical Applications of HMP Shunt

Glucose – 6 – Phosphate Dehydrogenase (G-6-PD) Deficiency

- There are about 400 million people all over the world suffering from the deficiency of the key enzyme Glucose – 6 – P dehydrogenase. The deficiency of this enzyme makes the individuals susceptible to hemolytic anemia.

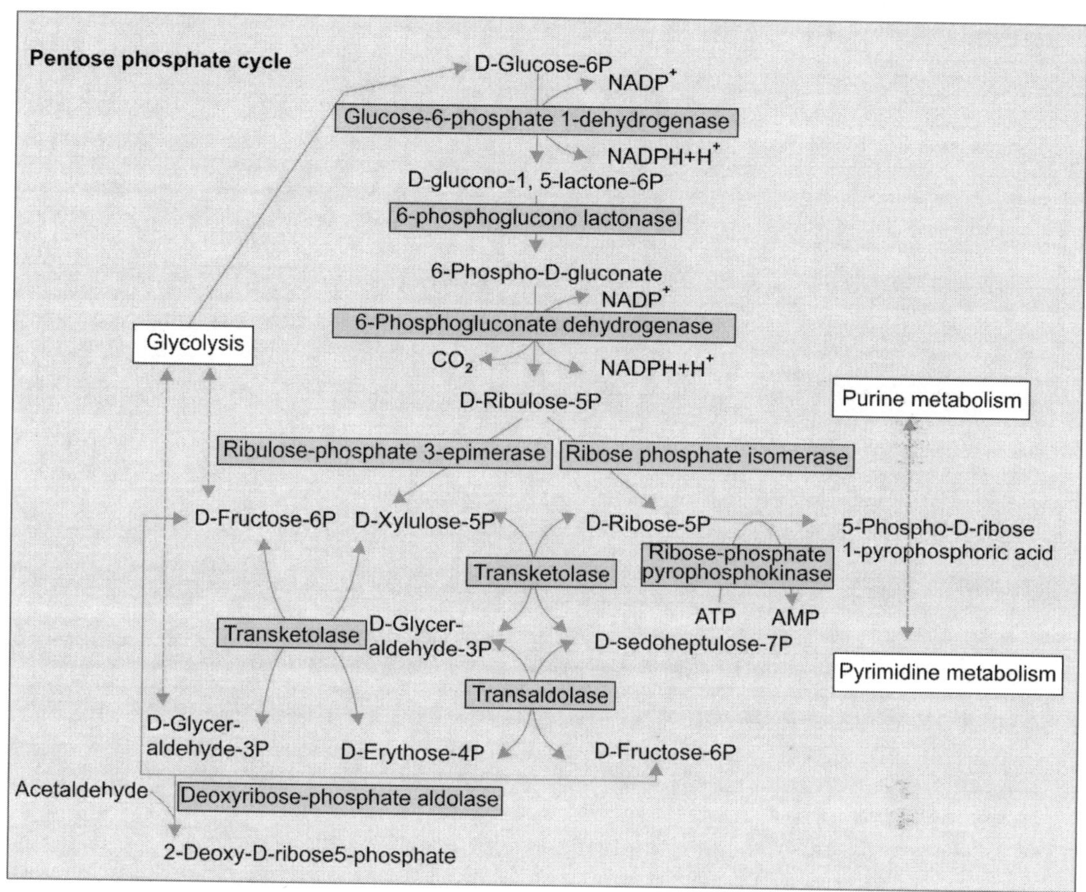

Fig. 10.21 HMP shunt – Complete pathway

- Most G–6–PD deficient individuals are asymptomatic; only the combination of G–6–PD deficiency and certain environmental factors produces the clinical manifestations.
- The RBCs of such individuals are at a constant risk of free radical damage on consumption of oxidant drugs like—antimalarial drugs like—Primaquine and divicine and also sulfa drugs. These drugs would enhance the production of reactive oxygen species and cause the RBCs to rupture.
- However, these individuals are resistant to malaria (Fig. 10.22).

Favism

- Fava beans have the same effect as that of the oxidant drugs on individuals with G–6–Pdh deficiency.
- An advantage of G–6–PD deficiency is that the individuals are resistant to malaria, as the parasite thrives in RBCs which are not quite stable.

Uronic Acid Pathway

- It is an alternative minor pathway of glucose metabolism and is not for energy production. It exists in the liver.

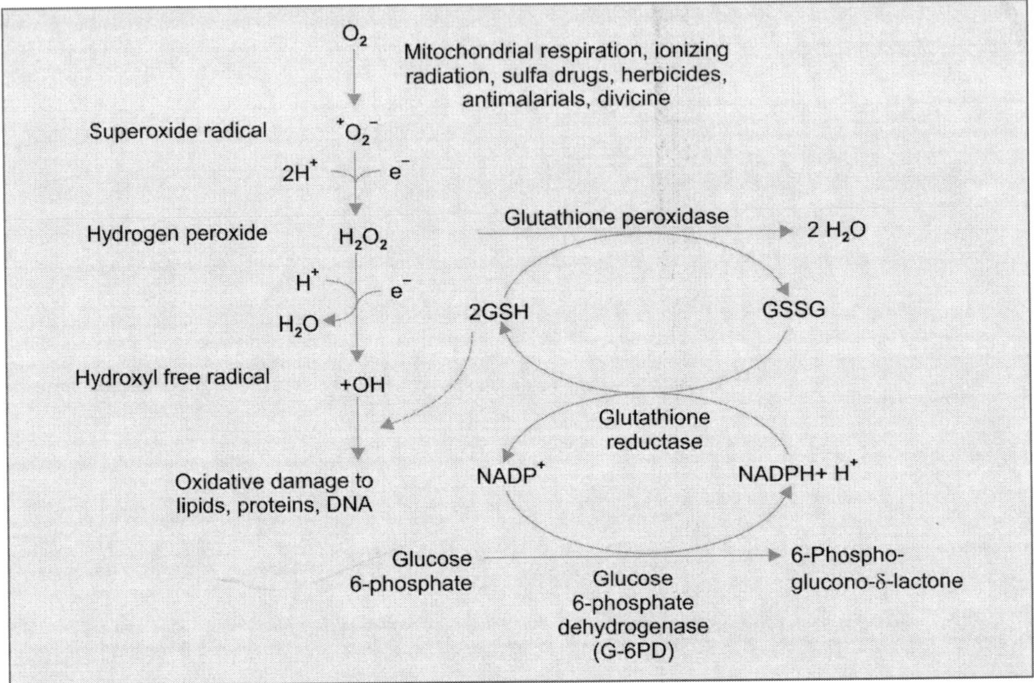

Fig. 10.22 Role of HMP shunt NADPH

- The pathway is as shown in the Figure 10.23.
- This pathway is unique because it synthesizes—
  - UDP glucuronate – principle conjugating agent
  - Ascorbate in all mammals with exception in humans, higher primates, guinea pigs and bats.
- The UDP glucose is oxidized in this pathway to generate UDP – glucuronate, which is formed by the oxidation of the primary alcoholic group of UDP glucose.
- UDP glucuronate has great significance in the:
  - Conjugation of drugs – glucuronidation
  - Conjugation of steroids including steroid hormones
  - Conjugation of bilirubin – Bilirubin diglucuronide
  - As component of mucopolysaccharide
- The UDP glucuronate is further hydrolyzed to glucuronate that undergoes still further reduction to L – gulonate. L – gulonate then is oxidized to L – ascorbate in the presence of L – gulonolactone oxidase.
- This enzyme was lost by humans and higher primates during the course of evolution and their failure to synthesize ascorbic acid. This enzyme is also deficient in fruit bats and guinea pigs as their diet is predominantly rich in vitamin – C, thus they too lost it during the course of evolution probably.
- Ascorbate can interconvert to dehydroascorbate and is completely catabolized to the L – gulonate in humans is therefore further decarboxylated to L – xylulose, which converts to D – xylulose via its reduction to xylitol and then hydration.

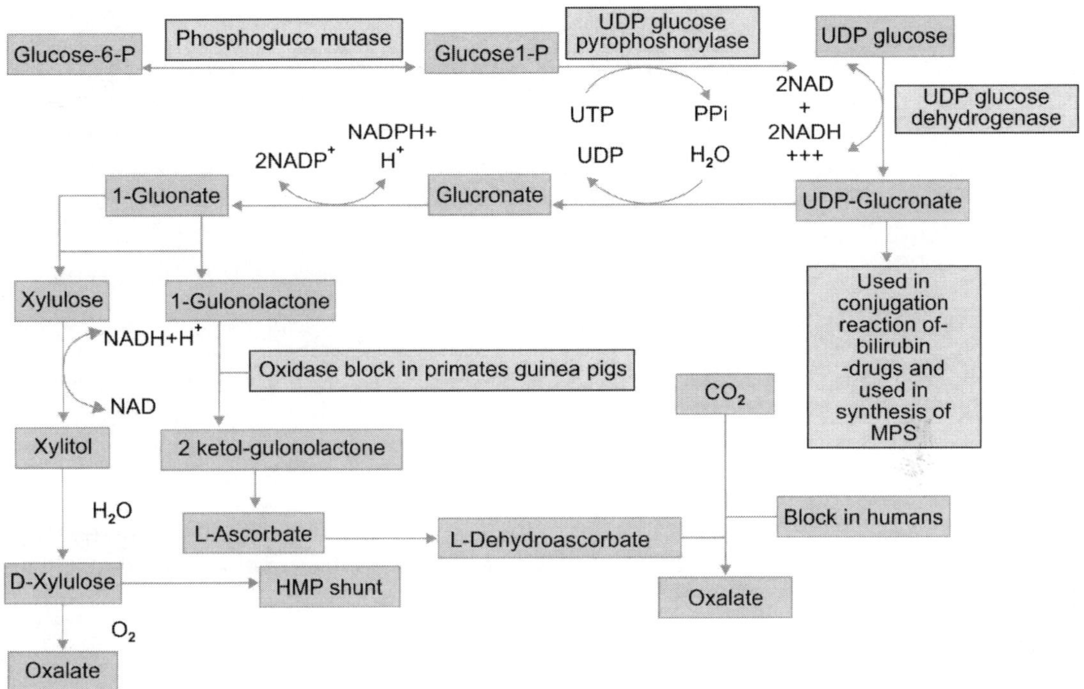

Fig. 10.23 Uronic acid pathway

- D – xylulose then enters the HMP shunt to further metabolized. Some of it is oxidized to oxalate to be excreted in urine.

Fructose Metabolism

Introduction

- The major source of dietary fructose is sucrose which upon hydrolysis yields equimolar amounts of glucose and fructose. Fructose also occurs in honey and in a large variety of fruits; hence, time name fructose, which means fruit sugar.
- Dietary fructose is absorbed by the GLUT 5 transporter and is carried to the liver via the hepatic portal vein. At the liver fructose is glycolyzed much more rapidly than glucose.
- Defects in fructose metabolism are much more common than those of other sugars.

Pathway of Fructose Metabolism

- For fructose to enter the intermediary metabolism, it has to be activated by phosphorylation that is carried out by hexokinase and fructokinase. However, hexokinase has a lower affinity for fructose than for glucose. So fructose is predominantly phosphorylated by fructokinase to fructose – 1 – P (Fig. 10.24).
- Principal organs where this enzyme is active are—liver and muscles.
- The pathway to utilization of fructose differs in muscle and liver.

At Liver

- Liver has the enzyme fructokinase. This enzyme phosphorylates the dietary fructose to F–1–P.
- F–1–P by the action of aldolase – B (F–1–P aldolase) splits F–1–P into glyceraldehyde and DHAP. DHAP enters the normal glycolytic pathway and glycerol kinase phosphorylates glyceraldehyde into glyceraldehyde – 3 – P to facilitate its entry into glycolysis.
- The affinity of aldolase B for fructose–1–P is much poorer than that of fructose–1,6–biphosphate, thus fructose–1–P accumulates in fructokinase—expressing tissues. Thus, aldolase B is the rate-limiting enzyme for fructose metabolism (but not glucose).

Fructose is Rapidly Removed from Circulation of Diabetics

- Dietary fructose gets phosphorylated as F–1–P which is a substrate for aldolase B at liver.
- Thus, the key regulatory step of glycolysis catalyzed by PFK – 1 gets bypassed, leading to a rapid glycosylation and removal of fructose from circulation.
- Besides, the regulation of phosphorylation of fructose by fructokinase is poorly regulated.

Fructose Floods the Metabolic Pathways by Triglycerides

- High fructose in diet floods the metabolic pathways by triglycerides. This because the rapid glycolysis causes a high availability of substrate for triglyceride formation—glyceraldehyde

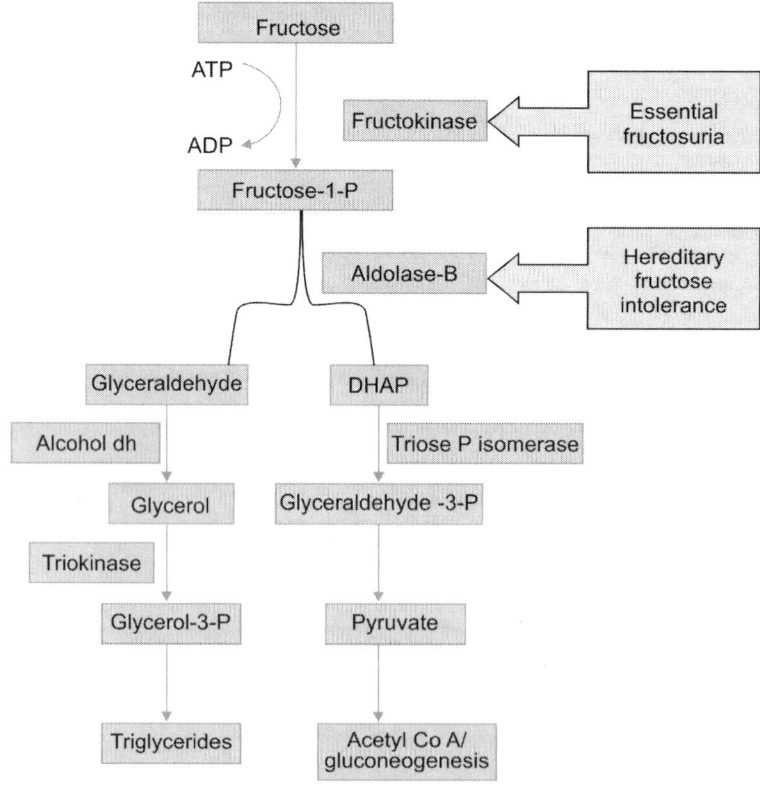

Fig. 11.24 Fructose metabolism

– 3 – P via enzymatic reaction catalyzed by alcohol dh converts to glycerol, which then is phosphorylated to glycerol – 3 – P by the glycerol kinase enzyme. The fatty acids are synthesized form the high amount of pyruvate converting to acetyl CoA.

- This also increases the risk of nonalcoholic fatty liver disease in individuals with obesity, insulin resistance and DM – 2.
  - The diets rich in fructose cause hypertriglyceridemia and hyperuricemia because the high availability of glycerol acts as a substrate for TGs. Simultaneously, the rate of activity of aldolase – B is not in sync with that of fructokinase, causing an accumulation of Pi in the liver. This will reduce the synthesis of ATP from ADP.
- Eventually the accumulated ADP is catabolized to cause hyperuricemia.

Polyol Pathway

- The polyol pathway works in the seminiferous tubules, lens of eyes, in Schwann cells of peripheral nerves, RBCs, ovaries, kidneys, etc. This pathway synthesizes fructose from glucose via an enzyme catalyzed pathway; the enzyme being aldose reductase (Fig. 10.25).
- The polyol pathway is also responsible for the synthesis of fructose at the seminiferous tubules as fructose serves as the fuel source for the sperms.
- The diabetic patients have an elevated level of circulating glucose, which can freely permeate these cells like lens of eye and nerves.
- Once within these cells the glucose follows the polyol pathway to synthesize sorbitol.
- Sorbitol being osmotically active causes damage to these tissues leading to cataract of eyes (turbidity in the lens of eye) and neuropathy of diabetes (Fig. 10.26).

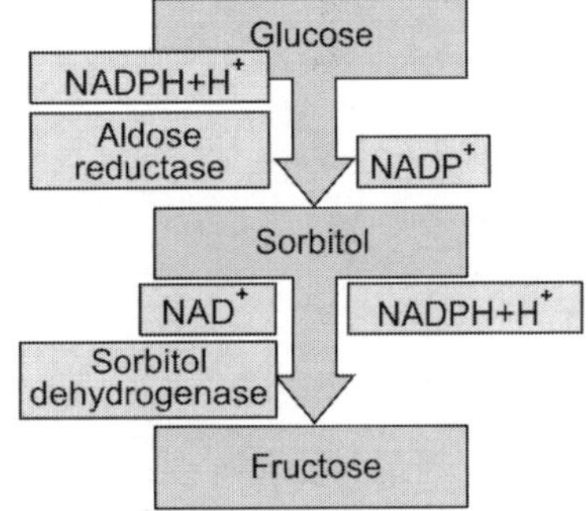

Fig. 10.25 Polyol pathway

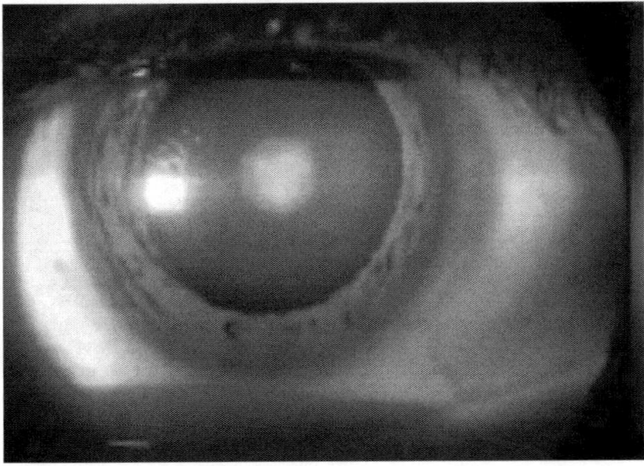

Fig. 10.26 Diabetic cataracts

At Muscles

- Muscle and adipose tissue contains only hexokinase can phosphorylate fructose to F–6–P which is a direct glycolytic intermediate. However, hexokinase has a very low affinity to fructose compared to glucose. So it is not a significant pathway for fructose metabolism, unless it is present in very high concentration blood.

Inherited Disorders of Fructose Metabolism

- Disorders of fructose metabolism are seen due to the defects of enzymes fructokinase and aldolase – B.
- Deficiency of fructokinase causes a benign condition—*Essential fructosuria*, where fructose accumulates in urine.
- Deficiency of Aldolase –B cause a severe condition—*Hereditary fructose intolerance*.
- This condition is characterized by severe damage to liver and kidneys owing to the accumulation of F–1–P.

Galactose Metabolism

Introduction

- Dietary galactose is primarily obtained from the hydrolysis of milk sugar lactose by the enzyme lactase at the intestinal brush border.
- Galactose is also absorbed by the GLUT5 transporter and is carried to the liver via the portal circulation.
- At the liver galactose is converted to glucose enzymatically.
- Some galactose is also derived by the normal wear and tear of the tissue glycolipids.

Pathway of Galactose Metabolism

- For the galactose to enter the intermediary metabolism, it must be converted to galactose – 1 – P.
- The enzyme galactose kinase is present in almost all the tissues and causes the phosphorylation of galactose to galactose – 1 – P.
- Galactose – 1 – P is then converted to UDP galactose by an exchange reaction with UDP glucose catalyzed by *galactose – 1 – P UDP glucose transferase (GPUT)*.
- The UDP galactose then in the presence of *galactose – 4 – epimerase* enzyme epimerises to UDP glucose and enters the glycogenic pathway and through which it may add up to BSL as and when required (FIg. 10.27).

Galactosemias

- Inherited disorders of galactose metabolism are the galactosemias.
- Galactosuria is the excretion of galactose in the urine, which may be caused by inherited defects in galactokinase, uridyl-transferase (the most common) or 4–epimerase.
- These can occur due to the defect in either galactokinase or GPUT or galactose – 4 – epimerase.

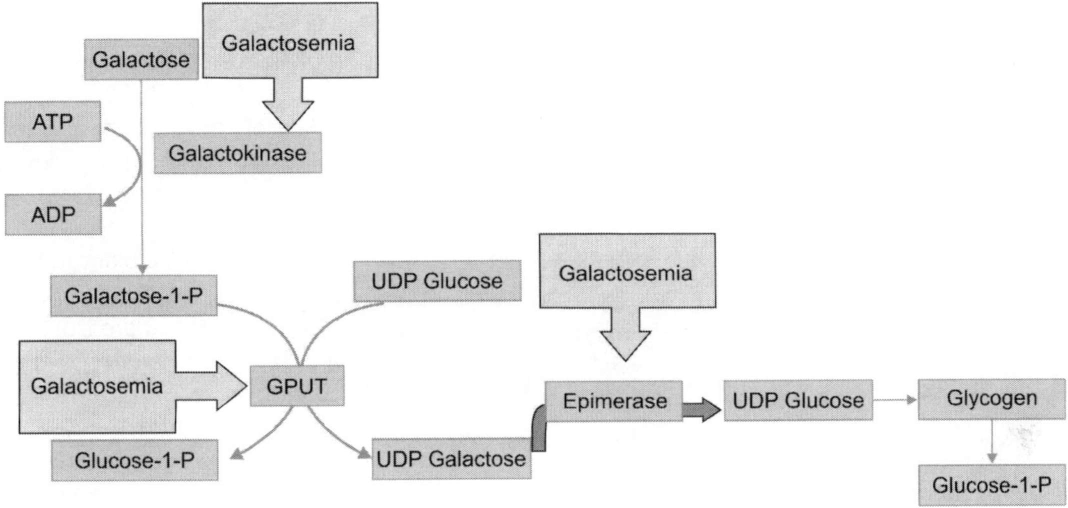

Fig. 10.27 Pathway of galactose metabolism

- Classical galactosemias occur due to defect in GPUT enzyme.
- This causes an accumulation of galactose – 1 – P in a variety of tissues as galactokinase is present in almost all tissues.
- The accumulated galactose – 1 – P is reduced to the sugar alcohol galactitol.
- Galactitol being osmotically active cause osmotic damage to the tissues where it accumulates like the lens of eye—cataract.
- Also accumulation of galactose–1–P depletes the liver of Pi and finally liver failure and mental retardation result.

Symptoms of Galactosemia

- Infants with galactosemia can develop symptoms in the first few days of life if they eat formula or breast milk that contains lactose:
  - Convulsions
  - Irritability
  - Lethargy
  - Poor feeding (baby refuses to eat formula containing milk)
  - Poor weight gain
  - Yellow skin and whites of the eyes (jaundice)
  - Vomiting
- Cataract and mental retardation are other major complications that are seen if not managed.
- Management can be done by giving infants the diet that is free of galactose like artificial milk preparations of soy protein.
- These cases treated by giving galactose-free diet are able to form UDP–galactose from UDP–glucose by galactose epimerase, which explain their normal growth and development.

Synthesis of Lactose at Mammary Gland

- At the mammary gland during lactation, the UDP–galactose in presence of lactose synthase combines with glucose to form lactose.
- Some individuals have hereditary lactose intolerance due to the lack of enzyme lactase. Such individuals are unable to digest the dietary lactose and if consume lactose they suffer from—
  - Abdominal cramps
  - Flatulence
  - Discomfort.

A Quick Look at the Carbohydrate Metabolism

- Dietary carbohydrates are digested in mouth and intestines to be hydrolyzed to simplest sugars—Monosaccharides.
- Monosaccharides are absorbed at the intestinal brush border by glucose transporters—SGLT1 – glucose and Na; GLUT5 – fructose and galactose and GLUT2 transports all three monosaccharides to blood stream.
- At liver all monosaccharides other than glucose convert to glucose.
- Glucose is the principal fuel source of brain, CNS and RBCs.
- Glucose is glycolyzed to produce ATP (50%).
- Total ATP generated in aerobic glycolysis is 8 and in anaerobic is 2 ATP.
- Anaerobic glycolysis occurs in skeletal muscles during strenuous exercise and in RBCs at all times.
- Key enzymes of glycolysis are hexokinase, PFK–1 and pyruvate kinase.
- Glycolysis is regulated reciprocally to gluconeogenesis.
- Pyruvate is the end product of aerobic glycolysis and lactate is end product of anaerobic glycolysis.
- Pyruvate is oxidatively decarboxylated to acetyl CoA by pyruvate dh.
- Acetyl Co A is then oxidized in CAC to generate 12 ATP per acetyl CoA.
- Overall one mol of glucose on complete oxidation by glycolysis and CAC gives 38 ATP.
- Excess of glucose is stored as glycogen at liver (5% by weight) and muscles (1% by weight).
- Glycogenesis is synthesis of glycogen and glycogenolysis is breakdown of glycogen to glucose –1– P.
- Glycogen has glucose units linked by glycosidic linkage alpha –1–4 in straight chain and alpha –1–6 at branch point.
- Glycogen metabolism is regulated by the covalent modification of key enzymes glycogen synthase (inactive in phosphorylated state) and phosphorylase (active in phosphorylated state).
- The BSL is maintained during fasting (upto 12 hours) by hepatic glycogenolysis.
- When hepatic glycogen is exhausted, BSL is maintained by hepatic gluconeogenesis.
- Gluconeogenesis is the new glucose synthesis from noncarbohydrate sources.
- Key enzymes of gluconeogenesis are glucose – 6 – Phosphatase, fructose 1,6, bisphosphatase, PEPCK and pyruvate carboxylase.
- Regulation of gluconeogenesis is by allosteric and covalent modification of PFK –2 and other enzymes of glycolysis.
- HMP shunt is an alternative oxidative pathway of glucose which does not generate energy but produces the reducing power as NADPH for reductive biosynthesis.
- Other alternative pathway for glucose metabolism is uronic acid pathway that synthesizes glucuronic acid for conjugation of drugs, steroids, steroid hormones, and also as component of MPS.
- Other monosaccharides—Fructose and galactose are metabolized at liver to form glucose and add up to glucose.

CHAPTER

11

Lipid Metabolism

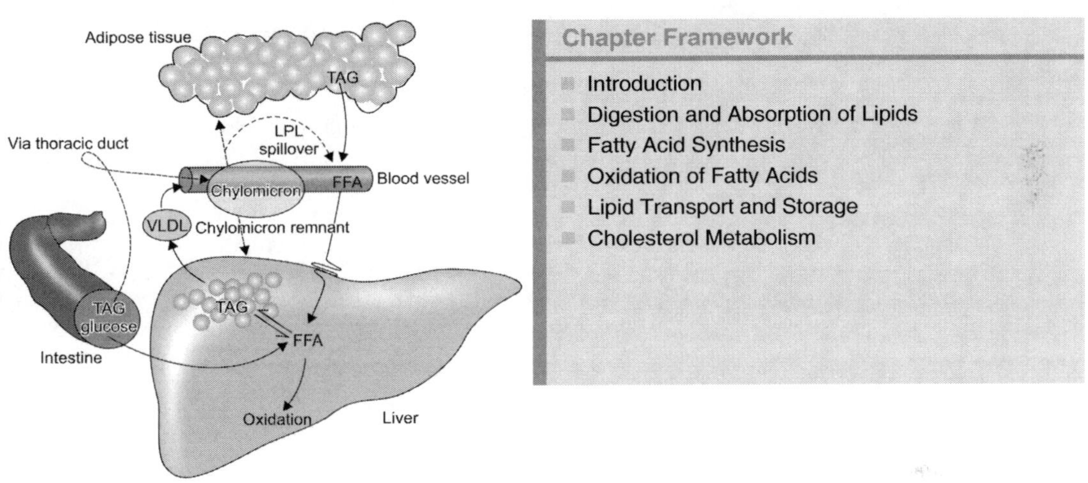

Chapter Framework

- Introduction
- Digestion and Absorption of Lipids
- Fatty Acid Synthesis
- Oxidation of Fatty Acids
- Lipid Transport and Storage
- Cholesterol Metabolism

Introduction

Lipid metabolism includes:

- The de novo synthesis of fatty acids via the FA synthase complex from excess carbohydrates.
- The biosynthesis of cholesterol.
- The synthesis of triglycerides at adipose tissue for storage.
- The mobilization of fatty acids from adipose tissue for oxidation.
- The transport of various lipids of endogenous and exogenous origin.
- The oxidation of fatty acids by β – oxidation for production of energy.

The dietary lipids are digested, absorbed and transported via chylomicrons to various body tissues to be utilized for structural purposes, energy production or for storage. Lipids are endogenously synthesized and transported from liver via lipoprotein particle (VLDL).

Digestion and Absorption of Lipids

Dietary Lipids

- Dietary fats are the most important cooking medium, providing taste and palatability to our food. Dietary fats include vegetable oils (sunflower, peanut, olive oil, etc.), butter and ghee.
- Chemically, the dietary fats provide us with triglycerides, cholesterol, essential fatty acids and fat soluble vitamins.

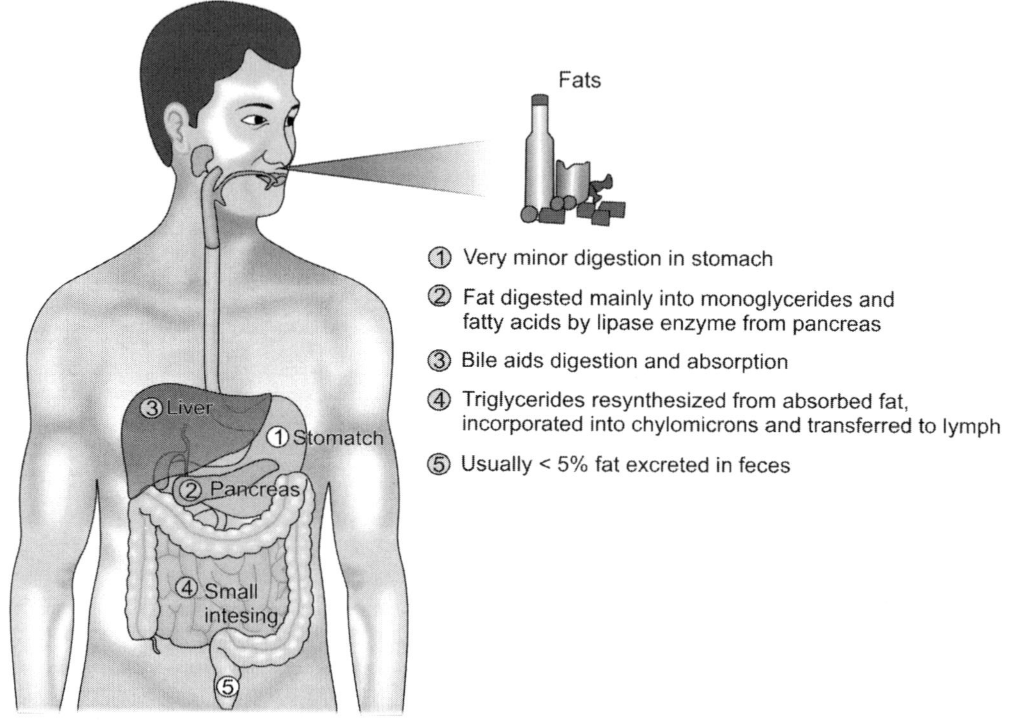

Fig. 11.1 Digestion and absroption of dietary lipids

- The digestion of dietary fat takes place in three phases, known as the gastric, duodenal, and ilial phases. These involve crude emulsification in the stomach, lipolytic breakdown by lipases and solubilization with bile salts in the duodenum and, finally, absorption into the epithelial cells or enterocytes lining the walls of the small intestine or ileum.
- One of the major challenges in the digestion and absorption of dietary fats is their insolubility in water and that the dietary triglycerides are too large to be absorbed directly into circulation. These are overcome by the emulsification of the fat in our stomach by the bile salts of bile juice.

Process of Digestion

At mouth

- Dietary lipids are slightly digested at mouth by the lingual lipase. This enzyme hydrolyses the dietary triglycerides of short chain saturated fatty acids. The enzyme is secreted by the Ebner's glands of the buccal cavity. It is one of the key components that make the digestion of milk fat in new born possible. Lingual lipase can penetrate into the milk fat globule, which makes this lipase vital to the digestive process of milk fat in new born babies. It hydrolyzes dietary triglycerides, forming diacylglycerols and free fatty acids.
- Lingual lipase has a low pH optimum, which makes it possible for this lipase to remain active even when pH levels are low. Thus, when the food bolus moves from mouth to the stomach,

some of the lipid digestion continues at the core of the bolus, till the pH drops down too acidic to stop its activity.

Gastric Phase (Fig. 11.2)

- The digestion by the lingual lipase continues at stomach till the pH at the core of the bolus drops too low. The stomach secretes another preduodonal lipase–gastric lipase. Gastric lipase is an acidic lipase secreted by the gastric chief cells in the fundic mucosa in the stomach.
- It has a pH optimum of 3–6. However, it acts at the small intestine. It also hydrolyzes the saturated short and medium chain fatty acid triglycerides.
- Together both these preduodenal lipases digest about 30% of the saturated short and medium chain triglycerides. In neonates, this may be as high as 50%.

Duodenal Phase (Fig. 11.2)

- The gastric chyme is acidic in nature. When it pours into the anterior part of the duodenum it stimulates the secretion of secretin and the partially digested fat induces release of cholecystokinin.
- Secretin causes secretion of bicarbonate rich pancreatic juice, thus neutralizing the acidic gastric chyme and making an environment suitable to pancreatic lipase.
- Cholecystokinin on the other hand induces secretion of the pancreatic enzymes.
- Also cholecystokinin induces the contraction f the gallbladder such that bile is poured alon with the pancreatic juice.
- The bile contains: Bile salts, cholesterol and a phospholipid called lecithin - major function of bile is emulsification of dietary fat.

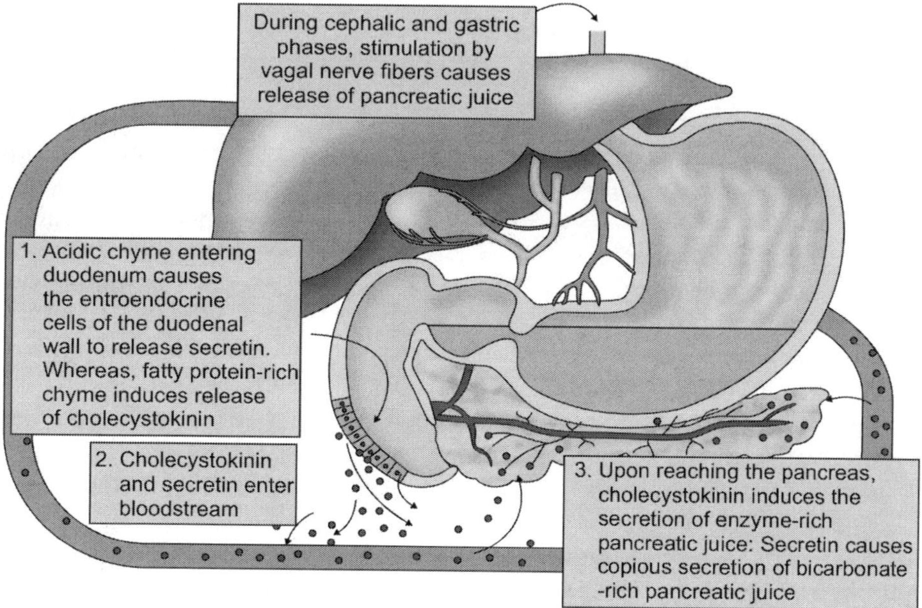

Fig. 11.2 Secretion of secretin and cholecystokinin

- Emulsification of the dietary fat breaks down the large fat globules into smaller ones thus increasing the surface area for the enzyme activity (Fig. 11.3).
- Among the pancreatic lipolytic enzymes, the pancreatic lipase is the most significant. Besides there is also secretion of a pancreatic colipase, phospholipase and cholesterol esterase.
- The colipase is an important enzyme as it helps anchor the pancreatic lipase on to its substrate triglycerides.
- Dietary triglycerides are hydrolyzed by the pancreatic lipase into 2, 3–di-acylglycerol and free fatty acids and then further hydrolysed to give 2 – monoacylglycerol.

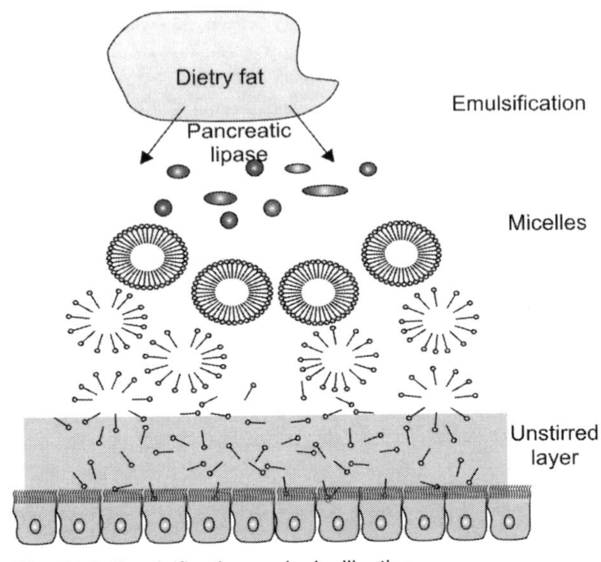

Fig. 11.3 Emulsification and micellization

- Dietary cholesterol esters are hydrolyzed into free cholesterol and fatty acids by cholesterol esterase.
- Dietary phospholipids are digested by phospholipases secreted in pancreatic juice. Phospholipases hydrolyzes the phospholipids into fatty acid and lysolecithin.

Ileal Phase

Micellization and Absorption of Dietary Lipids

- The bile salts along with phospholipids form micelles that have a peripheral layer of bile salts and the digested lipids occupy the central core of it. The lipids at the core are the monoglycerides, fatty acids, fat soluble vitamins and cholesterol (Fig. 11.4).
- Micelles are much smaller than emulsion droplets (4–7 nm versus 1 μm for emulsion droplets). Micelles are necessary because they transport the poorly soluble monoglycerides and fatty acids to the surface of the enterocyte where they can be absorbed.
- Micelles are constantly breaking down and reforming. They carry the nonpolar monoglycerides and fatty acids to the brush border.
- Because of their nonpolar nature, monoglycerides and fatty acids can just diffuse across the plasma membrane of the enterocyte.
- Some of the medium chain and short chain fatty acids simply diffuse across the cell membrane of the mucosal cell without micellization.
- Within the enterocyte, the monoglycerides are re-esterified to triglycerides and these then are secreted with chylomicrons into the lacteals.
- Cholesterol and FAs occupy the core of the micelles and are absorbed into the enterocyte to be secreted with chylomicron.
- End products of phospholipid digestion combine with the bile salts and form the micelles and are absorbed into the enterocytes and secreted with chylomicrons.
- During absorption the bile salts remain out of the enterocytes, only the end products of lipid digestion are absorbed.

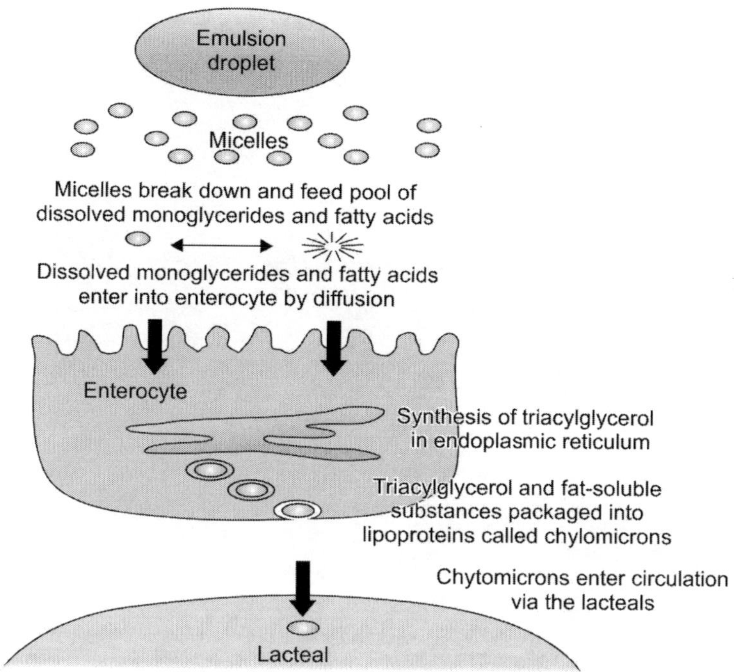

Fig. 11.4 Micellization and absorption of dietary fats

Fatty Acid Synthesis

Introduction

- Fatty acids are synthesized by the condensation of acetyl CoA units repetitively to form palmitate and other even chain fatty acids.
- Fatty acids are needed for:
  - The synthesis of triglycerides to be stored at adipose tissue
  - The synthesis phospholipids
  - The synthesis of sphingolipids
- Fatty acids are primarily synthesized in the cytosolic fraction of cells.
- The predominant tissues where this pathway is active are adipose tissue and to a little extent in liver.
- The prerequisition of fatty acid synthesis is the availability of the substrate (acetylCoA and NADPH).

Transfer of Acetate Units from Mitochondrial Acetyl CoA to the Cytosol

- Mitochondrial acetyl CoA is produced by the oxidation of pyruvate, and by the oxidation of fatty acids, ketone bodies, and certain amino acids. The coenzyme A portion of acetyl CoA, however, cannot cross the mitochondrial membrane; only the acetyl portion is transported to the cytosol (Fig. 11.5).

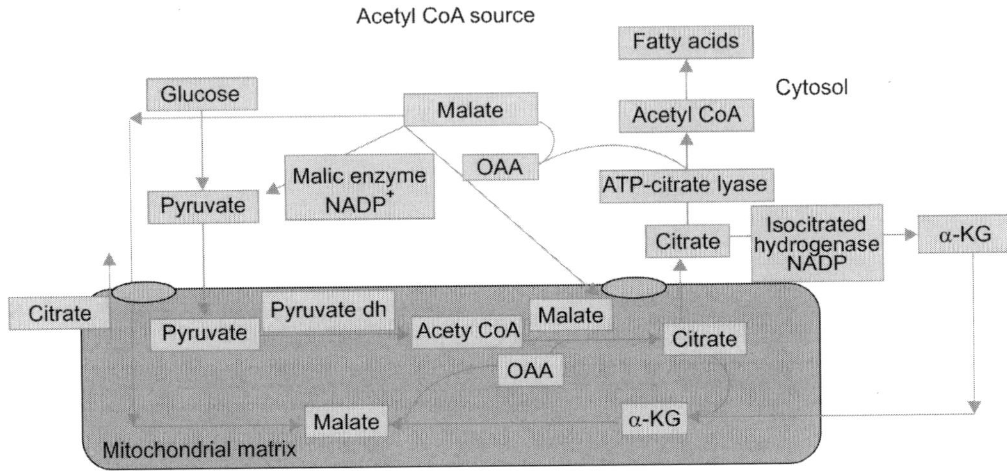

Fig. 11.5 Sources of acetyl CoA and NADPH +H+ for fatty acid synthesis

Sources of NADPH

- NADPH+H+ is derived from:
  - Two dehydrogenases of HMP shunt
  - Malic enzyme – This enzyme is a cytosolic enzyme that oxidises malate to pyruvate in cytosol using NADP+ as a coenzyme.
  - Cytosolic isocitrate dh.

Pathway of Fatty acid Synthesis

- The process of fatty acid synthesis is divided into:
  - *Initiation*
  - *Pathway*
  - *Elongation.*

Initiation

- The initiation of fatty acid synthesis occurs with the carboxylation of acetyl CoA to malonyl CoA in the presence of the key regulatory enzyme of fatty acid synthesis – *acetyl CoA carboxylase.*
- The enzyme is a multi-subunit enzyme that needs biotin as a coenzyme for its activity. It is an allosterically regulated enzyme, with citrate and ATP being the positive modifiers and long chain fatty acids as the negative modifier.

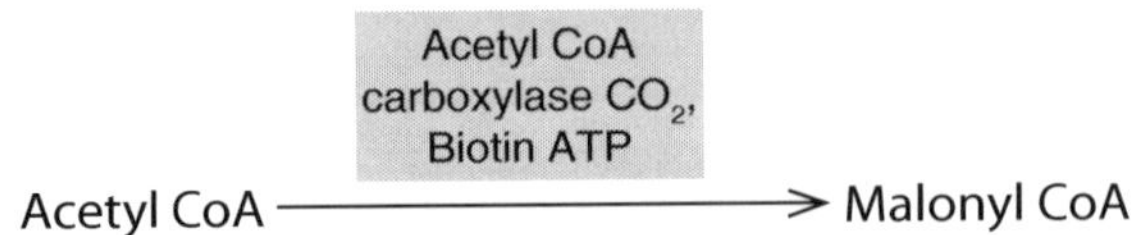

- The carboxylation occurs in the presence of HCO_3^- ions that donate CO_2.

Pathway

- The synthesis of fatty acid requires another multienzyme complex – *Fatty Acid Synthase complex.*
- The multienzyme complex is made up of two identical subunits (Fig. 11.6).
- Each subunit contains seven enzymes and an acyl carrier protein (ACP).
- ACP contains 4′-phosphopantetheine as a prosthetic group which has got a free sulphydryl (SH) group to which intermediates of fatty acid synthesis are bound.
- Condensing enzyme – Ketoacyl synthase has got a cysteine residue whose sulphydryl group binds acetyl (or acyl) group.
- The two subunits are arranged in a head to tail manner such that condensing enzyme cysteine residue of one subunit faces the ACP of the second subunit and vice versa.
- The two functional units synthesize two fatty acid molecules simultaneously.
- The process begins with the binding of acetyl CoA to cysteine residue of the ketoacyl synthase of both the subunits in the presence of acetyl transcylase. Then the malonyl CoA binds to the SH group of Acyl carrier Protein (ACP) in the presence of malonyl transacylase. This enzyme molecule with acetyl and malonyl groups attached is termed as the acetyl – malonyl enzyme.
- The acetyl group from subunit 1 shifts to the malonyl group on second subunit and with the decarboxylation of malonyl group, acetyl group condenses with it forming the 3 – ketoacyl enzyme (condensing enzyme).
- There is reduction of 3 – ketoacyl enzyme by NADPH+H^+ dependent enzyme – 3 – ketoacyl reductase to form 3- hydroxyacyl enzyme.
- NADPH + H^+ is provided by the HMP shunt (mainly), isocitrate dh (cytosolic) and malic enzyme.
- 3 – hydroxyacyl enzyme is then dehydrated by the hydratase enzyme in the fourth step to give 2,3 – unsaturated acyl enzyme.

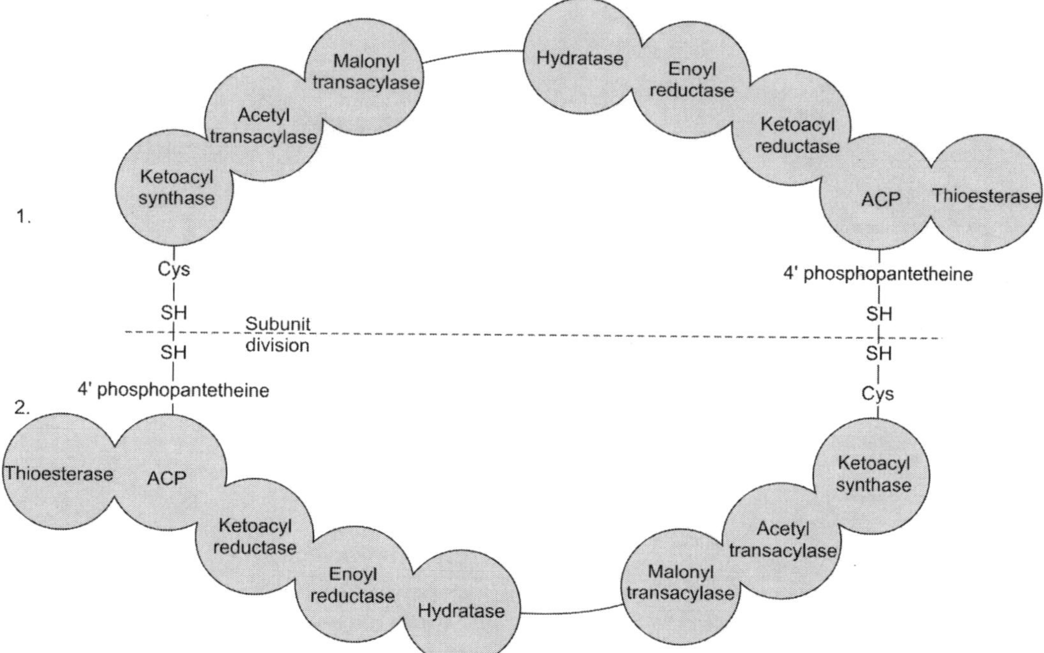

Fig. 11.6 Fatty acid synthase complex

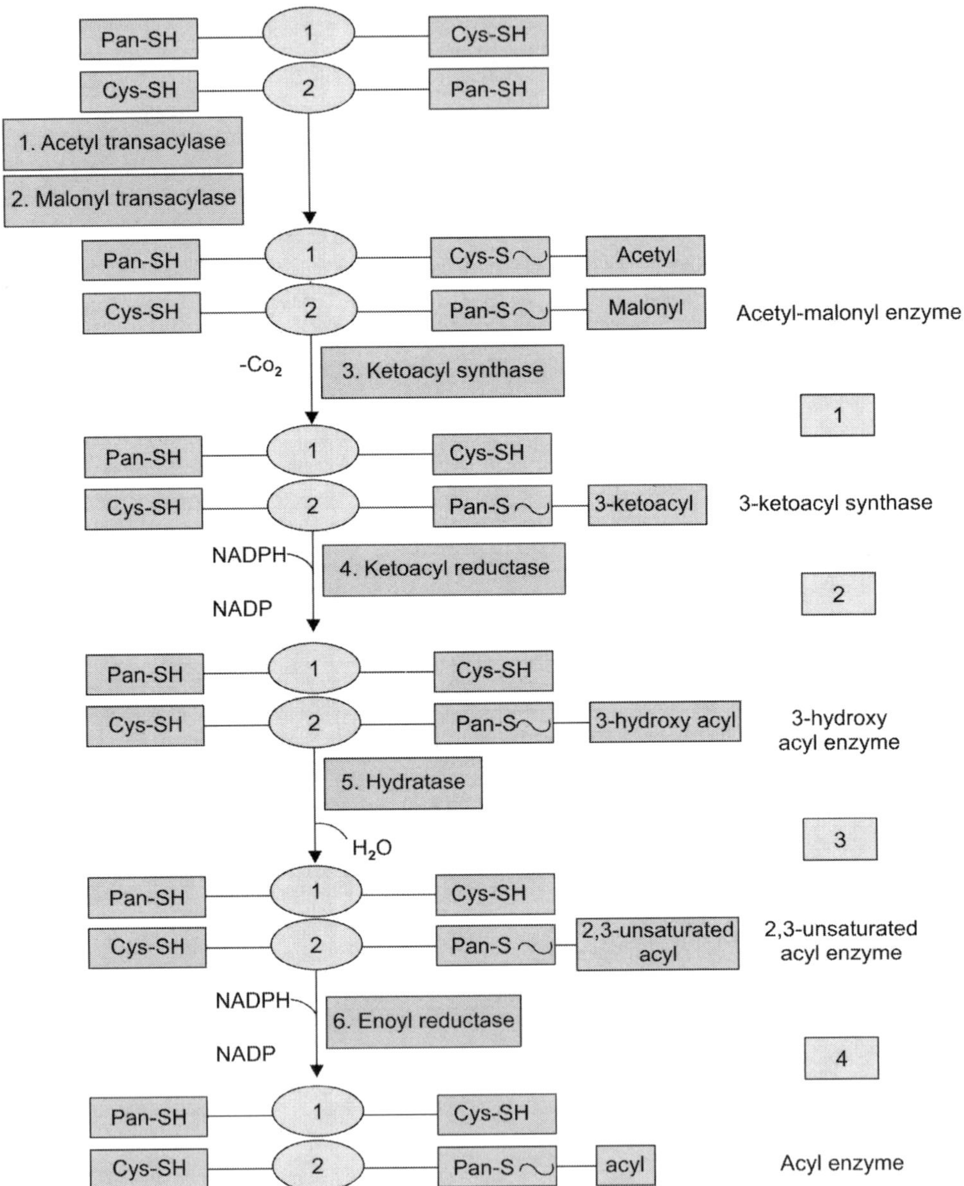

Fig. 11.7 Steps of fatty acid synthesis

- Finally the 2, 3 – unsaturated acyl enzyme is saturated by the enzyme enoyl reductase (NADPH+H^+ dependent) to give a saturated acyl enzyme derivative.
- These steps are repeated (step 1–4 of Figure 11.7) 7 times to give a 16 carbon residue attached to the FA synthase complex (2 residues one each on either ends).

- Once a palmitate residue is formed, the final enzyme of FA synthase – Thioesterase causes the release of the palmitate from the FA synthase complex.
- At the mammary gland, there is a different thioesterase specific for the C8, C10, C12 fatty acids which are present in the milk.
- For the synthesis of 16 – C palmitate, the steps 1 – 4 of Figure 11.7 are repeated 7 times.

Net reaction for palmitate synthesis is:

- 8 Acetyl CoA + 7 ATP + 14 NADPH + 14 H^+ ⟶ palmitate + 8 CoA + 7 ADP + 7 Pi + 14 $NADP^+$ + 6 H_2O

Elongation

- It occurs at the microsomal and mitochondrial fractions.
- Mitochondrial chain elongation is not very active and uses acetyl CoA as the donor of 2 – C units.
- Microsomal chain elongation is more active and uses malonyl CoA as the donor of 2–C units and NADPH+H^+ as the reducing power.
- Chain elongation occurs rapidly in well fed state and is abolished in fasting and diabetes mellitus.
- The process involves enzyme fatty acid elongase system, which acts similar to fatty acid synthase accept that the intermediates don't remain attached to a multienzyme complex.

Regulation of Fatty Acid Synthesis

Nutritional Status

- Lipogenesis occurs in the anabolic phase of metabolism.
- During the anabolic phase excess carbohydrate – glucose and intermediates like pyruvate, acetyl CoA and lactate convert to fats to be used in periods of deprivation like fasting or hibernation in other mammals.
- Thus lipogenesis is high during the well fed state.
- It is reduced in fasting conditions, in starvation, DM and feeding high fat diet.
- In all these conditions plasma fatty acid levels are high and there is an inverse relationship between plasma fatty acid levels and hepatic lipogenesis.
- When dietary fat is >10%, dietary carbohydrates will not be converted to fat.

Short-term Regulation (Allosteric)

- Acetyl CoA carboxylase is allosterically activated by citrate and inhibited by long chain acyl CoA.
- Citrate is high in well fed conditions indicating there is enough of substrate for lipogenesis.
- Acyl CoA when not esterified rapid enough, is high in plasma as in:
  - Lipolysis
  - High fat diet
  - DM
  - Fasting
  - Starvation.
- During these conditions, the high circulating fatty acids cause a feedback inhibition of their own synthesis, allosterically.

- High acyl CoA also inhibits the citrate transporter of mitochondrial membrane, so that no more citrate comes out of mitochondria to provide acetyl CoA as substrate.
- Acyl CoA also inhibits ATP/ADP exchange transporter of mitochondria, so the levels of ATP become high in mitochondria and Pyruvate dh is inhibited.
- Thus the availability of acetyl CoA reduces , further decreasing lipogenesis.

Long-term Regulation (Hormonal)

Insulin

- Increases glucose entry into adipose tissue, so increased substrate available for lipogenesis.
- Increases the esterification at liver.
- Increases the activity of Acetyl CoA, carboxylase and pyruvate dehydrogenase by covalent modification (dephosphorylation). So both the substrate of lipogenesis and the process of lipogenesis are increased.
- It inhibits lipolysis at the adipose tissue by inhibiting hormone sensitive lipase (reducing c – AMP)

Glucagon

- Increases lipolysis by increasing the concentration of c –AMP which activates hormone sensitive lipase.
- Inhibits *acetyl CoA carboxylase and pyruvate dehydrogenase* by phosphorylating, thus decreasing substrate availability.

Oxidation of Fatty Acids

Introduction

- Oxidation of fatty acids is a multi-step process occurring in various tissues during the catabolic phase of metabolism primarily to supply energy.
- The cellular site of fatty acid oxidation is mitochondria.
- Most fatty acids are oxidized by β-oxidation where there is a sequential removal of 2 carbon units in each cycle as acetyl CoA.
- Other pathways for oxidation of fatty acids are the α and omega oxidation pathways which are of minor significance.
- The cycle is repeated till whole fatty acid is completely converted to acetyl CoA, which then enters the CAC to be completely oxidized. Most common pathway of fatty acid oxidation is β-oxidation.
- Increased fatty acid oxidation is seen in conditions like uncontrolled diabetes mellitus, starvation and it leads to ketosis (excessive production of ketone bodies).

Activation of Fatty Acid

- A fatty acid is activated prior to entering the β-oxidation pathway by cytosolic enzyme *Thiokinase.*
- *Thiokinase* are of various types depending upon the C chain length (Fig. 11.8).

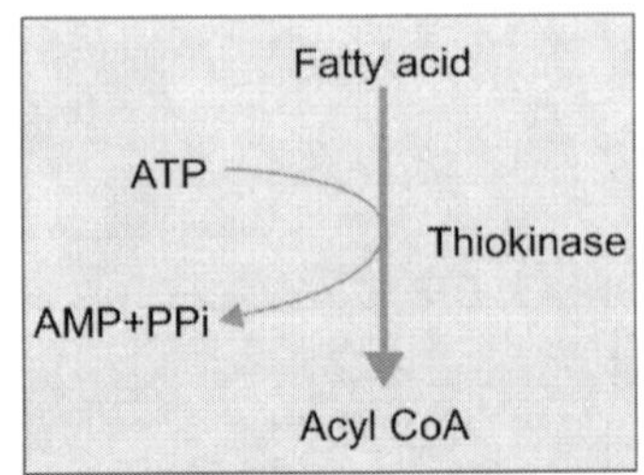

Fig. 11.8 Activation of fatty acid

Transport of Fatty Acids from Cytosol to Mitochondria

- Since the oxidation of fatty acids occurs in the mitochondria, thus a fatty acid has to be transported into the mitochondria. The short chain fatty acids can cross over into the mitochondria easily. However, the medium and long chain fatty acids require a special carrier system – *Carnitine transport system* (Fig. 11.9).
- Carnitine (β-hydroxy-γ-trimethylammonium butyrate), is widely distributed and is particularly abundant in muscle.
- Carnitine palmitoyl transferase 1 (CPT1) conversion of the long chain acyl-CoA to long chain acylcarnitine allows the fatty acid moiety to be transported across the inner mitochondrial membrane via carnitine translocase (CAT), which exchanges long chain acylcarnitines for carnitine.
- An inner mitochondrial membrane CPT2 then converts the long chain acylcarnitine back to long chain acyl-CoA. The long chain acyl-CoA enters the fatty acid β-oxidation pathway.

β-Oxidation (Figs 11.10 and 11.11)

- The four main enzymes involved in β-oxidation are: acyl-CoA dehydrogenase, enoyl-CoA hydratase, hydroxy acyl-CoA dehydrogenase, and ketoacyl-CoA thiolase (Fig. 11.10).
- Acyl-CoA dehydrogenase creates a double bond between the second and third carbons down from the CoA group on acyl-CoA and in the process produces a $FADH_2$.
- Next, enoyl-CoA hydratase removes the double bond just formed, in the process of adding a hydroxyl group to the third carbon down from the CoA group and hydrogen on the second carbon down from the CoA group.
- Hydroxyacyl-CoA dehydrogenase removes the hydrogen in the hydroxyl group just attached and in the process produces a NADH.
- In the final step, ketoacyl-CoA thiolase attaches a CoA group on to the third carbon down from the CoA group resulting in the formation of two molecules, an acetyl-CoA and an acyl-CoA that is two carbons shorter.

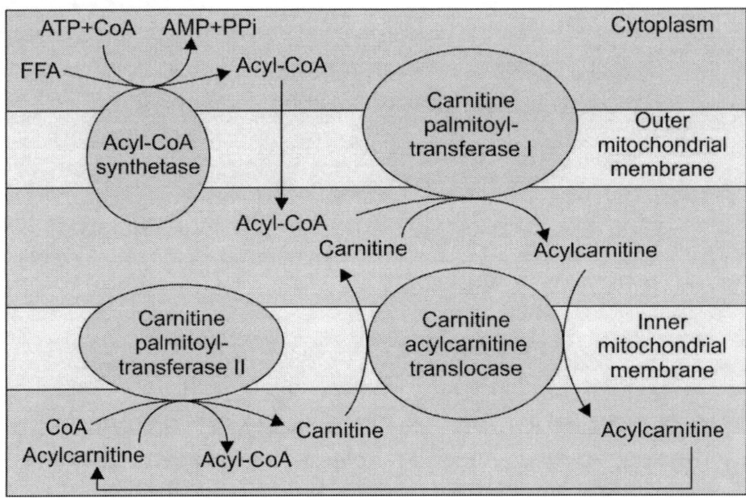

Fig. 11.9 Carnitine transport of fatty acids

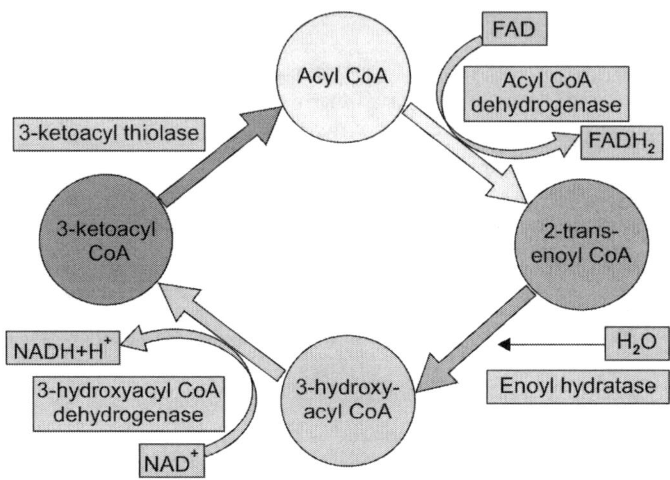

Fig. 11.10 β-oxidation pathway

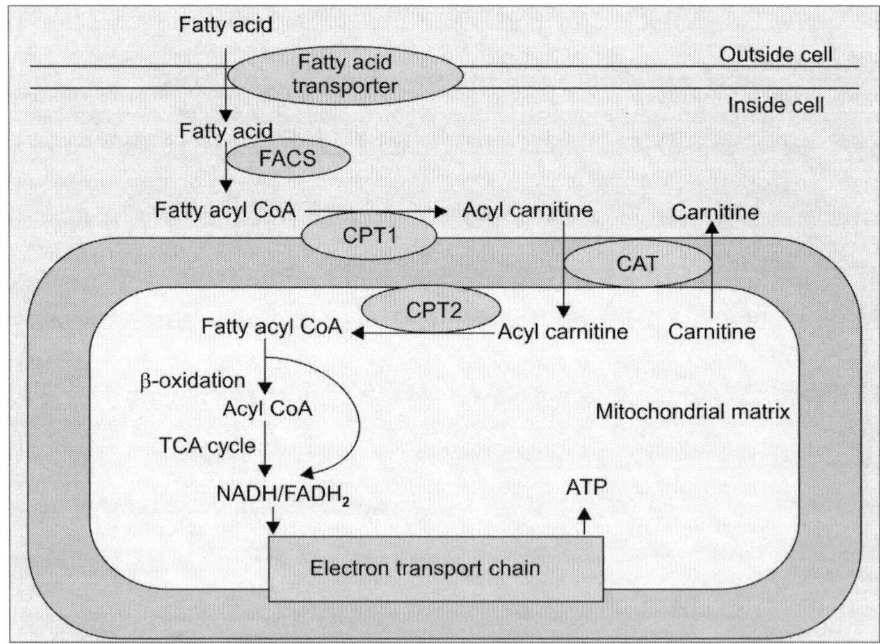

Fig. 11.11 An overview of β-oxidation

Fate of Acetyl CoA of β-Oxidation and Energetics of β-Oxidation

- This cycle goes on till the complete fatty acid molecule is oxidised to acetyl CoA units.
- If a palmitic acid is β-oxidised (C16), there will be 8 acetyl CoA units generated.
- There will be 7 β-oxidation cycles needed to release these 8 acetyl CO A units.
- Each acetyl CoA then enters the CAC.

- One β-oxidation cycle gives:
  - 1 $FADH_2$ i.e. 2 ATP
  - 1 $NADH+H^+$ i.e. 3 ATP
  - Total 5 ATP generated via respiratory chain per β–oxidation cycle
  - 7 cycles will give = 7 × 5 = 35 ATP
  - 8 acetylCoA in CAC = 12 × 8 = 96 ATP
  - Total ATP produced from 1 palmitic acid = 131
  - 2 ATP used in activation = 131 – 2 = 129 ATP
  - The acetyl CoA formed due to β-oxidation cannot enter the gluconeogenic pathway, because of lack of insulin
  - So in prolonged fasting or starvation the fatty acids oxidized to acetyl CoA liberate energy but do not synthesize glucose
  - Moreover, due to lack of OAA, the CAC is not properly established in prolonged fasting and starvation thus acetyl CoA is not completely oxidized.

Peroxisomal Oxidation of Fatty Acids

- A modified form of beta oxidation is seen in peroxisomes where the very long chain fatty acids (C_{22}, C_{24}, etc.) are oxidized upto octanoyl CoA and then further this octanoyl CoA is beta oxidized.
- The flavoproteins linked dehydrogenase step is associated with the production of H_2O_2 and is not linked to the respiratory chain. Thus, the peroxisomal dehydrogenation does not generate energy.
- This pathway is important for the shortening of the cholesterol side chain during bile acid synthesis. Besides, the peroxisomes are also involved in the synthesis of ether glycerolipids, cholesterol and dolichol.

Oxidation of Odd Chain Fatty Acids

- Odd chain fatty acids are oxidized by beta oxidation till 3 – C propionyl CoA is left.
- Fate of propionyl CoA is as shown in Figure 11.12.

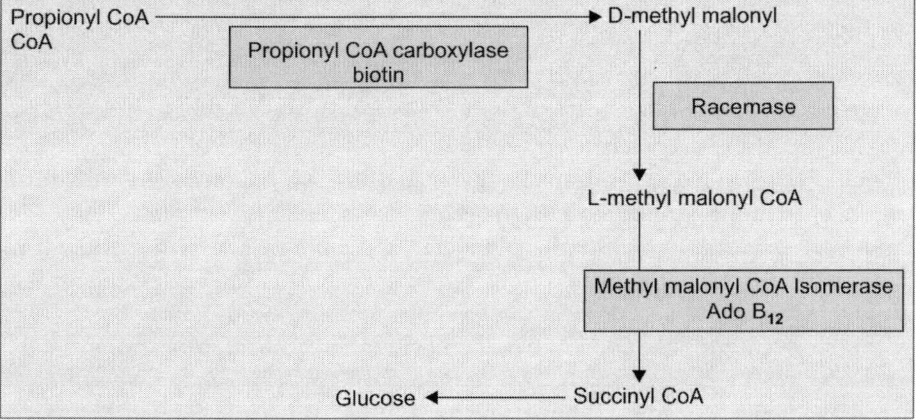

Fig. 11.12 Fate of propionyl CoA

Oxidation of Unsaturated Fatty Acids

- Oxidation of unsaturated fatty acids also occurs by β-oxidation untill a double bond is reached.
- Unsaturated fatty acids are also oxidized by β-oxidation but two additional enzymes are needed to deal with the double bonds.
- Double bonds in naturally occurring fatty acids have a *cis* conformation which, on hydration forms the D-isomers of hydroxyacyl CoA.
- At the double bond, two additional enzymes act:
  - Enoyl CoA isomerase – changing cis to trans configuration.
  - β-hydroxy acyl CoA epimerase – isomerises the L – isomer of β-hydroxy acyl CoA to D isomer, then β-oxidation proceeds.

α Oxidation

- Alpha oxidation pathway is present in brain. It is responsible for the oxidation of branched chain fatty acid phytanic acid, metabolic product of phytol, which occurs as a constituent of chlorophyll.
- Phytanic acid is a significant constituent of milk lipids and animal fats, and normally it is metabolized by an initial a hydroxylation followed by dehydrogenation and decarboxylation. β-oxidation cannot occur initially because of the presence of the 3methyl group.
- One carbon atom is removed at a time in the form of carbon dioxide and then β-oxidation can proceed.

ω Oxidation

- Another minor oxidative pathway is omega (ω)-oxidation in which the ω-carbon (CH_3) is converted into a carboxyl group and, then, b-oxidation starts.
- Two carbon atoms are removed successively from both the ends until a 6-carbon or 8-carbon dicarboxylic acid is left which is excreted in urine.
- The 6-carbon product is adipic acid, and the 8-carbon product is suberic acid from both the ends.

Ketone Bodies Synthesis (Ketogenesis)

- The liver constantly synthesizes low levels of ketone bodies—ketogenesis; their production becomes much more significant during fasting when ketone bodies are needed to provide energy to the peripheral tissues.
- The conditions when excessive fatty acids are oxidized are uncontrolled diabetes mellitus, starvation, etc. During prolonged fasting, at the liver acetyl CoA produced by the fatty acid breakdown (β-oxidation) inhibits the pyruvate dehydrogenase enzyme and activates the pyruvate carboxylase (key enzyme of gluconeogenesis). This causes the disruption of CAC and thus ketosis occurs.
- The compounds categorized as ketone bodies include – acetoacetate, acetone and β-hydroxy butyrate. The synthesis involves the condensation of 2 acetyl CoA to give acetoacetyl CoA catalyzed by thiolase enzyme as shown in Figure 11.13.
- Next the acetoacetyl CoA gets another acetyl CoA to condense in the presence of HMG CoA synthase and forms HMG CoA (3 – hydroxy – 3 – methyl glutaryl CoA).

- HMG CoA is then lysed to produce the ketone body acetoacetate with the elimination of acetyl CoA.
- Acetoacetate acts like the parent ketone body that can be decarboxylated spontaneously to acetone and be dehydrogenated to β-hydroxy butyrate by the enzyme β-hydroxy butyrate dehydrogenase (a NAD^+ dependent enzyme).
- The normal blood levels of ketone bodies are about 3 mg/dL and these are excreted via urine (acetoacetate and β-hydroxy butyrate) and with expired air (acetone).

Acetyl CoA

Thiolase

Acetoacetyl CoA

HMG-CoA synthase

Hydroxy-b-methylglutaryl CoA

HMG-CoA lyase

Acetoacetate

D-β hydroxybutyrate dehydrogenase

Acetone+CO_2 D-β hydroxybutyrate

Fig. 11.13 Ketone bodies synthesis

Oxidation of Ketone Bodies

- Liver has the enzymatic machinery to synthesize ketone bodies however; it lacks the enzymes that oxidize them.
- Ketone bodies are oxidized by the extra – hepatic tissues as fuel sources.
- Normally very less amount of ketone bodies are oxidized by extrahepatic tissues.
- They are used in proportion to their concentration in the blood by extrahepatic tissues, such as the skeletal and cardiac muscle and renal cortex. Brain too can oxidize ketone bodies and use them as fuel source.

Ketosis

- In conditions of prolonged fasting and starvation, insulin levels are reduced and glucagon is high, which activates the hormone sensitive lipase to cause excessive lipolysis and fats are lipolysed to provide energy.
- Liver picks up 30% of the circulating fatty acids under all circumstances.
- During prolonged fasting and starvation, there are high levels of fatty acids, so more are picked up by liver and oxidized by β-oxidation. (Fig. 11.14)
- β-oxidation causes an over production of acetyl CoA, more than can be oxidized in the CAC. So the acetyl CoA condenses to form the ketone bodies in excess.
- These ketone bodies are released in circulation, when the levels exceeds 12 mmol/l they are excreted in urine (*ketonuria*) and by lungs (fruity smell, *Kaussamaul respiration)*
- The increased levels of ketone bodies in blood are called *ketonemia.*
- These ketone bodies are excreted as Na and K salts, thus causing electrolyte depletion, reduced alkali reserve and acidosis – *Ketoacidosis.*
- These are osmotically active so excreted with lots of water.

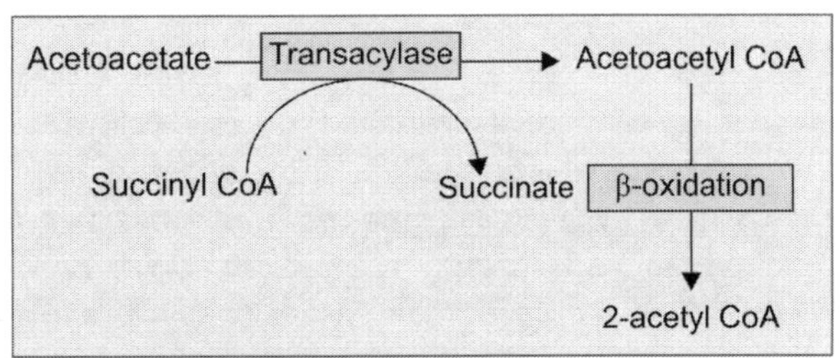

Fig. 11.14 Oxidation of ketone bodies

Adverse Effects of Ketosis

- The ketone bodies are acidic in nature and have to be excreted as their Na and K salts via urine. Thus their excessive excretion leads to a loss of the alkali reserve ($NaHCO_3$) of the body and causes (Fig. 11.15)
  - Ketoacidosis
  - Electrolyte imbalance
  - Fluid depletion
- All the above abnormalities cause severe clinical complications leading to enzyme dysfunction, organ dysfunction, CNS impairment, coma and finally if not treated death.

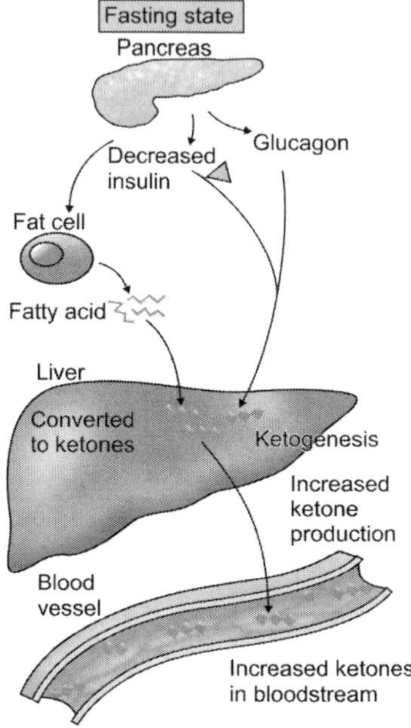

Fig. 11.15 Overview of ketosis

Regulation of Fatty Acid Oxidation and Esterification

- The regulation of fatty acid oxidation occurs at three levels:
  - At the level of entry of fatty acid into the mitochondria
  - Allosteric control
  - Hormonal control.

At the Level of Entry into Mitochondria

- The entry of fatty acids into the liver mitochondria is guarded by the regulation of the CPT -1 transporter by malonyl CoA.
- The liver picks up approximately 30% of the circulating fatty acids under all circumstances and is blessed with an unlimited capacity to esterify the incoming fatty acid to triglycerides. However, under conditions of high plasma fatty acids such as prolonged fasting, starvation, uncontrolled diabetes mellitus—The high levels of acyl CoA entering the liver inhibits the key regulatory enzyme of fatty synthesis (acetyl CoA carboxylase).
- This reduces the concentration of malonyl CoA and removes its inhibition on CPT -1 thus more and more fatty acids enter the mitochondria for oxidation and less is available for esterification.
- When the plasma fatty acid levels are low, the amount of fatty acid picked up by the liver shall also be low (i.e. low acyl CoA) which will remove the inhibition of acyl CoA on malonyl CoA and thus the CPT – 1 is blocked for the fatty acids to enter oxidative pathway and would be esterified.

Allosteric Control

- The key enzyme of fatty acid synthesis is allosterically modified by acyl CoA (negative modifier). High levels of it would inhibit the enzyme.
- The activity of the enzymes of fatty acid β-oxidation is affected by the level of the products of their reactions. Each of the β-oxidation enzymes are inhibited by the specific fatty acyl-CoA intermediate it produces. Interestingly, 3-ketoacyl-CoA can also inhibit enoyl-CoA hydratase and acyl-CoA dehydrogenase. β - Oxidation can also be allosterically regulated by the ratio of NADH/NAD^+ and acetyl-CoA/CoA level. A rise in the NADH/NAD^+ or acetyl-CoA/CoA ratios results in inhibition of fatty acid β-oxidation. Increases in the acetyl-CoA/CoA ratio have specifically been shown to lead to feedback inhibition of ketoacyl-CoA thiolase.

Hormonal Control

- The oxidation of fatty acids is affected by the ratio of insulin/glucagon.
- During fasting the reduced insulin/glucagon ratio phosphorylates and covalently modifies the enzyme acetyl CoA carboxylase such that the enzyme is inactivated leading to a reduction in concentration of malonyl CoA which relieves the inhibition on CPT – 1 and thus fatty acids are oxidized.
- Conversely during well fed conditions the serum insulin increases which dephosphorylates acetyl CoA carboxylase to activate it and increase the concentration of malonyl CoA which inhibits the CPT – 1.

Clinical Aspects of Fatty Acid Oxidation (Fig. 11.16)

Carnitine Deficiency

- Carnitine deficiency may be seen:
  - Patients of liver diseases – reduced synthesis
  - Patients of hemodialysis – carnitine gets removed form blood
  - During pregnancy – demand is more
  - In malnutrition or in pure vegans.
- Such individuals will be unable to oxidize the long chain fatty acids and thus there is accumulation of long-chain fatty acids and branched chain acyl residues in toxic amounts.
- Genetically carnitine deficiency is seen when there is a congenital lack of CPT-1 leading to an inability of the tissues to oxidize fatty acids. Thus the energy supply for gluconeogenesis is not available and causes hypoglycemia.
- Similarly, CPT – 2 deficiencies is seen on cardiac and skeletal muscles with symptoms of muscle weakness, cardiomyopathy and myoglobinuria on severe exercise.

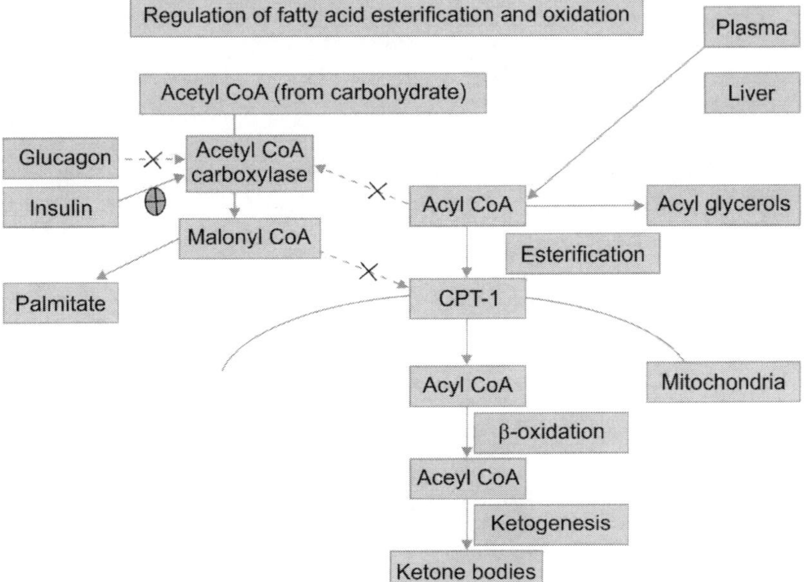

Fig. 11.16 Regulation of fatty acid oxidation and esterification

Medium Chain FA Dehydrogenase (MCAD) Deficiency

- This is one of the commonest inborn errors of fatty acid oxidation.
  It causes a decrease in fatty acid oxidation and severe hypoglycemia (because the tissues cannot obtain full energetic benefit from fatty acids and, therefore, must now rely on glucose).
- Infants are particularly affected by MCAD deficiency, because they rely for their nourishment on milk, which contains primarily MCADs.
- Treatment includes carbohydrate rich diet.

Refsum's Disease

An inherited defect in this pathway produces ***Refsum's disease***. Large amounts of phytanic acid accumulate in the body in Refsum's disease leading to neurological abnormalities with management involving dietary restriction of the fatty acid to check the disease progression.

Lipid Transport and Storage

Introduction (Fig. 11.17)

- Lipids are hydrophobic in nature and cannot be transported in an aqueous medium like plasma without being converted into more hydrophilic forms. Thus all lipids (endogenously synthesized and dietary) are made suitable for transport by converting them into ***Lipoproteins.***
- The lipoproteins are lipid – protein complexes which have a characteristic organization suitable for the transport of all lipids.

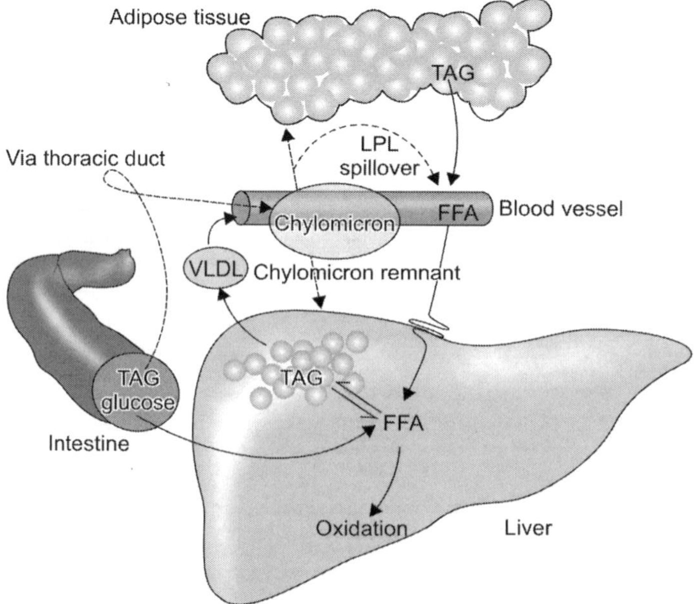

Fig 11.17 An overview of lipoprotein metabolism

Structure and Classification of Lipoproteins (Table 11.1)

- Structurally lipoproteins comprise of a peripheral coat of amphipathic lipids – bilayer of phospholipids and cholesterol and a central core of hydrophobic lipids as shown in Figure 11.18.

Table 11.1 Types of apoproteins

Apo A1	HDL, chylomicron	Activator of LCAT and ligand for HDL
Apo B_{100}	LDL, VLDL, IDL	Ligand for LDL receptor
Apo $B_4$8	Chylomicrons, chylomicrons remnants	Ligand for chylomicron remnant receptor
Apo CII	VLDL, HDL, chylomicrons	Activator of LPL
Apo CI	VLDL, HDL, chylomicrons	Activator of LCAT
Apo C III	VLDL, HDL, chylomicrons	Inhibitor of LPL
Apo E	VLDL, HDL, IDL, chylomicrons and chylomicron remnant	Ligand of chylomicron remnant and LDL receptor

- The peripheral coat of amphipathic lipids also has apoproteins embedded in it. Some of the apoproteins are embedded right through the thickness of the amphipathic lipid coat – they are termed as the *integral apoproteins (apo – B_{100}, apo – B_{40})*. These apoproteins cannot be exchanged amongst different lipoprotein classes.
- Others do not extend throughout the thickness of the peripheral coat but are attached to the surface of it – they are termed as the *peripheral apoproteins (apo – C, apo – E)*. These apoproteins can be exchanged between different lipoprotein classes.

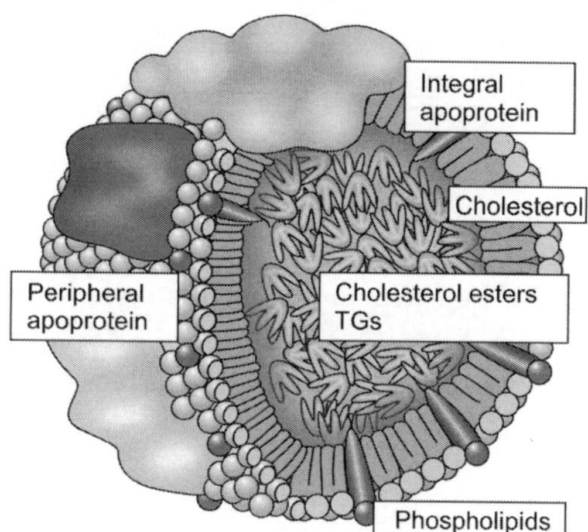

Fig 11.18 Structure of lipoprotein

- Functions of apoproteins
  - They serve as ligands for recognition by specific cellular receptors for, e.g. – apo- B_{100} is the ligand for LDL receptor.
  - They act as cofactors for the enzymes of lipoprotein metabolism for, e.g. apo – CII acts as the activator of enzyme lipoprotein lipase.
  - They provide polarity to lipoproteins.
- Apo B-100 is one of the longest single polypeptide chains known, having 4536 amino acids. Apo B-48 (48% of B-100) is formed from the same mRNA as apo B-100 after the introduction of a stop signal by an RNA editing enzyme.
- *The lipoproteins can be classified on the basis of:*
  - Density
  - Electrophoretic mobility

- As the amount of lipid increases in a lipoprotein, its density decreases and hence they are named as:
  - Chylomicrons
  - High density lipoprotein (HDLc)
  - Intermediate density lipoprotein (IDL)
  - Low density lipoproteins (LDLc)
  - Very low density lipoprotein (VLDL)
- Based upon the electrophoretic mobility the lipoproteins can be classified as (Fig. 11.19):
  - Alpha lipoproteins (HDLc)
  - β-lipoproteins (LDLc)
  - Pre – β-lipoproteins (VLDL)
  - Chylomicrons
- These names correspond respectively to the positions of the plasma proteins on electrophoresis.

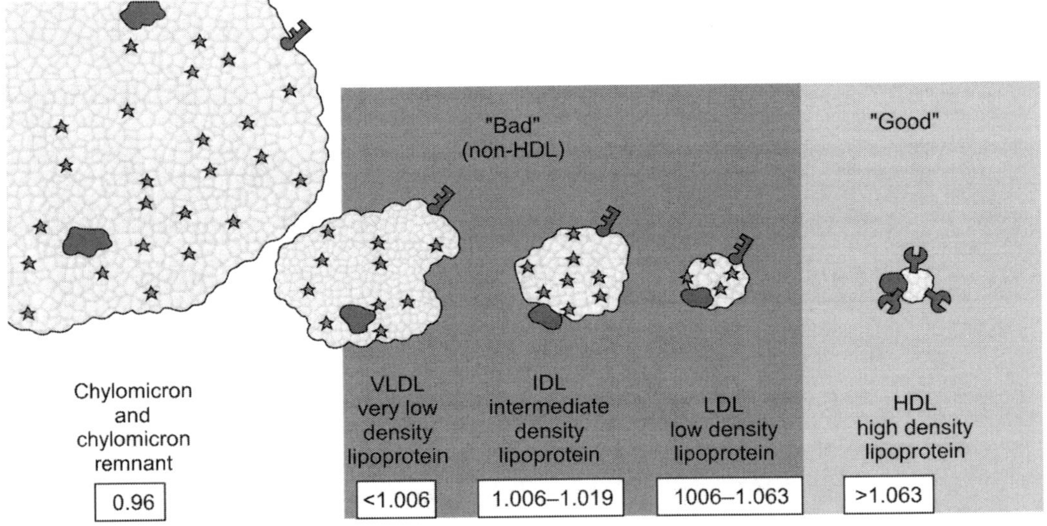

Fig. 11.19 Classification of lipoprotein

Chylomicrons Transport and Clearance (Fig. 11.20)

- Chylomicrons are synthesized and secreted by the intestinal mucosal cells as chyle draining the lymphatics of intestines. They are responsible for the transport of all dietary lipids like – triglycerides (predominantly), cholesterol esters, fat soluble vitamins, etc.
- The dietary lipids once absorbed at the intestinal mucosal cells, the monoacylglycerol re-esterifies to form triglycerides and cholesterol re-esterifies to cholesterol esters. The fat soluble vitamins are also esterified to their ester forms.
- The rough endoplasmic reticulum synthesizes apo – B_{48}. The dietary lipids are processed at the smooth ER and incorporate the apo – B_{48} with these lipids to form lipoprotein complexes – chylomicrons.
- These chylomicrons particles are further glycosylated at the smooth ER and then released into lacteals as nascent chylomicrons, particulate lipids of chyle.

- The lacteals open into the circulation via the thoracic duct and here they acquire the complete compliment of the apoproteins i.e. these nascent chylomicrons receive from HDL_C the apo – C – II and apo – E. This is so because Lipid metabolism is extremely dynamic. At the same time lipoproteins are processed to modify their nonpolar lipids, particles are interacting with each other, exchanging surface materials, apolipoproteins, and nonpolar lipids. HDL is an important reservoir for components cast off during the metabolism of other lipoproteins as well as lipids discarded by cells.

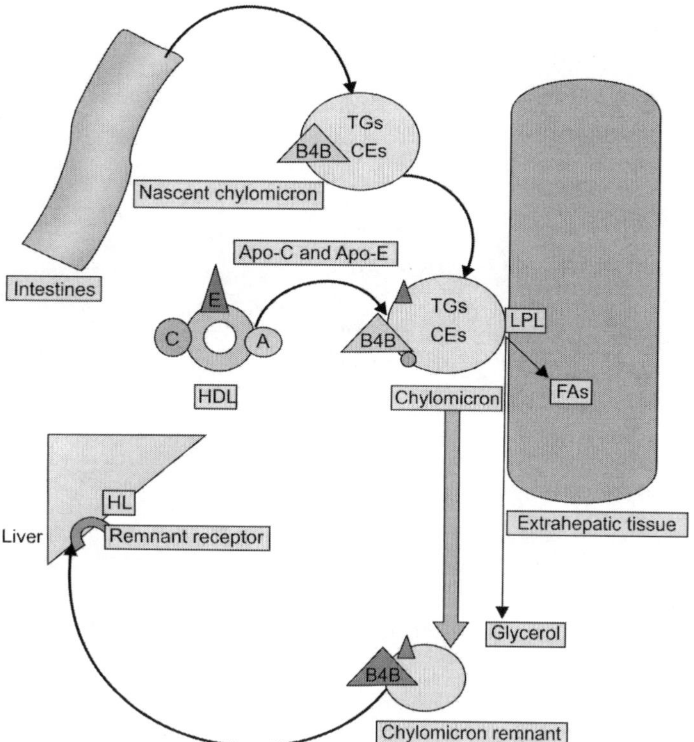

Fig. 11.20 Chylomicron metabolism

- The mature chylomicrons are then carried over to different peripheral tissues and organs going about distributing the absorbed lipids for utilization and storage.
- The triglycerides of chylomicrons get hydrolysed by the enzyme lipoprotein lipase (LPL) into free fatty acids and glycerol.
- The enzyme lipoprotein lipase is present bound to the walls of the blood capillaries, anchored to the endothelium by the proteoglycan chains of heparin sulfate and is found in tissues heart, adipose tissue, spleen, renal medulla, aorta, diaphragm, lactating mammary gland and neonatal liver but not in adult liver.
- At the adult liver is present another lipase – hepatic lipase, which is specific for chylomicron remnants and HDL_C metabolism but not with chylomicrons or VLDL.
- The enzyme LPL requires apo – C – II and phospholipids as cofactors for its optimal activity.
- The activity of LPL hydrolyses the TGs stepwise into diacylglycerol and FAs, monoacylglycerol and FAs and finally glycerol and FAs.
- The FFAs are transported in plasma bound to albumin; however bulk is transported into the tissue for oxidation as fuel or for storage as in adipose tissue.
- *The Km for Heart LPL is low than that of adipose tissue therefore during starvation, the fatty acids from TGs would be picked up more by the heart as a fuel source than being stored at adipose tissue. Thus the TGs are directed to heart during starvation.*
- The chylomicron remnants are cholesterol rich particles having the apo – E and apo –B_{48}. These are then finally picked up by the remnant receptor that recognises the apo – E as a ligand.

Synthesis, Transport and Metabolism of VLDL (Fig. 11.21)

- The synthesis of VLDL particles is also similar except that the site of synthesis is liver than intestines. The VLDL particles are transported from the liver to the extrahepatic tissues distributing endogenously synthesized triglycerides.
- The nascent VLDL particles have the apoprotein battery comprising of apo – C-II, apo – E, apo – B_{100}.
- It further receives its share of apo – C – II and apo – E from HDLc particle.
- VLDL reaches the extrahepatic tissues where in the presence of LPL, apo –C – II and phospholipids the TG store gets hydrolysed releasing the FAs to be taken up by the tissue and the glycerol into the circulation to be finally picked up by the liver as a gluconeogenic precursor.
- The LPL hydrolyses at one go about 30% of the TG content of VLDL making the resultant IDL richer in cholesterol. The apo – proteins apo – E is also lost back to the HDLc particles leaving behind apo – B_{100} and apo – C – II with IDL particles.
- These IDL particles are further carried to the extra hepatic tissues losing their TG content still further to the action of LPL and convert to the cholesterol rich LDLc particles.
- Another fate of IDL particles is that they may be directly picked up by the remnant receptor via the apo –E ligand. However, the major fate is conversion to LDLc particles.

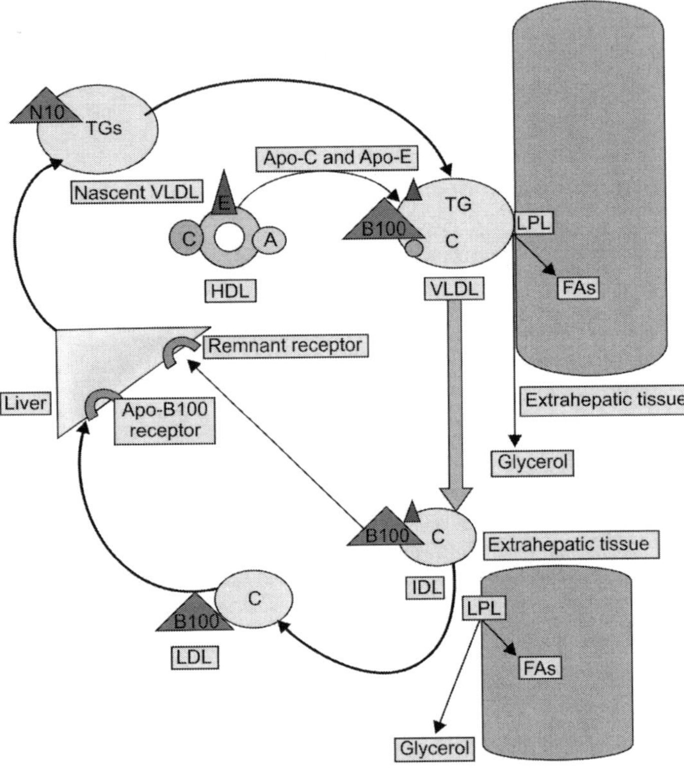

Fig. 11.21 VLDL and LDL transport

HDLc Metabolism

- HDLc is the 'good cholesterol'. It is synthesized at the intestines and liver with bilayer of phospholipids, limiting amounts of cholesterol, apo – A_1 and enzyme LCAT (lecithin – cholesterol acyl transferase). (Fig. 11.22)
- The nascent HDLc is discoid in shape when secreted. The liver nascent HDLc has the complete set of its constituent apoproteins i.e. apo – A_1, apo – C – I, C – II, C – III and apo – E.

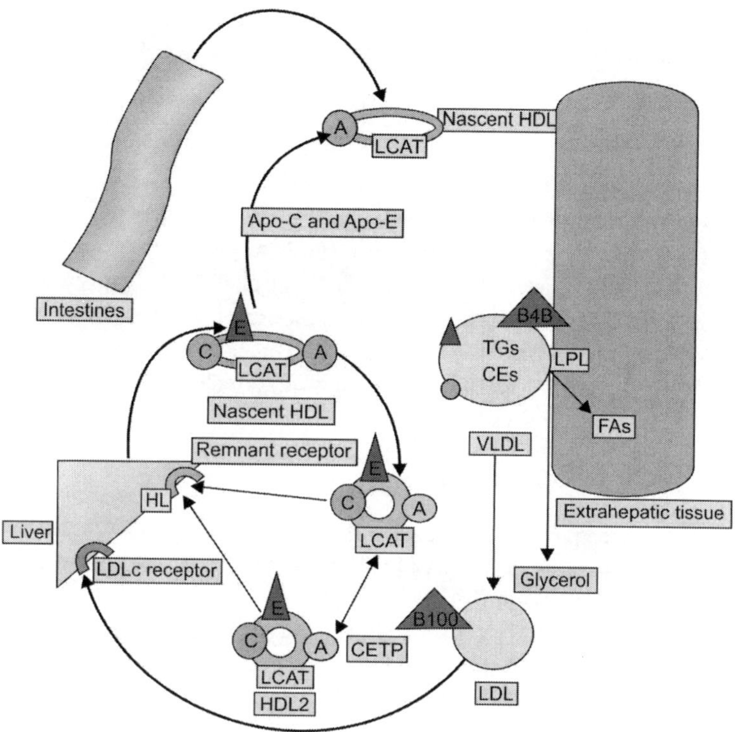

Fig. 11.22 HDLc metabolism

- Intestinal nascent HDLc does not have the complete set of apoproteins, rather has only apo – A_1 associated with phospholipids, limiting amounts of cholesterol and LCAT enzyme. However, it receives its complete set of apoproteins by transfer from the liver HDLc.
- As the HDLc is transported to various extrahepatic tissues in circulation, it exchanges free cholesterol from these tissues and from cholesterol rich lipoproteins like IDL, LDLc, chylomicron remnants to esterify it into cholesterol esters.
- The cholesterol esterification is carried out by the PUFA from C2 of phospholipids catalysed by LCAT with the release of lysolecithin in circulation.
- The cholesterol esters occupy the central core of HDLc and gradually this discoid HDLc particle acquires a spherical shape owing to the central occupancy of CEs.
- These spherical HDLc particles are the HDL_3 particles. These are responsible for the *reverse cholesterol transport – transport of cholesterol from tissues to liver.*
- The reverse cholesterol transport by HDLc is of great significance as it helps scavenge the free cholesterol present in tissues and in cholesterol rich lipoproteins like chylomicron remnants and LDLc such that it gets esterified to CEs and finally at the liver gets oxidised to bile salts.
- Thus HDLc is also termed as 'good cholesterol' since it scavenges the free cholesterol of LDLc (bad cholesterol) and chylomicron remnants.

- The HDL_3 particles receive more n more cholesterol from tissues via an ATP binding cassette transporter – 1 (that hydrolyses ATP for the binding of substrate) and converts to less dense HDL_2.
- The HDL_2 prevents feedback inhibition of CEs on LCAT by a protein – cholesterol ester transfer protein (CETP). This CETP transfers the CEs to VLDL in exchange for TGs making the HDL_2 particles richer in TGs and the VLDL particles richer in CEs.
- The plasma concentration of HDL_2 is inversely proportional to the risk of CVDs.
- HDL_2 reconverts to HDL_3 by either transferring its CEs to liver via a class B scavenger receptor (which picks up only the CEs and not the HDL particle). Or HDL_2 is hydrolysed by hepatic lipase to release phospholipids and TGs. Apo – A_1 is also released and some of it binds with minimum amounts of phospholipids and cholesterol to form pre-β-HDL.
- The pre β-HDL is most potent form in causing an efflux of cholesterol from tissues. An -excess of apo – A_1 is removed by kidneys.

Cellular Cholesterol Homeostasis

- Cholesterol is transported in plasma lipoproteins VLDL, IDL and LDLc.
- Cells need cholesterol for the synthesis of cell membranes, steroid hormones (adrenal gland and gonads), bile acids (liver cells), etc (Fig. 11.23).
- The cells pick up cholesterol via clathrin coated pits – LDLc receptors. These receptors are highly regulated and increase or decrease in number on the cell membrane depending upon the cellular cholesterol demand.

Increased Cellular Demand of Cholesterol

- When the cellular demand of cholesterol is high:
  - There occurs an up-regulation of the LDLc receptors causing increased uptake of LDLc particles. The LDLc receptors are taken in along with the LDLc particles. Once within the cell,

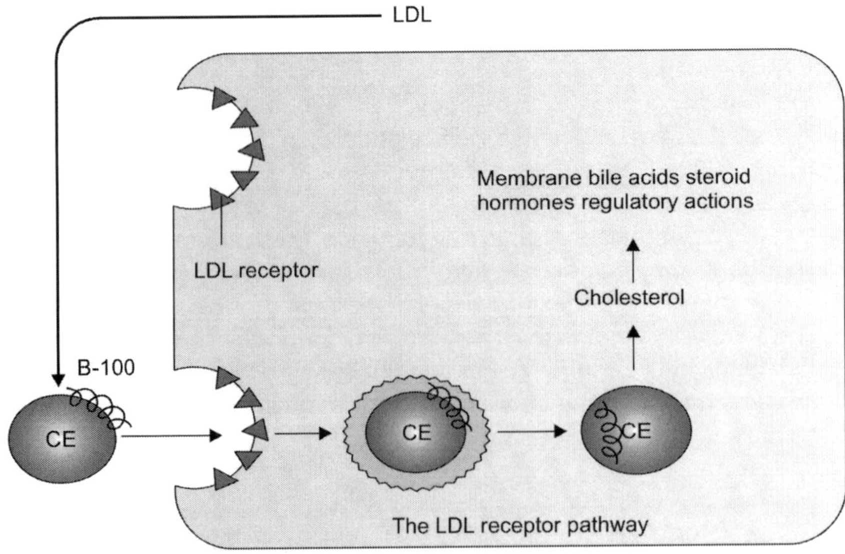

Fig. 11.23 Cholesterol homeostasis

these fuse with lysosomes forming an endosome where the LDLc is hydrolysed to release its cholesterol content to the cellular cholesterol pool and the receptors are released to occupy the cell membrane again, i.e. the receptors are recycled.
  - There is increased synthesis of cholesterol (all nucleated cells can synthesize cholesterol).
  - Some cholesterol is picked up by receptor free path directly from LDL and VLDL shown in Figure 11.24.
  - Cholesterol may be released by the increased activity of enzyme acyl cholesterol esterase (Fig. 11.24).
- The cholesterol taken up may be utilized for the cell membrane synthesis or steroid hormone synthesis or bile acid synthesis, etc.

Reduced Cellular Demand of Cholesterol

- When the cellular demand of cholesterol is reduced –
  - There is down – regulation of LDLc receptors due to feedback inhibition by the cellular pool of cholesterol.
  - Reduced biosynthesis of cholesterol due to feedback inhibition by the cellular pool of cholesterol.
  - More n more cholesterol gets esterified by the increased activity of acyl cholesterol acyl transferase (ACAT).
  - Some of the cholesterol is directly taken up by the HDLc particles under the effect of LCAT (Fig. 11.24).

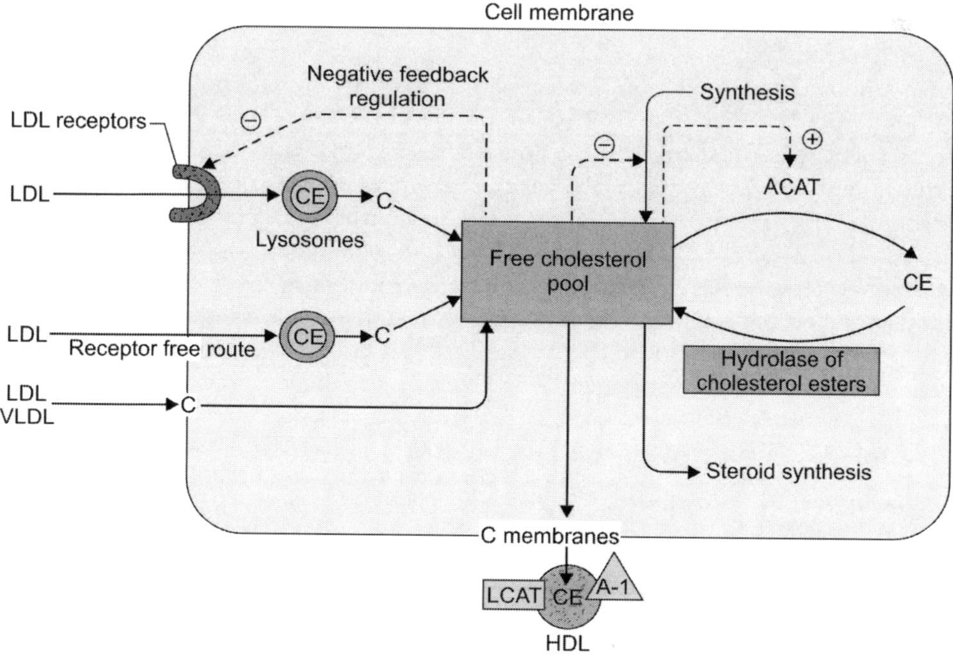

Fig. 11.24 Cellular cholesterol balance

Adipose Tissue Metabolism

- Fat is the largest energy reserve in mammals. Most tissues are involved in fatty acid metabolism, but three are quantitatively more important than others: adipose tissue, skeletal muscle and liver. Each of these tissues has a store of triacylglycerol that can be hydrolyzed (mobilized) in a regulated way to release fatty acids.
- Adipose tissue is the store house of lipids. It stores lipids as triacylglycerol (neutral lipids). The lipid content of the tissue is an important source of energy under conditions of unavailability of carbohydrates such as prolonged fasting or diabetes mellitus or starvation.
- The adipose tissue homeostasis of TGs is maintained hormonally.
- Adipose tissue fat storage is stimulated and fat mobilization suppressed, by insulin, leading to a drive to store energy in the fed state.
- The hormones epinephrine and glucagon, secreted in response to low blood glucose levels, activate the enzyme adenylyl cyclase in the adipocyte plasma membrane which produces the intracellular second messenger cyclic AMP (c-AMP). Cyclic AMP–dependent protein kinase (PKA) phosphorylates perilipin A (a protein coating the lipid droplets in adipose tissue).
- The phosphorylated perilipin causes hormone-sensitive lipase in the cytosol to move to the lipid droplet surface, where it can begin hydrolysing triacylglycerols to free fatty acids and glycerol.
- The fatty acids thus released (free fatty acids, FFA) pass from the adipocyte into the blood, where they bind to the blood protein serum albumin.
- Bound to this soluble protein, the otherwise insoluble fatty acids are carried to tissues such as skeletal muscle, heart, and renal cortex. In these target tissues, fatty acids dissociate from albumin and are moved by plasma membrane transporters into cells to serve as fuel.

Brown Adipose Tissue

- Brown adipose tissue metabolism comes into action when heat generation is required as in arousal from hibernation in bears or for protection against cold by shivering in new born infants. This is so because the brown adipose tissue has an abundance of mitochondria which oxidises the stored fat as a fuel. However, the brown adipose tissue also has a unique protein – *thermogenin* present in its mitochondria. This protein acts as a physiological uncoupler and thus oxidation occurs in mitochondria without phosphorylation – generating heat and very little energy is trapped as ATP. This is known as thermogenesis.
- Though not a prominent tissue in humans, it is present in normal individuals, where it could be responsible for "diet-induced thermogenesis." It is noteworthy that brown adipose tissue is reduced or absent in obese persons.

Clinical Implications of Lipid Transport

Fatty Liver

- Fatty infiltration of liver with endogenously synthesized triglycerides is termed as fatty liver. The liver cells lose their normal functional capacity due to fatty infiltration.

Causes of Fatty Liver

- *Increased plasma FFA* as in DM, starvation, high fat feeding—There is increased influx of Fatty acids into the liver, which get esterified, more than the amount that can be secreted as VLDL causing fatty infiltration of liver – Fatty liver.
- *Metabolic block* in the synthesis and secretion of the VLDL particles. Block in lipoprotein synthesis from apo protein and lipid—A defect may occur in the incorporation of lipids and apo proteins in the smooth ER.
- *Block in apoprotein synthesis*—As in protein malnutrition, or deficiency of essential amino acid methionine as it donates methyl groups for the synthesis of choline (a component of Phospholipids)
- *Inhibition of protein synthesis* like puromycin, CCl_4, ethionine.
- *Block in phospholipid synthesis due to deficiency of lipotropic factors*—Choline acts as lipotropic factor. A lipotropic factor prevents the deposition of fat in hepatocytes. A deficiency of choline causes defect in the synthesis of phospholipids, which are important constituent of lipoprotein's outer layer.
- *Defect in secretion of lipoprotein particle*—Orotic acid causes a block in secretion of lipoprotein particles from hepatocytes causing fatty infiltration.
- *Chronic alcoholism* – Ethanol is metabolized by alcohol dehydrogenase. (Fig. 11.25)
  - Increased levels of acetaldehyde are important source of activated acetyl group as acetyl CoA, which are important substrates for Fatty acids at liver, causing increased levels of TGs and Fatty liver.
  - High NADH+H^+ causes reduced CAC, net effect would be reduced oxidation of fatty acids and increased esterification, causing fatty liver.

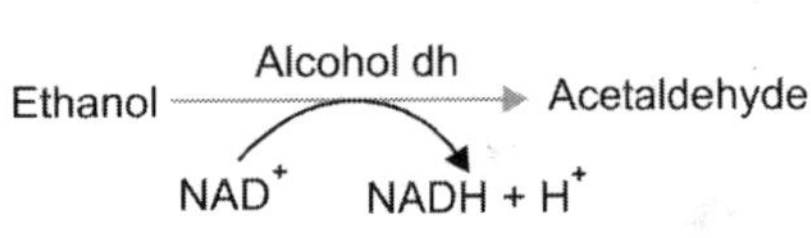

Fig. 11.25 Alcohol metabolism

Effect of Fatty Liver

- Fatty infiltration of liver causes a compromised functional ability of the liver cells.
- There is cirrhosis of liver.
- Liver gets fibrosed.
- Jaundice may occur.

Cholesterol Metabolism

Introduction

- Cholesterol is the principal animal sterol present in all animal cells. All nucleated cells can synthesize it. It is synthesized by virtually all tissues in humans, although liver, intestine, adrenal cortex, and reproductive tissues, including ovaries, testes, and placenta, make the largest contributions to the body's cholesterol pool. Our body synthesizes almost 1000 mg /day in a man of 68 kg. Total body cholesterol content is 35 gm (FIg. 11.26).

- Dietary sources of cholesterol include animal products like eggs, milk, butter, liver, meat, etc. Endogenous synthesis is inversely related to the dietary intake. A high intake decreases the endogenous synthesis.
- Cholesterol is eliminated from the liver as unmodified cholesterol in the bile, or it can be converted to bile salts that are secreted into the intestinal lumen
- It is present as either as cholesterol esters (70%) or as unesterified cholesterol (30%). Cholesterol is esterified by the PUFA at the C3 hydroxy group.
- It circulates in blood as a component of various lipoproteins.
- It is required for the formation of biological membranes, steroid hormones, vitamin D, bile salts and as component of myelin sheath.
- However an excess of cholesterol can be harmful as hypercholesterolemia has been associated with atherosclerosis and peripheral vascular diseases like CADs, hypertension, stroke, etc.

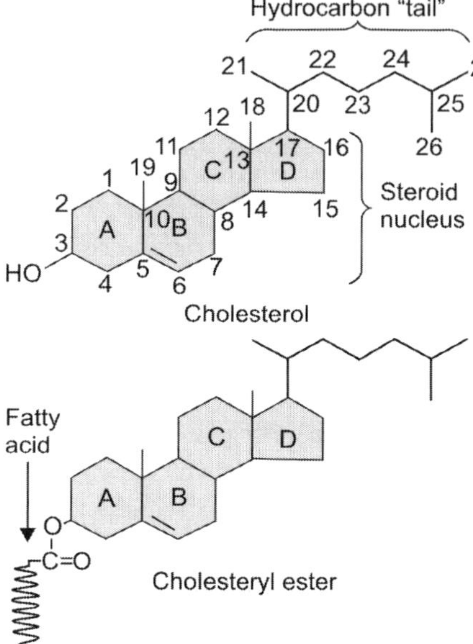

Fig. 11.26 Structure of cholesterol and cholesterol ester

Biosynthesis of Cholesterol (Figs 11.27 and 11.28)

- The principal sites of cholesterol biosynthesis are liver and intestines. The liver cells synthesize almost 10% of the total cholesterol synthesized along with intestines.
- All the carbon atoms for the synthesis of cholesterol are provided by acetyl CoA.
- ATP, NADPH, molecular oxygen and components of the microsomal hydroxylase system are also required besides the enzymes of cholesterol synthesis.
- The reactions can be divided into four stages:
  - Conversion of three molecules of acetyl CoA into 6-carbon compound, mevalonate.
  - Conversion of mevalonate into 5-carbon isoprenoid units.
  - Conversion of 6 isoprenoid units into a 30-carbon compound, squalene.
  - Conversion of squalene into cholesterol.
- The synthesis of cholesterol is extramitochondrial and steps till the synthesis of squalene are carried out in cytosol.
- The synthesis of mevalonate is the rate regulating step of the whole pathway being regulated by feedback inhibition of product of the pathway – cholesterol. This step also serves as the site of action of cholesterol lowering drugs – statins.
- There are a few isoprenoid compounds that arise form Farnesyl pyrophosphate like dolichol and ubiquinone.
- Squalene is the first 30 C intermediate formed during the pathway and it cyclises to give the first cyclic sterol lanosterol. But before it cyclises, squalene is oxidized in the membranes of ER by a mixed function oxidase – *Squalene epoxidase,* into Squalene 2,3 - epoxide in the presence of NADPH and O_2.
- Squalene 2, 3- epoxide is cyclized to lanosterol – The first cyclic structure of the pathway; by an oxidosqualene lanosterol cyclase.

- The steps from lanosterol to cholesterol are carried out in the membranes of ER. These steps involve the removal of extramethyl groups, shifting of double bonds and saturation of the side chain (Fig. 11.28).

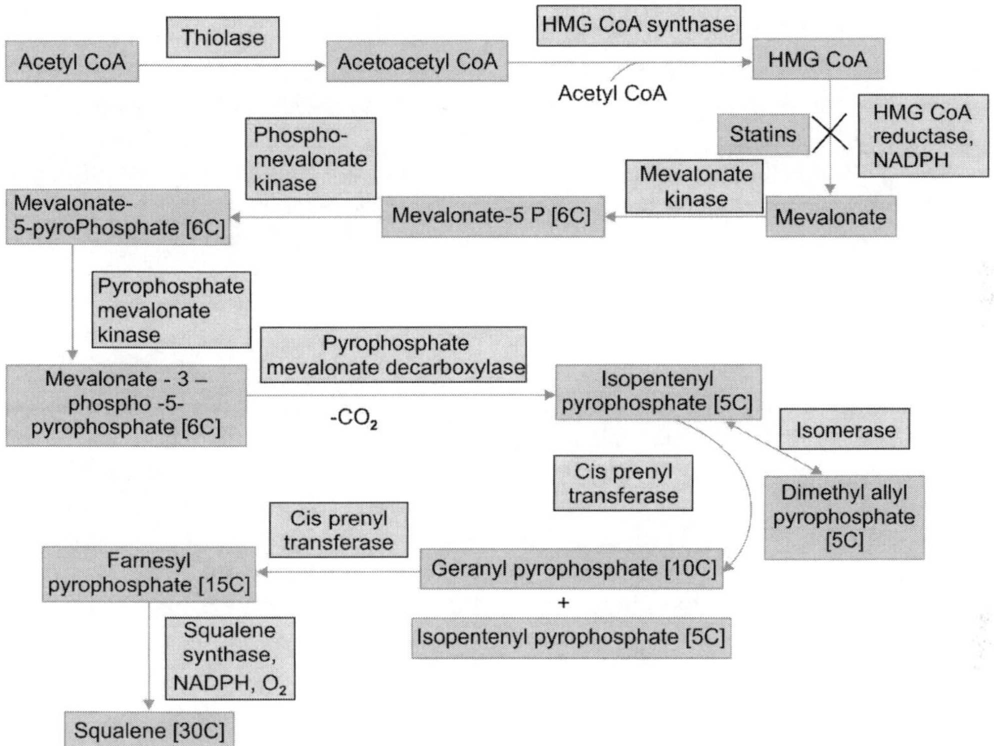

Fig. 11.27 Cholesterol synthesis pathway—Synthesis of squalene

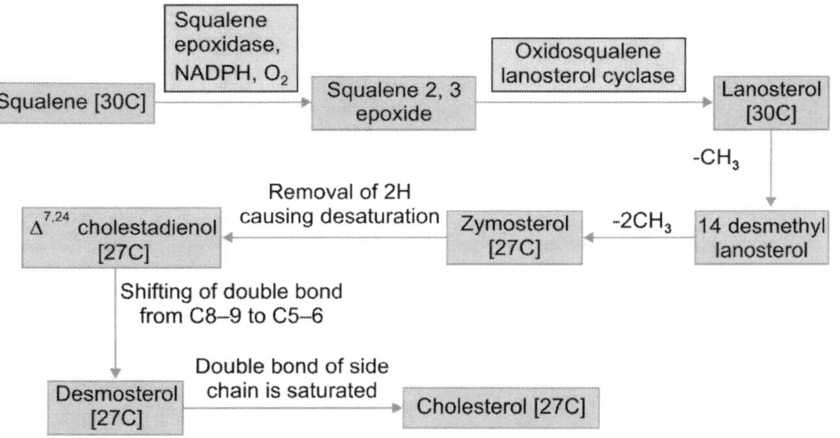

Fig. 11.28 Biosynthesis of cholesterol—Squalene to cholesterol

Regulation of Cholesterol Synthesis

The key regulatory enzyme of cholesterol biosynthesis is HMG CoA reductase. It is subject to different types of regulatory mechanisms like:

1. *At gene Level:* The activity of HMG CoA reductase is regulated at genetic level by the transcription factor – SRE activation and inhibition. The SRE is present just upstream the HMG CoA reductase gene. When the levels of cholesterol are low, a SRE binding protein (present bound to ER membrane) is released. This SREBP then binds and activates the SRE factor which increases the transcription and translation of HMG CoA reductase. Thus cholesterol synthesis is enhanced. Conversely, when the levels of cholesterol are high, the SREBP release from ER is inhibited and so the SRE is not activated reducing the overall rate of transcription and translation of HMG CoA reductase decreasing the synthesis of cholesterol (Fig. 11.29 label 1).
2. *Feedback inhibition*: The enzyme HMG CoA reductase is also regulated by product feedback inhibition. (Fig. 11.29 label 2)
3. *Covalent modification*: The enzyme HMG CoA reductase is a covalently modified enzyme that is active in dephosphorylated form and inactive in phosphorylated form.
   The covalent modification of the enzyme is regulated hormonally by insulin and glucagon via a c – AMP dependent protein kinase pathway. A reductase kinase catalyses phosphorylation of the active enzyme and makes it inactive.
   - Protein phosphatase dephosphorylates the inactive enzyme and makes it active.
   - Insulin activates protein phosphatase which converts the inactive HMG CoA reductase into the active form, and increases cholesterol synthesis.
   - Glucagon activates reductase kinase which converts the HMG CoA reductase into the in active form, and decreases cholesterol synthesis.

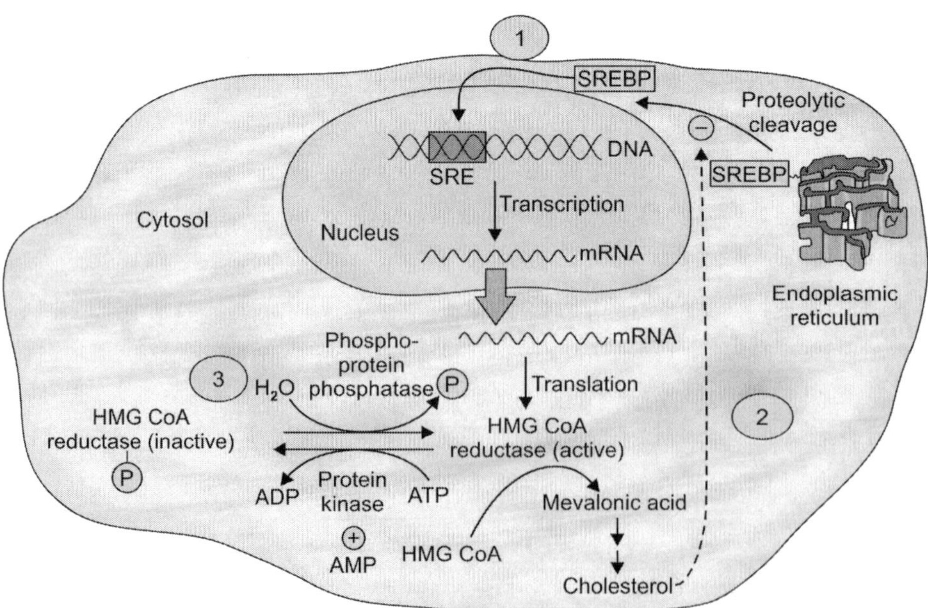

Fig. 11.29 Regulation of cholesterol synthesis

4. *Dietary regulation of cholesterol biosynthesis*
   - Increased dietary intake of cholesterol decreases endogenous synthesis of cholesterol.
   - It has been proposed that cholesterol or some metabolite of cholesterol, when present in excess, represses the synthesis of HMG CoA reductase.
   - This decreases the rate of cholesterol synthesis.

Catabolism (Fate) of Cholesterol

- The major pathway for the catabolism of cholesterol is its conversion into bile acids and bile salts.
- Cholesterol is converted into 7- α -hydroxycholesterol by 7- α -hydroxylase, a microsomal enzyme which requires oxygen, NADPH, cytochrome P-450 and ascorbic acid for its activity.
- Most of 7- α -hydroxycholesterol is converted into cholic acid which can combine with glycine to form glycocholic acid, and with taurine to form taurocholic acid.
- Some 7-α-hydroxycholesterol is converted into chenodeoxycholic acid which can form glycochenodeoxycholic acid and taurochenodeoxycholic acid.
- Most of the bile salts entering the intestine are reabsorbed into portal blood, brought to liver, and are re-excreted into the intestine by the liver (enterohepatic circulation of bile salts).
- The bile salts which are not reabsorbed are partly converted into various sterols – mainly coprostanol by the intestinal bacteria and are excreted.

Clinical Implications of Hypercholesterolemia (Table 11.2)

Hypercholesterolemia and Atherosclerosis

- The normal serum cholesterol is 150 – 220 mg/dL. However, raised levels of serum cholesterol have been a characteristic feature of a number of clinical conditions – both genetic as well as secondary to some disease.
- *Primary hypercholesterolemia* as in seen in some familial hyper cholesterol emic disorders. In these there is some genetic defect which leads hypercholesterolemia.
- *Secondary hypercholesterolemia* is seen to occur secondary to diseases like Diabetes mellitus, Obstructive Jaundice, Hypothyroidism, etc.
- *Cholesterol is transported as component of the plasma lipoproteins – HDLc (good cholesterol), LDLc (bad cholesterol) and chylomicron remnants.*
- Hypercholesterolemia has been long proposed cause of atherosclerosis.
- *Atherosclerosis* is defined as the deposition of cholesterol and cholesterol rich lipoproteins in the intima of medium and large sized arteries. The cholesterol rich lipoproteins primarily getting deposited are the LDLc particles and the chylomicron remnants.
- Simply deposition of these lipoprotein particles is not that harmful, the major damage is incurred on the oxidation of these particles in the intimal layer. It is the oxidized LDLc which further attracts the macrophages for scavenging the oxidised LDLc. However, the protective mechanism of the body works against it and these macrophages engulf more n more of oxidised LDLc, oxidising it still further and themselves convert into the foam cells whose maximum cytoplasm is occupied by the lipid droplets hence the name foam cells.
- These foam cells attract more macrophage secrete growth factors that stimulate the intimal layer to fibroses and form a layer around these cells – *fibrofatty plaque* is formed.

Table 11.2 Genetic defect in lipoprotein metabolism—Hypo and hyperlipoproteinemias

Name of disease	*Defect*	*Biochemical effect and symptoms*
Abetalipoproteinemia	No chylomicrons, VLDL or LDL formed due to defective lo	Blood TGs low, liver accumulates TGs, fat malabsorption, early death
Familial α-lipoprotein deficiency	Low or absent HDL	Hypertriglyceridemia as apo-GII is absent, atherosclerosis in elderly
Type-I	Deficiency of LPL	Slow clearance of chylomicrons and VLDL, low LDL and HDL. No increased risk of CHD
Type-IIa	Defective LDL receptors	Raised LDL and hypercholesterolemia
Type-III (Broad β-disease)	Defective apo-E	Increased chylomicrons and VLDL hypercholesterolemia, xanthomas and atherosclerosis
Type-IV (Hypertroglyceridemia)	Overproduction of VLDL, associated gluocose intolerance, hyperinsulinemia	Hypercholesterolemia, due to raised VLDL seen in obesity, DM – II, alcoholism
Type-V	Defect in LPL and apo - CII	Hypertrigyceredemia, low LDL and HDL
Familial hyperalpha lipoproteinemia	Increased HDL	Rare condition and beneficial to health
Hepatic lipase deficiency	Deficiency of hepatic lipase	Accumulation of HDL and VLDL remanants, atherosclerosis, CHD
LCAT deficiency	HDL remains as nascent discs	Plasma cholesterol esters and lysolecithin low
Wolman's disease	Deficiency of cholesterol ester hydrolase	Reduced clearance of LDL, hypercholesterolemia and atherosclerosis

- This fibrofatty plaque obliterates the lumen of the blood vessel, reducing the flow of blood through it and the blood flows with jerk in it causing hypertension.
- At times these fibro fatty plaques may also get calcified, hardening the arteries raising the blood pressure which may cause intravascular thrombosis.
- Such plaque when present in coronary arteries may cause myocardial infarction; if in cerebral artery may cause stroke.
- The plaque can also get dislodged from the vessel wall and float freely in the circulation. Such a plaque if stuck up at any vital organ artery will cause failure of that organ for, e.g. renal artery – renal failure.
- Serum TG is also a major risk factor for atherosclerosis and CHD as the major TG transporting lipoprotein particle VLDL is metabolized to LDLc.
- Management of serum cholesterol.

Maintenance of normal blood cholesterol level is a must as hypercholesterolemia leads to atherosclerosis. There are various measures for reducing the serum cholesterol to normal value.

Changes in Food Habits and Lifestyle

Lifestyle Changes

Initial monitoring of serum cholesterol can be done by means of changes in lifestyle, i.e. leading more active life as opposed to sedentary life. Stress free lifestyle, moderate exercise should be done to reduce obesity.

Food Habits should be Changed

- PUFA should be taken in a moderate amount and such that ratio of ω-6 to ω -3 is 4. Intake of PUFA is important good cholesterol HDL esterifies free cholesterol of tissues and of BAD cholesterol LDL by using these PUFA. Once esterified, the cholesterol esters are carried by HDL to liver to be metabolized to bile acids which are finally excreted via GIT in feces. ω-3 fatty acids are present in fish liver oils and a proper ratio of ω -6 and ω-3 fatty acids is seen in cereals and pulses.
- Dietary fibers—Green leafy vegetables should be consumed as plant sterols absorb dietary cholesterol.
- Reduce the intake of sugar and artificially sweetened drinks as they have fructose which by passes the control point of glycolysis to flood the lipid pathways.

Diabetes should be Under Control

- DM is an important cause of secondary hypercholesterolemia since the disease is primarily concerned with a defect in carbohydrate metabolism due to insulin deficiency.
- Lack of insulin leads to an enhanced mobilization of fats raising the levels of VLDL and eventually LDLc. Thus Diabetics should closely monitor their blood sugar levels.

Avoid Cigarettes Smoking

Cigarettes should be avoided as nicotine activates the hormone sensitive lipase that causes lipolysis raising the plasma FFAs which are β-oxidized to acetyl CoA a precursor for cholesterol synthesis.

Drugs

- Hypocholesterolmic drugs are given to patients who do not respond to dietary and lifestyle changes.
- Important Hypocholesterolmic drugs include –
  - *Statins* – As they inhibit HMG CoA reductase.
  - *Cholestyramine resin* – Binds to bile salts and prevents their enterohepatic circulation leading to loss of bile salts of faces. Thus more and more blood cholesterol is converted in bile salts for maintaining a constant pool of bile salts thus blood cholesterol level is reduced.
  - *Nicotinic acid* – Large doses of nicotinic acid reduces the secretion of apo – B100 containing lipoproteins.
  - *Clofiberate and gemfibrozil* – Increase the activity of LPL and reduce serum TG and VLDL.

The new-kids on the block:

Lp (a)

- Lp (a) is 1 mol of apo – A attached to 1 mol of LDLc. It is highly atherogenic and are important in early age atherosclerosis. It inhibits the thrombolysis by interfering with the plasminogen activation.
- Lp(a) is particularly high in the Indian population making them more susceptible to atherosclerotic risk at an early age than their Caucasian counterparts.

CVD risk ratios

- The ratios of total cholesterol/HDL and apo – B/apo –A_1 are the modern day tools for CVD risk evaluation.
- These ratios add an edge to the traditional lipid profile.

Table 11.3 Serum lipid profile and CVD risk ratios

Adult value	*Desirable*	*Borderline*	*High risk*
Cholesterol	<200 mg/dL	200–240 mg/dL	>240 mg/dL
Triglycerides	<200 mg/dL	200–400 mg/dL	400–1000 mg/dL
HDL–Cholesterol	>60 mg/dL	35–45 mg/dL	<35 mg/dL
LDL–Cholesterol	<130 mg/dL (<100 mg/dL if the patient has CHD)	130–160 mg/dL	>160 mg/dL
Total Cholesterol/ HDL	< 4.0	5.0	> 6.0
Apo – B/apo –A1	0.4	1	1.4

A Quick Look at the Lipid Metabolism

- Dietary lipids are the cooking medium and supply EFAs and fat soluble vitamins.
- Dietary lipids digestion begins at the mouth with the lingual lipase and continues with gastric lipase at stomach and finally at intestines with pancreatic lipase.
- Bile salts emulsify the dietary lipids helping digestion and in absorption of dietary lipids via micellization.
- All dietary lipids are transported via chylomicrons.
- De novo synthesis of fatty acids takes place in the cytosol of certain tissues like liver, adipose tissue, mammary gland, brain, etc.
- Key regulatory enzyme of FA synthesis is acetyl CoA carboxylase.
- De novo synthesis of FAs occurs on a FA synthase complex using NADPH and acetyl CoA as a substrate.
- Elongation of FAs occurs in the microsomal fractions.
- FAs oxidised by beta oxidation mainly to produce ATP and acetyl CoA.
- One Palmitate gives 131 ATP.
- The a-oxidation occurs in brain and oxidises phytanic acid but does not produce ATP.
- Removal of omega carbon followed by oxidation is omega oxidation of FAs.
- Ketone bodies are synthesized by partial oxidation of FAs.
- Excessive production of ketone bodies causes ketosis, ketonuria and ketoacidosis.
- The control over the fate of FAs between esterification and oxidation is regulated at the entry by CPT – I and hormonally by insulin and glucagon – insulin enhances esterification and glucagon oxidation.
- Lipids are transported in blood as lipoprotein complexes – HDL, IDL, LDL, VLDL and chylomicrons.
- Cholesterol synthesis is regulated by HMG CoA reductase at gene level, by feedback inhibition and, covalent modification and by dietary intake of cholesterol.

Contd...

Contd...

- LDL is the bad cholesterol as it has the tendency to deposit in the intimal layer and get oxidized to form atherosclerotic plaques.
- HDL is the good cholesterol and it scavenges the free cholesterol from tissues and cholesterol rich lipoproteins to carry it to liver – reverse cholesterol transport.
- Hypercholesterolemia can occur genetically – primary hypercholesterolemia and it can also be secondary to other diseases – secondary hypercholesterolemia.
- Hypercholesterolemia increases the risk of CVDs.
- Management of hypercholesterolemia is by – lifestyle changes, dietary changes, exercise, stress free life, low fat meal, high fibre meal, avoid cigarette smoking and artificially sweetened drinks.
- Last option should be drug – Hypocholesterolmic drugs.

CHAPTER

12

Amino Acid Metabolism

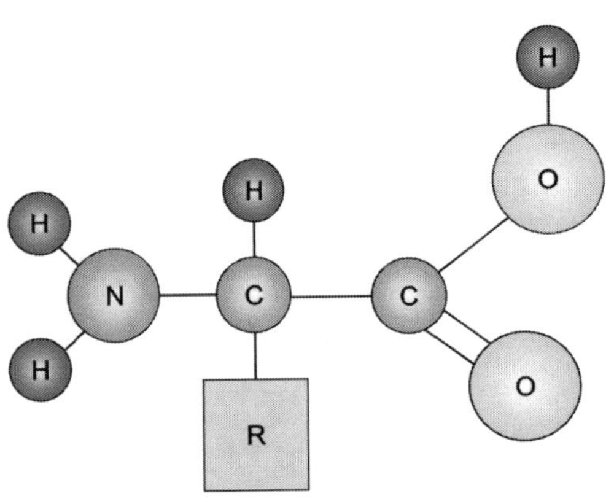

Chapter Framework

- Digestion and Absorption of Proteins
- Catabolism of Amino Acids—Fate of Amino Nitrogen: Ammonia Transport and Urea Cycle
- Catabolism of Carbon Skeleton of Amino Acids—Aliphatic Amino Acids
- Catabolism of Carbon Skeleton of Amino Acids—Aromatic Amino Acids
- Catabolism of Carbon Skeleton of Amino Acids—Branched Chain Amino Acids

Introduction

Amino acids are the building units of all proteins. Dietary proteins are digested into the simplest unit amino acid which is then absorbed to be transported via blood circulation to different tissues. The amino acids are dynamic in nature, i.e. the amino acids are utilized for the synthesis, repair and regeneration of tissue proteins and any excess of the amount utilized will be catabolized to urea and excreted.

There are 20 different amino acids in the human body of which 8 are essential, 2 semi – essential and rest are nonessential. All these amino acids—NH_2 group has a common fate on catabolism, i.e. form urea. However the carbon skeletons are varied and so are their fates. The following sections would discuss the fate of various amino acids once digested and absorbed.

Digestion and Absorption of Proteins

Dietary Proteins

- Proteins in diet are the principal source of nitrogen and sulfur for the human body. The major dietary protein sources include animal products—meat, egg, milk and plant products like legumes, pulses and nuts, etc.
- The dietary proteins are primarily utilized for the tissue protein formation, needed in tissue growth and repair and are poor sources of energy.

- Good quality dietary proteins with all essential amino acids should exist in our daily diet, since proteins are not stored in our body as carbohydrates (glycogen at liver and muscles) and lipids (triglycerides at adipose tissue).
- A daily intake of good quality proteins insures a state of nitrogen balance in a healthy adult.

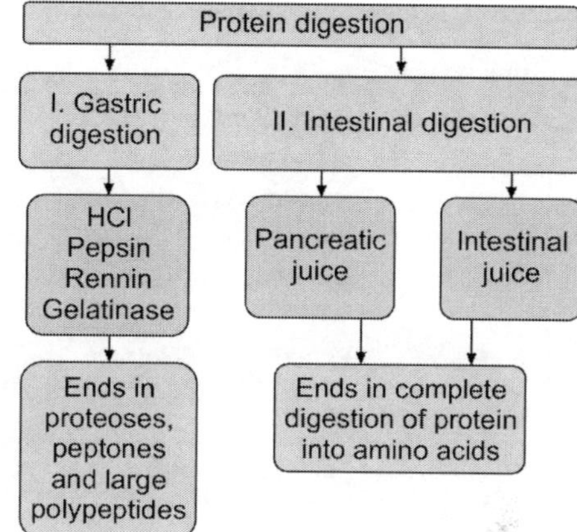

Fig. 12.1 Proteins digestion

Digestion of Proteins (Figs 12.1 and 12.2)

- Digestion of dietary proteins can be categorized as mainly the gastric phase and the duodenal–ileal phase, since there is no proteolytic enzyme in the oral cavity.
- The digestive enzymes of proteins—proteolytic enzymes act like biological scissors cutting the peptide bonds in a highly specific way.
- The enzymes splitting internal peptide bonds of proteins are known as *endopeptidases* and those removing the amino acids from terminal ends sequentially are termed as the *exopeptidases—(amino peptidases—removing amino acids from amino terminal end and carboxy peptidases—removing amino acids from carboxy terminal end).*

Gastric Phase

- Stomach secretes gastric juice that is highly acidic (pH 1–3). HCl contributes to the acidity of the gastric juice. Besides, HCl the gastric juice mainly contains proteolytic enzymes— Pepsinogen and rennin.

Role of HCl

1. HCl has bactericidal effect on the food ingested.
2. HCl causes the denaturation of the dietary proteins disrupting the quaternary, tertiary and secondary structure of proteins.

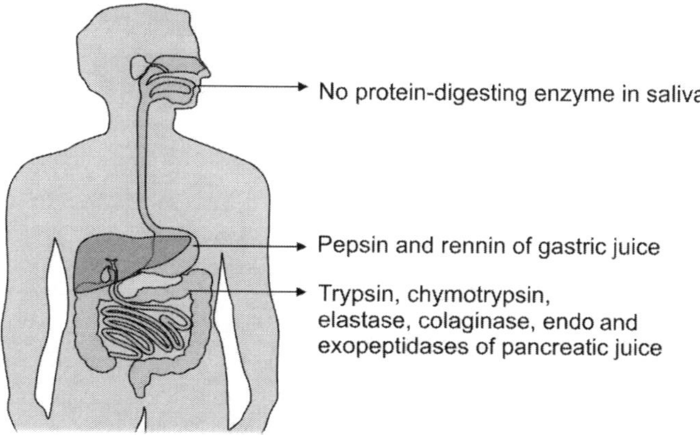

Fig. 12.2 Digestion of proteins in the gut

Table 12.1 Proteolytic enzymes

Endopeptidases		*Exopeptidases*	
Enzyme Name	*Site of Action*	*Enzyme Name*	*Site of Action*
Pepsin	Aromatic amino acids (Phe, Tyr, Trp,) and Acidic amino acids (Asp and Glu)	Amino peptidase	Successive amino terminal ends amino acids removal
Trypsin	Peptide bonds where carboxyl groups contributed by Lys and Arg	Carboxypeptidases	Successive carboxy terminal amino acids removal
Chymotrypsin	Peptide bonds formed by amino acids – Phe, Tyr, Trp; Leu, Met, Asp, His		
Elastase	Peptide bonds formed by small non-polar amino acids like Ala, Ser, Gly		

3. It also activates pepsinogen to pepsin at a pH of ~ 3.5. Pepsin is an endopeptidases and it splits denatured proteins into proteoses, peptones and large polypeptides.

Intestinal Phase (Fig. 12.3)

- The acidic gastric chyme when reaches the first part of small intestine, it stimulates the secretion of regulatory hormones and peptides—secretin and cholecystokinin (CCK).
- These together stimulate release of alkaline pancreatic juice containing bile and pancreatic proteolytic enzymes namely—trypsinogen, chymotrypsinogen, procarboxypeptidases A and B, proelastases, collagenases.
- The proteolytic enzymes are secreted in zymogenic form so as to protect the pancreas and gut-wall against autolysis.
- The zymogenic enzymes are activated as shown in the reactions:

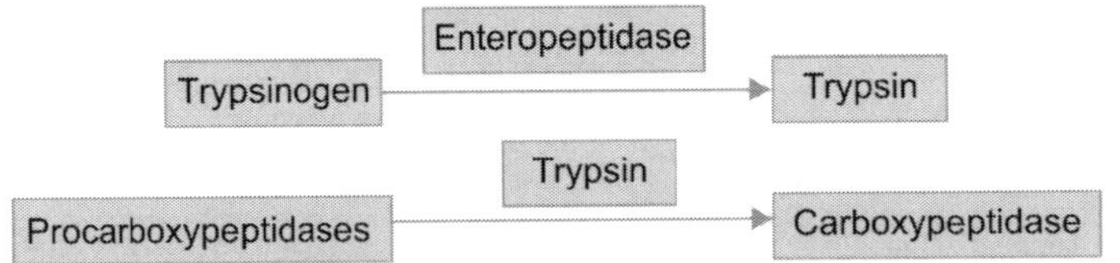

- These exopeptidases (carboxy and amino peptidases) attack peptide bonds at the carboxy C-terminal end of polypeptides to release free amino acids.
- Several peptidases are produced by the brush border of the small intestine, including the ileum, enabling peptide digestion and amino acid absorption to occur in the distal small intestine. Some of these peptidases include—
  - Amino peptidases, which vary in specificity and cleave amino acids from the amino N-terminal end of oligopeptides
  - Dipeptidylaminopeptidases, some of which are magnesium-dependent and hydrolyze N-terminal amino acids from dipeptides.
  - Tripeptidases, which are specific for selected amino acids and hydrolyze tripeptides to yield a dipeptide and a free amino acid.

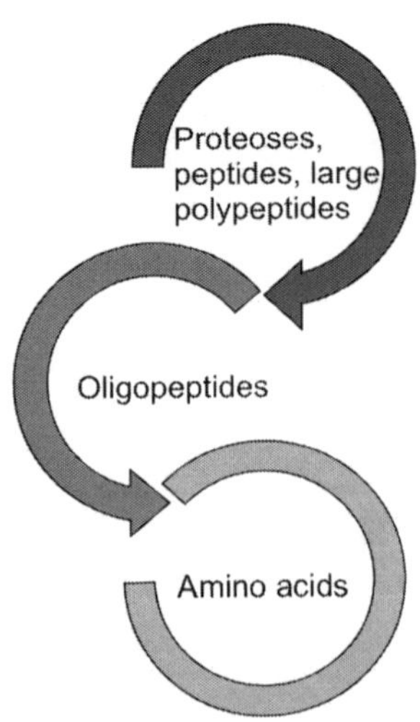

Fig. 12.3 Intestinal digestion of proteins

- The pancreatic digestion of proteins ends at the amino acids—The simplest unit building up the proteins.

Absorption of Amino acids

- The absorption of amino acids is similar to that of monosaccharides, i.e. it follows the sodium-dependent secondary active transport.
- Absorption of amino acids occurs along the entire intestinal mucosal layer however maximum part of it occurs at the proximal part of small intestine.
- The amino acids are mainly transported via a sodium-dependent transporter as shown in Figure 12.4.
- The amino acids bind to the transporter first followed by the sodium molecule. Once the sodium–amino acid co-transporter complex forms, a conformational change in the complex results in the delivery of the sodium and amino acid into the cytoplasm of the enterocyte. Lastly, sodium is pumped out of the cell by Na^+/K^+-ATPase.

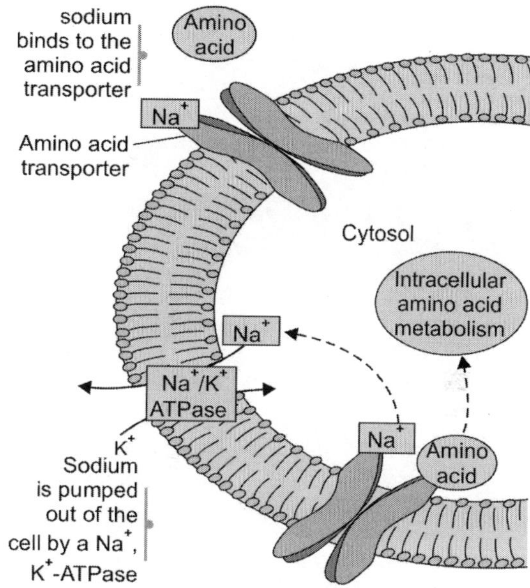

Fig. 12.4 Absorption of amino acids

- The rate of absorption of amino acids is affected by the hydrocarbon side chain, charge on the amino acid and the nutritional significance.
  - The increase in size of hydrocarbon side chain increases the rate of absorption, so branched chain amino acids are absorbed faster.
  - The neutral amino acids are absorbed faster.
  - The essential amino acids are absorbed at a faster rate than nonessential ones.
- The neutral amino acids have yet another transport mechanism—γ-glutamyl cycle (Meister's cycle) at the intestinal brush border.
- In the γ-glutamyl cycle, glutathione acts as a carrier of selected neutral amino acids into cells.
- The Meister's cycle is typical for the absorption of neutral amino acids and is present in the intestinal mucosal layer. Glutathione acts as a carrier of the amino acids as shown in Figure 12.5.
- The transport of the amino acids across the basolateral membrane of the enterocyte into the interstitial fluid occurs by diffusion and sodium independent pathway.
- Many of the amino acids absorbed following protein digestion are used by the intestinal cells for energy or synthesis of proteins and other nitrogen-containing compounds including:
  - Structural proteins for new intestinal cells
  - Nucleotides
  - Apo-proteins necessary for lipoprotein formation
  - New digestive enzymes
  - Hormones
  - Nitrogen-containing compounds.
- In addition, amino acids may be partially metabolized either to other amino acids or to other compounds that may be released into portal blood.

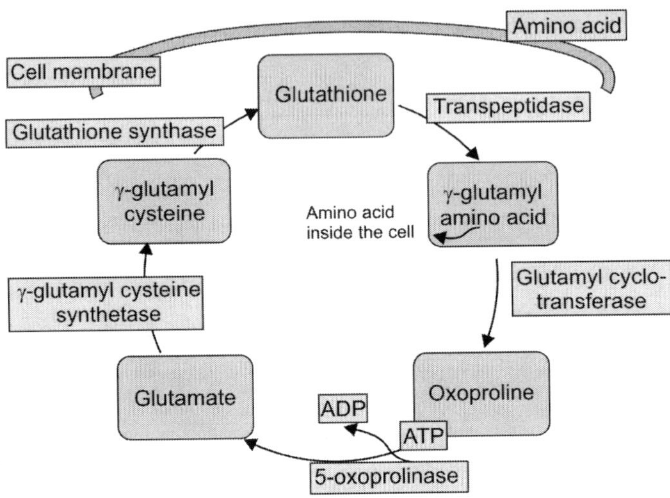

Fig. 12.5 Meister's cycle

Catabolism of Amino Acids—Fate of Amino Nitrogen: Ammonia Transport and Urea Cycle

Introduction

A constant pool of amino acids is maintained in our body (100 gram) (Fig. 12.6). Amino acids are derived from diet, endogenous synthesis and protein turnover. Proteins in our body are continuously undergoing turnover (1–2%) daily. This rate of turnover is high in tissues undergoing structural modifications like the uterine tissues during pregnancy, skeletal muscles in starvation, skin, GIT mucosa, etc. The proteins are not stored in our body like the storehouses of glycogen or triglycerides. Thus in lack of a storehouse of proteins, we lack a source of constant supply of amino acids for future use. In lieu of this constant turnover of tissue proteins we need to consume good quality proteins (with all essential amino acids) in our diet daily. These would help us sustain the tissue proteins and any amino acid in excess of the tissue demand would be completely catabolized.

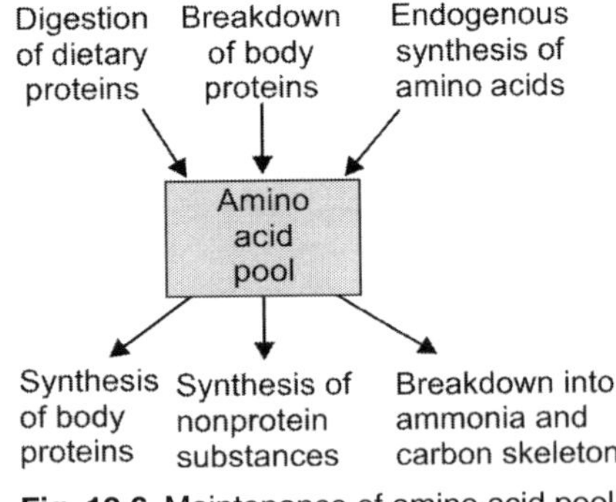

Fig. 12.6 Maintenance of amino acid pool

Liver is the principal organ that takes up amino acid after meals from the portal blood (50–65%). The liver cells have a high capacity for the uptake and catabolism of amino acids, especially those that have not been utilized for protein synthesis or synthesis of other nitrogenous compounds. The amino acid oxidation at liver accounts for almost 50% of the energy supply of the liver, needed for gluconeogenesis or urea synthesis.

- In human beings, disposal of amino groups of amino acids involves four steps:
  - Transfer of amino groups of different amino acids to α-keto glutarate to form glutamate.
  - Oxidative deamination of glutamate and release of ammonia.

  - Transport of ammonia to liver.
  - Synthesis of urea in liver.
- The carbon atom of urea is provided by carbon dioxide, one of the nitrogen atoms comes from ammonia and the other from aspartate (NH_2–CO–NH_2; Urea).

Fate of the –NH_2 Group of Amino Acid

- The –NH_2 group of an amino acid protects it from oxidation and therefore has to be removed prior to oxidation.
- The –NH_2 group of amino acids is removed by transamination and deamination to give aspartate and ammonia—the ultimate sources of nitrogen of urea.

Transamination

- Transamination is the process of interconversion of a pair of α-amino acid and α-keto acids in the presence of enzymes transaminases and coenzyme pyridoxal phosphate.
- This is a reversible reaction and plays significant role in the synthesis of nonessential amino acids.
- All amino acids except Lys, Thr, Pro, Hydroxy proline undergo transamination. These enzymes are found in the cytosol of cells throughout the body—Especially those of the liver, kidney, intestine, and muscle.
- During amino acid catabolism, the transamination of amino acids pools up the amino groups of amino acids into α-keto glutarate to form glutamate.
- There are several transaminases, each transferring the α-amino group of a specific amino acid to α-keto acid which is generally α-keto glutarate.
- The enzyme is named after the amino acid donating the amino group, e.g. alanine aminotransferase (glutamate pyruvate transaminase) and aspartate aminotransferase (glutamate oxaloacetate transaminase).
- The two most important aminotransferase reactions are catalyzed by alanine aminotransferase and aspartate aminotransferase—SGPT and SGOT. (Figs 12.7 to 12.9)
- SGPT has α-keto acid – amino acid pair as—α-KG and alanine.
- SGOT has α-keto acid – amino acid pair as—α-KG and aspartate.

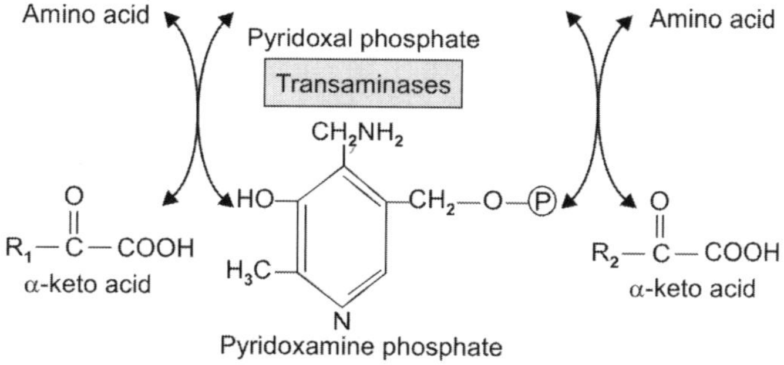

Fig. 12.7 Transamination

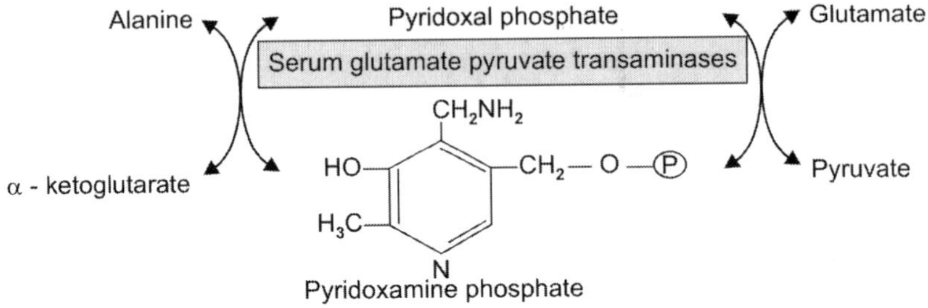

Fig. 12.8 Transamination by SGPT/ALT

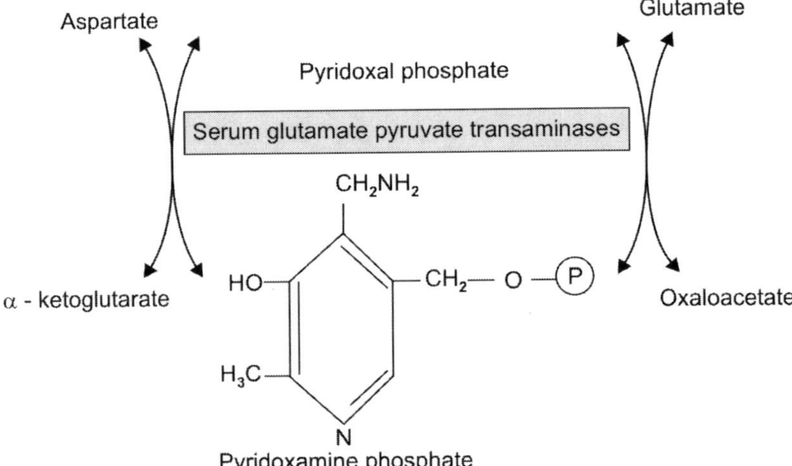

Fig. 12.9 Transamination by SGOT/AST

- The reaction is readily reversible. However, during amino acid catabolism, this enzyme (like most aminotransferases) functions in the direction of glutamate synthesis. Thus, glutamate, in effect, acts as a "collector" of nitrogen from amino acids.
- During amino acid catabolism, AST transfers amino groups from glutamate to oxaloacetate, forming aspartate, which is used as a source of nitrogen in the urea cycle.

Oxidative Deamination (Fig. 12.10)

- Oxidative deamination reactions involve only the removal of an amino group, with no direct transfer to another compound. Some amino acids that are more commonly deaminated include glutamate, histidine, serine, glycine, and threonine.
- However, many of these same amino acids also can be transaminated.
- The amino groups are concentrated in glutamate, which is the only amino acid that can undergo oxidative deamination at a significant rate.
- Oxidative deamination of glutamate is catalyzed by glutamate dehydrogenase.
- Glutamate dehydrogenase can use NAD^+ as well and $NADP^+$ as coenzyme.
- $NADP^+$ is probably used for synthesis of glutamate from α-ketoglutarate and NAD^+ for oxidative deamination of glutamate.

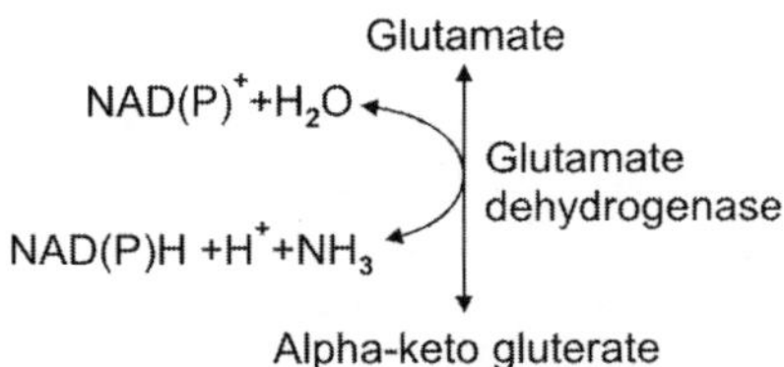

Fig. 12.10 Oxidative deamination

- Thus, the sequential action of transamination (resulting in the collection of amino groups from other amino acids onto α-keto glutarate to produce glutamate) and the subsequent oxidative deamination of that glutamate (regenerating α-keto glutarate) provide a pathway whereby the amino groups of most amino acids can be released as ammonia.
- Some ammonia can be liberated from amino acids by the actions of L-amino acid oxidase and D-amino acid oxidase.

Nonoxidative Domination

Nonoxidative domination of α-NH_2 groups of Ser and Thr is carried out by dehydratases without use of NAD^+/$NADP^+$.

a. Ser $\xrightarrow[\text{PLP}]{\text{Ser Dehydratases}} \text{Pyruvate} + NH_4^+$

b. Thr $\xrightarrow[\text{PLP}]{\text{Thr Dehydratases}} \alpha\text{-keto butyrate} + NH_4^+$

Fate of Ammonia

Since ammonia is extremely toxic, it is immediately removed from the circulation and converted to less toxic metabolites. The NH_4^+ released by domination has 3 fates:

- Formation of glutamine
- Formation of glutamate
- Formation of urea.

Transport of Ammonia

- The complete enzyme system for the synthesis of urea is present only in liver.
- Though liver is the major site for catabolism of amino acids as well, some ammonia is produced in other tissues also which must be transported to liver without causing ammonia intoxication.
- Normal concentration of ammonia in blood is 10 to 80 µg/dL
- Even a small rise in blood ammonia level, which may occur if hepatic function is impaired or if a portacaval shunt is formed, may damage nervous tissue.

Transport of Ammonia to the Liver

- Two mechanisms are available in humans for the transport of ammonia from the peripheral tissues to the liver for its ultimate conversion to urea. The first, found in most tissues, uses *glutamine synthase* to combine ammonia with glutamate to form glutamine—Nontoxic transport form of ammonia.

- The glutamine is ported in the blood to the liver where it is cleaved by glutaminase.
- Second transport mechanism, used primarily by muscle, involves transamination of pyruvate (the end-product of aerobic glycolysis) to form alanine. Alanine is transported by the blood to liver, where it is converted to pyruvate, again by transamination to produce glutamate and free ammonia. The pyruvate synthesizes glucose, which can enter the blood and be used by pathway called the glucose-alanine cycle.

Ammonia Transport from Various Tissues

- Glutamate, which is formed by transamination of α-ketoglutarate in many tissues, transports the amino groups of various amino acids to liver in a nontoxic form.

Ammonia Transport from Brain (Fig. 12.11)

- Since brain tissue is extremely sensitive to ammonia, it possesses a mechanism for immediate detoxification of ammonia.
- Ammonia is combined with glutamate to form glutamine by glutamine synthetase.
- A constant supply of glutamate is required for this reaction, which is formed mainly from α- ketoglutarate, an intermediate of citric acid cycle.

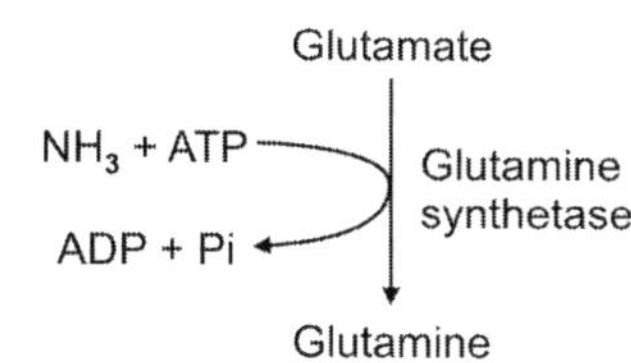

Fig. 12.11 Ammonia transport from brain

Transport of Glutamine

- Glutamine released into circulation can be taken up by liver and kidneys wherein glutaminase converts it into glutamate and ammonia.
- Thus, ammonia can be transported from brain in the form of nontoxic glutamine.

$$\text{Glutamine} + H_2O \longrightarrow \text{Glutamate} + NH_3$$

Ammonia Transport from Muscles

- In muscles, amino groups of many amino acids are transferred to pyruvate forming alanine.
- Alanine is transported to liver where pyruvate is reformed, and the amino group of alanine is transferred to α-ketoglutarate (Fig. 12.12).
- Thus, glucose-alanine cycle not only transports pyruvate from muscles to liver for gluconeogenesis but also transports the amino groups of amino acids from muscles to liver.

Transport of Ammonia from the Intestines

- Significant quantities of ammonia are formed in the intestine by the action of bacterial enzymes on amino acids and urea.
- Catabolism of dietary purines and pyrimidines also liberates ammonia.
- All this ammonia is released into portal blood. Liver extracts all the ammonia when portal blood passes through it.

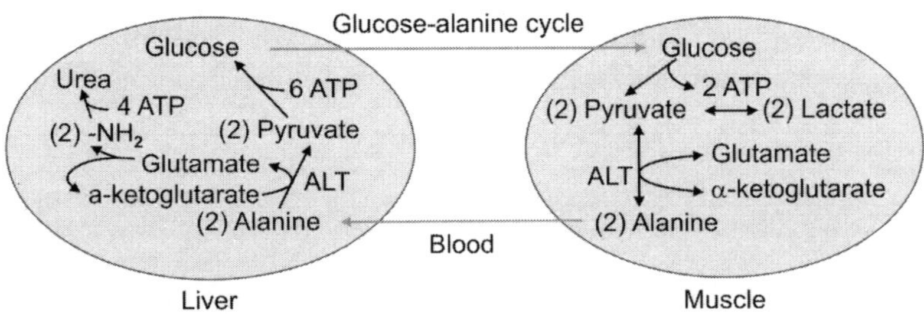

Fig. 12.12 Glucose-alanine cycle dual role as ammonia transport and gluconeogenesis

Synthesis of Urea

- Ammonia is converted into nontoxic urea in liver by a cyclic sequence of reactions known as urea cycle or Krebs-Henseleit's cycle (Fig. 12.13).
- Urea is released into circulation, and is excreted by the kidneys in urine.

Hepatic encephalopathy

- Life-threatening neurological abnormalities can occur in severe liver diseases, e.g. cirrhosis of liver.
- Disturbed hepatic architecture can lead to the formation of portacaval shunt, where portal blood which is rich in ammonia mixes with systemic blood.
- Decrease in the number of functioning liver cells impairs the ability of liver to convert ammonia into urea.
- All this can result in severe hyperammonemia.
- Hyperammonemia causes encephalopathy manifesting as:
  - Blurring of vision
  - Slurring of speech
  - Tremors
  - Hepatic coma and death.
- Brain possesses a mechanism for immediate detoxification of ammonia by synthesis of glutamine from glutamate and ammonia.
- Glutamate required for this reaction is formed from α-ketoglutarate, an intermediate of citric acid cycle.
- Excessive removal of α-ketoglutarate can result in impairment of citric acid cycle limiting the production of ATP
- Apart from energy deficit, increased synthesis of γ-aminobutyric acid (GABA) from glutamate and inhibition of uptake of some amino acids by brain cells due to increased level of glutamine cause encephalopathy.

- An adult man excretes about 30 gram of urea per day which accounts for nearly 90% of the nitrogen excretion.

Significance of Urea Cycle

- It converts toxic NH_3 to less toxic urea.
- It synthesizes semi-essential amino acid arginine.
- Fumerate and aspartate link urea cycle to TCA cycle.
- Ornithine formed in urea cycle is a precursor of nonessential amino acid proline and of polyamines spermine and spermidine.

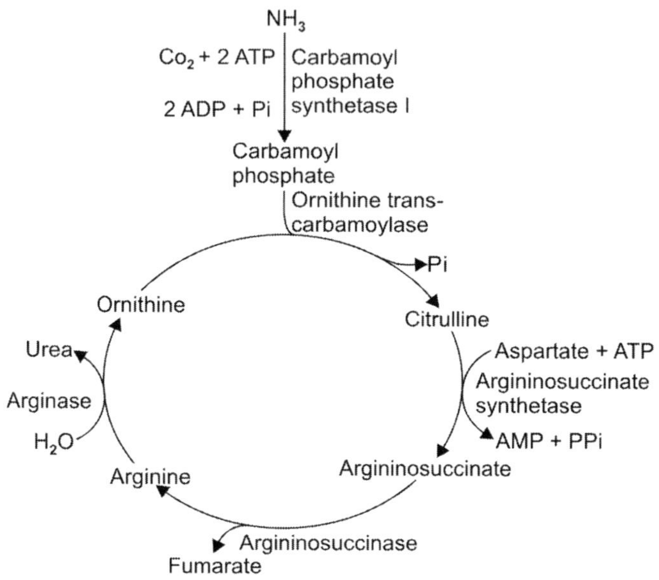

Fig. 12.13 Urea cycle

Regulation of Urea Cycle

- Glutamate dehydrogenase, which provides ammonia for urea synthesis, is an allosteric enzyme.
- It is inhibited by ATP and GTP, and is activated by ADP and GDP.
- Thus, a decrease in energy content increases the catabolism of amino acids and synthesis of urea.
- Mitochondrial carbamoyl phosphate synthetase is also an allosteric enzyme.
- It is activated by N-acetyl glutamate which is formed by transfer of the acetyl group from acetyl CoA to glutamate.

Inborn Errors of Urea Cycle (Table 12.1)

- These disorders are very rare.
- *Clinical features*, which are common to all though varying in severity, are vomiting, distaste for protein-rich foods, lethargy, irritability, ataxia and mental retardation.

Table 12.1 Inborn errors of urea cycle

Disorder	*Deficient enzyme*
Hyperammonemia, type I	Carbamoyl phosphate synthetase
Hyperammonemia, type II	Ornithine transcarbamoylase
Citrullinemia	Arginiosuccinic acid synthetase
Argininosuccinic aciduria	Argininosuccinase
Hyperargininemia	Arginase

- Small and frequent meals, low in protein, help in preventing sudden and excessive rise in blood ammonia and lead to improvement.

Catabolism of Carbon Skeleton of Amino Acids – Aliphatic Amino Acids

Introduction

- The amino acids can be classified as per their carbon skeleton into:
  - Aliphatic – Gly, Ala, Met, Cys, Ser, Thr
  - Aromatic – Phe, Trp, His
  - Acidic – Asp, Glu
  - Basic – Arg, Lys, Asn, Gln
  - Branched chain – Val, Leu, Isleu
  - Imino acid – Proline and Hydroxyproline
- Those amino acids that are not utilized for synthesis of proteins or other nitrogenous products are catabolized.
- The catabolic end-products of these amino acids may be—
  - *Glucogenic:* Such amino acid carbon skeletons on catabolism breakdown into intermediates of CAC or gluconeogenesis and thus can convert to glucose. Therefore these amino acids are termed as glucogenic amino acids, e.g. – Glycine, alanine, valine, proline, aspartate, glutamate, arginine, histidine, etc.
  - *Ketogenic:* Such amino acids carbon skeletons on catabolism breakdown to produce ketone bodies—acetone or acetoacetate or β-hydroxy butyrate, e.g. Leucine.
  - *Gluco-Ketogenic:* The carbon skeletons of such amino acids one portion is catabolized to ketone bodies and the other half is catabolized to ketone bodies, e.g. – Phenylalanine, tryptophan, etc.

Glycine

- Glycine (Gly) is a nonessential amino acid, i.e. it can be synthesized in our body enzymatically.

Synthesis of Glycine

- Glycine can be synthesized in our body from two different reactions:
  - *From Serine:* The carbon skeleton of serine is catabolized in the presence of serine hydroxy methyl transferase and THFA such that the 1–C unit is transferred to THFA forming N_5 N_{10} methylene THFA and what remains is glycine.

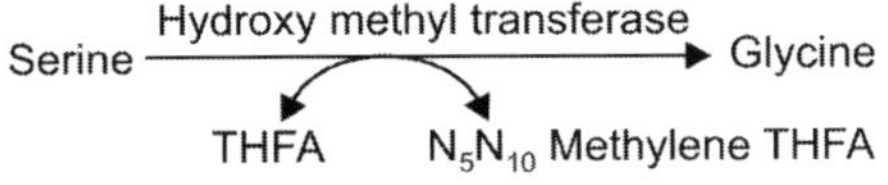

– Glycine cleavage system (glycine synthase)

$$\text{Glycine} \xrightarrow[\text{PLP, THFA, lipoamide (S–S)}]{\text{Glycine synthase}} CO_2 + NH_4^+ + N_5, N_{10} \text{ Methylene THFA}$$

- Glycine cleavage system is a multi-enzyme complex with activities of—
  - Glycine decarboxylase for decarboxylation.
- Amino methyl transferase for transfer of methylene group to THFA and a lipoamide dehydrogenase to regenerate oxidized lipoic acid this is a reversible reaction thus both synthesis of glycine and catabolism of glycine occurs by this reaction.

Catabolism of Glycine

Catabolism of glycine occurs in 3 ways:

- **Glycine synthase system** *(see in synthesis of Glycine)*
- Glycine oxidase causing oxidative deamination

$$\text{Glycine} \xrightarrow[\text{Glycine oxidase}]{H_2O \;\; H_2O_2} \text{Glyoxalate} \rightarrow \text{Oxalate} \rightarrow \text{Excreted}$$

$$\text{Glyoxalate} \rightarrow \text{Formate} \rightarrow N_{10} - \text{formyl THFA}$$

Functions of Glycine

Heme Synthesis

- Glycine is required for the synthesis of heme. It is an important reactant for the key regulatory enzyme of heme synthesis—ALA synthase.

$$\text{Glycine + Succinyl} \xrightarrow{\text{CoA—ALA synthase } B_6PO_4} \text{ALA} \longrightarrow \text{Heme}$$

Creatine Synthesis (Fig. 12.14)

- Glycine is required for the synthesis of creatine—A nitrogenous compound present in muscles as creatine phosphate. Creatine phosphate stores high energy phosphate and releases it during muscle contraction for conversion of ADP to ATP.
- The reaction involves not just glycine but also arginine and methionine. The reaction is seen in Figure 12.14.
- The creatine – P after release of the high energy phosphate converts into a cyclic anhydride —*Creatinine* nonenzymatically.

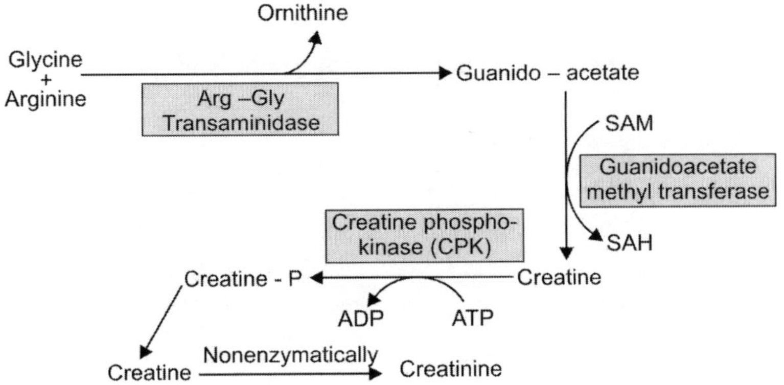

Fig. 12.14 Biosynthesis of creatine

- Excretion of creatinine is a function of the glomerular filtration rate and its estimation helps assess the renal function.

Glutathione

- Glutathione is a tripeptide – γ – glutamyl-cysteinyl-glycine. It is an active cofactor for enzymes having thiol (-SH) groups at their active sites since, it helps maintain these groups in a reduced form.
- Glutathione is also a component of peroxidases group of enzymes, e.g. Glutathione peroxidases, where it helps scavenge the peroxy-free radicals.

Conjugation of Bile Acids

- The primary and secondary bile acids—Cholic acid, chenodeoxycholic acid and deoxycholic, lithocholic acids respectively are secreted as the conjugates of glycine.

Detoxification

- Glycine helps in the detoxification of benzoic acid present as food preservatives. Glycine conjugates with benzoic acid and converts to less toxic hippuric acid that is excreted in urine.

Collagen

- Collagen is the most abundant protein. It has a triple helix structure (*see* chapter no. 3). The triple helix structure is stabilized due to the presence of glycine after every two amino acids. This is a unique feature of collagen that every third amino acid is glycine. This is important too because only a small molecule like glycine can accommodate in the limited area present down the center of the triple helix.

Protein Synthesis

- Glycine is the component of various proteins like tissue proteins, hormones, enzymes, etc.

Inborn Errors of Glycine Metabolism

Primary Hyperoxaluria

- It is an inborn error with a defect involving a failure to catabolize glyoxalate, which therefore gets oxidized into oxalate. An excess of oxalate is excreted in urine and oxalate deposits in urinary tract—Uriolithiasis, in kidneys—Nephrocalcinosis, and early mortality from renal failure or hypertension.

Clinical Features

- Urolithiasis
- Nephrocalcinosis
- Recurrent urinary tract infections
- Death in childhood/early adult life due to renal failure or hypertension.

Glycinuria

In this there is a defect in renal tubular reabsorption of glycine the plasma levels of glycine are normal. However due to defective renal tubular reabsorption there is excretion of glycine in urine and tendency to form oxalate stones.

Nonketotic Hyperglycenemia

- It is characterized by the defect in multi—enzyme complex—*glycine cleavage system.*
- It is named so to differentiate from the ketoacidosis seen in defects of branched chain amino acids, where the glycine levels are elevated due to unknown reasons.
- Defective glycine cleavage causes hyperglycenemia and show symptoms of mental insufficiency with the patients' hardly surviving infancy.
- Neurologic symptoms are seen because glycine is an inhibitory neurotransmitter.

Sulfur-containing Amino Acids

- Sulfur-containing amino acids include—cysteine, cystine and methionine. Cystine is formed by the condensation of two cysteine amino acid residues at their –SH groups.
- Out of the three S-containing amino acids, cysteine and cystine are nonessential amino acids and methionine is essential amino acid.

Synthesis of Cysteine

- Cysteine is synthesized by transfer of the sulfur atom derived from methionine to the hydroxyl group of serine. As long as the supply of methionine is adequate, cysteine is nonessential. Cysteine is synthesized from methionine and serine (*as shown in pathway*).
- Homoserine is deaminated to a-ketobutyrate by homoserine deaminase.

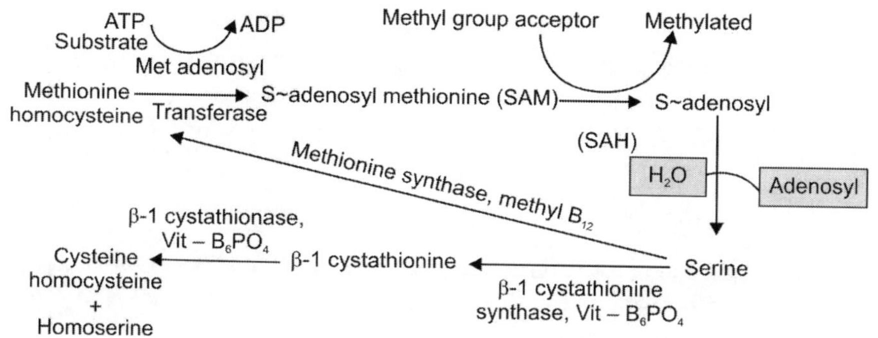

Fig. 12.15 Metabolism of methionine

- Ketobutyrate is converted into propionyl CoA.
- Propionyl CoA is then converted into succinyl CoA via methyl malonyl CoA.

Catabolism of Cysteine

- Cysteine, derived from the sulfur of homocysteine and a molecule of serine, is metabolized in several ways. The pathway chosen is determined by the needs of the cell.
- The major metabolite is cysteine sulfinate, which is further metabolized to sulfite and pyruvate, or to Hypotaurine and taurine. Two major pathways are:
  - Transamination
  - Direct oxidative pathway
    - *Transamination:* Cysteine is transaminated in the presence of transaminases as shown in pathway below.

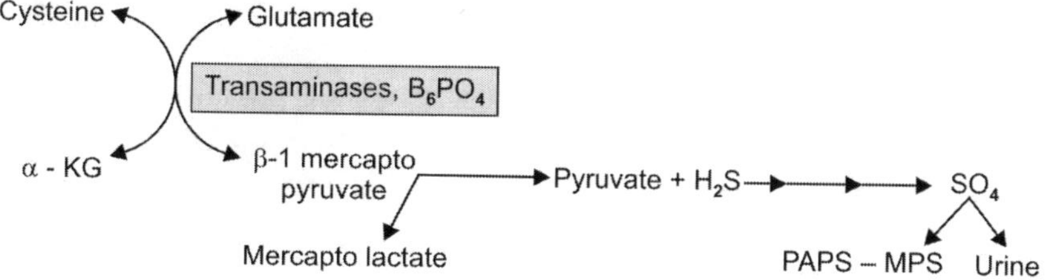

- The cysteine is catabolized to SO_4 which is excreted as urinary SO_4 and also synthesizes phospho-adenosyl phosphosulfate—which is a component of mucoploysaccharides.
- Direct oxidative pathway.
- Cysteine undergoes direct oxidation in the presence of a dioxygenase—Cysteine dioxygenase to cysteine Sulfinate and then transaminated and desulfurated sequentially to pyruvate. The pyruvate can then be completely oxidized.
- During catabolism of cystine, it is first reduced to cysteine by *cystine reductase* and further cysteine is catabolized as shown in pathway below.

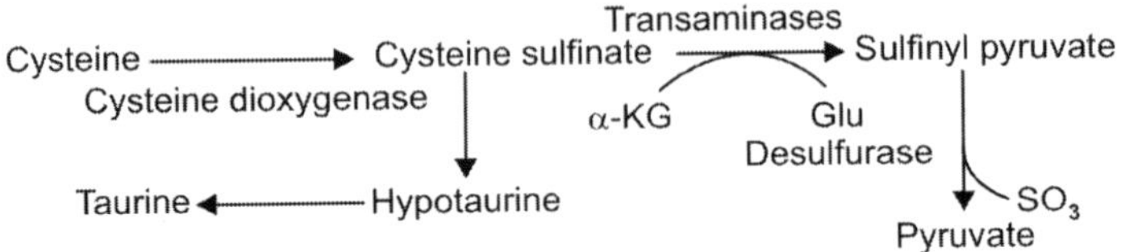

Functions of Cysteine

- Cysteine is glucogenic in nature and thus adds up to blood glucose via gluconeogenesis.
- Cysteine is the most important dietary source of sulfur.
- Cysteine is present in taurine, insulin, CoA, GSH and vasopressin.
- Taurine is an abundant intracellular free amino acid. It probably plays a necessary role in brain development and forms conjugates with bile acids and may enhance bile flow increasing cholesterol clearance by the liver. Taurine may also play a role in removing toxic intermediates, in regulating intracellular calcium, and, because of its abundance, in osmoregulation.
- Cysteine is important in detoxification mechanisms.

Inborn Errors of Metabolism of S-containing Amino Acids

There are several disorders of cysteine metabolism.

Cystinuria

- The renal tubular cells have three types of transporters for amino acids transporting:
  - Type-I
  - Type-II—Lysine, ornithine, arginine
  - Type-III—Cystine, ornithine, lysine, arginine (COLA)
- In cystinuria, the defect is in the type-III transporter. Cystine, lysine, arginine, and ornithine are excreted. Apart from cystine calculi, cystinuria is benign.
- *Management*—Treatment is limited to removal of stones, prevention of precipitation by drinking large amounts of water or alkalinizing the urine to solubilize cystine, or formation of soluble derivatives by conjugation with drugs.

Cystinosis

- It is much more serious. Here cystine accumulates in the lysosomes. The defect is believed to be in the cystine transporter of lysosomal membranes. Cystine accumulates in the lysosomes of spleen, bone marrow, cornea, liver, lymph nodes and WBCs.
- The stored cystine forms crystals in many cells, with a serious loss of function of the kidneys, usually causing renal failure within ten years.
- Clinical manifestations include:
  - Photophobia
  - Itching in eyes
  - Headache
  - Hepatomegaly.

Homocystinuria

- Homocysteinurias are a set of autosomal recessive disorders occurring due to defect in conversion of homocysteine to methionine. There are four types of homocystinurias as shown in Figure 12.16.

Signs and Symptoms of Homocystinurias

- Mental retardation
- Growth failure
- Flat foot and Charley Chaplin gait
- Skeletal deformities—Kyphosis, scoliosis and arachinodactyly.
- Eye manifestations—Ectopia lentis (Subluxation of lens), myopia and glaucoma.
- Vascular changes
- Thrombosis—Homocysteine causes activation of Hageman factor leading to intravascular thrombosis.
  - Death occurs in the second or third decade of life.
  - Diagnosis can be done using chromatographic technique, where an abnormal spot of homocysteine is seen in patients.

Management

- Management of these patients is done by giving a diet low in methionine and rich in cysteine.

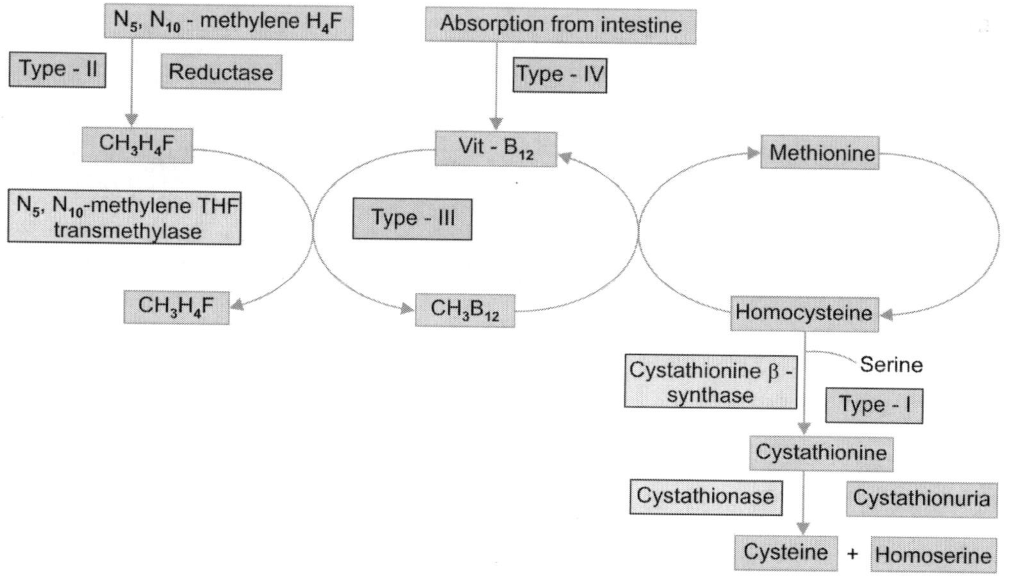

Fig. 12.16 Homocystinurias

Serine (Ser) and Threonine (Thr)

- Serine is a nonessential amino acid and is synthesized denovo from the glycolytic intermediate 3 – phosphoglycerate.
- Serine is catabolized to intermediates of gluconeogenesis (glucogenic in nature) or Ser is deaminated by Ser dehydratase forming pyruvate.
- Ser synthesizes important compounds line betaine, choline, ethanolamine and is precursor for the synthesis of selenocysteine—*An unusual amino acid present in certain proteins like glutathione peroxidase.*
- Threonine is an essential amino acid and it is catabolized by a Thr dehydratase similar to Ser.

Catabolism of Carbon Skeleton of Amino acids—Aromatic Amino Acids

Introduction

- Aromatic amino acids include phenylalanine, tyrosine, tryptophan and histidine; of which phenylalanine and tryptophan are essential, histidine is semi-essential and tyrosine is nonessential.

Phenylalanine (Phe)

- Phe has two important roles to play—Protein synthesis and tyrosine synthesis. The Phe spared of both these functions is completely catabolized. The catabolic breakdown of phenylalanine gives rise to both fumerate and acetoacetate thus it is both glucogenic as well as ketogenic in nature. Tyrosine is synthesized from Phe by its hydroxylation. Various inborn errors of metabolism of Phe are shown in Figure 12.17.

Inborn Errors of Phenylalanine Metabolism

- Inherited disorders of metabolism occur due to a defective or a deficient gene which is responsible for the synthesis of a key regulatory enzyme. As a Result there occurs a block in the pathway using the accumulation of substrates and alternative metabolites of the substrates. These might be toxic to the cells and tissues of the body leading to the clinical symptoms of the inherited disorders.

Phenylketonuria (PKU)

Etiology

- It is an inherited disorder (autosomal recessive) of Phe metabolism characterized by the inability to form tyrosine. It occurs due to—
  - Defect in phenylalanine hydroxylase—Classical PKU (Type I)
  - Defect in H2 biopterin reductase—Atypical PKU (Type II and III)
  - Defect in synthesis of H2 biopterin—(Type IV and V PKU)

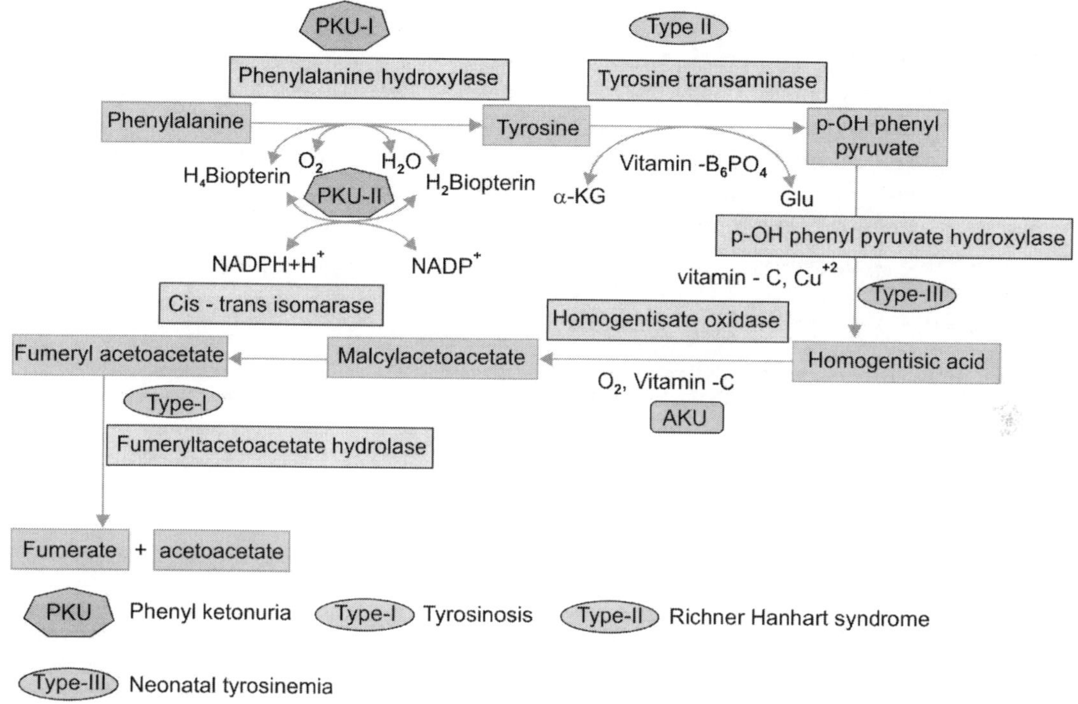

Fig. 12.17 Phenylalanine metabolism and inborn errors

Abbreviation: PUK; Phenyl ketonuria, Type-I; Tyrosinosis, Type-II Richner Hanhart syndrome; Type III Neonatal tyrosinemia

Occurrence

- 1 in 11,000 births
- Due to the defective enzyme, there is accumulation of Phe which converts to alternative metabolites phenyl lactate, phenyl acetate, phenyl acetyl glutamine and phenyl pyruvate which are toxic to body tissues.
- The disease gets its name due to high levels of urinary ketone—phenyl pyruvate.

Clinical Symptoms

- Mental retardation—It is the most characteristic feature of PKU patients. Almost 1% of patients in mental hospitals have PKU.
  - The IQ of such patients is low and ranges from 25 to 50. There is defective myelination of nerves and the weight of brain is below normal.
  - Neurological symptoms besides mental retardation, there are seizures, tremors, difficulty in walking and talking.
- Hypopigmentation—PKU patients have lighter skin; have gray or blue eyes due to lack of synthesis of melanin. This is because tyrosine is not there or is low therefore no synthesis eczema is seen.
- Mousy odor in urine due to phenyl lactates.
- PKU mothers/pregnant ladies with PKU have high blood levels of Phe causes the abnormal development of fetus.

Diagnosis

- Early detection of PKU is necessary.
- DNA probes aid prenatal diagnosis of defects in phenylalanine hydroxylase or di hydro biopterin reductase.
- Diagnosis can be done by detection of urinary Phe and alternative metabolites by $FeCl_3$ test which give an olive green color with phenyl pyruvate.
- Blood Phe level can be detected using *Guthrie test*. However, blood levels do not increase until the 1st week after birth.

Management

- PKU mothers should take diet low/without Phe to prevent damage to fetus.
- Infants once detected with PKU should be given artificial milk preparations low or no Phe to prevent irreversible brain damage. Such a diet is continued till the age of 6 year as after this age the normal diet can be resumed because by then the blood brain barrier is mature and no Phe can cross this barrier.

Alkaptonuria (AKU)

- AKU is an AR disorder. It is one of the Garrod's Tetrads. Other three are essential pentosuria, cystinuria and albinism.

Etiology and Symptoms

- It occurs due to defect in enzyme homogentisate oxidase (Fig. 12.17). Thus, there is accumulation of homogentisic acid in blood and is excreted in urine. Such urine on standing turns black due to oxidation of homogentisic acid by atmospheric oxygen.
- The blood homogentisic acid gets oxidized to benzoquinone acetate which polymerizes to black colored alkapton bodies and gets deposited in:
  - Intervertebral disks
  - Ear pinna cartilages—darkened ear pinna
  - Joints.
- This is termed as *ochronosis*. It occurs in third or fourth decade of life and has symptoms like backache, joint pain and arthritis develops due to tissue damage.

Treatment

- It is a benign condition and is not life-threatening so not treated. In later stages arthritis may be managed.

Tyrosinemia

Type – I Tyrosinemia/Tyrosinosis

Acute *Tyrosinosis*

- Defect in fumaryl acetoacetate hydrolase.
- Acute hepatic failure and death in the 1st year of life.

Chronic Tyrosinosis

- Chronic condition is milder than acute, cirrhosis of liver and death occurs by age 10.

Symptoms

- Increased blood and urine tyrosine.
- Increased Met in blood.
- Excretion of all metabolites of Tyr like tyramine, N – acetyl tyrosine.

Type II Tyrosinemia/Richner-Hanhart Syndrome

- Defect in tyrosine transaminase.

Symptoms

- Elevated blood and urinary tyrosine.
- Elevated blood and urinary p – OH Phe pyruvate,
- No elevated Met.
- Eye manifestations—eye lesions, corneal erosions.
- Skin manifestations—lesions of skin on palms and soles.

Type III Tyrosinemia/Neonatal Tyrosinemia

- Defect in p – hydroxy phenyl pyruvate hydroxylase.
- High serum tyrosine in premature infants as the liver is immature.
- In term infants low birth weight.
- As the liver matures accumulated tyrosine is metabolized and serum levels to adult levels.

Specialized Products of Tyrosine

Melanin

- Melanin is the pigment of hair, skin and iris.
- It is derived from a Greek word "Melano" meaning black.
- Melanin acts as a natural sunscreen/filter against the UV rays of the solar spectrum.
- It is synthesized and stored in the melanosomes of melanocytes of skin/hair/iris and provides them color respectively.
- The color of the skin depends upon the
  - Conc. of melanin.
  - Distribution of melanosomes.
  - Oxidation state of melanin.

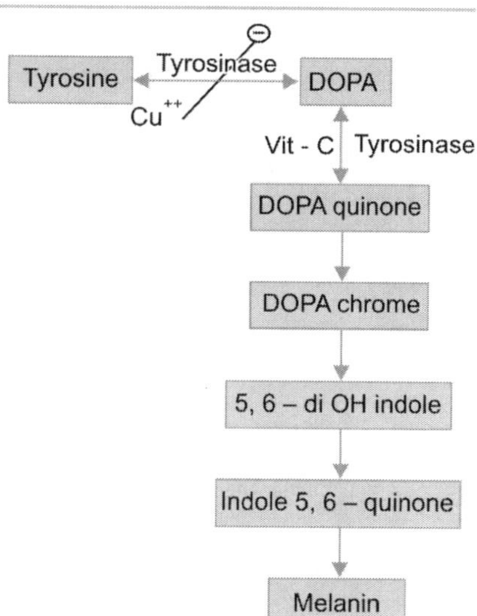

Fig. 12.18 Biosynthesis of melanin

Synthesis of Melanin (Fig. 12.18)

- The synthesis of melanin occurs from tyrosine. Tyrosine is oxidized to dihydroxy phenylalanine (DOPA) by the mixed function oxidase—tyrosinase that uses Cu as a cofactor rather than tetrahydrobiopterin.

- DOPA is further oxidized by tyrosinase to DOPA quinone. Beyond DOPA quinone all the further reactions are nonenzymatic spontaneous reactions where DOPA quinone is sequentially decarboxylated to dopachrome, then 5,6 dihydroxy indole, Indole 5,6 – quinone and finally melanin.

Albinism

- It is a heritable clinical disorder characterized by hypomelanosis.
- It is of 2 types:
  - *Type I—Tyrosinase negative*

    There is a total absence of the enzyme leads to lack of melanin in skin, hair and iris.

    Eye manifestations—There are oculocutaneous manifests. Iris is golden yellow and there is reduced visual acuity.

    Skin and hair manifestations—hair blonde

    Skin—In Caucasians – Milky white

    —in Orientals – Slightly tanned

    Due to lack of melanin, the patients on exposure to sun develop rashes on skin and are prone to skin cancer. Such kids are called Surajmukhi Children.
  - *Type II—Tyrosinase positive*

    The melanocytes are unable to take up tyrosine therefore no melanin synthesized but if tyrosine is injected into them then in-vitro melanin is synthesized. The skin of such albinos is slightly tanned, nail brownish and iris gray/blue.

Catecholamines (Fig. 12.19)

- Catecholamines include—DOPA, dopamine, epinephrine, and norepinephrine.
- Catecholamines are synthesized from tyrosine.
- Catecholamines are secreted by the adrenal medulla. They act as hormones and are important neurotransmitters too.

Parkinson's disease

Parkinson's disease occurs due to a deficiency of dopamine secreting cells in brain. The motor symptoms of Parkinson's disease result from the death of dopamine-generating cells in the substantia nigra. It is treated early on with levodopa or dopamine agonists.

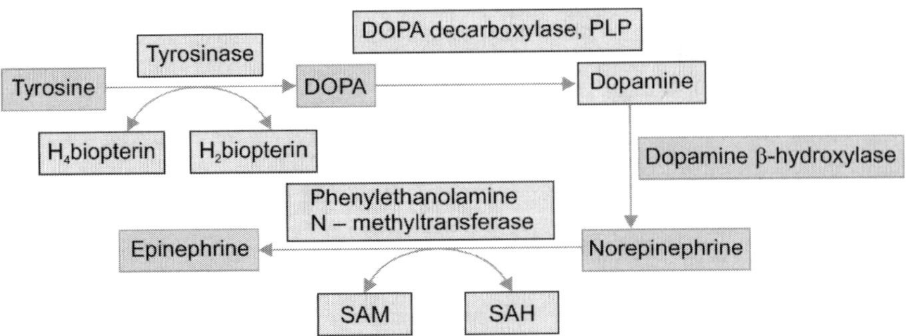

Fig. 12.19 Biostnthesis of catecholamines

Catabolism of Catecholamines (Fig. 12.20)

- Catecholamines are catabolized to vanillylmandelic acid as shown below. About 15% of the norepinephrine gets catabolized, rest being picked up again by the sympathetic adrenergic neurons.
- The excretion of vanillylmandelic acid is enhanced in conditions like—Pheochromocytoma where there is tumor of the chromaffin cells.

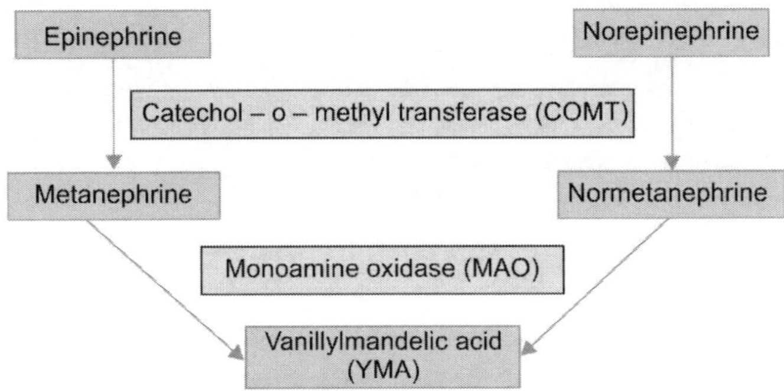

Fig. 12.20 Catabolism of catecholamines

Thyroid Hormones

- Thyroid hormones are iodinated tyrosines. Thyroid gland secretes three hormones—T_3, T_4 and reverse—T_3.
- T_3 is 3, 5, 3′—triiodothyronine.
- T_4 is 3, 5, 3′, 5′ - tetraiodothyronine.
- Reverse T_3 is 3′, 5′, 3—triiodothyronine.
- Tyrosine is iodized in the thyroid gland in a stepwise manner.

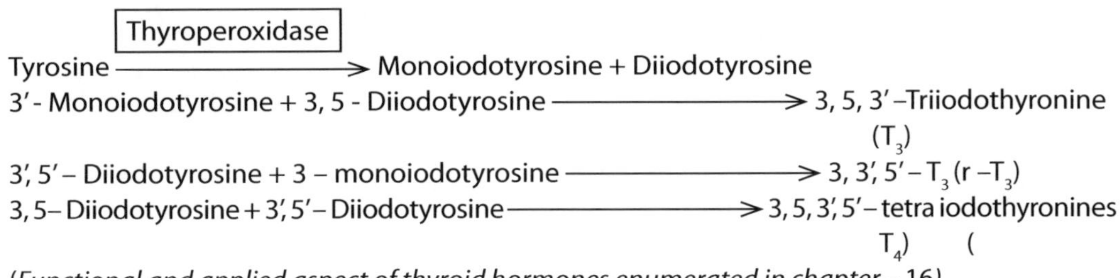

(Functional and applied aspect of thyroid hormones enumerated in chapter – 16*)*

Tryptophan (Trp)

- Tryptophan is an essential amino acid and needs to be consumed in daily diet.
- It is important in protein synthesis and is also gives rise to specialized products like—Niacin, serotonin and melatonin.
- Catabolism of Trp gives rise to acetoacetate and alanine, thus it is both a ketogenic as well as glucogenic.

- The catabolic pathway of Trp is unique in that it shunts to give rise to niacin about 3% of the Trp follows this route. 60 mg of Trp can synthesize 1 mg of niacin.
- Another branch point in tryptophan catabolism (major fate—97% of Trp follows this route) is the catabolism of Trp by the heme enzyme—Trp pyrrolase (Fig. 12.21), Trp pyrrolase/ Tryptophan dioxygenase is induced by glucocorticoids and glucagon. It is found in liver.
- N- formyl kynurenine formed by the Trp pyrrolase enzyme is further catabolized by kynurenine formylase to kynurenine.
- Kynurenine is hydroxylated by the kynurenine hydroxylase enzyme using NADPH as the coenzyme.
- Beyond 3-hydroxy kynurenine, the activity of kynurenase enzyme in conjunction with vitamin B_6 splits apart an alanine residue (thus Trp is glucogenic) and 3-hydroxy anthranilic acid is formed.
- A deficiency of vitamin-B_6 leads to a block in the enzyme activity at kynurenase. This causes the accumulated substrate 3-hydroxy anthranilic acid that oxidizes to xanthurinic acid (xanthurenate).
- 3-hydroxy anthranilic acid is normally further catabolized sequentially to 2-amino muconate semialdehyde which follows through a major route (97%) to acetyl CoA. Thus, Trp is ketogenic in nature too.
- About 3% of the 2-amino muconate semialdehyde is converted to niacin coenzymes via a quinolinate (detail pathway in Chapter 6).

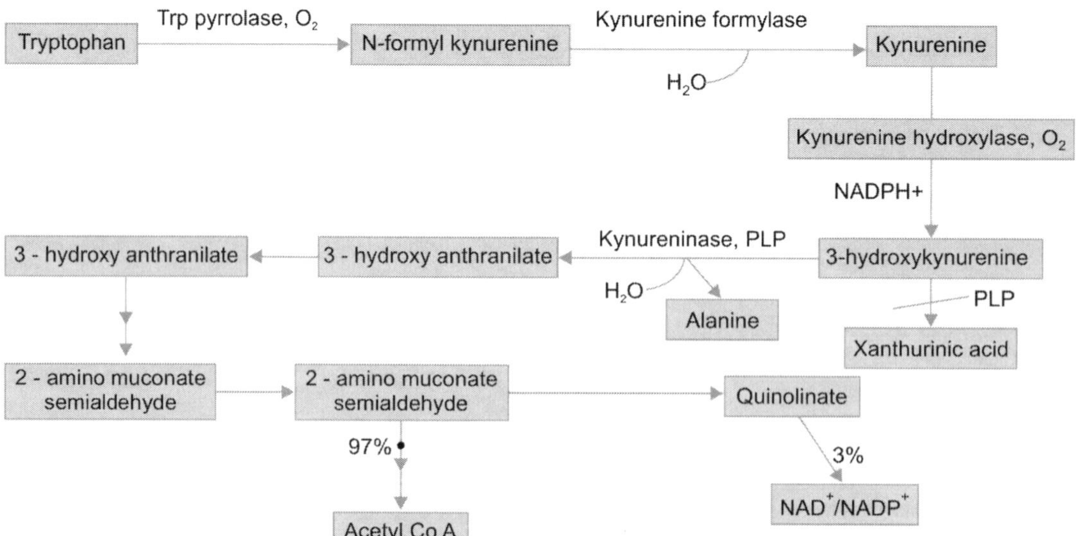

Fig. 12.21 TRP metabolism

Specialized Products of Tryptophan

Serotonin and Melatonin

- Tryptophan can synthesize two important specialized products—Serotonin and melatonin (Fig. 12.22).
- Serotonin is synthesized by the hydroxylation, followed by decarboxylation of tryptophan as shown in Figure 12.22.
- Serotonin is an important biogenic amine that is secreted by the mast cells, platelets, lungs, spleen and brain.
- At the blood vessels this serotonin causes vasoconstriction and bronchoconstriction by contracting the smooth muscles of blood vessels and bronchioles.
- At brain, serotonin acts like an important neurotransmitter that induces sleep.

Protein-rich Meal induces Wakefulness

- After a protein-rich meal, there are high levels of circulating amino acids in blood. This causes a sort of 'traffic jam' at the blood brain barrier and bulky amino acids like Trp cannot be taken up by the brain. Thus serotonin synthesis is reduced causing alertness rather than sleep induction.

Carbohydrate-rich Meal induces Sleep

- After a carbohydrate-rich meal, the blood sugar level rises causing the secretion of insulin. This will clear the amino acids from blood circulation, more taken being taken up by the muscles and thus there is less competition for Trp at the blood brain barrier which is readily taken up. The Trp in brain synthesizes serotonin and induces sleep.
- Strangely, extra serotonin appears to lead to sleepiness in females, but only calmness in males.

Melatonin synthesis:

- Serotonin can be further acetylated and methylated sequentially to give melatonin. Melatonin is a hormone secreted by the pineal gland.
- This hormone is responsible for the regulation of our sleep and wake cycle.
- It is secreted in circadian rhythms and is synthesized mostly at night.
- Melatonin induces sleep by inhibition of synthesis and secretion of neurotransmitters— GABA and dopamine.

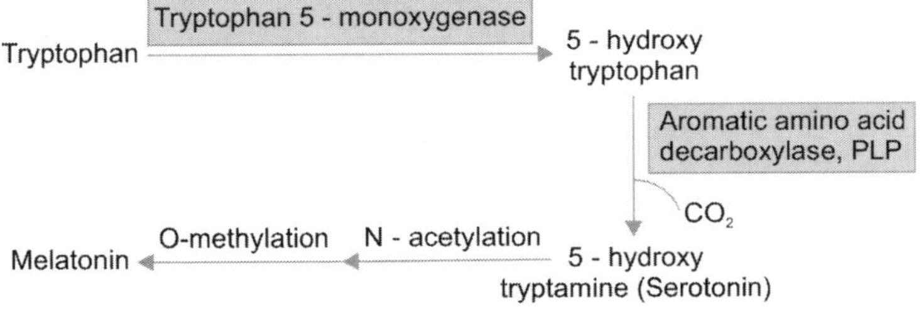

Fig. 12.22 Synthesis of serotonin and melatonin

Niacin

- Trp synthesizes niacin coenzymes—NAD^+ and $NADP^+$. These are synthesized during the catabolism of carbon skeleton of Trp (as shown in Figure 12.21).

Inborn Errors of Tryptophan Metabolism

Hartnup's Disease

Etiology

- Hartnup's disease is an inborn error of tryptophan metabolism. The defect in this disease is in the renal tubular reabsorption and intestinal absorption of dietary tryptophan and other neutral amino acids.
- As a result of the defective transport of Trp at renal tubules and intestines, the synthesis of niacin, serotonin and melatonin is adversely affected.

Symptoms

- There is niacin deficiency leading to pellagra like symptoms.
- The serotonin synthesis is reduced and leads to neurological symptoms characteristic of Hartnup's disease—with bizarre behavior and tendency of self-mutilation.
- Aminoaciduria also is seen due to failure of transport of amino acids from kidneys.

Treatment

- Treatment is done by administration of nicotinic acid orally, which would relieve the pellagra-like symptoms. However, the aminoaciduria persists.

Carcinoid Syndrome

Etiology

- Carcinoid syndrome occurs due to tumor of the argentaffinoma cells of the intestines. These cells normally synthesize and secrete serotonin that helps maintain the normal gut motility.
- However, the tumors of argentiffoma cells over-synthesize and secrete serotonin. For this a large amount of tryptophan is diverted towards serotonin synthesis and less is available for the synthesis of niacin.

Symptoms

- Niacin deficiency causes pellagra-like symptoms.
- The over secretion of serotonin at gut causes increased gut motility—Diarrhea, hot flushes, fluctuating hypertension.

Catabolism of Carbon Skeleton of Amino Acids: Branched Chain Amino Acids

Introduction

- There are three branched chain amino acids (BCAA)—Valine, leucine and isoleucine. All the three are nutritionally essential amino acids and must be supplemented in daily diet for an optimally health life and overall growth and development.
- The metabolism of BCAA is unusual since it starts in the muscles (as there is a larger concentration of BCAA transaminases in muscles than in liver).

Catabolism of Branched Chain Amino Acid's Carbon Skeleton

- The initial few steps of the metabolism are identical for all three BCAAs but eventually they completely catabolize to give different products (Fig. 12.23).
- The process begins with the transamination of the BCAAs to their respective α-keto acids. Since the concentration of BCAA transaminases is higher in muscles than in liver, the process is initiated in the muscles and thus these BCAA are excellent sources of energy.
- The second step is oxidative decarboxylation of the BCAA α-keto acids to their acyl CoA residues. The enzyme is branched chain α-keto acid dehydrogenases that is similar to the pyruvate dh complex in activity, coenzyme requirement and regulation.
- The activity of this enzyme complex is higher in liver and lower in muscles during well-fed state—Indicating higher oxidation of dietary BCAA by liver. Conversely during fasting the reverse happens, i.e. the levels of this enzyme are higher in muscles than in liver diverting the BC keto acids to muscles for oxidation as sources of energy.
- The third common enzyme activity is the dehydrogenation of the acyl CoA residues of the BC α-keto acids to give their unsaturated acyl CoA derivatives.
- Beyond these unsaturated acyl CoA derivatives, the fate of the three amino acids is different; such that on complete catabolism, valine gives succinyl CoA, isoleucine gives acetyl CoA and succinyl CoA and leucine gives acetoacetate.
- The succinyl CoA eventually enters the gluconeogenic pathway to produce glucose and acetyl CoA gives ketone bodies. Thus valine is glucogenic, isoleucine is both gluco and ketogenic and leucine is purely ketogenic.

Inborn Errors of BCAA Metabolism

- Enzyme deficiencies in catabolism of branched chain amino acids are not common. In general, they produce acidosis in newborn infants or young children.

Maple Syrup Urine Disease (MSUD)

- The most common abnormality of BCAA metabolism is MSUD.
- It occurs due to the deficiency or mutation in the branched chain keto acid dehydrogenase enzyme. (step – 2 in metabolism of BCAA)
- The defect causes an accumulation of the branched chain keto acids leading to acidosis and their excretion in urine.

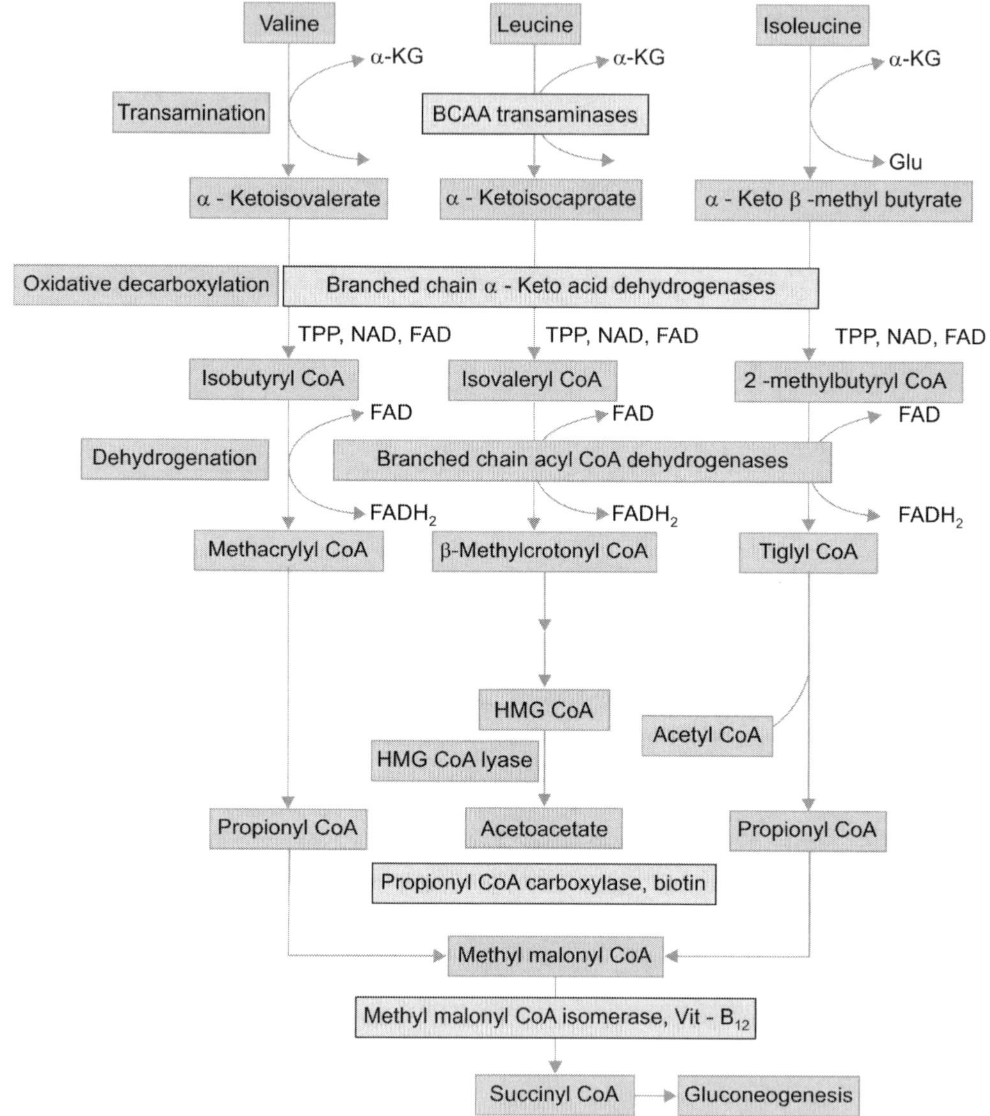

Fig. 12.23 BCAA metabolism

- The excretion of these branched chain keto acids in urine gives the urine its typical odor of *burnt sugar* hence the name—Maple Syrup Urine Disease.

Symptoms

The symptoms start appearing in the first week antenatally:

- The infant is difficult to feed
- Vomiting is frequent
- Acidosis
- Severe mental retardation in surviving cases
- If not treated coma and early death.

Diagnosis

Early diagnosis should be done to avert dire consequences. Early diagnosis is done enzymatically assessing the levels of BCAA metabolic enzymes.

Treatment

Since these amino acids are essential, their metabolically low levels are maintained such that their blood levels never exceed the metabolic demand. The infants are fed with diet deficient in BCAAs by artificial milk preparations.

Some other inborn errors of lower frequency are:

- Intermittent branched chain ketonuria due to slightly defective α-keto acid decarboxylase.
- Isovaleric acidemia due to defect in enzyme isovaleryl CoA dehydrogenase.

Biogenic Amines

Introduction

- Biogenic amines are organic poly cations derived from aromatic or cationic amino acids.
- Amino acids are decarboxylated by amino acid decarboxylases to give biogenic amines like:
  - Histidine gives histamine
  - Tryptophan gives tryptamine/Serotonin
  - Tyrosine gives epinephrine, norepinephrine and dopamine
  - Arginine and ornithine give polyamines spermine and spermidine
  - Cadaverine from lysine.
- These biogenic amines are formed as a result of normal metabolism in humans and all of them have important roles to play.
- In humans, biologic amines are involved in brain activity, the regulation of body temperature and stomach pH, gastric acid secretion, the immune response, and cell growth and differentiation, etc.

Histamine

Site of Synthesis and Secretion

- Histamine is present in all tissues; however, the important tissues involved in synthesis and secretion of histamine include the mast cells, lungs, spleen, platelets, gastric mucosa cells, etc.
- At hypothalamus of brain it acts like a neurotransmitter and its levels vary with the circadian rhythms.
- Histamine is a biogenic amine synthesized from histidine amino acid. Histidine gets decarboxylated by a histidine decarboxylase enzyme in the presence of PLP as a coenzyme.

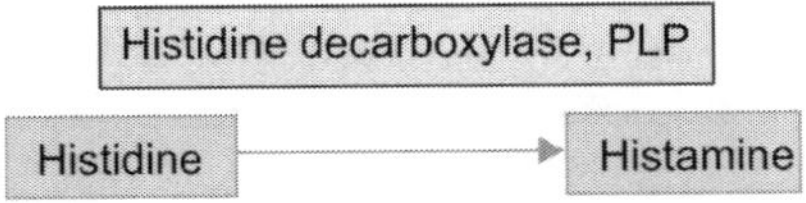

Functions of Histamine

- It causes vasodilation.
- It is an intermediate of allergic reactions.

- It increases vascular permeability.
- It is an excitatory neurotransmitter.
- It stimulates the secretion of gastric juice, thus the H_2 receptors of gastric mucosa are the site of action of the antacid drugs.

Tryptamine/Serotonin

Site of Synthesis and Secretion

- Serotonin is secreted by the mast cells, basophils, platelets, lungs, spleen, by brain cells at hypothalamus, limbic system, cerebellum, spinal cord, GIT and retina.
- Tryptophan gets decarboxylated by to give tryptamine/serotonin (*See* Fig. 12.22). Serotonin is an important biogenic amine and has one $-NH_2$ group (monoamine).

Functions of Serotonin

- Serotonin increases the blood pressure due to its vasopressive effect.
- Serotonin at the intestinal cells is responsible for the stimulation of peristalsis.
- Serotonin released at brain causes mood depression and induces sleep.
- Serotonin is an inhibitory monoamine at brain.
- Serotonin has also been found to be responsible for pain perception.
- It causes platelet aggregation.

Catecholamines (Dopamine, Epinephrine and Norepinephrine)

Site of Synthesis and Secretion

- Catecholamines include dopamine, epinephrine and norepinephrine.
- They are synthesized form tyrosine (as shown on page 321) at adrenal medulla. Adrenal medulla has 90% cells secreting epinephrine and 10% cells secreting norepinephrine.
- Most of the epinephrine is secreted by the adrenal medulla (80%) and is stored in the chromaffin cells.
- Most of the norepinephrine is secreted in tissues innervated by sympathetic nerves (80%) in situ or is transported to the site of via circulation from the adrenal medulla.
- The half-life of catechol amines is about 2 minutes.
- Normal blood levels of catecholamines are:
  - Epinephrine—3 µg/dL
  - Norepinephrine—30 µg/dL
  - Dopamine—3.5 µg/dL

Functions of Catecholamines

- Functions of epinephrine and norepinephrine are similar except that the effect of epinephrine is more prolonged (10 times) than that of norepinephrine owing to the slower degradation and removal of former.
- The effects of epinephrine and norepinephrine are dependent upon the type of tissue receptors; however a few generalized functions for these two are:

- *Effect on metabolism*—Epinephrine increases the BMR and the overall oxygen consumption (i.e. it is a calorigenic hormone).
- *Effect on carbohydrate metabolism*—Epinephrine increases the rate of glycogenolysis thus increasing the BSL (discussed in chapter 10).
- *Effect on lipid metabolism*—Epinephrine and norepinephrine causes lipolysis of the stored fat from adipose tissue in the presence of glucocorticoid hormone.
- Epinephrine and norepinephrine cause generalized *vasoconstriction.*
- Epinephrine has a positive *chronotropic* effect (Increase heart rate), *ionotropic* effect (force of contraction of heart), increase excitability and conductivity of heart muscle. Thus increasing the overall activity of heart. This along with vasoconstrictor action leads to hypertension when excessive amounts are secreted in certain conditions like *Pheochromocytoma.*
- Rate and force of respiration are also increased by epinephrine along with *bronchodilator effect.*
- Dopamine is secreted at adrenal medulla, dopaminergic neurons of basal ganglia where it acts like a neurotransmitter.
- General functions of dopamine are:
  - Vasoconstriction by causing release of epinephrine.
  - Increased systolic blood pressure.
  - Vasodilation in mesentery.
- *Deficiency of dopamine in basal ganglia causes Parkinsonism.*

Polyamines

Site of Synthesis and Secretion of Polyamines

- Polyamines are biogenic amines with multiple $-NH_2$ groups. Classically, polyamines are a family of molecules (i.e. putrescine, spermine, and spermidine) derived from ornithine according to a decarboxylation/condensative process (Fig. 12.24).
- These are ubiquitous in all human cells.
- More recently, it has been demonstrated that arginine can be metabolized according to the same pathway leading to agmatine formation.
- Agmatine is transformed into carbamilputrescine by agmatine imino hydroxylase (AIH). Finally, carbamilputrescine is converted into putrescine.
- In the second pathway, arginine is converted into ornithine and then ornithine is converted into putrescine by ornithine decarboxylase (ODC).
- Cadaverine is synthesized from lysine in a one-step reaction with lysine decarboxylase (LDC).

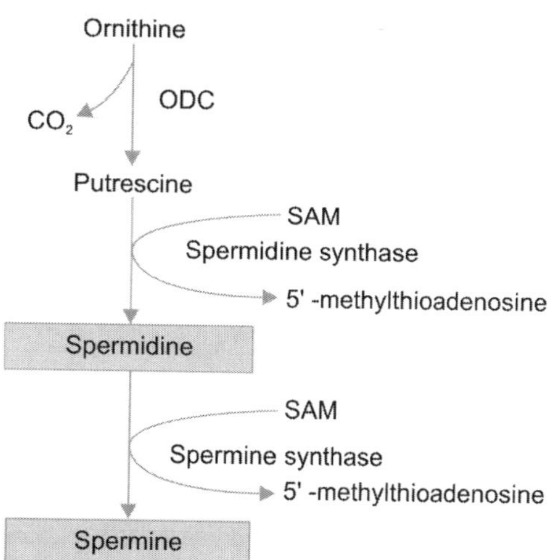

Fig. 12.24 Biosynthesis of polyamines

Functions of Polyamines

- *Role in cellular growth*—Although their exact functions have not yet been identified, it is clear that the polyamines play important roles in a number of cellular processes such as replication, transcription, and translation. These roles are exerted by specific interactions that can only be mediated by the cationic polyamines. Proper cell development depends on polyamines, as they have a profound stabilizing effect on a cell DNA. Young children need polyamines for growth—far more than adults.

- *Role in nervous system*—They are also critical to the healthy function of the nervous system.
- *Role in apoptosis:* There is also evidence suggesting a role for polyamines in programmed cell death (apoptosis). Polyamine deficiency under certain circumstances, result in programmed cell death or apoptosis. This is so because in polyamine deficiency, the DNA is destabilized, making it vulnerable to nuclease attack paving way for apoptosis.
  - *The key enzyme of polyamine synthesis—Ornithine decarboxylase is being now explored as a potent site for drug action to cure cancer. This is because of high rates of turnover of the enzyme in malignancy due to the increased rate of cell division.*
  - Polyamines are catabolized completely to CO_2 and NH_2.

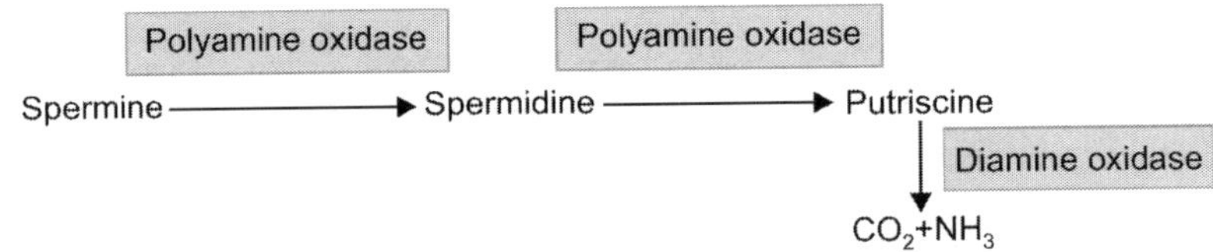

- These end-products of polyamine catabolism are excreted in urine. In cancerous tissues the increased rate of turnover of cancer cells increases the concentration of polyamines in body fluids.
- The blood and urinary levels of polyamines are used for detection of cancer and for follow up of the cancer therapy.

A Quick Look at the Amino Acid Metabolism

- Dietary proteins are digested to yield amino acids which get absorbed via secondary active transport and the meister's cycle.
- The amino acids are used as the building blocks of the body proteins.
- The amino acids are transaminated to pool up their amino groups into glutamate.
- Ammonia is transported as glutamate and glutamine to liver where deamination occurs to releases NH3 and urea is synthesized.
- Urea cycle occurs at liver mitochondria.
- Carbon skeleton of some amino acids is glucogenic—glycine, alanine, valine, serine, threonine, etc.
- Carbon skeleton of some amino acids is both glucogenic and ketogenic like—tryptophan, isoleucine, etc.
- Leucine is purely ketogenic amino acid.
- Glycine participates in synthesis of—heme, creatine and glutathione.
- Glycine is useful in conjugation of bile acids.
- Cysteine, cystine and methionine are S-containing amino acids.
- Active methionine is S – adenosyl methionine, which is useful in trans methylation reactions.
- Aromatic amino acid phenylalanine is used for protein synthesis and for tyrosine synthesis.
- Tyrosine is important precursor of thyroid hormones, melanin, catecholamines.
- Tryptophan is a precursor of niacin, serotonin and melatonin.
- Inborn errors of amino acid metabolism occur due to genetically defective genes of amino acid metabolism like PKU, AKU, cystinosis, cystinuria, glycinuria, albinism, etc.
- Biogenic amines are synthesized from the decarboxylation of amino acids.
- Important biogenic amines are histamine, serotonin, GABA, putrescine, spermdine, spermine.

CHAPTER

13

Purine and Pyrimidine Metabolism

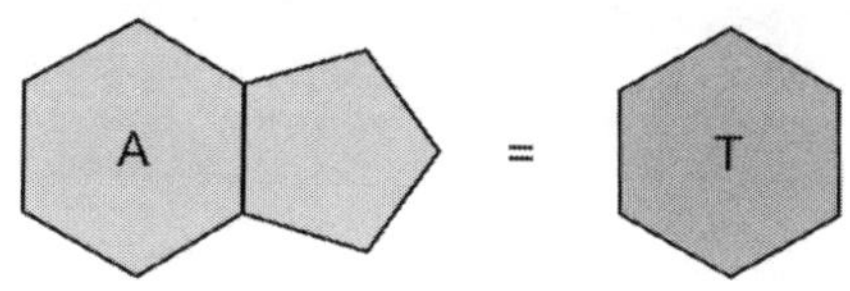

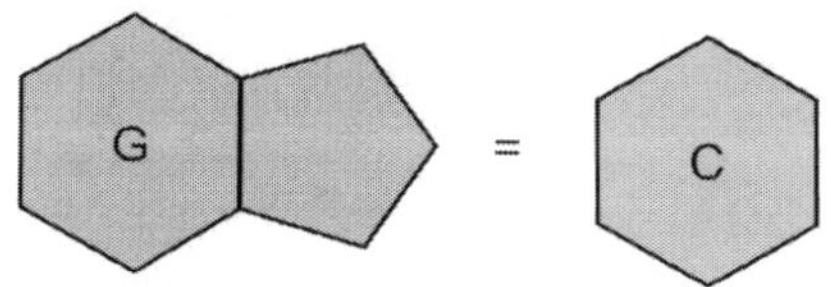

Chapter Framework

- Purine Metabolism
  - Introduction
  - Digestion and Absorption of Nucleotides
  - Purine Biosynthesis—De novo and Salvage
  - Purine Catabolism
  - Disorders of Purine Metabolism
- Pyrimidine Metabolism
  - Pyrimidine Biosynthesis—De novo and Salvage
  - Pyrimidine Catabolism and its Inherited Disorders

Introduction

- Purines and pyrimidines are essential constituents of animal and plant cells and are contained in various compounds. It is interesting to consider that some of these compounds are very stable, e.g. DNA, while others are rapidly turned over, e.g. ATP, NAD, NADP, etc. The purine and pyrimidine nucleotides are essentially required for the synthesis of genetic material DNA and also as a component of RNA. If there is a defect in their synthesis, both DNA replication and protein synthesis would be adversely affected.
- The synthesis of purine and pyrimidine nucleotides is highly significant to all the cells of body since these are constantly required for the multiplication of the cells as part of DNA.
- Besides this there are several nucleotide coenzymes—NAD, NADP, FAD, ATP, GTP, c-AMP, c- GMP, etc. that have significance in the metabolic activities and their regulation in a cell.
- The metabolism of nucleotides is complex because the molecules are large and composed of several different parts.
- The purine nucleotides on catabolism give end product uric acid that is sparingly soluble in water and pyrimidine nucleotides produce water-soluble end products.
- Defects in the catabolism of nucleotides, genetic or acquired cause metabolic disorders.
- Nucleotide metabolism is also important because it serves as a target for the development of several important pharmaceuticals.

Digestion and Absorption of Polynucleotides

- The dietary purine and pyrimidine nucleotides are present in all the organic food as nucleoproteins. These are present in all the cells as component of genetic material DNA and RNA.
- The dietary nucleoproteins are hydrolyzed by the gut proteolytic enzymes releasing nucleic acids. The nucleic acids are further hydrolyzed by nucleases to give polynucleotides that are digested by the oligonucleotidases enzymes of pancreatic juice into mononucleotides.

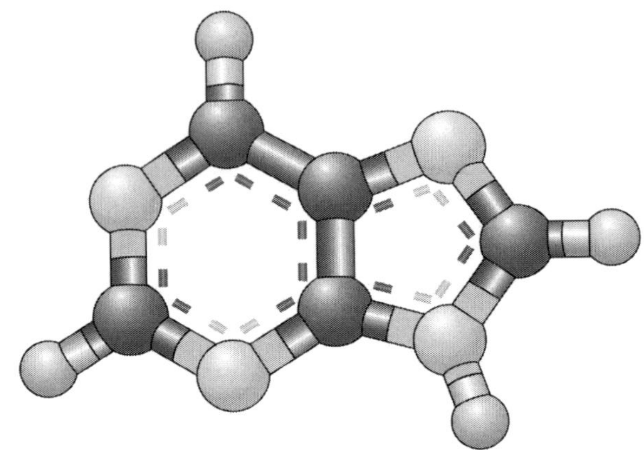

Fig. 13.1 Structure of purine ring

- The mononucleotides are either absorbed into the blood or are hydrolyzed by phosphodiesterase to free purines and pyrimidines that are absorbed into the circulation (Fig. 13.1).
- These dietary purines and pyrimidines although absorbed in the blood, these are not utilized by the body for the synthesis of new nucleic acid molecules—DNA or RNA. Instead these purine and pyrimidine bases are completely catabolized to their catabolic end products and excreted in urine.

Purine Metabolism

Introduction

- The body's demand for purine and pyrimidine nucleotides is fulfilled by the biosynthesis of both these nucleotides either by:
  1. De novo synthesis
  2. Salvage pathway.

Purine Biosynthesis

De Novo Synthesis

This is the most important pathway of purine nucleotide synthesis.

- The various atoms of the purine ring are contributed by different amphipathic intermediates like glycine, N_5, N_{10}- methylene H_4F, N_{10} formyl H_4F, CO_2, aspertate and glutamate (Fig. 13.2).
- This pathway starts with PRPP and slowly builds the purine base on the ribose phosphate molecule by essentially adding one atom at a time until the molecule inosine monophosphate (IMP) is constructed, which is the parent nucleotide giving rise to both AMP and GMP. The pathway is reproduced below (Fig. 13.3A).
- Phosphoribosyl pyrophosphate synthase (PRPP synthase) is the key regulatory enzyme of purine de novo synthesis. However, PRPP synthase is a common enzyme of both purine and pyrimidine synthesis.

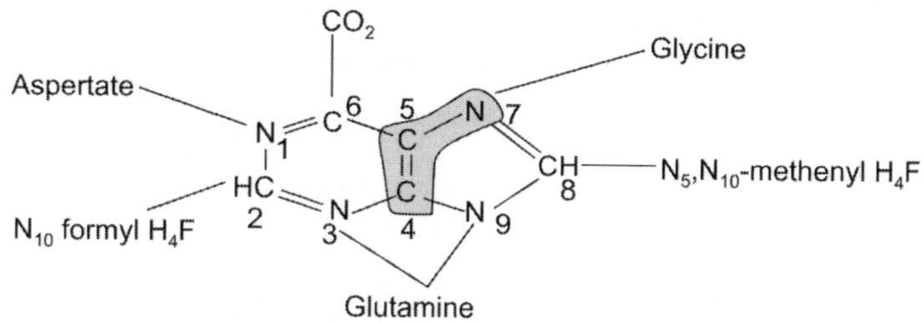

Fig. 13.2 Amphipathic contributors of the purine ring

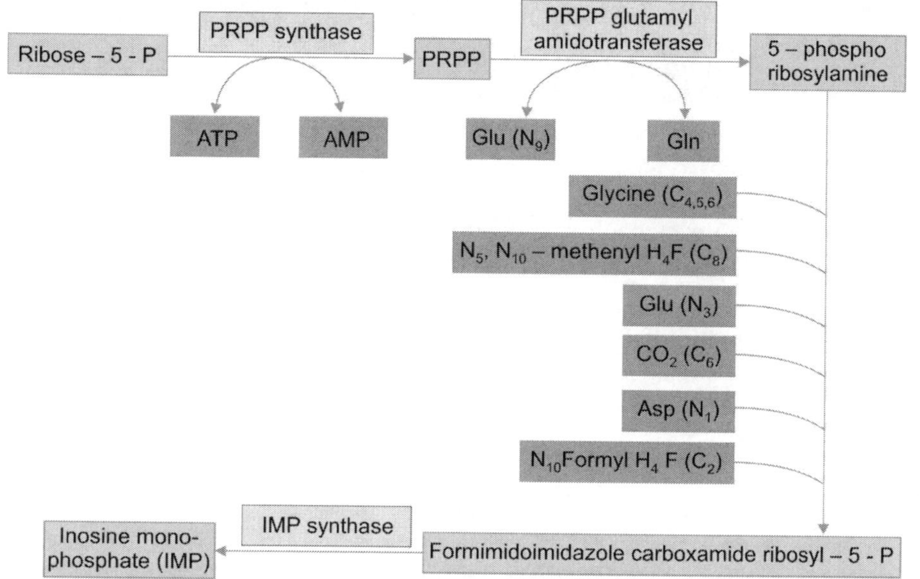

Fig. 13.3A De novo synthesis of parent purine nucleotide IMP

- PRPP glutamyl amido transferase is the first committed enzyme of this pathway. It is the first enzyme unique to purine biosynthesis, thus it is termed as the first committed enzyme of purine biosynthesis.
- The IMP converts to AMP by condensing with aspertate in the presence of adenylosuccinate synthase giving Adenylo succinate. Adenylo succinate is hydrolyzed in presence of adenylo-succinase to release the carbon skeleton of aspertate as fumerate and NH_2 group is retained forming AMP. This reaction requires GTP (Fig. 13.3B).
- The IMP is oxidized in presence of a NAD requiring enzyme IMP dehydrogenase to form xanthosine monophosphate (XMP) which in the presence of ATP and Gln picks up NH_2 forming GMP (Fig. 13.3B).
- Since ATP is required for synthesis of GMP and GTP for synthesis of AMP, the cellular concentrations of ATP and GTP help regulate the levels of GMP and AMP respectively by cross-regulation.
- Overall, the de novo synthesis of purine nucleotides is quite an expensive affair, since it utilizes the amphipathic intermediates and high energy phosphates (5 ~P).

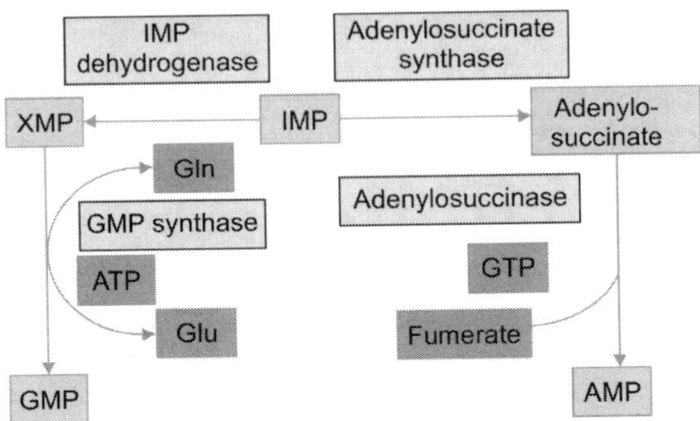

Fig. 13.3B Conversion of IMP to AMP and GMP

- The enzymatic steps of de novo synthesis are important sites of drug action. Most of the drugs are:
  - Antifolate drugs inhibiting reactions requiring folate derivatives. For example, methotrexate, 6 – mercaptopurine, mycophenolic acid.
  - Glutamine analogs inhibiting reactions requiring glutamine for transferring an amino group. For example, azaserine and diaznorleucine.
- This process primarily occurs at the liver and the rest of the tissues get these formed nucleotides via circulation.

Salvage Pathway

- Not all cells are capable of de novo synthesis of purine nucleotides. Certain cells like the erythrocytes, polymorph nuclear blood cells and brain cells cannot synthesize the purine nucleotides by de novo synthesis as they lack the enzymatic machinery necessary for it. These tissues use another pathway—*Salvage pathway.*
- Salvage pathway is a *saviour of energy and amphibolic intermediates.* This pathway converts the nucleosides obtained from cellular degradation into nucleotides.
- The pathway uses lesser energy as compared with the de novo synthesis.
- This process involves the:
  - *Phosphoribosylation of free purine nucleotides*: This process is catalyzed by two enzymes–
    - Adenosyl phosphoribosyl transferase (APRTase)
    - Hypoxanthine guanine phosphoribosyl transferase (HGPRTase)

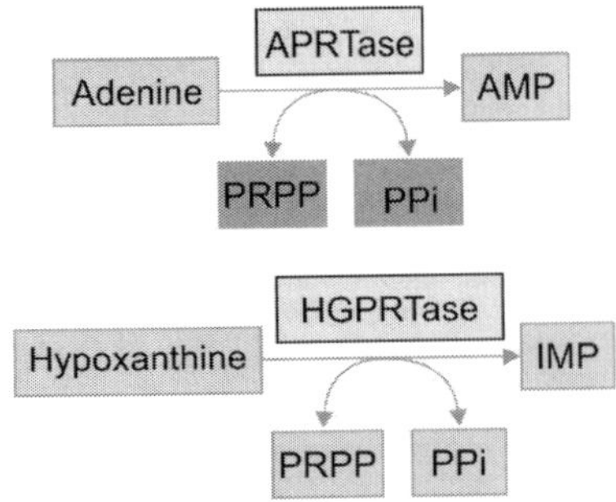

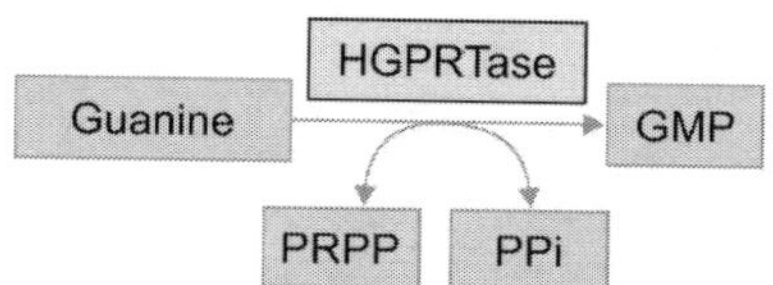

- Both the enzymes utilize PRPP as the donor of ribose – 5 – P unit for carrying out the Phosphoribosylation.
  - *Phosphorylation of purine nucleosides:* The purine nucleosides released during cellular turnover convert to the purine nucleotides by phosphorylation. There are two enzymes involved in this process –
    - **Adenosine kinase**

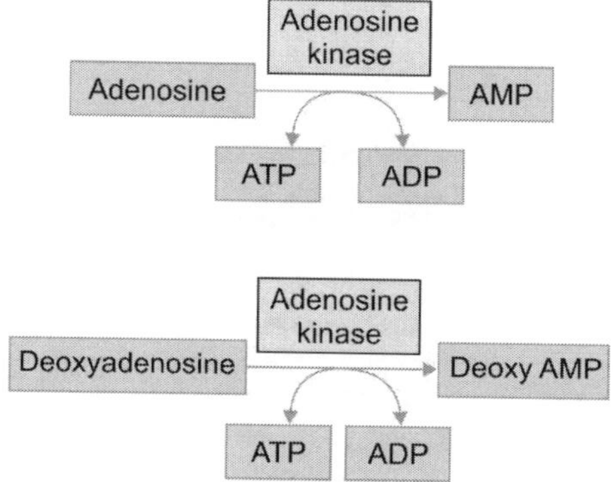

    - **Deoxycytidine kinase**

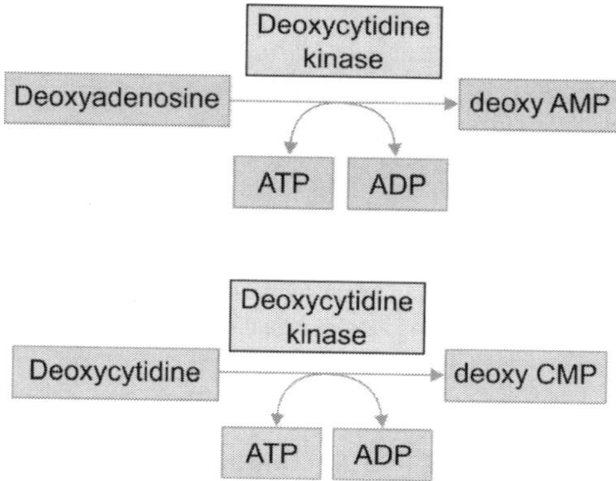

- The nucleotides thus synthesized in the de novo synthesis and salvage pathway are both ribose sugar derivatives and are present in RNA and some coenzymes. However, for the deoxy ribonucleotides of DNA, the enzyme ribonucleotides reductase causes the reduction of the ribose nucleotides with the thioredoxin as the H donor. Active thioredoxin (reduced) is regenerated by the enzyme thioredoxin reductase in presence of $NADPH+H^+$.

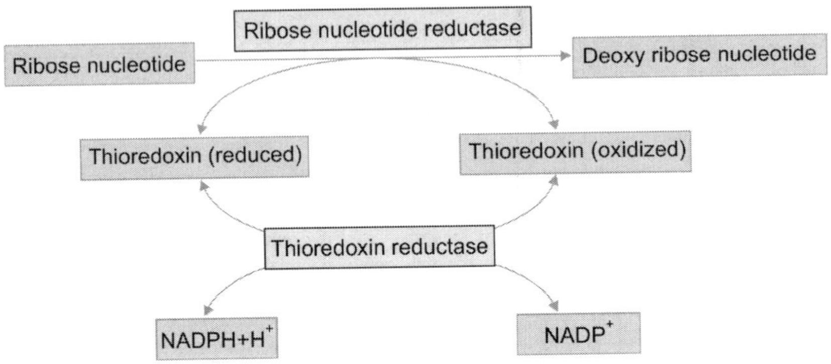

Regulation of Purine Biosynthesis

Regulation of De novo synthesis of Purines

- The de novo synthesis of the purine nucleotides requires of amphibolic intermediates and also high energy phosphates, thus the stringent regulation of this pathway is highly desirable and useful.
- The de novo synthesis is regulated at the bottle-neck of the pathway at the key enzyme–PRPP synthase.

Feedback Inhibition

- The enzyme PRPP synthase is regulated by feedback inhibition. The purine nucleotides AMP and GMP feedback inhibit the enzyme PRPP synthase.
- The enzyme is highly sensitive to the concentrations of PRPP, which in turn is dependent upon the availability of ribose – 5 – P.
- Similarly, the committed enzyme of de novo synthesis, PRPP glutamyl amidotransferase is feedback inhibited by the nucleotides GMP.

Cross–regulation of AMP and GMP Synthesis

- The synthesis of AMP and GMP from IMP has a cross-regulation by the high energy phosphates of these two nucleotides—ATP and GTP.
- Since ATP is needed for the synthesis of GMP from IMP and GTP for the conversion of IMP to AMP thus the concentrations of these two nucleotides would reciprocally regulate their synthesis.
- When the cellular concentration of ATP is high, the synthesis of GMP would occur conveniently and vice a versa.
- When the cellular concentration of GTP is high, the synthesis of AMP would occur and vice a versa.
- Thus, this cross regulation ensures a balanced production of AMP and GMP.

Allosteric Regulation

- The enzyme PRPP glutamyl amidotransferase is allosterically inhibited by GMP.
- AMP is an allosteric inhibitor of adenylosuccinate synthetase.
- Similarly, GMP is an allosteric inhibitor of IMP dehydrogenase.

Regulation of Salvage Pathway of Purine Biosynthesis

- The salvage pathway is regulated mainly by the availability of PRPP.
- The available PRPP is used primarily for salvage reactions, and secondarily for de novo synthesis.

Purine Catabolism

- Purines synthesized endogenously are catabolized to uric acid in liver and kidneys.
- The dietary purines on absorption are not utilized by the body rather they get completely catabolized to nitrogenous end product uric acid (Fig. 13.4).
- The uric acid must be eliminated from the body since humans lack the enzyme uricase. The uric acid thus produced is excreted via kidneys and gut.
- The total urate pool is about 1000 mg of which, 1/3rd is excreted by the gut (200 mg /day) and 2/3rd is excreted by the kidneys (600 mg/day approximately).
- It is probable that the elimination of urate via the alimentary tract is a passive process and varies with plasma urate concentrations. Under normal conditions, negligible amounts of

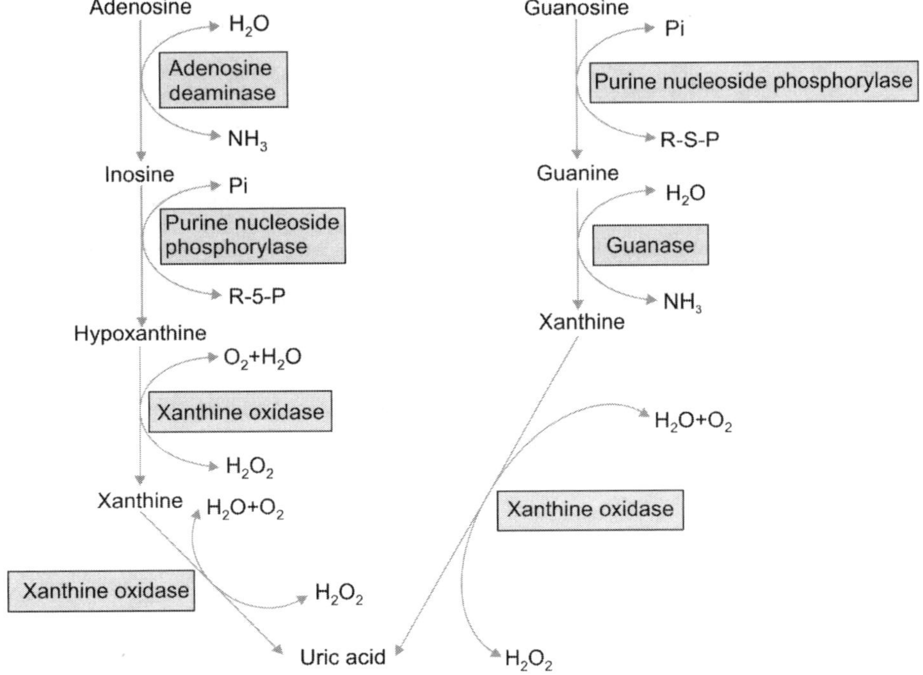

Fig. 13.4 Purine catabolism

urate are found in the feces because it is degraded by colonic bacteria. In a sterilized bowel, on the other hand, urate excreted into the lumen does not undergo uricolysis and may be found in the feces.

- Uric acid is a weak acid which is ionized at normal body pH and thus occurs in the blood or tissues in the form of the urate ion.
- When ionized, uric acid can form salts with various cations but 98% of extracellular uric acid is in the form of the monosodium urate. However, the proportion in the form of uric acid or urate is pH dependent so that the ratio between these two forms may vary considerably in urine.

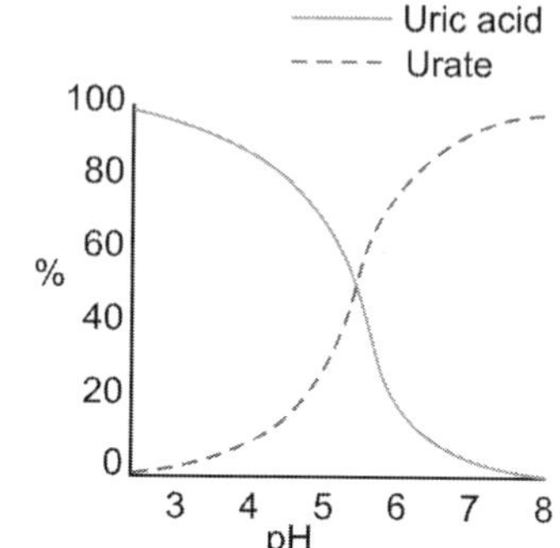

Fig. 13.5 Effect of pH on state of Uric acid; at pH 5.7 equal amounts of urate and uric acid exist

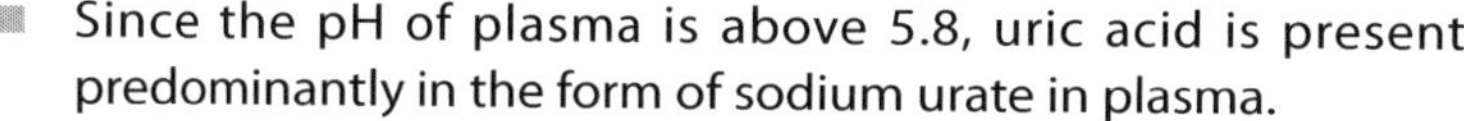

- Since the pH of plasma is above 5.8, uric acid is present predominantly in the form of sodium urate in plasma.
- The normal levels of serum uric acid in adult males are 5.5 mg/dL to 6.5 mg/dL and in females is 4 mg/dL to 6 mg/dL.
- Levels higher than 7 mg/dL is termed as hyperuricemia.
- Urate is considerably more soluble in plasma, synovial fluid and urine than in aqueous solutions. Even so, above a concentration of about 7.0 mg/dL (0.42 mmol/L), plasma is supersaturated with urate.
- Perhaps because this is often a stable situation and because of the other constituents of plasma, there may be no tendency to crystal formation. However, in individuals susceptible to formation of crystals, there is precipitation of urate crystals in synovial fluid of joints, leading *gouty arthritis*.
- The solubility of uric acid in urine rises exponentially as the pH increases above 4. Both urate and uric acid solubility fall with decreasing temperatures.

Disorders of Purine Metabolism

- The disorders of purine metabolism are more frequent than that of pyrimidine metabolism.
- The most important disorder of purine metabolism is *Gout*. Gout is predominantly a disease of adult males, with a peak incidence in the fifth decade.
- Gout is a disorder of crystal deposition in various body tissues. It occurs due to hyperuricemia. Uric acid being sparingly soluble in water gets precipitated as needle shaped birefringent crystals. These are birefringent, i.e. they appear yellow when the plane of polarized light is parallel to that of the crystal and blue when the plane of polarized light is perpendicular to it.
- Collection of these crystals is termed as *tophi*.

Clinical Features of Gout

- *Hyperuricemia*: A serum or plasma urate concentration greater than 7.0 mg/dl (0.42mmol/l) in males and 6.0 mg/dL (0.36 mmol/L) in females.
- *Acute gouty arthritis*: Sudden, intense inflammation in and around the joints (most typically, but not limited to, the big toe) and other areas of soft tissues such as the Achilles tendon (heel), olecranon bursa (elbow), helix of the ear.

- The crystals start depositing from the big toe of foot and gradually spread to other joints. This makes the joints painful and movement difficult.
- *Urolithiasis*: Uric acid stones in the kidney and urinary collecting system.
- *Chronic interstitial nephropathy*: Disease related to the deposition of monosodium urate monohydrate crystals in the substance of the kidney itself.

Types of Gout

Primary Gout

- Primary gout is a hyperuricemic condition due to some genetic disorder of purine metabolism.
- About 10% of patients with hyperuricemia are overproducers of uric acid of which no more than 10% (i.e. 1% of all hyperuricemic people) have primary identifiable inherited derangements in mechanisms regulating purine nucleotide synthesis de novo.

Etiology

- Primary gout occurs due to defect in the enzymes –
  1. PRPP synthase—Super active
  2. PRPP synthase—Resistant to feedback inhibition
  3. HGPRTase—Complete deficiency.
- The super active PRPP synthase or the PRPP synthase resistant to feedback inhibition shall lead to an overproduction and excessive catabolism of purines leading to hyperuricemia and primary gout.
- The complete deficiency of HGPRTase enzyme causes sparing of PRPP for de novo synthesis leading to over production and over catabolism of purines and gout.

Secondary Gout

- Secondary gout is the hyperuricemia occurring secondary to disorders other than that of purine metabolism.

Etiology

- Secondary gout is seen due to disorders characterized by an excessive cellular turnover leading to hyperuricemia and gout, for example, Cancer, Polycythemia vera, Psoriasis, etc.
- Secondary gout is also seen in patients of renal failure as they are unable to excrete the excessive uric acid.
- Secondary gout is also seen in lactic academia as lactic acid competes with uric acid for excretion.

Management of Gouty Arthritis

- *Avoid purine rich food like*: Fish like salmon, sardine, mackerel, meat extracts, beans, lentils, peas, asparagus, etc.

- *Avoid excessive alcohol*: This is so because, the alcohol is metabolized by alcohol dehydrogenase producing NADH and leads to lactic acidosis. The lactate then competes with uric acid for excretion.
- *Cold climate*: The cold climate reduces the solubility of both urate and uric acid appreciably causing the precipitation of crystals of uric acid or urate and acute gouty arthritis.
  - Thus individuals with hyperuricemia and high susceptibility to gout, on consuming purine rich diet and alcohol in cold climates or polar regions sleep symptomless at night. However, due to accumulation of uric acid and lacticacidemia, are woken up in early hours of the morning due to excruciating pain in the joints caused by the gouty arthritis.
- *Intake of water increased*: The increased intake of water washes out the excess of uric acid. Alkalinization of urine is another method for solubilising urate crystals of renal tubules.
- *Drugs*: Different types of drugs help manage gout:
  - Anti-inflammatory drug – Colchicine reduces pain.
  - Uricosuric drug – Probenicid causes elimination of uric acid via urine.
  - Suicide inhibitor – Allopurinol causes inhibition of xanthine oxidase.

Some of the other common inborn errors of purine metabolism are:

- Lesch - Nyhan syndrome
  - It occurs due to the partial deficiency of HGPRTase.
  - It is characterized by an overproduction hyperuricemia characterized by frequent episodes of uric acid lithiasis and a bizarre syndrome of self-mutilation.
- Adenosine deaminase deficiency
  - The defect is of adenosine deaminase enzyme.
  - It is associated with immunodeficiency where both the T – cells and B – cells are sparse and dysfunctional, i.e. there is severe combined immunodeficiency disease (SCID).
  - In lack of treatment (by bone marrow transplant or gene therapy) the infants die of fatal infections.
- Purine nucleoside phosphorylase deficiency
  - This disorder occurs due to deficiency of purine nucleoside phosphorylase in T – cells but have apparently normal B – cell function.
  - Due to this defect there is accumulation of d ATP and d GTP which inhibits the enzyme ribonucleotides reductase and thus the cells are depleted gradually of DNA precursors.

Pyrimidine Metabolism

Introduction

- The dietary pyrimidines are not utilized by the tissues for DNA synthesis or for the formation of coenzymes. Thus, the pyrimidines needed for the tissue repair, regeneration and new tissue synthesis is all synthesized either de novo or by salvage pathway similar to purines.
- The major pathways for pyrimidines synthesis are:
  a. De novo synthesis
  b. Salvage pathway

De novo Pyrimidine Synthesis

- The de novo synthesis of the pyrimidine ring involves a step wise addition of the various atoms of the pyrimidine ring by amphibolic intermediates (Fig. 13.6).
- Five of the first six enzyme activities of pyrimidine biosynthesis reside on multifunctional polypeptides; this increases the overall efficiency of the biosynthesis.
- The synthesis of pyrimidine nucleotides begins with the condensation of CO_2 with glutamine amino group in the presence of ATP such that a carbamoyl phosphate is synthesized, similar to that of urea cycle. The enzyme is carbamoyl phosphate synthase – II (CPS – II).
- However, the enzyme CPS – II is cytosolic and not mitochondrial like CPS – I of urea cycle.
- The reaction differs from that of urea cycle since the amino group donor is glutamine and not NH_4^+.
- Further the different atoms of the pyrimidine ring are added sequentially to form the Orotic acid (Fig. 13.8).
- Orotate then combines with PRPP to form the OMP which through decarboxylation gives rise to UMP, the first pyrimidine nucleotide.
- UMP is phosphorylated sequentially to UTP using ATP.
- UMP gives rise to the other pyrimidine nucleotides – CMP and TMP as shown in Figure 13.8.
- d-UMP is synthesized by the deamination of d-CMP by d-CMP deaminase. This appears to be a major pathway for the formation of d-UMP which then eventually is methylated to TMP by accepting 1 – C unit from N_5, N_{10} – methylene H_4F (Fig. 13.7).

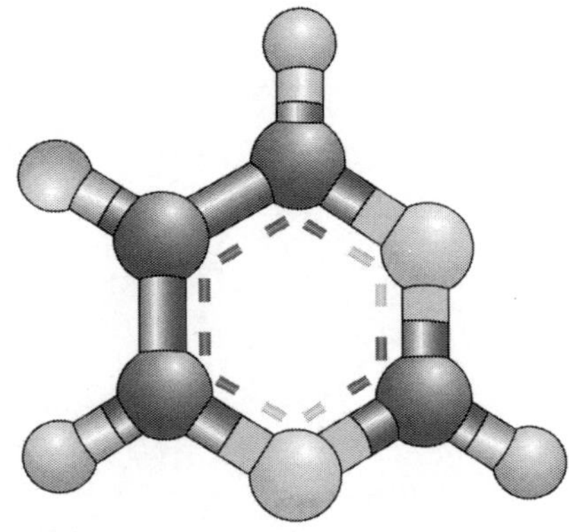

Fig. 13.6 Pyrimidine ring

Salvage Pathway of Pyrimidine Nucleotide Biosynthesis

- The mammalian cells reutilize few free pyrimidines but salvage the pyrimidine ribonucleosides by phosphorylating them in the presence of respective kinases.
- The different kinases are:
  - Uridinecytidine kinase
  - Deoxycytidine kinase
  - Thymidine kinase

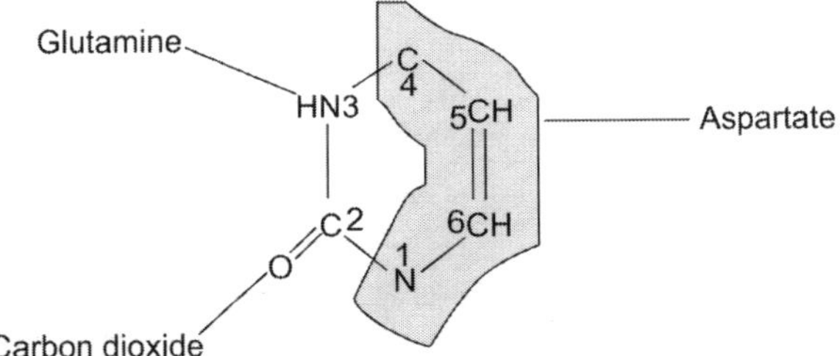

Fig. 13.7 Amphibolic intermediates contributing pyrimidine ring atoms

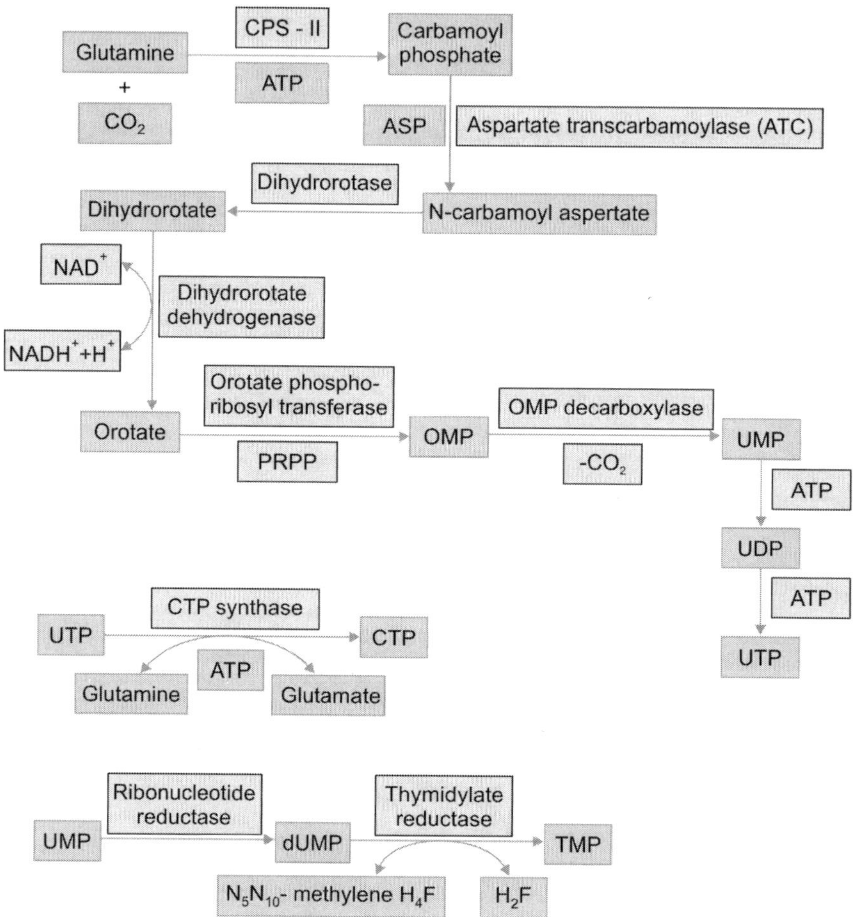

Fig. 13.8 Pyrimidine biosynthesis pathways

Regulation of Pyrimidine Biosynthesis

- The regulation of pyrimidine nucleotides biosynthesis is carried out allosterically at the enzymes-
  - CPS – II
  - ATC
- CPS – II is allosterically inhibited by the UTP and purine nucleotides and is activated by PRPP.
- ATC is inhibited by CTP and activated by ATP.
- Besides this the first three and last two enzymes are regulated by coordinate repression, derepression.

Coordinated Regulation of Purine and Pyrimidine Biosynthesis

- The biosynthesis of purines and pyrimidine nucleotides is coordinately regulated mole for mole.
- PRPP synthase the enzyme that provides PRPP for both pathways is feedback inhibited by both purines and pyrimidines.

Catabolism of Pyrimidine Nucleotides

- Unlike the purine rings, which are not cleaved in human cells, the pyrimidine ring can be opened and degraded to highly soluble structures, such as β-alanine, and β-aminoisobutyrate.

Disorders of Pyrimidine Metabolism

- Since the end products of pyrimidine catabolism are highly water-soluble, pyrimidine overproduction results in few clinical signs or symptoms.
- In severe overproduction of PRPP, there is overproduction of pyrimidine nucleotides as well and increased excretion of β-alanine.
- Since N_5, N_{10} – methylene H_4F is required for thymidylate synthesis, disorders of folate and vitamin B_{12} metabolism result in deficiencies of TMP.
- Orotic acidurias occur due to defect in enzymes of pyrimidine biosynthesis.
  - Type – I orotic aciduria occurs due to deficiency of orotate phosphoribosyl transferase and OMP decarboxylase.
  - Type – II orotic aciduria occurs due to deficiency of OMP decarboxylase.

Signs and symptoms of orotic acidurias
- Abnormal growth
- Megaloblastic anemia
- Excretion of large amounts of orotic acid in urine.

Management of orotic acidurias
- Feeding uridine rich diet reduces excretion of orotic acid in urine and improves anemia.

A Quick Look at the Purine and Pyrimidine Metabolism

- Dietary purines and pyrimidines are not utilized rather are completely catabolized.
- Purines and pyrimidines required by the body are biosynthesized by—De novo synthesis (from amphibolic intermediates) or by salvage pathway (from purine and pyrimidine nucleosides).
- Purine biosynthesis is regulated by the feedback regulation of the key enzymes—PRPP synthase and PRPP glutamyl amidotransferase.
- Purines are catabolized to uric acid. Inherited defect of purine catabolism causes hyperuricemia and gout.
- Pyrimidines are catabolized to CO_2 and NH_3.
- Inherited defects of pyrimidine metabolism causes orotic acidurias.

Section – 4

Endocrinology

- An Introduction to Endocrinolgy
- Hormone Action
- Hormones of Pituitary and Hypothalamus
- Hormones of Thyroid Gland
- Hormones of Parathyroid Gland
- Hormones of Pancreas and Gut
- Hormones of Adrenal Gland
- Hormones of Gonads

CHAPTER

14

An Introduction to Endocrinology

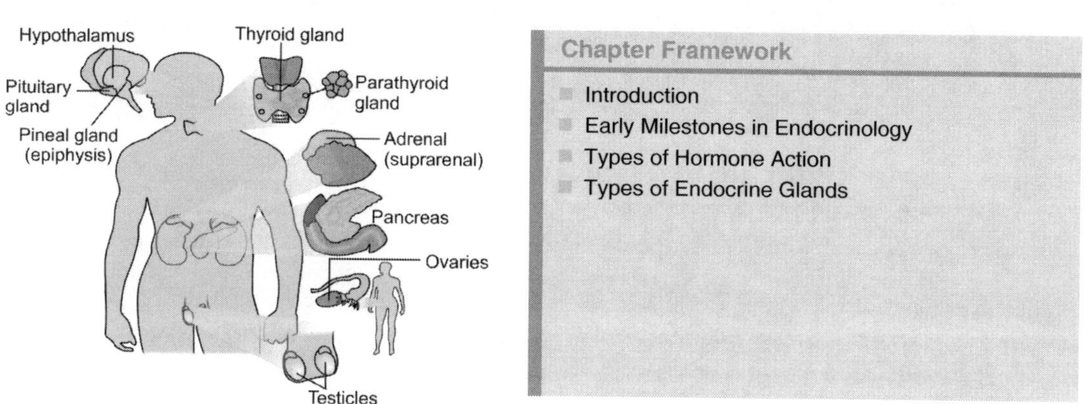

Chapter Framework

- Introduction
- Early Milestones in Endocrinology
- Types of Hormone Action
- Types of Endocrine Glands

Introduction

- Endocrinology is the study of endocrine glands, their diseases and their secretions— *Hormones.*
- The study of endocrinology began in China. The Chinese were isolating sex and pituitary hormones from human urine and using them for medicinal purposes by 200 BC.
- The ancient Indian scriptures too report of prevalence and treatment of diabetes in *Devik yuga to 10,000 BC,* by Maharishi Patanjali in *'Yogsutra'.*
- The birth of modern endocrinology can be said to have occurred in 1889 at the *Societe de Biologie* in Paris where Charles-Edouard Brown-Séquard, a professor at the College de France and one of the most distinguished physiologists of the nineteenth century presented his lecture on self-administration of animal testes extract that improved his physical strength, intellectual capacity and sexual potency.
- Within a short time proof was obtained for the existence of multiple chemical messengers, and a dynamic discipline was born—Endocrinology.
- Hormones are the chemical messengers secreted by the endocrine glands that execute the physiological functions of these glands.
- Some of the early milestones in the history of endocrinology are shown in Table 14.1.
- Ernest Starling is the first endocrinologist, having discovered the hormone 'secretin' in 1902 with Bayliss and coined the term 'hormone' in 1905. It comes from the Greek word *'hormacin'* meaning *'to excite'.*

Table 14.1 Early milestones in endocrinology

1889	Brown-Sequard self-administers testis extracts
1891	Murray treats myxoedema with thyroid extract
1894	Oliver and Schaefer describe epinephrine
1903	Bayliss and starling discover secretin
1904	Bouin and Ancel deduce role of the Leydig cell in male phenotypic differentiation
1909	MacCallum and Voetlin discover link between parathyroid glands and calcium metabolism
1913	Farmi and von den Velden treat diabetes insipidus with posterior pituitary extracts
1921	Evans and Long describe growth hormone
1922	Discovery of insulin by Banting and Best

- The hormones can be:
  - Autocrine—Acting on cells that secrete them.
  - Paracrine—Acting on cells present in close vicinity to them.
  - Endocrine—Secreted by endocrine glands and acting on cells present far from their site of release. (Fig. 14.1)
- Endocrine glands are ductless glands, i.e. they secrete their secretions—Hormones, directly into blood circulation and are then carried to the different organs via circulation.
- The different endocrine glands are:
  - Pituitary gland—Master gland
  - Thyroid gland
  - Parathyroid gland
  - Pancreas
  - Adrenal gland/Suprarenal gland
  - Testes
  - Ovaries.

Some other organs secreting hormones are:

1. Kidneys secreting angiotensin
2. Pineal gland secreting melanocyte secreting hormone
3. GI tract secreting few hormones from specialized cells of GI tract.

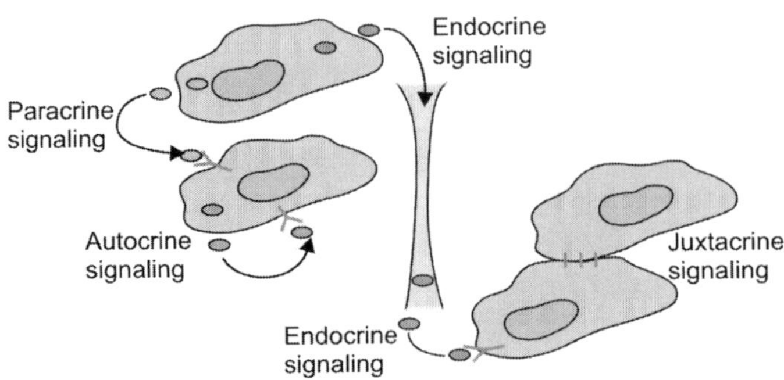

Fig. 14.1 Types of action of hormones

- This current section throws light on all the endocrine glands, their chemical messengers—Hormones, physiological roles of hormones, pathologies associated and the organ function tests that would help assess their normal or abnormal functioning.

A Quick Look at the Introduction to Endocrinology

- Endocrinology is the most dynamic principle of medicine.
- It involves the study of endocrine glands and their chemical secretions—Hormones.
- The important endocrine glands include—Pituitary, thyroid, parathyroid, pancreas, adrenals, and testes and ovaries.
- Other important organs secreting hormones are—Kidneys, pineal gland and GI tract.

CHAPTER

15

Hormone Action

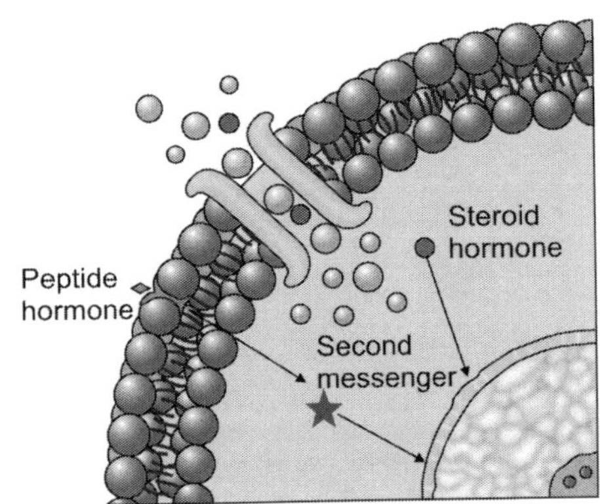

Chapter Framework

Introduction

- Cellular activities are coordinated by the exchange of ions and molecules between adjacent cells across gap junctions. This direct communication occurs between two cells of the same type, and the cells must be in extensive physical contact. The two cells communicate so closely that they function as a single entity. Such direct communication is highly specialized and relatively rare.
- Most communication between cells involves the release and receipt of chemical messages. Paracrine communication involves the use of chemical signals to transfer information from cell to cell within a single tissue.
- Endocrine communication is carried out by endocrine cells releasing chemicals called hormones.
- Hormones are chemical messengers synthesized by organisms that initiate biological responses by binding with high affinity and specificity to target cell receptors within the same individual. They are characterized by:
  - Endogenous synthesis
  - High affinity and specificity of binding to specific receptors on target cells
  - Initiates biological response.
- Thus, hormones exert their effects by modifying the activities of target cells, specific cells that possess the receptors needed to bind and "read" the hormonal message.
- They can be broadly classified into:
  - Amino acid derivatives
  - Peptide derivatives
  - Lipid derivatives.

Amino Acid Derivatives

- These are hormones that are derived from amino acids directly, e.g.
  - Derivatives of tyrosine
    - Catecholamines (epinephrine, norepinephrine, dopamine)
    - Thyroid hormones (dipeptides).
  - Tryptophan derivative
    - Melatonin

      (*Synthesis of amino acid derivative hormones has been discussed in amino acid metabolism with respective amino acids*).

Peptide Derivatives

- These are proteinaceous hormones which are synthesized as follows:
  - Synthesized on the ribosomes attached to rough-ER
  - All of them have ER targeting sequence on the N-terminus (signal peptide)
  - Synthesized as prohormones
  - Inactive molecules converted to active hormones in ER and Golgi, sometimes after secretion
  - Exocytosed from the cell
  - Work from the outside the cell (bind to surface receptors).
- Peptide hormones include:
  - Glycoproteins from anterior pituitary—More than 200 amino acids long, with carbohydrate side chains.
    1. Thyroid-stimulating hormone (TSH)
    2. Luteinizing hormone (LH)
    3. Follicle-stimulating hormone (FSH).
  - Steroid hormones and amino acid derivatives are included in group 1 hormones and group 2 hormones include all proteins and peptide hormones
  - Group 2 hormones including all the hormones secreted by the hypothalamus, heart, thymus, digestive tract, pancreas, and posterior lobe of the pituitary gland, as well as most of the hormones secreted by the anterior lobe of the pituitary gland (Table 15.1).
    a. Growth hormone (GH)
    b. ADH
    c. Oxytocin
    d. Prolactin (PRL)
    e. Peptides and small proteins
       1. Digestive tract hormones
       2. Pituitary hormones
       3. Pancreatic hormones

Lipid Derivatives

There are two classes of lipid derivatives:

- Eicosanoids—Derived from arachidonic acid e.g. leukotrienes, prostaglandins, prostacyclins and thromboxanes.

Table 15.1 General features of the steroid and polypeptide hormones

	Steroid Hormones (Group I)	*Peptide hormones (Group II)*
1.	Lipophilic	Hydrophilic
2.	Transport proteins present	No transport proteins
3.	Half—life few hours to days	Half-life few minutes
4.	Receptor intracellular	Receptor on plasma membrane
5.	Mediator—Hormone receptor complex	Mediator—Second messengers like cGMP, cAMP, Ca, metabolites of phosphoinositols, kinase cascades, e.g. Protein hormones

- Steroid hormones—Derived from cholesterol. e.g. androgens from testes, estrogen and progestins from ovaries, corticosteroids by adrenal cortex, calcitriol from kidneys.

- Hormone action at the cellular level begins with the association of the hormone and its specific receptor. All receptors, whether for polypeptides or steroid hormones have at least 2 functional domains—
  - Ist domain recognition domain binds the hormone.
  - IInd domain that generates a signal to couple hormone recognition to some intracellular function. This coupling is called signal transduction.

Signal Transduction for Steroid Hormones

- Steroid hormones can directly traverse the plasma membrane of cells to initiate their response via cytoplasmically located receptors called steroid hormone receptors.
- These receptors belong to intracellular receptor super family that transducer signals from some other hydrophobic biomolecules like thyroid hormones and retinoids.

Mechanism of Action of Steroid Hormones

- The steroid hormones and other group I molecules being lipophilic diffuse through the plasma membrane of all cells but bind their specific cytoplasmic receptors only in the target cells.
- The hormone receptor complex next undergoes a temperature and salt-dependent activation reaction (Fig. 15.1).
- This results in change in size, conformation and surface charges so that this H–R complex binds to the chromatin.
- The H–R complex binds to specific DNA sequences called hormone response elements (HRE) and activates or inactivates specific genes.
- By selectively affecting gene transcript and production of specific m RNAs, the amounts of different proteins is affected and so is the metabolic response.
- The gene which is affected should be present in transcriptionally active regions, i.e. should be susceptible to DNAase activity such that the DNA strands are opened up for binding of the transcription complex.
- Besides the gene to be activated/inactivated should have at least 2 regulatory sequences—HRE and a promoter element.
- HRE is the site of binding of the H–R complex and modulates frequency of transcription initiation.

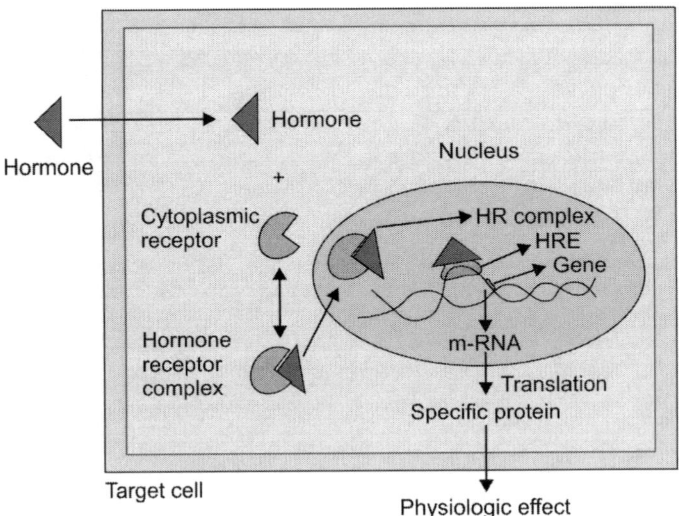

Fig. 15.1 Mechanism of action of steroid hormones

- Promoter element is present downstream HRE and it specifies the site of RNA polymerase II attachment, i.e. it determine the accuracy of transcription initiation.
- Both these regulatory sequences are always present upstream the gene.
- Genes controlled by several hormones will have a corresponding numbers of HREs.
- Although simple HREs transmit hormone response, in some genes the HREs require some transacting factors for their optimal activity. Such complexes of HREs and their transacting factors are called hormone response units (HRUs).
- The communication between the basal transcription complex and HRU is accomplished by one or more protein molecules called *coregulator,* e.g. CBP, b 300, etc.

Signal Transduction in Peptide Hormones

- Peptide hormones are the second group of hormones.
- Protein and peptide hormones are synthesized on r- endoplasmic reticulum of the different endocrine cells. They are usually synthesized first as larger proteins that are not biologically active-preprohormones and are cleaved to form smaller-prohormones in the endoplasmic reticulum.
- These are then transferred to the Golgi apparatus for packaging into secretory vesicles. In this process, enzymes in the vesicles cleave the prohormones to produce smaller, biologically active hormones and inactive fragments.
- These hormones cannot permeate the target cells rather these execute their physiological roles by binding to specific cell surface receptors on their target cells.
- The diverse effects of peptide and protein hormones upon their target cells are mediated by a series of biochemical events which link the primary site of peptide hormone action, the plasma membrane, with a variety of intracellular messages sent via the second messengers.

- The peptide hormones bind to the specific target cell receptors, which initiates:
  - Receptor associated changes in enzyme activity leading to alteration in transcription frequency and activity via specific cellular proteins.
  - Receptor associated changes in enzyme activity leading to generation of second messengers that will eventually cause the modulation of activity of the transcription factors at genetic level (Fig. 15.2).
- Second messengers are low molecular weight signaling molecules that carry messages of the hormonal activity from cell membrane to the nuclear level.
- The hormones have been classified based upon the type of second messengers they require for completing their function.
  - The second messenger is cAMP
    - α_2-adrenergic catecholamines
    - β-adrenergic catecholamines
    - Adrenocorticotropic hormone (ACTH)
    - Antidiuretic hormone (ADH)
    - Calcitonin
    - Human chorionic gonadotropin (hCG)
    - Corticotropin-releasing hormone (CRH)
    - Follicle-stimulating hormone (FSH)

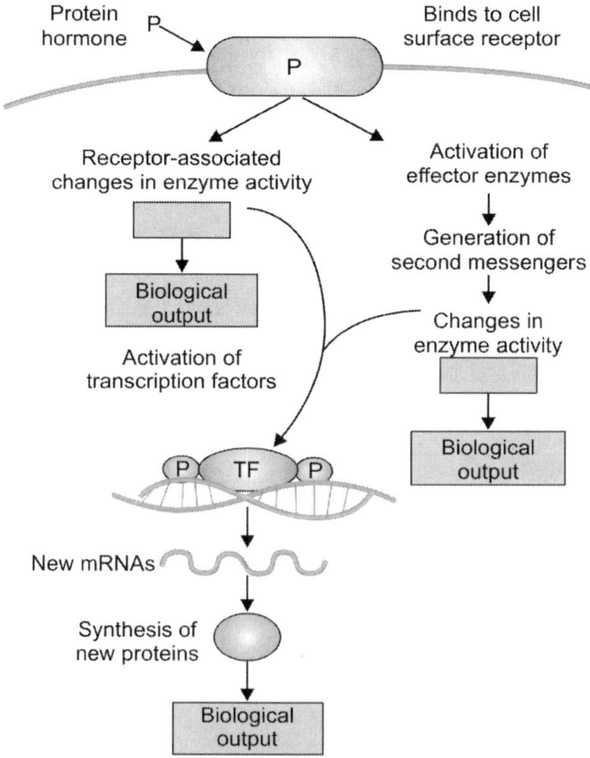

Fig. 15.2 Mechanism of action of peptide hormone

  - Glucagon
  - Lipotropin
  - Luteinizing hormone (LH)
  - Melanocyte-stimulating hormone (MSH)
  - Parathyroid hormone (PTH)
  - Somatostatin
  - Thyroid-stimulating hormone (TSH)
- The second messenger is cGMP
  - Atrial natriuretic factor (ANF)
  - Nitric oxide (NO)
- The second messenger is calcium or phosphatidylinositol (or both)
  - Acetylcholine (muscarinic)
  - α_1-adrenergic catecholamines
  - Angiotensin II
  - Antidiuretic hormone (vasopressin) (ADH)
  - Cholecystokinin
  - Gastrin
  - Gonadotropin-releasing hormone (GnRH)
  - Oxytocin
  - Platelet-derived growth factor (PDGF)
  - Substance P
  - Thyrotropin-releasing hormone (TRH)
- The second messenger is a kinase or phosphatase cascade
  - Chorionic somato mammotropin
  - Epidermal growth factor (EGF)
  - Fibroblast growth factor (FGF)
  - Insulin-like growth factors I and II (IGF – I and II)
  - Nerve growth factor (NGF)
  - Platelet- derived growth factor (PDGF)
  - Erythropoietin
  - Growth hormone (GH)
  - Insulin
  - Prolactin.

G-Protein-Coupled Second Messengers

- Some hormones bind to specific cellular receptors that cause signal transduction via a GTP-binding protein intermediary thus the name G-protein-coupled receptors.
- The structure of a G-protein-coupled receptor (GPCR) generally comprises seven α-helical trans-membrane domains, an extracellular N-terminus, and an intracellular C-terminus.
- GPCRs constitute one of the largest families of membrane proteins, and their main function is to transduce extracellular signals into intracellular reactions.
- G-proteins located within the cell are activated by G-protein-coupled receptors (GPCRs) that span the cell membrane.

- Signaling molecules (ligand/hormones) bind to a domain of the GPCR located outside the cell. An intracellular GPCR domain in turn activates a G-protein.
- The G-protein activates a cascade of further signalling events that finally results in a change in cell function. G-protein-coupled receptor and G-proteins working together transmit signals from many hormones, neurotransmitters, and other signalling factors.
- There are two classes of G-proteins. The first function as monomeric small GTPases whiles the second function as heterotrimeric G-protein complexes.

Heterotrimeric G-protein Complexes

- The Heterotrimeric G-proteins have 3 subunits—α, β and γ. The trimeric G-proteins are named for their ability to bind guanosine nucleotides (GTP/GDP) (Fig. 15.3).
- Receptor-activated G-proteins are bound to the inside surface of the cell membrane. They consist of the G_{α} and the tightly associated $G_{\beta\gamma}$ subunits.
- The complex is anchored to the plasma membrane through prenylated groups on the β γ subunits and by myristoylated groups on α-subunits.

Activation

- When a hormone/ligand activates the G-protein-coupled receptor (Gs), it induces a conformational change in the receptor that causes an exchange of GDP for GTP on the G_{α} subunit.
- In the traditional view of heterotrimeric protein activation, this exchange triggers the dissociation of the G_{α} subunit, bound to GTP, from the $G_{\beta\gamma}$ dimer and the receptor.
- Both G_{α}-GTP and $G_{\beta\gamma}$ can then activate different *signaling cascades (or second messenger pathways)* and effector proteins, while the receptor is free to activate the next G-protein.
- Displacement of GDP by GTP causes α-subunit to dissociate from the trimeric complex and to associate with other intracellular signalling proteins. The α-subunit binds to and activates the effector (E).

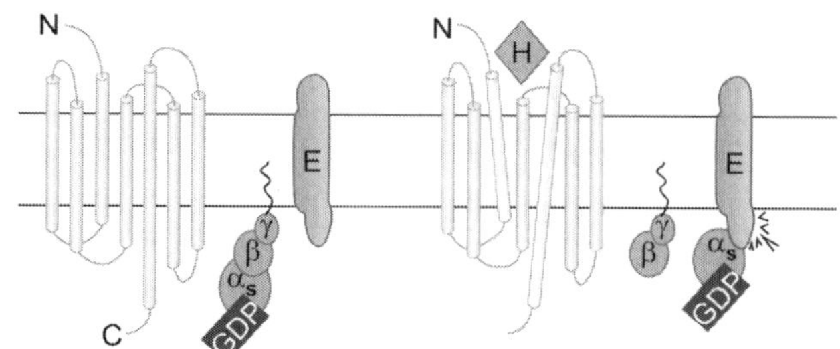

Fig. 15.3 G-protein-coupled receptors

- Effector can be adenylyl cyclase, Ca^{2+}, Na^+, or Cl^- channels (α_s), or it could be a K^+ channel (α_i), phospholipase-C β (α_q), or cGMP phosphodiesterase (α_t).
- The βγ subunit can also have direct actions on E.

Termination

- The G_α subunit will eventually hydrolyze the attached GTP to GDP by its inherent enzymatic activity (GTPase), allowing it to re-associate with $G_{\beta\gamma}$ and starting a new cycle.
- A group of proteins called regulator of G-protein signaling (RGSs), act as GTPase-activating proteins (GAPs), and specific for G_α subunits, act to accelerate hydrolysis of GTP to GDP and terminate the transduced signal.
- In some cases, the effector itself may possess intrinsic GAPs activity, which helps deactivate the pathway.
- Some of the G-protein-coupled receptors are inhibitory in nature (G_i) and such receptors when bound to a hormone will inhibit the effector molecule.

Monomeric G-protein Complexes

- Certain small GTPases also bind GTP and GDP and are involved in signal transduction.
- These proteins are homologous to the alpha (α) subunit found in hetero trimers, but exist as monomers.
- They are small (20-kDa to 25-kDa) proteins that bind to GTP.
- This family of proteins is homologous to Ras GTPases and is also called the Ras superfamily GTPases.

Second Messengers of GPCRs

- The GPCRs can use different types of second messengers as the effectors.
- Some of the second messengers are discussed below:

cAMP

- Certain hormones like ACTH, FSH, HCG, LH, PTH, TSH, etc. have the G-protein-coupled receptors that activate the membrane bound effector—Adenyl cyclase.
- The G-protein that stimulates the adenyl cyclase is termed as G_s.
- The activated adenyl cyclase leads to the synthesis of cAMP which in turn activates the cAMP-dependent protein kinases (Fig. 15.4).
- The active protein kinases then execute the hormonal functions by carrying out various biochemical reactions.
- cAMP initiates a cascade of biochemical reactions, i.e. a few molecules of cAMP activate a large number of other enzyme proteins, thus amplifying the overall effect of the hormone molecule.
- The G-protein that inhibits adenyl cyclase is termed as G_i.
- On the binding of a hormone to the G_i, the adenyl cyclase is inhibited and so are the generation of the cascading reactions.
- Cholera toxin catalyzes the ADP ribosylation of α_s so that it loses its intrinsic GTPase activity. As results, there is a permanent activation of G–protein leading to an increase in cAMP concentration in intestinal mucosal cells.

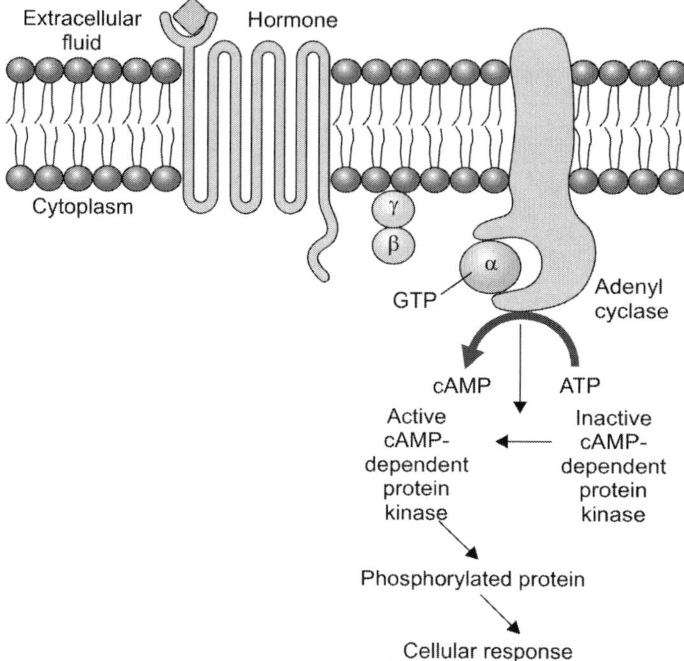

Fig. 15.4 Mechanism of action of cAMP-dependent GCPRs

- This causes phosphorylation of Cl^- channels causing large efflux of electrolytes and water into the gut and causes the severe diarrhea characteristic of cholera.
- The type of action carried out by the cAMP-dependent G-protein receptors varies from one tissue to another depending upon its intracellular enzymatic machinery.

Protein Kinase A (PKA)

- PKA is a multimeric enzyme comprising of 2 catalytic (c) and 2 regulatory (R) subunits.
- R_2C_2 form is the inactive form. Binding of 4 cAMP to R subunit leads to the release of catalytically active C^- subunits, which can then phosphorylate and modulate key enzymes. e.g. Regulation of glycogenesis and glycogenolysis (see Chapter – 10 and Fig. 10.9)
- Due to such a multilayered signal transduction there is amplification of the original signal so that binding of a few hormone molecules causes release of a large number of sugar molecules.

Cell Membrane Phospholipids Second Messengers/Phosphatidyl Inositol—Ca^{++}

- Hormones like insulin, GnRH, gastrin, cholecystokinin, etc. use Ca^{++} and phosphatidyl inositol as second messengers.
- These hormones bind to the cellular receptors activating the coupled G-proteins that activate enzyme phospholipase C (Fig. 15.5).
- Phospholipase C hydrolyzes the phosphatidyl inositol bisphosphate (PIP_2) into inositol triphosphate (IP_3) and Di acyl glycerol (DAG).

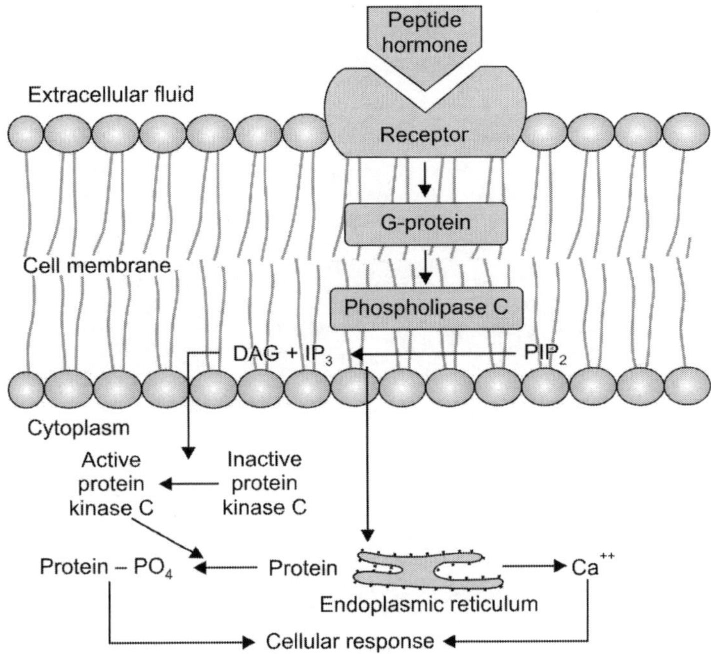

Fig. 15.5 Membrane phospholipids as second messenger producers

- The IP_3 causes release of Ca^{++} from intra cellular sources like r-ER and mitochondria. The released Ca^{++} in turn carries out specific functions like smooth muscle contraction and cellular secretions.
- Ca^{++} binds to a cellular protein calmodulin (it has 4 Ca binding sites) and activates a number of cellular calmodulin-dependent kinases.
- These kinases are further responsible for the activation or inhibition of proteins involved in cellular response to the hormone, e.g. myosin kinase acts directly on muscle protein myosin to cause smooth muscle contraction.
- The DAG causes activation of a protein kinase C that phosphorylates cellular proteins leading to specific cellular responses.

Tyrosine Kinase and Other Cascading Protein Kinases

- Hormones like insulin, EGFs, PDGF, Growth hormones, IGFs, etc. bind to their specific cellular receptors and initiate the phosphorylation of tyrosine residues (normally tyrosine residues in mammalian tissues occurs with a very low frequency $<0.03\%$).
- Most of the hormones involved in tissue growth, differentiation and inflammatory response either have an intrinsic tyrosine kinase activity or are associated with proteins which themselves have tyrosine kinase activity.
- The activation of tyrosine kinase then initiates a cascade of events involving different protein kinases, phosphatases and other regulatory proteins (Fig. 15.6).
- The hormones like growth hormone, cytokines, prolactin, erythropoietin also involve the tyrosine kinase activity. However, in these hormone receptors the tyrosine kinase activity is not inherent of the receptors but the binding of the hormone to the receptor causes an activation of cytoplasmic tyrosine kinases like Tyk2, Jak1 and Jak2.

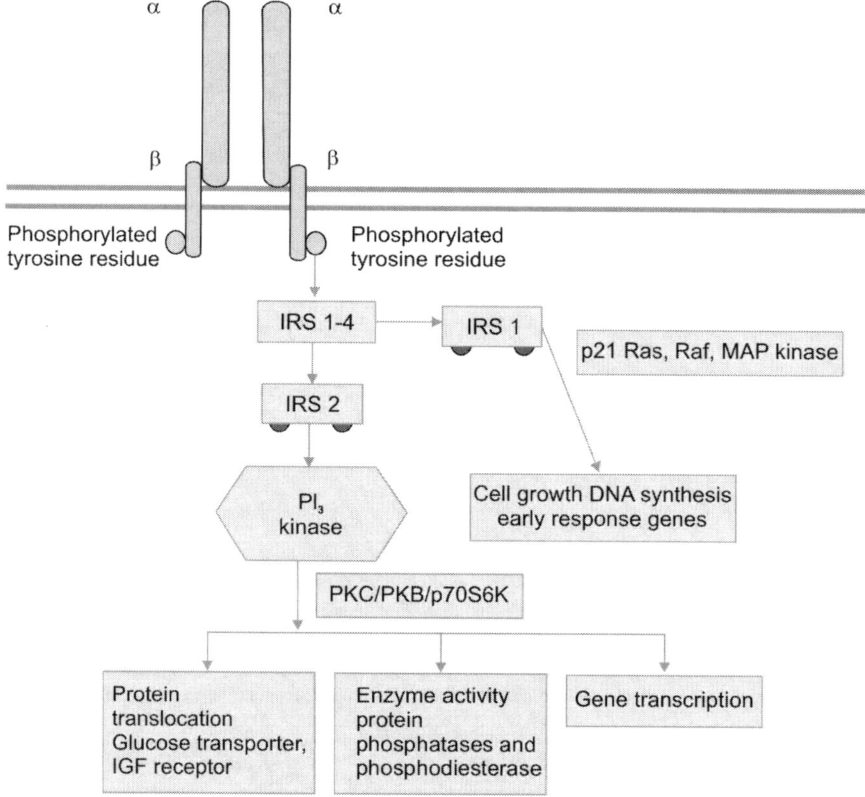

Fig. 15.6 Tyrosine kinase activity of peptide hormones

- Such proteins then phosphorylate one or more cytoplasmic proteins like STAT protein (signal transducers and activators of transcription).
- The STAT protein on phosphorylation dimerizes and translocates to nucleus binding specific DNA sequences and causing gene expression.
- Certain other cytosolic proteins may also activate the PI3 kinase or the MAP kinase pathway.
- Looking at the above description, it is obvious that there is quite cross-talk among the different hormone action pathways and that be it the steroid hormones or the peptide hormones, they do influence the gene expression for carrying out the physiologic role of the hormone.

A Quick Look at the Hormone Action

- Steroid hormones act by crossing-over into the target cell and binding to specific genetic sequences on the DNA leading to the physiologic effect of the hormone.
- Peptide hormones act by binding to specific cellular receptors and by signal transduction via G-protein-coupled receptors and second messengers.
- The important second messengers include—cAMP, Ca, phosphotidyl inositol, cGMP, protein kinases.

CHAPTER

16

Hormones of Pituitary and Hypothalamus

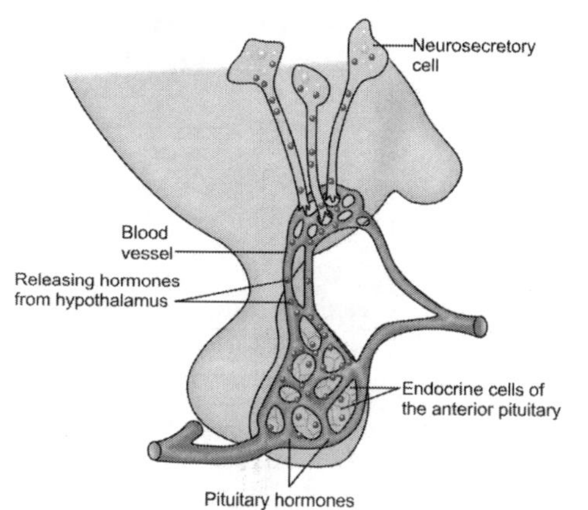

Chapter Framework

Introduction

- Pituitary (*Hypophysis)* is the master endocrine gland, situated in the *sella turcica*—a bony cavity at the base of the skull.
- The gland is the size of a pea approximately weighing 0.5 g to 1 g.
- The gland comprises of three sections:
  - Anterior pituitary (*Adenohypophysis).*
  - Intermediate lobe *(Pars Intermedia)- almost absent in humans.*
  - Posterior pituitary *(Neurohypophysis)*
- The gland is connected via a hypothalamo-hypophysial portal system to the hypothalamus.
- The hypothalamus receives signals from the different sections of brain (as in response to pain, pleasure, depression, or blood concentrations of electrolytes, nutrients, water, etc.) and secretes in response to these specific *hypothalamic releasing and inhibitory hormones*.
- The hypothalamic releasing and inhibitory hormones are transported via the hypothalamo – hypophysial portal vessels to the pituitary.
- Pituitary secretes various peptide hormones in response to the hypothalamic hormones (Fig. 16.1).
- The different hormones secreted by the pituitary are:
  - Anterior pituitary secretes 6 different peptide hormones.
    - Growth hormone—Secreted by somatotropes and stimulates overall growth and affects metabolism of carbohydrates, lipids and proteins.

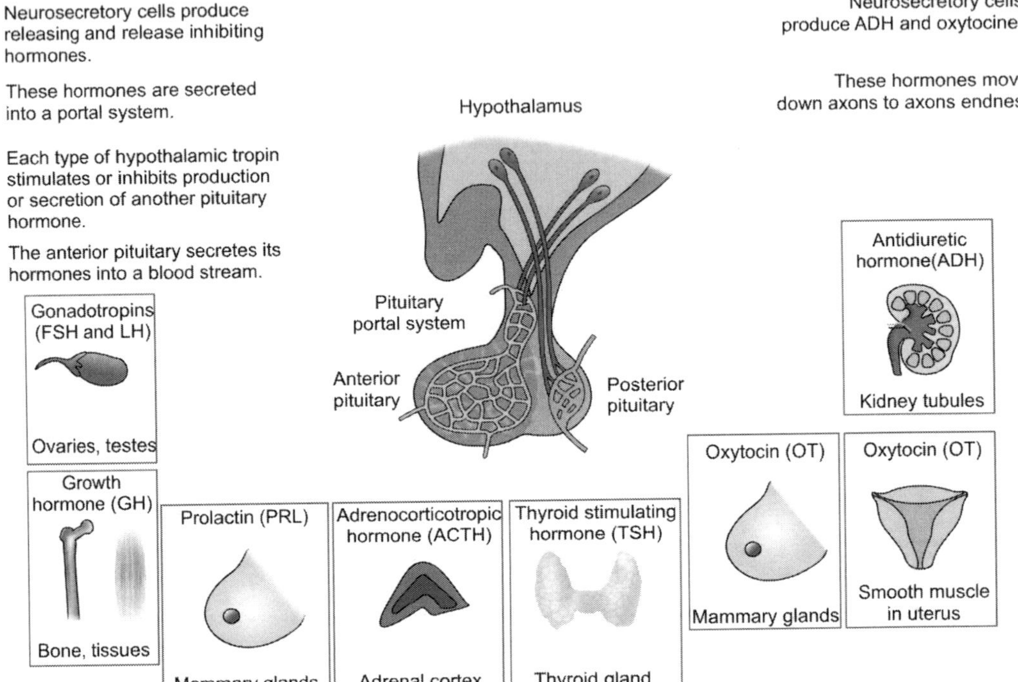

Fig. 16.1 Pituitary-hypothalamic hormones and their action

- Adrenocorticotropin hormone (ACTH)—Secreted by corticotropes and stimulates adrenal cortex for secretion of hormones.
- Thyroid-stimulating hormone (TSH)—Secreted by thyrotropes and stimulates thyroid gland for secretion of thyroid hormones.
- Follicular-stimulating hormone (FSH)—Secreted by gonadotropes and stimulates development of ovarian follicles and spermatogenesis regulation.
- Luteinizing-hormone (LH)—Secreted by gonadotropes and stimulates production of ovarian hormones and testis hormones.
- Prolactin—Secreted by lactotropes and stimulates milk production and secretion.

– Posterior Pituitary
  - Anti-diuretic hormone (ADH)/ Vasopressin—Act on kidney tubules for reabsorption of water and have vasopressive action.
  - Oxytocin—Act on smooth muscles of uterus and is important during labor and milk ejection.

- The hypothalamus releases tropin hormones, i.e. the hormones which regulate secretion of pituitary hormones. The different tropin hormones are:
  – Thyrotropin releasing hormone (TRH)—Stimulates secretion of TSH by thyrotropes.
  – Corticotropin releasing hormone (CRH)—Stimulates secretion of ACTH by corticotropes.
  – Growth hormone releasing hormone (GHRH)—Stimulates secretion of GH by somatotropes.
  – Growth hormone release inhibitory hormone (GHIH)—Inhibits secretion of GH by somatotropes.

- Gonadotropin releasing hormone (GnRH)—Stimulates secretion of FSH and LH by gonadotropes.
- Prolactin inhibiting hormone—Inhibits secretion of prolactin by the lactotropes.

Growth Hormone – Prolactin – Chorionic Somatomammotropin = One Hormone Group

- The hormones—GH, prolactin and chorionic somatomammotropin (secreted by placenta) are grouped as one family based on their structural homology.
- All three hormones range from 19 to 199 amino acids in peptide chain length and have considerable homology in structure that each has 2 homologous disulfide bonds and also share common antigenic determinants.
- There is 85% homology in prolactin and GH.

Growth Hormone

- The GH is 191 amino acids in length, synthesized by the somatotropes of anterior pituitary.
- Although, there is considerable homology in the GHs of humans and bovine and procine GHs, but functionally the later are not active in humans, rather the GHs from higher primates have functional capabilities in humans.
- The GH binds to its target cell surface receptors and activates a JAK2 tyrosine kinase activity.
- The auto-phosphorylation of the tyrosine residues on the receptor leads to activation of several cellular signaling pathways like the STAT protein phosphorylation, IRS phosphorylation, phospholipase-C activation and MAP kinase activation. (as shown in Chapter 15 Figures 15.5 and 15.6)
- These signaling pathways cause the effect of the hormone.

Physiological Roles of Growth Hormone

- *Metabolic roles:* Growth hormone enhances body protein, uses up fat stores, and conserves carbohydrates.
  - GH increases protein synthesis by enhancing the rate of transcription and translation.
  - GH Increases the mobilization of fats from adipose tissue, thus increasing the plasma FFAs.
  - GH reduces the glucose utilization overall.
- *Skeletal effects*:
  - GH enhances the new bone deposition and growth of the bones overall since it enhances the protein synthesis and deposition by the chondrocytes and osteocytes. GH particularly stimulates the osteoblasts, so that the mature bones would continue to become thicker and thicker under the influence of GH throughout the life.
  - GH exerts its effects of skeletal growth via somatomedins (4 different types); especially somatomedin C. Deficiency of somatomedin C in African pygmies is the cause of their short stature.

Normal Levels

The normal concentration of growth hormone in the plasma of an adult is between 1.6 and 3 ng/mL. In a child or adolescent it is about 6 ng/mL.

Pathophysiology of Growth Hormone

- *Panhypopituitarism:* It shows an overall decreased secretion of all of the anterior pituitary hormones either congenitally or due to a tumor of anterior pituitary developing later in life.
  - Panhypopituitarism in adults causes hypothyroidism, suppression in secretion of hormones of adrenal cortex and gonadotropic hormones.
- *Dwarfism:* It could be due to panhypopituitarism or due to absence of somatomedin C as in African Pygmies – *Levi – Lorain dwarfs*. It is seen in childhood and the overall skeletal growth is reduced leaving the subject as a dwarf. Most of them are with panhypopituitarism so sexual development also does not occur. However, *Levi – Lorain dwarfs* have normal sexual maturity.
- *Gigantism:* Acidophilic cells tumor causes secretion of excessive GH. All body tissues grow rapidly, including the bones. If the condition occurs before adolescence, before the epiphyses of the long bones have become fused with the shafts, height increases so that the person becomes a giant.

Prolactin/Luteotropic Hormone/Lactogenic Hormone

- Prolactin is secreted by the acidophilic cells of anterior pituitary.
- Its structural homology to GH is already described.
- Its mechanism of action is also similar to that of GH, i.e. tyrosine kinase pathway.
- Functionally this hormone acts on breast tissue primed by female sex hormones and causes the breast tissue growth, especially during pregnancy for initiating and maintaining lactation.

Glycoprotein Family of Anterior Pituitary Hormones—TSH, FSH, LH

- Anterior pituitary secretes a group of glycoprotein hormones—TSH, FSH and LH.
- These hormones are grouped together considering the fact that all of these are:
  - Glycoproteins in nature.
  - Comprise of 2 subunits α and β.
  - The two subunits are joined together by non-covalent linkages.
  - The specific biologic activity of the hormone is inherent of the β–subunit which is highly conserved for each hormone.
  - The inter hormone and interspecies hybrids of these hormone subunits does not affect the biologic activity, e.g. TSH αLHβ will show LH activity and hTSHα mTSHβ will have mouse TSH activity.
  - The subunits are glycosylated with 2 oligosaccharide units each on α and β subunits.
  - All of these hormones execute their specific function via second messenger cAMP.
  - All these hormones are synthesized as preprohormones and get activated by further post-translational processing.

Thyroid-stimulating Hormone (TSH)

- It is heterodimer made up of subunits α and β.
- It has α subunit 89 amino acid and β subunits112 amino acids secreted by the thyrotropes.

- It principally stimulates the thyroid gland for the secretion of thyroid hormones for which it affects all aspects of T_3 and T_4 synthesis and secretion.

Follicular-stimulating Hormone (FSH)

- It is heterodimer made up of subunits α (89) and β (112).
- It is a gonadotropin hormone secreted by the anterior pituitary gonadotropes.
- FSH stimulates the follicular cells of the ovaries and the sertoli cells of the testes.

Luteinizing Hormone (LH)

- It is heterodimer made up of subunits α (89) and β (112).
- It causes ovulation and formation of corpus luteum.
- It stimulates production of estrogen and progesterone by ovaries.
- It stimulates testis for the secretion of testosterone.

Pro-opiomelanocortin Family (POMC)

- POMC family comprises of peptide hormones—ACTH, MSH and certain neurotransmitters and neuromodulators like endorphins.
- The POMC gene gets expressed in the anterior lobe of pituitary and in the intermediate lobe.
- The POMC molecule is translated as a 285 amino acid long precursor molecule.
- The precursor molecule gets processed in such a way that three different peptides are formed, namely—ACTH, MSH and LPH (luteotropin hormone).
- As is clear from the Figure 16.2, processing of POMC gives rise to the various peptides.
- Out of the POMC peptides the ACTH has an inherent MSH activity and vice versa.
- ACTH is responsible for the stimulation of adrenal cortex and MSH regulates our sleep-wake cycle.

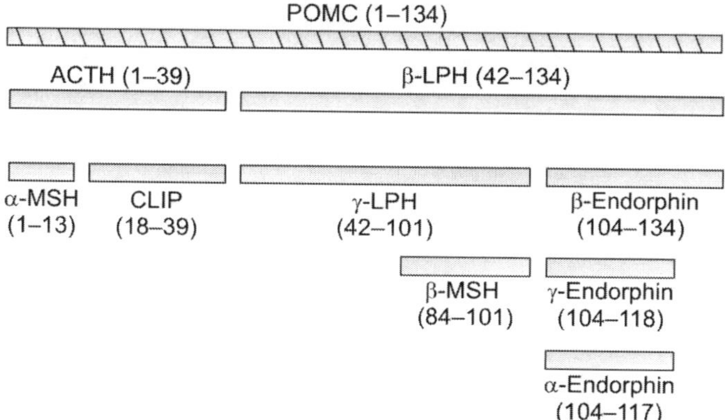

Fig. 16.2 Processing of POMC to give different peptide hormones and neuromodulators

Hormones of Posterior Pituitary

- The posterior lobe of pituitary secretes two very important peptide hormones—Oxytocin and vasopressin.
- Oxytocin acts on the breast tissue and uterine tissue for milk ejection and during labor respectively.
- Vassopressin/ADH makes the renal tubules permeable to water so that there is water reabsorption and prevents diuresis.
- Both these hormones are nonapeptides with a slight variation in their amino acid sequences.
- These hormones have Ca and phosphatidyl inositol as second messengers.

A Quick Look at the Hormones of Pituitary

- Pituitary is the master gland regulating the activity of all the other endocrine glands.
- Its activity is regulated by hypothalamic hormones reaching pituitary by a pituitary-hypothalamo-portal tract.
- Hypothalamus secretes the tropin hormones that stimulate or inhibit release of pituitary hormones. (CRH, GHRH, GHIH, Prl IH, TRH, GnRH)
- Anterior pituitary secretes—GH, ACTH, FSH, LH, TSH and prolactin.
- Posterior pituitary secretes—ADH and Oxytocin.
- GH acts via somatomedin C.
- GH excess causes gigantism and deficiency causes dwarfism (Pygmies or Levi – lorain dwarfs).

CHAPTER

17

Hormones of Thyroid Gland

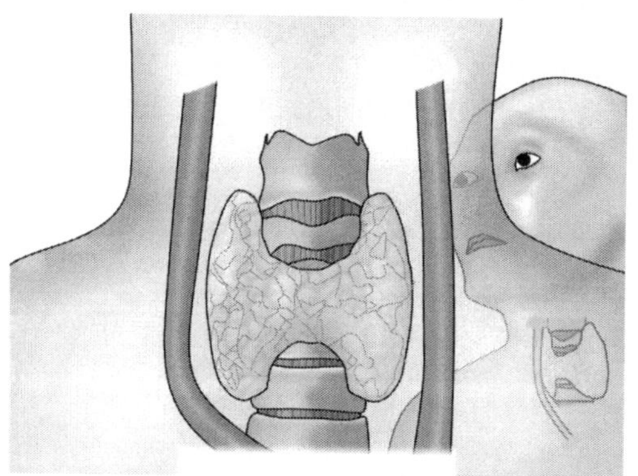

Chapter Framework

- Introduction
- Biosynthesis and Section of Thyroid Hormones
- Functions of Thyroid Hormones
- Pathophysiology of Thyroid Hormones
  - Hypothyroidism
  - Hyperthyroidism

Introduction

- The thyroid gland was the first endocrine gland to be recognized.
- It is a butterfly-shaped gland present in the neck region located immediately below the larynx on each side of and anterior to the trachea.
- It is one of the largest endocrine gland weighing approximately 15 g to 20 g in an adult.
- The gland synthesizes and stores large quantities of less active prohormones which are converted into its most active form in the target tissues.
- The physiologically active hormones secreted by the thyroid gland and found in the blood stream are triiodothyronine (T_3) and tetraiodothyronine/thyroxine (T_4).
- These two hormones are amino acid derivatives—They are iodinated tyrosines.
- The two hormones are under the feedback control of the anterior pituitary hormone TSH and hypothalamic hormone TRH (Thyrotropin releasing hormone) that stimulates the pituitary for secretion of TSH.
- The hormones are stored in the gland bound to a colloid—Thyroglobulin.
- Another hormone secreted by the C-cells of thyroid gland is calcitonin, which regulates calcium metabolism (*Calcitonin is discussed in chapter 18 with hormones of parathyroid)*

Biosynthesis and Secretion of Thyroid Hormones

- Thyroid hormones are synthesized by the gland following entrapment of iodide, conversion to iodine and coupling of iodine with tyrosine, followed by the coupling of two iodinated tyrosine molecules (Fig. 17.1).

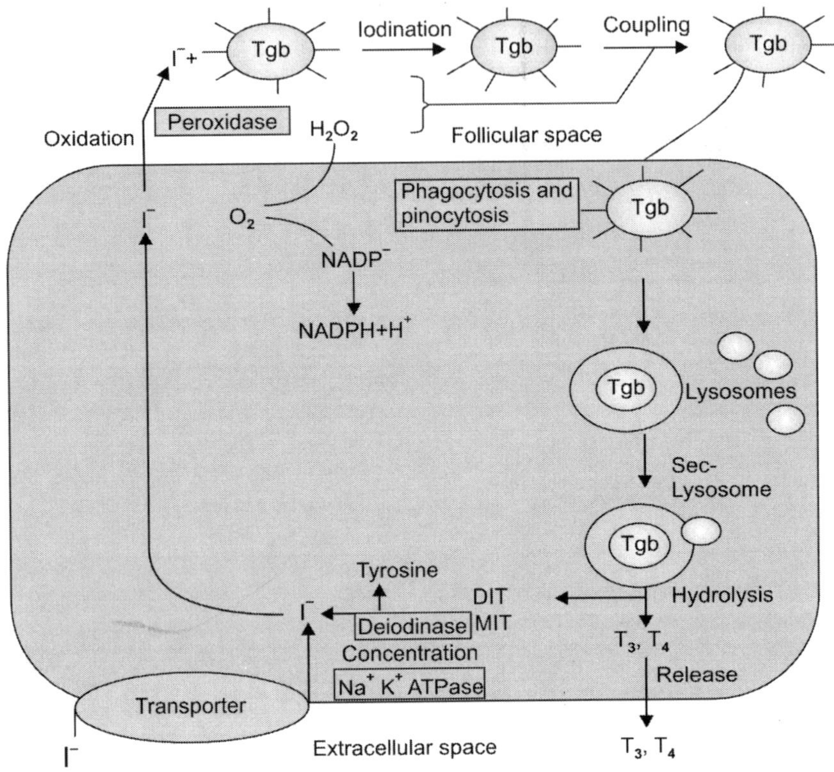

Fig. 17.1 Biosynthesis of thyroid hormones

- T_3 and T_4 so formed are attached to thyroglobulin for storage and are released as needed as protease splits them from the globulin.
- Thus thyroglobulin is the precursor of T_3 and T_4 and is stored in the extracellular colloid.
- The various steps of thyroid hormone synthesis are:
  - *Concentration:* Iodine molecules are trapped by the follicular cells by a Na^+-K^+ ATPase iodide pump. In a normal gland, the iodide pump concentrates the iodide to about 30 times its concentration in the blood.
  - *Oxidation:* The iodide ions concentrated by the follicular cells are oxidized to either nascent iodine (I°) or to I_3^- that enables this active iodine to bind to tyrosine residues and form the iodotyrosines—Mono iodotyrosine (MIT) and Di-iodotyrosines (DIT). The oxidation reaction is catalyzed by the enzyme peroxidases—Thyroperoxidase and H_2O_2. This enzyme is present at the apical surface of the follicular cells where this reaction is carried out.
  - *Iodination/Organification of Thyroglobulin:* The thyroid gland secretes glycoprotein thyroglobulin. It is synthesized on the r-ER and is glycosylated at the golgi apparatus to be finally secreted at the apical surface of the follicular cells. Each thyroglobulin has about 70 tyrosine residues. The thyroglobulin molecule gets iodinized in the presence of an enzyme *iodinase*. The process occurs within seconds as soon as the thyroglobulin is released form the golgi apparatus. This forms MIT and DIT.

- *Coupling:* The MIT and DIT are coupled in the presence of thyroperoxidase to form the thyroid hormones (Fig. 17.2):
  - Triiodothyronine (T_3)—Coupling of MIT and DIT. Chemically, it is 3, 5, 3'- triiodothyronine.
  - Tetraiodothyronines (T_4)—Coupling of 2 DIT. Chemically, it is 3, 5, 3', 5' – tetraiodothyronine.
  - Reverse T_3 – Chemically, it is 3, 3', 5' – triiodothyronine. It is an inactive derivative.
  - The iodothyronines thus formed are part of the thyroglobulin molecule which is stored in the follicular cells lumen. Several weeks supply exists in the thyroid gland.

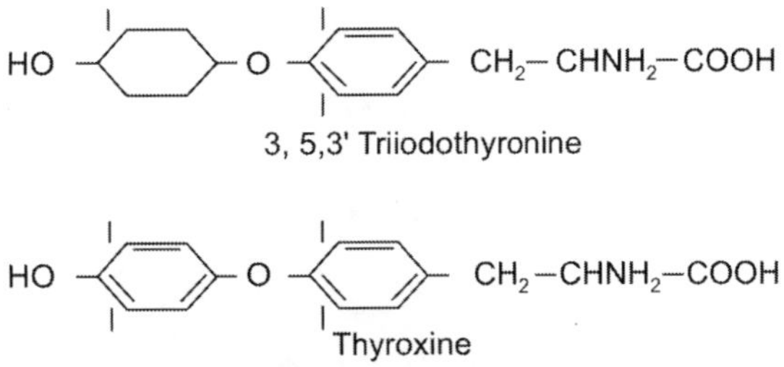

HO – (ring, I) – O – (ring, I, I) – CH_2–$CHNH_2$–COOH

3, 5,3' Triiodothyronine

HO – (ring, I, I) – O – (ring, I, I) – CH_2–$CHNH_2$–COOH

Thyroxine

Fig. 17.2 3,5,3'-triiodothyronine and thyroxine

- *Release of thyroid hormones:* The thyroid hormone is released in response to the TSH from anterior pituitary. The stimulation of the thyroid gland by TSH enhances all aspects of thyroid hormones biosynthesis and secretion. The apical surface of the gland engulfs the thyroglobulin by phagocytosis and pinocytosis. Within the follicular cell the phagosome fuses to the lysosome to form phagolysosome. The hydrolytic enzymes of the phagolysosome release the T_3 and T_4 at the basal end of the cell into the blood circulation.
  - Of the total circulating thyroid hormones 7% is T_3 and 93% is T_4. The T_4 gets deiodinized as it reaches the different target tissues.
  - To form normal quantities of thyroxine, about 50 milligrams of ingested iodine in the form of iodides are required each year, or about 1 mg/week. When iodine supplies are sufficient, the T_4:T_3 ratio is about 7:1. To prevent iodine deficiency, common table salt is iodized with about 1 part sodium iodide to every 100,000 parts sodium chloride.

Functions of Thyroid Hormones

- The functions of these two hormones are qualitatively the same, but they differ in rapidity and intensity of action. Triiodothyronine is about four times as potent as thyroxine, but it is present in the blood in much smaller quantities and persists for a much shorter time as compared to that of thyroxine.
- These hormones have nuclear receptors and they increase the transcription of a number of genes by attaching to the specific DNA sequences. All the effects of thyroid hormones are a result of this transcription and translation of specific genetic sequences (Fig. 17.3).

Metabolic role of Thyroid Hormones

- Thyroid hormones increase the metabolic activity of all the tissues of the body. The excessive secretion of thyroid hormones raises the BMR 60–100% above normal and less secretion reduces the BMR by 40–50%.
- The metabolic activity is raised since thyroid hormones increase the number and activity of mitochondria, increase the active transport of ions across cell membrane (Na^+-K^+ ATPase) thus increasing the heat production.

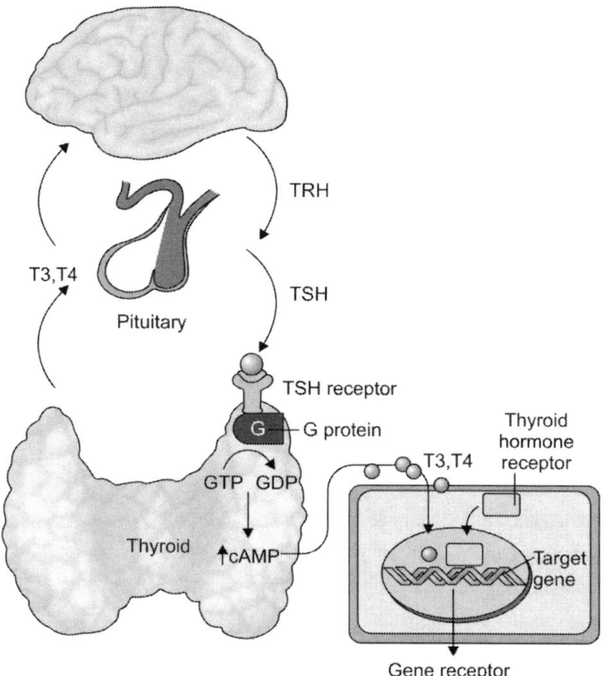

Fig. 17.3 Mechanism of action of thyroid hormone

Effect on Carbohydrate Metabolism

- Thyroid hormones stimulate all aspects of carbohydrate metabolism, i.e. uptake of glucose, utilization of glucose by glycolysis and CAC, storage as glycogen and production of glucose by gluconeogenesis and glycogenolysis.

Effect on Lipid Metabolism

- Thyroid hormones enhance all aspects of fat metabolism in – particular they increase the mobilization of lipids from storehouse raising the plasma FFAs, increases the oxidation of fats.
- Increased thyroid hormones cause excessive breakdown of cholesterol, thus reducing serum cholesterol and converse is seen in reduced secretion of thyroid hormones.

Vitamins Requirement Raised

- Since thyroid hormones raise the metabolic rate thus the demand of vitamins is also raised since they are the coenzymes of the various metabolic reactions.

Effect on Cardiovascular System (CVS)

- Thyroid hormones increase the cardiac output, tissue blood flow, heart rate, heart strength and respiration.

CNS

- Thyroid hormones are required for proper brain development as they increase the rate of cerebration.

Effects on Other Endocrine Glands

- Increased thyroid hormone increases the rates of secretion of most other endocrine glands, but it also increases the need of the tissues for the hormones.

Effect on Sexual Function

- Thyroid hormones are important for the normal sexual functions as lack of thyroid hormones can lead to loss of libido in men and menorrhagia or polymenorrhea in women.

Pathophysiology of Thyroid Disorders

Hypothyroidism

- Hypothyroidism is characterized by reduced thyroid hormone secretion and activity.
- It occurs due to:
  - *Autoimmune thyroiditis:* Presence of autoantibodies against the thyroid gland itself.
  - *Endemic goiter:* Endemic areas with low or deficient levels of iodine in soil, like the hilly areas of show patients of enlarged goitres owing to the lack of Iodine. Such patients are unable to synthesize thyroid hormones which lead to an unabated secretion of TSH that stimulates the gland constantly for more thyroid hormone synthesis and secretion. Thus making the gland hypertrophied and enlarged. The defect can also be with the various steps of iodine concentration, oxidation or coupling genetically; leading to a reduced thyroid hormone synthesis and secretion.
  - *Myxedema:* It is hypothyroidism due to any of the above-mentioned causes in adulthood. It is characterized by bagginess under the eyes and swelling of the face (due to formation of excessive tissue gel comprising of hyaluronic acid and chondroitin). The edema is nonpitting edema.
  - *Cretinism:* It is the hypothyroidism seen in fetal life, infancy or childhood. It occurs due to the congenital lack of the thyroid gland in such infants or due to iodine deficiency or due to defect in thyroid gland to synthesize thyroid hormone. This condition is characterized especially by failure of body growth and by mental retardation.
  - *Surgical removal of the hyperactive gland can also lead to hypothyroidism.*
    - In the above conditions the levels of thyroid hormones are lower than normal and TSH is higher than normal.

Signs and Symptoms of Hypothyroidism

- Reduced BMR up to 50%.
- Leatharginess and sluggishness due to lack of energy. Mental sluggishness.
- Weight gain due to edema.

- Reduced gut motility leading to constipation.
- Reduced cardiac output, blood volume.
- Dry skin, coarse hair, husky voice.
- Hypercholesterolemia due to reduced catabolism of cholesterol and tendency of atherosclerotic CVDs.

Hyperthyroidism

- Hyperthyroidism is characterized by over activity of the thyroid gland secreting more than normal levels of the hormones T_3 and T_4.
- It occurs due to:
  - *Grave's disease/Toxic goitre/Thyrotoxicosis:* It is characterized by autoimmunity, i.e. autoantibodies are seen that stimulate the gland for hypertrophying it rather than causing its atrophy. These are *thyroid-stimulating immunoglobulins (TSIs)* which cause a continuous stimulation of the TSH receptors (for more than 12 hrs rather than a normal of approximately 1 hr) resulting in hyperthyroidism. It also feedback inhibits the secretion of TSH.
  - *Thyroid adenoma:* A localized tumor of the thyroid gland itself is seen in this condition that secretes excessive amounts of thyroid hormones.
    - *In both the above conditions the levels of thyroid hormones are higher than normal and TSH is feedback inhibited.*

Signs and Symptoms of Hyperthyroidism

- BMR is raised by 50–100% above normal depending upon the severity.
- Fine muscle tremors and muscle weakness are seen.
- Weight loss.
- Excessive gut motility leading to diarrhea.
- Insomnia or sleeplessness.
- Exophthalmos or protruding eyeballs due to edematous swelling of retro-orbital muscles tissue and degeneration in extraocular muscles.
- Intolerance to heat.
- Reduced serum cholesterol due to increased rate of catabolism.
  - *Thyroid function tests are discussed in Practical Biochemistry section*

A Quick Look at the Hormones of Thyroid

- Thyroid is the largest endocrine gland, secreting T_3 and T_4.
- The thyroid hormones are regulated by the hypothalamic and pituitary hormones TRH and TSH.
- Thyroid hormones are iodinated tyrosines.
- Thyroid hormones raise the metabolic activities of all the cells of the body and affect the metabolism of carbohydrates, lipids and proteins.
- Hypothyroidism due to autoimmunity or endemic goiter causes reduced BMR, edema, weight gain, hypercholesterolemia, constipation, letharginess, hoarse voice, dry skin, etc.
- Hyperthyroidism due to toxic goiter or thyroid adenoma causes raised BMR, muscle tremors, heat intolerance, hypercholesterolemia, insomnia, weight loss, exophthalmos, etc.

CHAPTER

18

Hormones of Parathyroid Gland

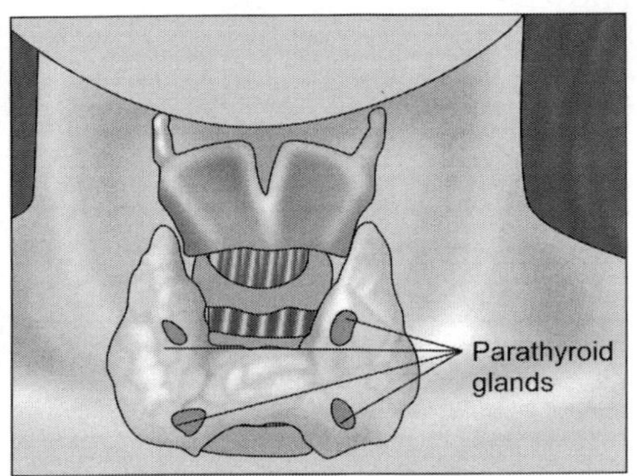

Chapter Framework

Introduction

- There are four parathyroid glands in humans; they are located immediately behind the thyroid gland —One behind each of the upper and each of the lower poles of the thyroid (Fig. 18.1).
- The parathyroid gland of the adult human being contains mainly chief cells and moderate number of oxyphil cells.
- The chief cells secrete the hormone parathyroid hormone.

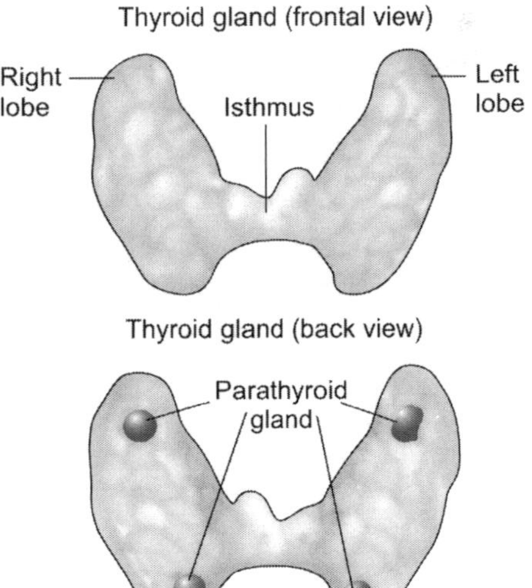

Fig. 18.1 Anatomical position of parathyroid gland

Structure of Parathyroid Hormone (PTH)

- PTH is first synthesized on the ribosomes in the form of a pre-pro-PTH, a polypeptide chain of 115 amino acids.
- This is cleaved first to a pro-PTH with 90 amino acids, then to the hormone itself with 84 amino acids by the endoplasmic reticulum and golgi apparatus.
- Finally is packaged in secretory granules in the cytoplasm of the cells.

- PTH_{1-34} has full biologic activity, and the region PTH_{25-34} is primarily responsible for receptor binding. The second messenger for PTH is c – AMP. Thus PTH acts via GCPRs.
- Smaller compounds with 34 amino acids adjacent to the N terminus of the molecule have also been isolated from the parathyroid glands that exhibit full PTH activity.
- Because the kidneys rapidly remove the whole 84-amino acid hormone within minutes but fail to remove many of the fragments for hours, a large share of the hormonal activity is caused by the fragments.
- Cathepsin B cleaves PTH into two fragments: PTH_{1-36} and PTH_{37-84}.
- PTH_{37-84} is not further degraded; however, PTH_{1-36} is rapidly and progressively cleaved into di and tri-peptides.

Secretion of PTH

- PTH is secreted in response to the plasma Ca levels.
- When the levels of Ca drop (normal – 9 – 11 mg/dl) the hypocalcemic blood circulating through the parathyroid gland stimulates the gland for the secretion of PTH.
- Conversely when the levels of plasma Ca are raised above the normal value, there is feedback inhibition of the secretion of PTH.

Functions of PTH

- The overall action of PTH is to increase plasma Ca^{++} levels and decrease plasma phosphate levels (Fig. 18.2).

Action on Bones

- PTH acts directly on the bones to stimulate Ca^{++} resorption. At the bones PTH increases the osteoclastic activity causing bone resorption that adds up to the plasma calcium level.

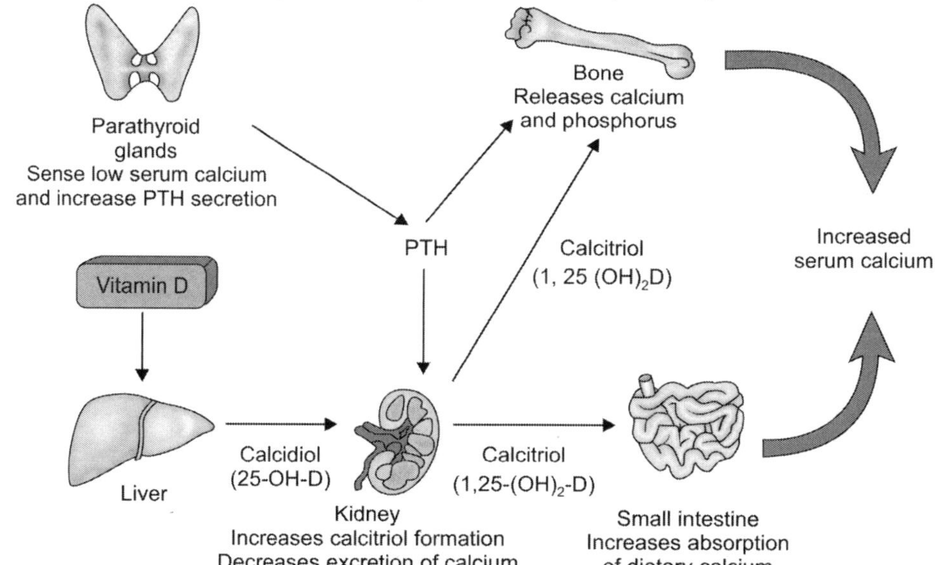

Fig. 18.2 Functions of PTH

Action on Kidneys

- At the Kidneys, PTH stimulates Ca^{++} re-absorption in the distal tubule of the kidney and inhibits re-absorption of phosphate (thereby stimulating its excretion) i.e. PTH causes excretion of phosphorous and reabsorption of Ca raising the serum Ca and reducing the levels of P.

Action on Intestines

- PTH also acts indirectly on intestine by stimulating 1, 25-(OH)2-D synthesis. PTH increases the activity of the kidney enzyme—1-α-hydroxylase thus increasing the synthesis of calcitriol (active vitamin – D). Calcitriol in turn increases the absorption of dietary Ca via a protein calbindin synthesized by the intestines.

Regulation of PTH Secretion

- When Ca^{2+} falls, cAMP rises and PTH is secreted.
- 1, 25-$(OH)_2$-D inhibits PTH gene expression, providing another level of feedback control of PTH.
- Despite close connection between Ca^{2+} and PO_4, no direct control of PTH is exerted by phosphate levels.

Calcitonin

- Calcitonin is synthesized and secreted by the parafollicular cells of the thyroid gland.
- They are distinct from thyroid follicular cells by their large size, pale cytoplasm, and small secretory granules.
- The target cell for calcitonin is the osteoclast.
- Calcitonin acts via increased cAMP concentrations to inhibit osteoclast motility and cell shape and inactivates them.
- The major stimulus of calcitonin secretion is a rise in plasma Ca^{++} levels. Calcitonin is a physiological antagonist to PTH with regard to Ca^{++} homeostasis and acts to decrease plasma Ca^{++} levels.
- The major effect of calcitonin administration is a rapid fall in Ca^{2+} caused by inhibition of bone resorption.
- While PTH and vitamin D act to increase plasma Ca^{++}; only calcitonin causes a decrease in plasma Ca^{++}.
- More important role of calcitonin is in control of bone remodeling. It is used, clinically, in treatment of hypercalcemia and in certain bone diseases in which sustained reduction of osteoclastic resorption is therapeutically advantageous.
- Chronic excess of calcitonin does not produce hypocalcemia and removal of parafollicular cells does not cause hypercalcemia since PTH and vitamin D3 regulation dominate.

Calcium Homeostasis

- Maintenance of a normal serum calcium level (9–11 mg/dL) is a tightly controlled homeostatic mechanism. The homeostasis is regulated by PTH, Calcitonin and vitamin-D (Fig. 18.3).
- There is a constant flux of Ca in the ECF (900 mg) into and out of it.

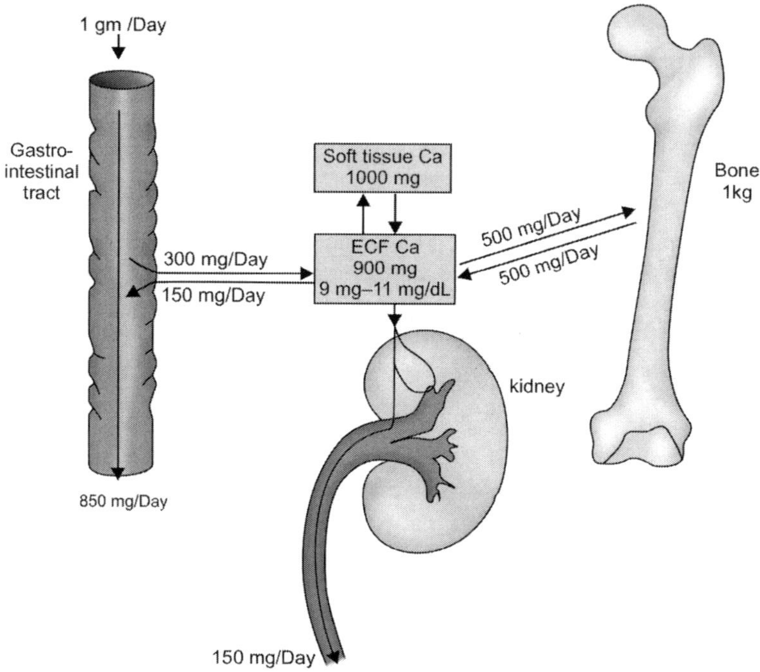

Fig. 18.3 Homeostatic balance of Ca at ECF

Flux of Ca into ECF

- The major source of flux of Ca into the serum is via the gut as absorbed Ca (300 mg/day).
- Bones are dynamic connective tissue and are constantly being deposited and dissolved. The dissolution of bones adds up to serum Ca (500 mg/day).
- Some Ca is taken up by the soft tissues (1,000 mg is present in the soft tissues).

Flux of Ca out of ECF

- Ca is removed from the ECF by the constant process of bone deposition and remodeling (500 mg/day). About 1 kg Ca is present in the bones. Bones are the major storehouse of Ca.
- Kidneys also remove Ca from the ECF with a daily excretion of 150 mg/day.
- Some Ca is deposited in the soft tissues.
- About 150 mg/day is secreted into gut with digestive juices.

Hormonal Regulation of Calcium Homeostasis (Fig. 18.4)

- Blood ionized calcium concentrations are remarkably stable in healthy individuals because of the homeostatic system involving the actions of the three calciotropic hormones on the target organs of bone, gut, and kidney.

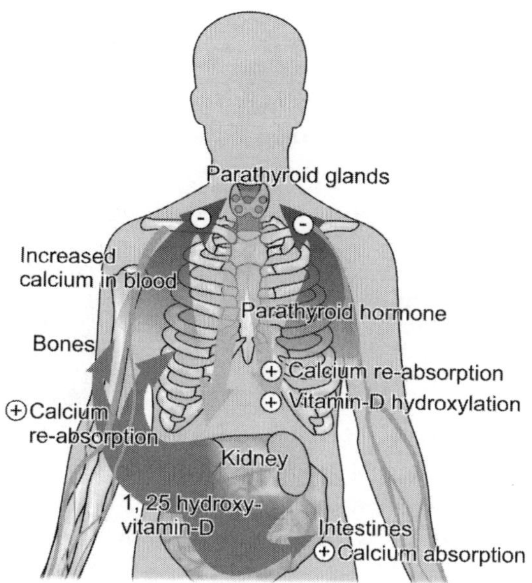

Fig. 18.4 Calcium homeostasis by PTH, calcitonin and vitamin-D

Action of PTH

- The Parathyroid hormone is secreted in response to a receding serum Ca level (hypocalcemia). This hormone's main target tissue is the bone, which under the influence of this hormone gets dissolved due to an increased osteoclastic activity. This process continues till the osteoclasts reach the haversian canals and then these osteoclasts get transformed back to the osteoblasts.
- The osteoclasts continue to eat up the bone matrix, releasing Ca and P into the circulation.
- Secondly, the PTH acts on the distal convoluted tubules of the kidneys causing re-absorption of Ca and an excretion of the P.
- Thirdly, the PTH increases the synthesis of active vitamin-D—Calcitriol that will enhance the absorption of dietary Ca at the gut and re-absorption of Ca at renal tubules.
- Thus the serum Ca level is raised to normal.
- If the serum Ca levels are high—Hypercalcemia is seen; it leads to a feedback inhibition of the secretion of the PTH from the parathyroid gland thus eliminating all its effect and will no longer add up to the serum Ca level.

Action of Calcitonin

- Calcitonin decreases the serum Ca level as it inhibits the osteoclastic activity at the bones.
- Calcitonin acts on the renal tubules and causes excretion of Ca and re-absorption of P.
- Under hypercalcemic conditions, calcitonin is secreted for the excretion of excess Ca and maintenance of normal Ca levels.
- Conversely under hypocalcemic conditions the calcitonin secretion is reduced to maintain the level of Ca.

Action of Vitamin-D

- Vitamin-D (calcitriol) enhances the serum Ca by:
  - Increasing the absorption of dietary Ca at the gut.
  - Increasing the re-absorption of filtered Ca at the distal renal tubules.

Pathophysiology of Parathyroid Gland

Hypoparathyroidism

- It is characterized by a reduced secretion of PTH.
- It could be due to:
  - Accidental surgical removal of one or more of the parathyroid glands during partial thyroidectomy.
  - Genetic/Primary hypoparathyroidism seen in autoimmune destruction of the gland.
- Symptoms include muscle cramps and tetany due to hypocalcemia. Severe and acute hypocalcemia causes the paralysis of respiratory muscles, laryngospasm and convulsions.
- Long-standing hypocalcemia causes cataracts, cutaneous changes and calcification of basal ganglia.
- Pseudohypoparathyroidism is an inherited disorder where the PTH produced is biologically active however; there is an end-organ resistance to its action. It can occur due to defect in Gs protein and a defective step beyond formation of cAMP.
- Symptoms are similar to hypoparathyroidism with additional developmental abnormalities like short stature and mental retardation.

Hyperparathyroidism

- It occurs due to an excessive production of PTH.
- The over-production of PTH could be due to:
  - Parathyroid adenoma
  - Parathyroid hyperplasia
  - Ectopic production of PTH or PTH-related peptide (PTHrp).

PTHrp is a small peptide similar in structure and action to PTH as it stimulates the PTH receptors. PTHrp is produced by some cancerous tumors. Its action causes hypercalcemia of malignancy.

- Symptoms of hyperparathyroidism include:
  - Extensive bone resorption.
  - Kidney stones.
  - Nephrocalcinosis.
  - Recurrent urinary tract infections.
  - Reduced renal function.

(Parathyroid function tests have been discussed in detail in the Practical Biochemistry section.)

A Quick Look at the Hormones of Parathyroid

- Parathyroid gland is present behind each of the upper and lower two lobes of thyroid gland.
- They secrete PTH.
- PTH secreted as a preprohormones is eventually matured to PTH.
- PTH acts via cAMP.
- Target tissues of PTH—Bones, kidneys and gut.
- PTH acts on target tissues such that it raises the serum Ca levels and reduces the P levels.
- PTH along with calcitonin and calcitriol helps maintain a Ca homeostasis.
- Calcitonin is secreted by the C cells of thyroid gland and it acts such that it reduces serum Ca level.
- Hypoparathyroidism causes tetany, muscular spasms, laryngospasm and paralysis of respiratory muscles.
- Hyperparathyroidism causes hypercalcemia and calcification of soft tissues including nephrocalcinosis, recurrent urinary tract infections.

CHAPTER

19

Hormones of Pancreas and Gut

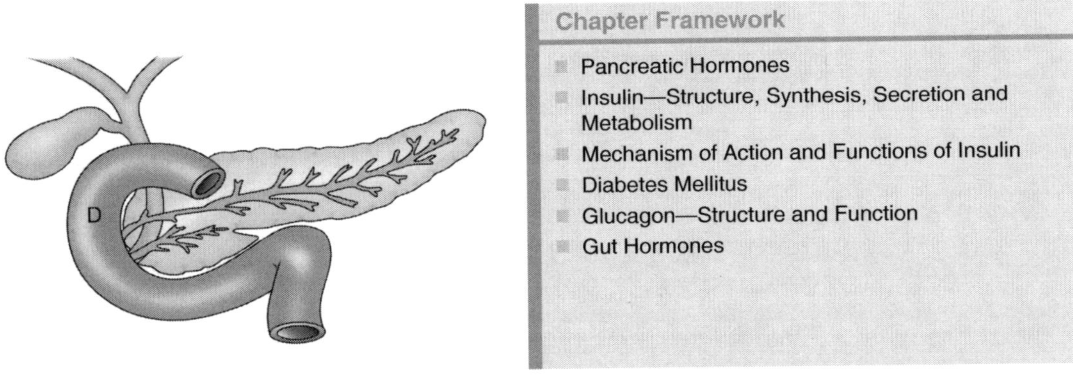

Chapter Framework

- Pancreatic Hormones
- Insulin—Structure, Synthesis, Secretion and Metabolism
- Mechanism of Action and Functions of Insulin
- Diabetes Mellitus
- Glucagon—Structure and Function
- Gut Hormones

Pancreatic Hormones

- Pancreas is a unique gland as it has both endocrine and exocrine actions. The exocrine portion is comprised of acinar cells that secrete the enzyme rich pancreatic juice.
- The endocrine portion is the islets of Langerhans, which secrete two important glucoregulatory hormones—Insulin and glucagon.
- There are about 1 – 2 million islets of Langerhans in the human pancreas.
- Each islet is composed of β-cells (60%) secreting Insulin, α-cells (25%) secreting glucagon, delta cells (10%) secreting Somatostatin (Fig. 19.1).

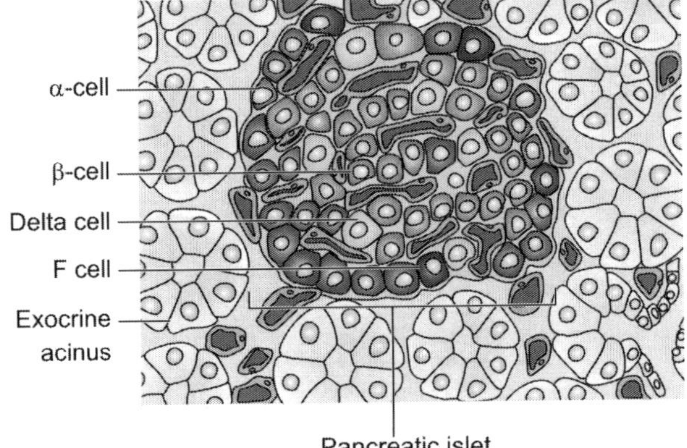

Fig. 19.1 Islets of Langerhans

- In addition to these cells, another small group of cells are the PP cells that secrete pancreatic polypeptide.
- Islets are highly vascularized; although islets comprise only 1 to 2% of the mass of the pancreas, they receive about 10 to 15% of the pancreatic blood flow.

Insulin—Structure, Synthesis, Secretion and Metabolism

Structure of Insulin

- Insulin is a peptide hormone secreted by the pancreatic β-cells. It was discovered by FG Banting and C Best in the year 1921 from dogs pancreas. It was used to keep diabetic dogs alive and later used in the 1922 for treating a 14-year-old diabetic boy.
- Insulin was first prepared in laboratory in the year 1939 by Michael Katsoyannis, making insulin the first ever hormone to be completely synthesized in laboratory and also paved way for the treatment of otherwise fatal diabetes.
- Structurally insulin is composed of two peptide chains (A – 21 and B – 30 amino acids long) linked up by two inter-chain and one intra-chain disulfide linkages.

Synthesis of Insulin

- It is initially synthesized as a preprohormone—Preproinsulin by the pancreatic β-cells.
- This preproinsulin is synthesized at the r – ER of the β-cells and has a 23 amino acid long leader sequence that directs it into the ER cisternae and then is removed once inside the cisternae.
- This produces a proinsulin molecule that provides for the necessary conformation of the mature insulin molecule and for the formation of disulfide bonds.
- Starting from the amino terminal end, proinsulin has B – chain sequences followed by Connecting peptide sequences and finally A – chain sequences (Fig. 19.2).
- This proinsulin is transferred to the golgi apparatus where it folds in specific configuration such that disulfide bonds are formed between
  - A7 and B7
  - A20 and B19
  - A6 – 11
- This proinsulin molecule then undergoes site specific cleavage such that a connecting peptide is cleaved off and mature insulin molecule with two peptide chains A and B is formed.
- Most of the proinsulin is converted to mature insulin, however some (approximately 1/6th) may remain as proinsulin and converts to mature insulin during release.
- The mature insulin is packaged as hexamers with Zn ions in secretory granules and is stored in the pancreatic β-cells. Proinsulin is also packed with Zn ions.

Secretion of Insulin

- Insulin is secreted in response to rising blood glucose level, amino acids, fatty acids, ketoacids and parasympathetic stimulation. Insulin secretion is inhibited by low blood glucose, epinephrine and sympathetic stimulation.

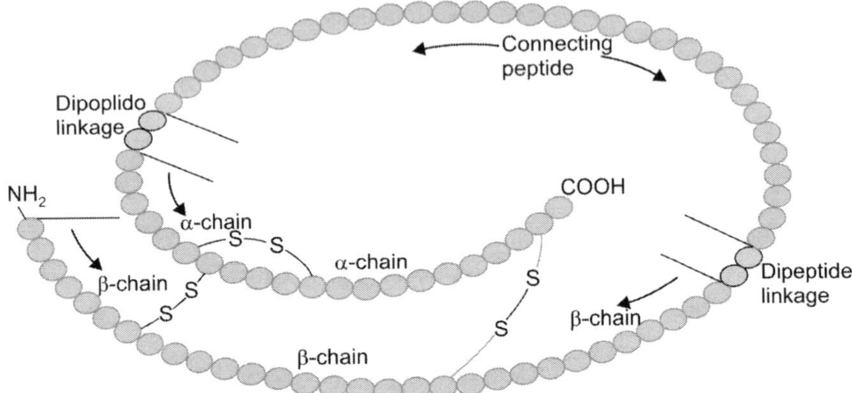

Fig. 19.2 Structure of proinsulin

- The secretion of insulin parallels that of the blood glucose rise.
- β-cells are excitable cells. In low glucose they are hyperpolarized and in high glucose they fire action potentials that depolarize their membrane. This is because glucose is oxidized to produce ATP. The raised ATP/ADP then causes the inhibition of ATP sensitive K^+ channels blocking the exudation of K^+ ions hyperpolarising the β cells membranes (Fig. 19.3).
- The hyperpolarized β-cells membranes causes calcium channels to open and entry of calcium leads to exocytosis of insulin.

Metabolism of Insulin

- Once an insulin molecule has docked onto the receptor and effected its action, it may be released back into the extracellular environment, or it may be degraded by the cell.
- The two primary sites for insulin clearance are the liver and the kidney.
- The liver clears most insulin during first-pass transit, whereas the kidney clears most of the insulin in systemic circulation.

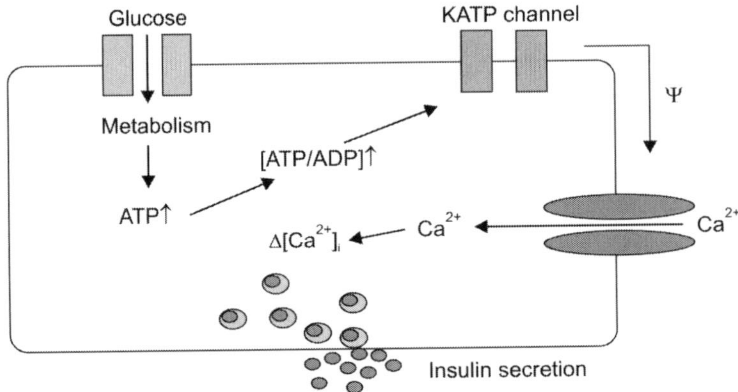

Fig. 19.3 Secretion of insulin

- Degradation normally involves endocytosis of the insulin-receptor complex, followed by the action of insulin-degrading enzyme.
- Most insulin molecules are degraded by:
  - Insulin specific protease, cleavage insulin proteolytically between amino acids residues 16 and 17 of B chain.
  - Hepatic glutathione-insulin transhydrogenase that reduce the disulfide bonds then the individual A and B chains are rapidly degraded.
    - An insulin molecule produced endogenously by the pancreatic beta cells is estimated to be degraded within about one hour after its initial release into circulation (insulin half-life 4–6 minutes).

Mechanism of Action of Insulin

- Insulin is peptide hormone that binds to its target cell receptors and executes its biologic functions via signal transduction.
- The signal transduction in insulin molecule is carried out by the inherent tyrosine kinase activity of the insulin receptors (Discussed in detail in Chapter 15)
- Binding of insulin to its receptors activates tyrosine kinase that transfer phosphate group from ATP and phosphorylate tyrosine residues on the β-subunits of the receptors (autophosphorylation).
- Further the phosphorylated tyrosine residues cause signal transduction by phosphorylation of number of intracellular proteins [insulin receptor substrates (IRS)] that finally cause insulin's biologic effects.

Functions of Insulin (Fig. 19.4)

Effects on Carbohydrate Metabolism

- *Increase uptake of glucose*: Insulin enhances the translocation of glucose transporters from cellular pool to the cell membrane especially at adipose tissue and skeletal muscles (GLUT4 transporter). Brain, RBCs, hepatocytes, intestinal mucosa, renal tubules and cornea have insulin independent glucose transporters.
- *Increases utilization of glucose*: Insulin increases the gene expression of enzymes of glucose oxidizing pathways like glycolysis, CAC. At the liver it stimulates pathways that store glucose like glycogenesis and inhibit pathways that add up BSL like glycogenolysis and gluconeogenesis as insulin reduces the gene expression of enzymes of these pathways. Thus, it has hypoglycemic effect.

Ingested glucose →
- 50% oxidation via glycolysis
- 30-40% stored as TG via lipogenesis
- 10% stored as glycogens in liver and muscles

Effects on Lipid Metabolism

- *Reduces the rate of lipolysis*: Insulin inhibits the key enzyme of lipolysis at adipose tissue, i.e. hormone sensitive lipase by causing its dephosphorylation thus reducing the rate of release of FFAs into blood circulation.

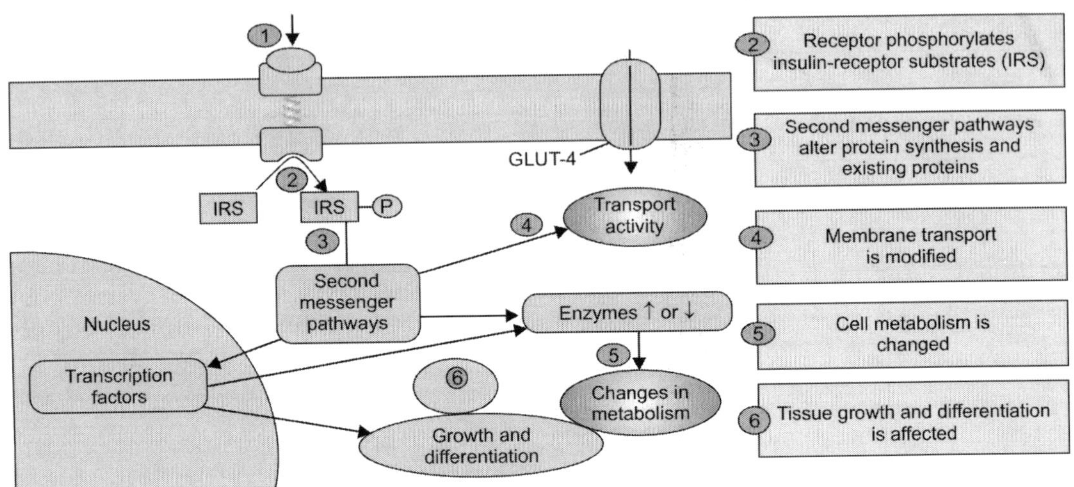

Fig. 19.4 Mechanism of action and functions of insulin

- *Increases the rate of lipogenesis*: Insulin increases the number and activity of key enzyme for lipogenesis, i.e. – acetyl CoA carboxylase, FA synthase, citrate lyase.
- Insulin also provides for the coenzyme and substrate for lipogenesis, i.e. glycerol – 3 – P and NADPH + H^+ from HMP shunt (mainly).
- *Increases the uptake of glucose into adipocytes*: The increased number of GLUT transporters on adipocytes in response to raised insulin levels causes more entry of glucose into the adipocytes.
- *Thus insulin has an anabolic effect on lipid metabolism.*

Effects on Protein Metabolism

- *Increased uptake of amino acids*: Insulin increases the uptake of amino acids at muscles and liver.
- *Increased rate of protein synthesis*: Insulin increases the rate of gene expression for various cellular proteins including metabolic enzyme proteins, or transporter proteins or the proteins for cellular growth and differentiation.
- *Reduce protein degradation*: Insulin reduces the rate of protein degradation.

Effects on Growth

- *Promotes growth of the fetus*: Insulin promotes cellular growth and tissue differentiation during embryogenesis thus promotes the growth of fetus.
- *Promotes postnatal growth by inhibiting protein degradation*: Postnatal growth is promoted by insulin since it works in synergy with the growth hormone for optimal growth. Insulin is also needed for promotion of IGFs (somatomedins) which are important for the normal growth.

Diabetes Mellitus (Fig. 19.5)

- Diabetes is a group of metabolic disorder due to actual or virtual deficiency of insulin characterized by raised blood sugar, polyuria, polydipsia and polyphagia.

- It is a chronic disorder where there is either reduced production of insulin by the pancreas due to autoimmune destruction of beta cells as in type – I DM or there is resistance to the insulin action (Insulin resistance) as in type – II DM.
- Lack of insulin causes:
  - *Hyperglycemia*: Due to the lack of insulin either absolute or due to resistance to its action, the target cells of insulin are unable to take up glucose and pathways producing glucose run unabated (like glycogenolysis and gluconeogenesis) leading to hyperglycemia.
  - *Glycosuria and polyuria*: The hyperglycemia (>180 mg/dl) causes osmotic diuresis as sugar is osmotically active, thus increasing the frequency of urination. (Fig. 19.5)
  - *Polydipsia*: Excessive urination causes intense thirst i.e. polydipsia.
  - *Polyphagia*: The loss of glucose in urine is not just responsible for polyuria but also it amounts for a considerable loss of calories that have not been trapped; thus more n more food is consumed for supplying the calories indicating more hunger or polyphagia.
  - *Weight loss*: There is weight loss despite of excessive consumption of food owing to the siphoning of the calories as sugar in urine and the use of body tissues as fuel source.
  - *Excessive fat mobilization*: Since insulin is lacking the utilization of glucose as a fuel source does not occur and the inhibitory effect of insulin on lipolysis is removed. Now the stored fats in adipose tissues are mobilized by lipolysis raising plasma FFAs that are oxidiszed for generating ATP.
  - *Ketosis*: Excessive fat oxidation causes generation of ketone bodies – acetone, acetoacetate and β-hydroxy butyrate. Under conditions of uncontrolled DM excessive production of ketone bodies causes ketonemia, ketonuria, ketosis, ketoacidosis and finally coma and death if not managed properly. Ketoacidosis occurs due to a depletion of the alkali reserve [$NaHCO_3$] since ketone bodies are excreted as Na salts.

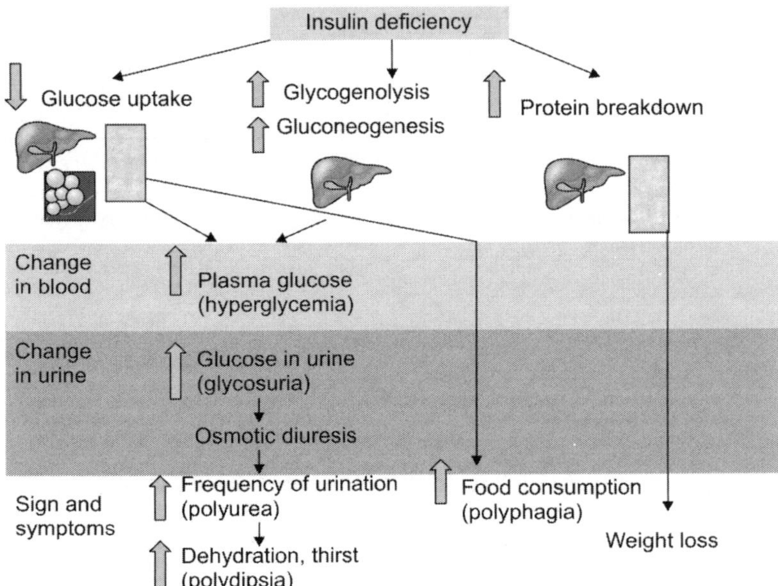

Fig. 19.5 Diabetes signs and symptoms

Types of Diabetes Mellitus (Table 19.1)

Type – I DM/Insulin Dependent DM (IDDM)

- It occurs due to autoimmune destruction of the pancreatic β-cells (auto anti insulin anti-bodies are present in these patient) or due to viral infection. Thus there is an absolute deficiency of insulin.
- It is an inherited disorder.
- It is seen in age group less than 20 years of age hence the name Juvenile DM.
- It comprises approximately 5 to 10 % of all the diabetics.
- It is characterized by severe hyperglycemia and severe ketosis.
- There is progressive weight loss as there is absolute lack of insulin causing uncontrolled lipolysis and tissue proteins are catabolized for providing amino acids as gluconeogenesis sources.
- Treatment is by giving exogenous insulin as subcutaneous injections for, e.g. – Levitin.

Type – II DM/Noninsulin Dependent DM (NIDDM)

- It is characterized by the down regulation of the insulin receptors thus there is resistance (Insulin resistance) to the action of insulin secreted by the β-cells—Noninsulin dependent DM.
- This is a chronic disease that is seen to occur with advancing age (age >40 years) in susceptible individuals thus the name Maturity onset DM.
- It is not genetic in origin.
- It comprises 90 to 95% of the diabetic patients.
- There is hyperglycemia but ketosis is mild unless it is uncontrolled.
- Its incidence increases with obesity as the insulin receptors are down regulated in obese subjects.
- The subjects have high plasma insulin levels (hyperinsulinemia); however the cells are resistant to the action of insulin, i.e. there is a state of Insulin resistance.
- Since the cells cannot bind to insulin, the action of insulin is not executed and leads to a state of hyperglycemia, glycosuria, polyuria, polydipsia and polyphagia. Ketosis is less frequent and is not severe unless the condition is uncontrolled. This is because the insulin has some functional capacity intact unlike type – I DM where there is an absolute deficiency of insulin causing excessive fat oxidation and ketosis.
- It is managed by lifestyle changes and drugs like Sulfonylurea drugs (Tolbutamide, Glyburide, etc.)

Secondary Complications of DM

Protein Glycosylation

- Hyperglycemia causes nonenzymatic addition of glucose to protein - glycation of protein, e.g. Glycated Hb (HbAc1) (Normal value is 3–5%).
- Glycation disturbs the normal functions of the proteins. For example glycation of collagen stiffens the extracellular matrix thus reducing the elasticity of vessel walls.

Table 19.1 Differences between Type – I and Type – II diabetes mellitus

IDDM (Type-I)	*NIDDM (Type-II)*
Onset - usually under 20 years of age	Usually over 40 years of age
Juvenile DM	Adult onset DM
10 % of diabetes are IDDM	90% of diabetes are NIDDM
Insulin synthesis not there due to auto-immune destruction of β-cells	Insulin synthesized but receptors down regulated
Genetically inherited	Not inherited
Auto-antibodies seen	Not seen
Obesity-uncommon	Common
Ketoacidosis-severe	Usually not there unless condition is uncontrolled
Treated by insulin injections given subcutaneously. Commercial name – Levitin	Treated by giving oral hypoglycemic drugs like Tolbutamide, Glyburide, etc.

Angiopathies

- Angiopathy is a term used for disease of blood vessels. The most common example is diabetes angiopathy.
- Macroangiopathy: It develop due to accumulation of fat and blood clots in a large blood vessel which blocks the vessel and causes ischemia of the of the organ concerned. It causes diseased like ischemic heart disease and stroke.
- Microangiopathy: It occurs due to high blood glucose which enters the endothelial cells lining the fine blood vessels. This excess glucose forms excess glycoproteins on their surface and cause thickening of and weakening of basement membrane.
- The vessels walls bleed and leak protein and slow down flow of blood then causing ischemia /gangrene of the tissue. It causes:
  - Diabetic nephropathy
  - Diabetic foot tissues not getting enough blood supply thus develops gangrene and ultimately foot might be amputated
  - Peripheral neuropathy
  - Diabetic retinopathy.

Diabetic Cataract

- Glucose can be reduced to sorbitol (in the lens of eye) which is osmotically active. Lens of eye is freely permeable to glucose but not to sorbitol. In diabetes, sorbitol is produced in excess owing to the hyperglycemia. This sorbitol causes osmotic damage to lens of eye, finally causing—Diabetes Cataract.

Diagnosis of Diabetes Mellitus

- Diabetes is diagnosed by analysing the fasting blood sugar sample. If the fasting BSL is >126 mg/dL on more than one occasion with or without presence of sugar in the urine sample is considered to be a confirmed case of diabetes.

- In patients with latent diabetes, i.e. those patients who have a normal fasting BSL but their postprandial BSL is on a higher range, are subjected to the glucose tolerance test (Discussed in Practical Biochemistry section in Chapter 45).
- These patients although do not have full blown diabetes at the moment however they are prone to develop it in few years' time.
- Nowadays only fasting BSL and post prandial BSL are taken for the diagnosis of diabetes mellitus.
- Since hyperglycemia causes glycosylation of the body proteins as discussed earlier, the values of glycated Hb are now being used as a diagnostic and prognostic tool in diabetics.
- A higher than normal glycated Hb denotes an uncontrolled state of glycemia over a duration of at least 120 days *(as the Hb once glycated cannot be converted back to normal and is destroyed at the end of the lifespan of RBCs).*

Insulinomas

- It is a rare condition where insulin secreting adenomas are present in the pancreatic β-cells and they secrete an excessive amount of insulin.
- Almost 10 to 15 % of these insulinomas is malignant and may have metastasis with large amount of insulin being secreted by both the primary and the secondary tumors.
- The excess amount of insulin causes severe hypoglycemia and can cause hypoglycemic shock. This occurs since in severe hypoglycemia the brain and CNS do not get sufficient glucose as a fuel source thus leading to brain dysfunction.

Glucagon

- Glucagon is a pancreatic peptide hormone secreted by the alpha cells of islets of Langerhans.
- It is a single polypeptide chain of 29 amino acids in length. It has immunologic and physiologic homology with the enteroglucagon and secretin hormones secreted by the gut mucosa.
- It is synthesized as a larger proglucagon molecule which is processed to give the final product as glucagon (Fig. 19.6).
- Only 30 to 40% is immunreactive glucagon in circulation, rest is inactive large precursor molecules. Glucagon circulates free in the plasma and does not have any transport protein.
- Glucagon is secreted in response to hypoglycaemia and its secretion is inhibited by glucose, amino acids, fatty acids, GIT hormones and neurotransmitters (Fig. 19.7).
- Glucagon acts via GCPRs and uses c – AMP as the second messenger.
- It is inactivated at the liver.

Functions of Glucagon

- It increases the gene expression of key – enzymes of glucose producing pathways like –
  - Gluconeogenesis—PEPCK, glucose – 6–phosphatase, pyruvate carboxylase.
  - Glycogenolysis—Phosphorylase (in liver but not in muscle).
- It increases the rate of lipolysis by increazing the concentration of c–AMP and activating the key enzyme hormone sensitive lipase.
- It increases the breakdown of proteins to release amino acids that are used as substrates of gluconeogenesis.

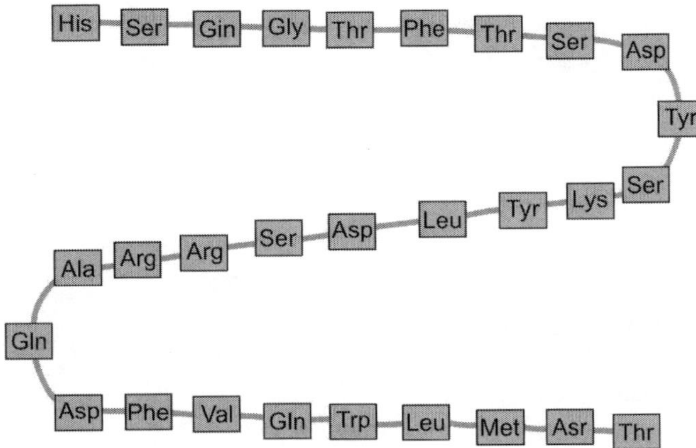

Fig. 19.6 Structure of glucagon

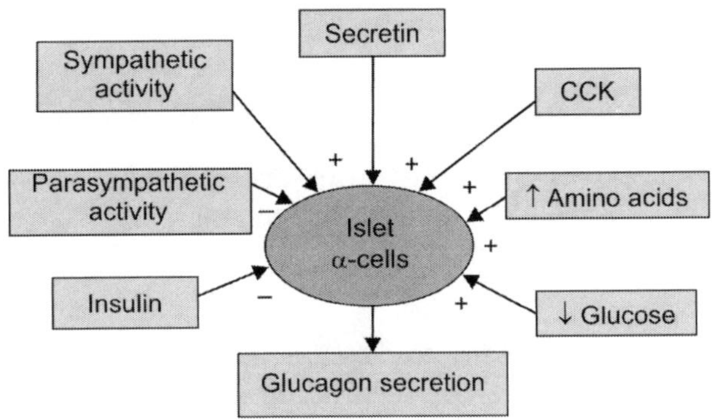

Fig. 19.7 Factors affecting glucagon secretion

Pathophysiology of Glucagon

- Glucagon excess and deficit are rare. Glucagon excess is seen in cancer of α-cells (glucagonomas).
- There is no report of glucagon deficit.

Insulin and Glucagon Balancing Act (Fig. 19.8)

- Insulin and glucagon are the pancreatic hormones that work to keep a balance in the BSL. Both these hormones are responsible for the maintenance of a normal BSL.
- During fasting conditions the low BSL stimulates the pancreatic α-cells for the secretion of Glucagon and the secretion of insulin is inhibited.

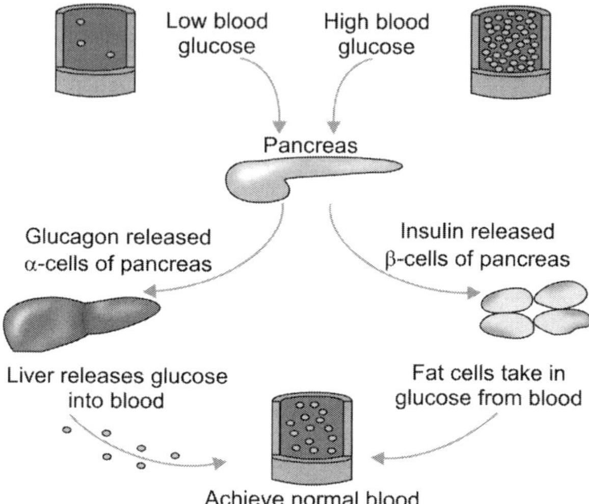

Fig. 19.8 Balance in the action of insulin and glucagon

- Glucagon raises the BSL to normal range by increazing rate of glycogenolysis and gluconeogenesis.
- Conversely after the meals when BSL rises, Insulin is secreted in response which reduces the BSL to normal by increasing glucose uptake and utilization.

Somatostatin

- It is a cyclic polypeptide hormone secreted by the delta cells of islets of Langerhans.
- Initially Somatostatin was discovered as a hormone secreted by the hypothalamus, where it inhibits the secretion of the anterior pituitary hormone – Growth hormone.
- Somatostatin is secreted as a preprohormones and is processed to give the active form comprizing of 28 amino acids.
- It works via the GCPRs and uses c – AMP as the second messenger.

Functions of Somatostatin

- Somatostatin inhibits the secretion of the other hormones of pancreas, i.e. insulin and glucagon by paracrine action.
- It decreases gastric emptying.
- It decreases secretion of gastrin hormone and thus the secretion of gastric juice is also reduced.
- It decreases the exocrine secretions of pancreas.
- It decreases the splanchnic blood flow.
- It reduces the absorption of glucose.
- In pharmacologic amounts it blunts the ketosis caused due to insulin deficiency as it inhibits the secretion of glucagon that may occur in insulinopenia.

Pancreatic Polypeptide

- It is a large polypeptide of 36 amino acids secreted by a group of pancreatic cells named the F – cells.
- Its function is unknown but its secretion has been observed to be raized in fasting, by protein rich meal, exercise, acute hypoglycemia and is reduced or inhibited by Somatostatin and IV glucose.

Gut Hormones

- The gastrointestinal tract has a crucial role in the control of energy homeostasis through its role in the digestion, absorption, and assimilation of ingested nutrients. Furthermore, signals from the gastrointestinal tract are important regulators of gut motility and satiety.
- Important gut hormones identified are:
  - Gastrin family including gastrin and CCK.
  - Secretin family including secretin, glucagon, gastric inhibitory peptide (GIP), vasoactive intestinal peptide (VIP), glicentin.
- *Gastrin* from the gastric antrum and the duodenum stimulates gastric acid and pepsin secretion.
- *Cholecystokinin (CCK)* from the duodenum and jejunum stimulates contraction of the gallbladder and the secretion of pancreatic enzymes.
- *Secretin* from the duodenum and jejunum stimulates the secretion of bicarbonate by the pancreas.
- *Gastric inhibitory polypeptide (GIP)* from the small bowel enhances insulin release and inhibits secretion of gastric acid.
- *Vasoactive intestinal polypeptide (VIP)* from the pancreas relaxes smooth muscles and stimulates bicarbonate secretion by the pancreas.
- Certain neurocrine secretions of the gut are:
  - Neurotensin
  - Bombesin like peptide
  - Substance – P
  - Somatostatin
- Little is known of the functions of these gut hormones mechanism of action but functionally these hormones act locally on local organs and affect various processes of the GIT like secretion of enzyme rich digestive juices, or gut motility.
- Some of these are also produced by brain and other neural tissue where they act as neuromodulators or neurotransmitters.

Pathophysiology

- *Gastrinomas* are gastrin-secreting endocrine tumors associated with Zollinger-Ellison syndrome. Hypergastrinemia results in increased hydrochloric acid (HCl) production with resultant recurrent peptic ulcers.
- *VIPomas* are rare tumors that secrete vasoactive intestinal peptide. This condition is associated with watery diarrhea, hypokalemia, and achlorhydria.

A Quick Look at the Hormones of Pancreas and Gut

- Pancreas has 60% β-cells, 25% α-cells and 10% delta cells.
- Pancreas secretes insulin, glucagon, Somatostatin, pancreatic polypeptide.
- Insulin is secreted by the pancreatic beta cells.
- Insulin is secreted in response to high blood glucose, amino acids, fatty acids, keto acids.
- Insulin is stored in pancreatic β-cells as hexamers bound to Zn ions.
- Insulin reduces the blood sugar level, increases glucose uptake, utilization, storage, fat storage, protein anabolism and reduces gluconeogenesis, glycogenolysis, lipolysis, protein catabolism.
- Deficiency of insulin causes DM (Type – I and II).
- Glucagon is secreted in response to hypoglycemia.
- It enhances the activities of enzymes that add upto BSL.
- Somatostatin inhibits secretion of pancreatic hormones by paracrine action.
- Important gut hormones are – Gastrin family and Secretin family responsible for regulating the secretion of digestive juices and gut motility.

CHAPTER

20

Hormones of Adrenal Gland

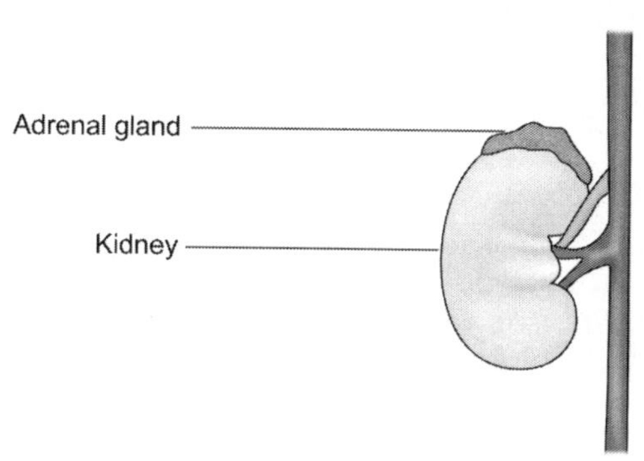

Chapter Framework

- Introduction
- Hormones of Adrenal Cortex
- Transport, Functions and Catabolism of Adreno-Corticoid Hormones
- Hormones of Adrenal Medulla
- Mechanism of Action and Functions of Catecholamines

Introduction

- Adrenal gland is also termed as the suprarenal gland because it is present on the superior poles of the two kidneys.
- The gland is divided into two parts—The peripheral cortical part known as the adrenal cortex (80%) and the central core termed as the adrenal medulla (20%).
- The adrenal cortex secretes the adrenocorticosteroid hormones namely the mineralocorticoids (by Zona glomerulosa), glucocorticoids (by Zona fasiculata) and adrenal androgens (by Zona reticularis).
- The adrenal medulla, lying in the center of the adrenal gland, is functionally related to the sympathetic nervous system and secretes the Catecholamines epinephrine and norepinephrine in response to stress.

Hormones of Adrenal Cortex

- Adrenal cortex synthesizes the steroid hormones – glucocorticoids and mineralocorticoids.
- The synthesis of all steroid hormones begins with cholesterol and is catalyzed by a series of regulated, enzyme-mediated reactions.
- The first reaction is the side chain cleavage of the steroid ring nucleus by a *STAR (1)* (Steroidogenic Acute Regulatory Protein) and *side chain cleavage enzyme in presence of Cytochrome P450 (SDCC450)* (2).
- This produces pregnenolone.
- Pregnenolone is produced in the mitochondria from where it is transported to the ER.

- At the endoplasmic reticulum pregnenolone is reduced by the *3–β-hydroxy steroid dehydrogenase (NADPH dependent)* (3) and progesterone is formed. The progesterone can synthesize both glucocorticoids and mineralocorticoids.
- This *17-α-hydroxylase (17, 20 – lyase)* (7) adds up a hydroxy group on 17 position of progesterone to give 17–α-hydroxy progesterone.
- Then 17-α-hydroxy progesterone is further hydroxylated by *21 hydroxylase* (4) to 11 – deoxycortisol which moves out of the ER to re-enter the mitochondria.
- The 11 – deoxycortisol then is finally hydroxylated at 11-position by *11 beta hydroxylase* (5) to give the active glucocorticoid hormone cortisol.
- Conversely the progesterone can also undergo 21-hydroxylation in presence of 21 alpha hydroxylase to give 11 – deoxy corticosterone and then further 11-hydroxylation to give the corticosterone and finally corticosterone is oxidized by *Corticosterone methyl oxidase* (6) to give active mineralocorticoid – Aldosterone (Fig. 20.1).

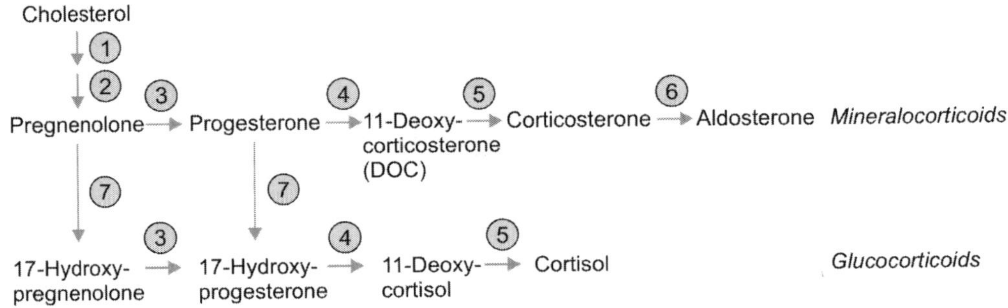

Fig. 20.1 Biosynthesis of adrenocorticosteroid hormones

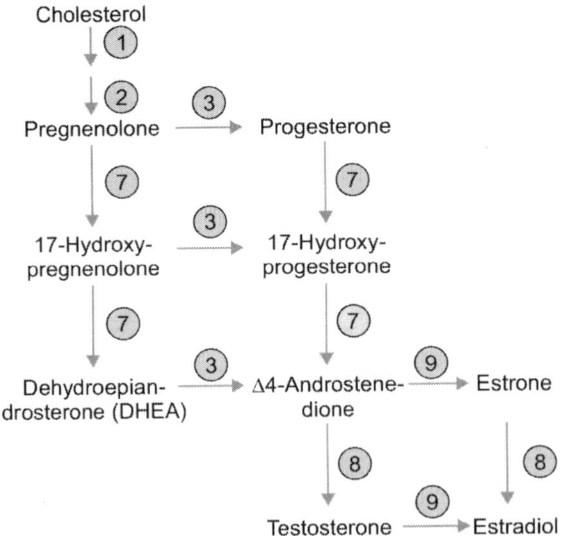

Fig. 20.2 Biosynthesis of adrenal androgens

Adrenal Androgens

- The adrenal androgens are synthesized as shown in the Figure 20.2 [Enzymes – 1,2,3 and 7 – same as in Figure 20.1 and 8 – 17 β-hydroxy steroid dehydrogenase; 9 – Aromatase].
- Several moderately active male sex hormones called adrenal androgens (the most important of which is dehydroepiandrosterone) are continually secreted by the adrenal cortex, especially during fetal life.
- Progesterone and estrogens, which are female sex hormones, are secreted in minute quantities.
- Normally, the adrenal androgens have only weak effects in humans. (Functions of androgens are discussed in Chapter 12)

Regulation of Secretion of Adrenal Cortex Hormones

- The secretory rates of CRF, ACTH, and cortisol are high in the early morning but low in the late evening, thus the plasma cortisol levels are high an hour before arising in the morning and a low around midnight.
- The secretion of the glucocorticoid hormones is regulated by a feedback mechanism by the pituitary – hypothalamic axis as shown in Figure 20.3.
- Aldosterone secretion is regulated by a renin – angiotensin system that is sensitive to the changes in blood pressure and electrolyte concentration (Fig. 20.4).

Mechanism of Action of Adrenal Steroid Hormones

- The adrenal steroid hormones bind to the intracellular receptors like the other steroid hormones (as discussed in Chapter 15).
- The glucocorticoid hormones have specific receptors that have well defined functional domains (Fig. 20.5):
  - Amino terminal domain—It has antigenic sites and also has a transactivation domain/activation function (τ1/AF1) that modulates the promoter.

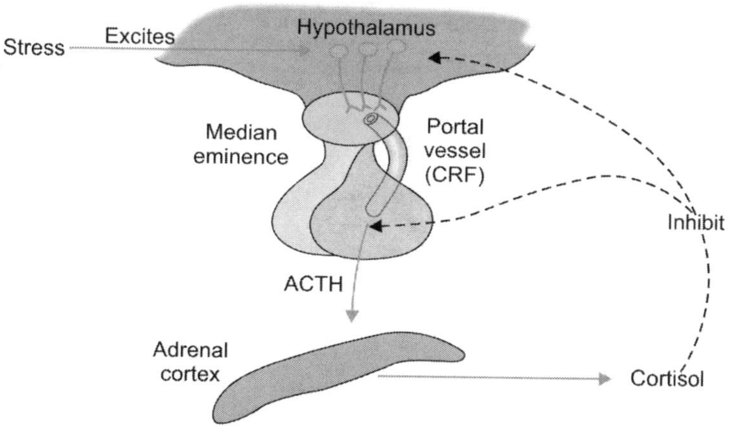

Fig. 20.3 Regulation of secretion of adrenal hormones

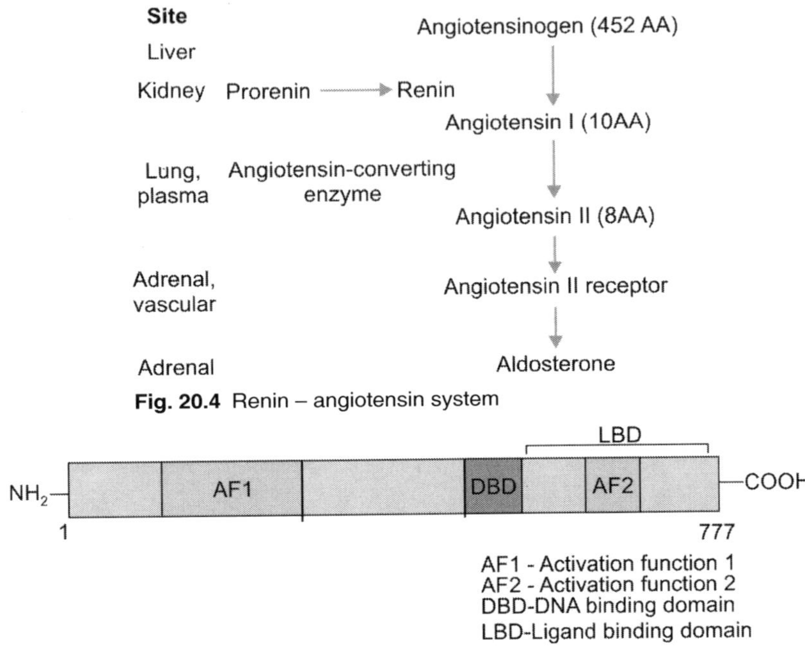

Fig. 20.4 Renin – angiotensin system

Fig. 20.5 Glucocorticoid receptor

- Carboxy terminal domain—It has the DNA binding region and a transactivation domain/ activation function (τ2/AF2). Besides these two sequences there is also a sequence that helps in dimerization of the receptor molecule such that it binds to the glucocorticoid response element (GRE).
  - The glucocorticoid hormone receptor belongs to the super family of steroid – Thyroid – retinoid family of hormones.
  - The glucocorticoid hormone regulates the gene expression.
- The hormone-receptor complex binds to the specific consensus sequences present upstream the transcription initiation site.
- Thus, the glucocorticoid hormones act as enhancers of gene expression.
- The mineralocorticoids also act in similar manner.

Transport, Functions and Catabolism of Adrenocorticoid

Transport

- The adrenal steroids need a plasma transport protein since these are lipophilic molecules.
- *Glucocorticoids* are transported bound to a protein *transcortin/corticosterone binding globulin (CBG).*
- Cortisol binds tightly with CBG and has a half-life of 1.5–2 hours.
- The unbound cortisol represents the biologically active form.
- *Aldosterone*—The major mineralocorticoid doesn't have any plasma transport protein however, it binds weakly to albumin. The other hormones with mineralocorticoid activity are corticosterone and deoxycorticosterone which bind to CBG.

Functions

Glucocorticoids (Cortisol)

- Glucocorticoids enhance the rate of gluconeogenesis so as to fight the stress situation and provide the brain cells enough fuel as glucose.
- It decreases the utilization of glucose by other body tissues.
- It increases the cellular protein catabolism to release amino acids as gluconeogenic precursors. However, the plasma proteins and liver proteins are increased by cortisol.
- Cortisol increases the mobilization of fatty acids from adipose tissue raising the plasma FFAs that are oxidised as fuel source under conditions of stress as glucose is spared.
- Cortisol inhibits the inflammatory process by decreasing capillary permeability, supressing immune system (T – cells reduced), reduce migration of WBCs to site of inflammation and reduces fever as it inhibits release of interleukin – 1.

Mineralocorticoids (Aldosterone)

- Aldosterone increases reabsorption of sodium (Na) and simultaneously increases secretion of potassium by the renal tubular epithelial cells.
- Although, there is reabsorption of Na at the renal tubules under the influence of aldosterone, however, the ECF Na does not increase markedly because Na reabsorption is followed by osmotic reabsorption of water. Also slight increase in Na causes the thirst centre to be stimulated.

Catabolism

- Both the adrenal steroid hormones are removed by conjugation with glucuronic acid at the liver and finally through the urine (20%), faeces (70%) and some through skin.

Pathophysiology of Adrenal Cortex

- *Addison's disease*: It is primary adrenal insufficiency due to atrophy of adrenal cortex. It is characterised by hypoglycemia, extreme sensitivity to insulin, stress intolerance, anorexia, weight loss, nausea and weakness due to lack of cortisol. These patients also have low blood pressure, reduced GFR and reduced plasma Na^+ with hyperkalemia (high K^+).
- *Secondary adrenal insufficiency* may occur due to tumor or infarction or infection causing reduced ACTH secretion which in turn reduces secretion of adrenocorticoids.
- *Cushing's syndrome*: It is due to excess of glucocorticoid hormones. It can occur due to ACTH secreting adenomas of pituitary or ectopic ACTH secreting adenomas or from adrenal adenomas. These patients have symptoms of hyperglycemia or glucose intolerance, muscle wasting, skin thinning, osteoporosis, lymphoid tissue involution, negative nitrogen balance and peculiar fat redistribution with typical abdominal obesity and a 'buffalo hump' (more fat over neck and shoulders). Some symptoms like hypernatremia, hypokalemia, edema, and hypertension are due to mineralocorticoid effects of cortisol.
- *Conn's syndrome (Primary aldosteronism):* It occurs due to small adenomas of glomerulosa cells. Its manifestations include – hypokalemia, hypernatremia and alkalosis. Owing to the high levels of aldosterone hormone, the plasma renin – angiotensin II levels are low or supressed.

- *Secondary aldosteronism*: It occurs due to renal artery stenosis that causes hyperplasia of the juxta-glomerular (JG) cells and high levels of renin and angiotensin II. It manifests symptoms similar to Conn's syndrome with exception of high renin – angiotensin.

Hormones of Adrenal Medulla

- The adrenal medulla, lying in the centre of the adrenal gland, is functionally related to the sympathetic nervous system and secretes the Catecholamines epinephrine and norepinephrine in response to stress.
- Adrenal medulla has the chromaffin granules that biosynthesize and stores the catecholamines.
- *Synthesis and catabolism of Catecholamines is discussed in Chapter 12.*
- The secretion of the catecholamines is neurally regulated. On neural stimulation, the chromaffin granules membranes fuse with the plasma membrane to release the catecholamines by exocytosis.
- The process is stimulated by β-adrenergic and cholinergic agents and inhibited by α-adrenergic agents.
- These are taken up again at neuronal ends if unused for conserving these.
- The catecholamines released from adrenal medulla do not have the reuptake mechanism so it circulates in the plasma and reaches the liver and skeletal muscles to carry out their effect and are then catabolized (as shown in Chapter 12).
- They are rapidly catabolized and have a half-life of a few seconds (10 – 30 second).

Mechanism of Action of Catecholamines

- The α-2 and beta adrenergic catecholamines use c – AMP as the second messenger and α-1 adrenergic use Ca and or phosphatidyl inositol as second messenger.

Functions

- Norepinephrine causes constriction of essentially all the blood vessels of the body, causes increased activity of the heart, inhibition of the gastrointestinal tract and dilation of the pupils of the eyes.
- Epinephrine has similar effects with few exceptions.
- It causes only weak constriction of the blood vessels in the muscles, in comparison with norepinephrine.
- It has a greater effect on cardiac stimulation than does norepinephrine.
- It has 5 to 10 times as great a metabolic effect as norepinephrine (epinephrine can increase the cellular metabolic rate by 100% above normal).
- Metabolically epinephrine and norepinephrine enhance the rate of hepatic glycogenolysis, gluconeogenesis, and lipolysis at adipose tissue raising plasma FFAs.

Pathophysiology of Adrenal Medulla

- Pheochromocytoma – tumors of adrenal medulla are seen to cause severe hypertension as they have a high norepinephrine to epinephrine ratio.

A Quick Look at the Hormones of Adrenal Gland

- Adrenal gland is present on the superior poles of both the kidneys.
- Adrenal gland has an outer cortex (80%) and inner medulla (20%).
- Adrenal cortex secretes glucocorticoids, mineralocorticoids and adrenal medulla secretes catecholamines.
- Important Glucocorticoid is cortisol.
- Important mineralocorticoid is aldosterone.
- The adrenocorticoid hormones are steroidal chemically and mechanism of action is that of steroid hormones involving intracellular receptors.
- Glucocorticoid enhances gluconeogenesis, reduces peripheral utilisation of glucose, increases protein catabolism, supresses immune response.
- Mineralocorticoid increases reabsorption of sodium and reduces reabsorption of potassium at renal tubules thus increasing excretion of potassium and reducing that of sodium.
- Excessive secretion of Adrenocorticoid causes – Cushing's syndrome and Conn's syndrome.
- Deficiency of adrenocorticoid hormones causes Addison's disease.
- Adrenal medullary hormones are secreted in excess in pheochromocytoma.

CHAPTER
21
Hormones of Gonads

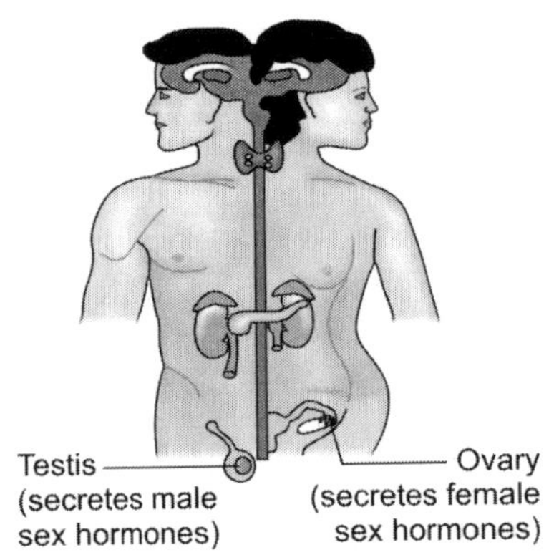

Chapter Framework

Introduction

- Gonads are the sex organs that secrete male and female sex hormones as well as synthesize the respective haploid gametes.
- The testes are the site of spermatogenesis and secrete the male sex hormones, namely testosterone which is responsible for the development of the male secondary sexual characteristics.
- The ovaries in females are the site of oogenesis and secrete the female sex hormones, namely estrogens and progesterone that are responsible for the female secondary sexual characteristics and the menstrual cycle.

Male Sex Hormones Biosynthesis

- The major male sex hormones are testosterone, androstenedione and dehydroepiandrosterone (DHEA), collectively termed as androgens, of which most important is testosterone.
- Testosterone is secreted by the interstitial cells of Leydig of the testis.
- Testosterone is a steroid hormone that regulates the male secondary sexual characteristics and the process of gametogenesis in the males.
- The synthesis of testosterone is same as shown in Figure 21.1 (androgen synthesis).

Transport and Metabolism of Testosterone

- Testosterone is secreted into the circulation on synthesis by the interstitial cells of Leydig. In the plasma it binds loosely to albumin and tightly to sex hormone binding globulin (SHBG).

- It has a plasma half-life of about 30 minutes during which duration it carries out its tissue specific actions or is completely catabolized.
- The testosterone that binds to the tissues is converted to dehydrotestosterone that eventually carries out the physiologic roles of testosterone.
- The testosterone that doesn't bind to the target tissues is degraded at liver into androsterone and DHEA and then conjugated with glucuronate to be excreted with bile in feces or urine.

Functions of Male Sex Hormones

- In the embryonic stage the secretion of testosterone by genital ridges causes the development of male fetus.
- Testosterone secretion by the testes causes the descent of testes into the scrotum by the last 2–3 months of gestation.
- Testosterone causes development of the secondary sexual characteristics in a male at puberty like:
  - Heaviness of voice.
  - Thickening of skin and acne development.
  - Facial and body hair growth.
  - Increased muscle and bone protein synthesis.
  - Increased Ca retention at bones making them stronger.
- It increases BMR.

Regulation of Secretion of Male Sex Hormones

- The secretion of the male sex hormones is under the feedback control of GnRH from the hypothalamus which in turn stimulates the anterior pituitary gonadotropins LH and FSH.
- GnRH stimulates the secretion of LH and FSH which cause respectively secretion of testosterone and spermatogenesis.

Pathophysiology

- Hypogonadism—It is lack of testosterone in males, if it occurs before puberty secondary sexual characteristics do not develop. In adults many features regress. Primary hypogonadism occurs due to failure of the testes to secrete testosterone. There are some cases where there is lack of receptors of testosterone thus although the levels of testosterone are normal, genetically male individual yet there is hypogonadism and feminization of the external genitalia.

Female Sex Hormones Biosynthesis

- The major female sex hormones are estrogens (esterone, estriol and estradiol) and progesterone secreted by the ovaries.
- The biosynthesis is as shown in the Figure 21.1.
- The biosynthesis is similar to that of the male sex sterol with an additional aromatase enzyme acting on testosterone and androstenedione to give the esterone and estradiol that can form estriol by a 16 α-hydroxylase. Thus the male and the female sex steroids differ mainly in an aromatization of the A ring of the sterol nucleus.

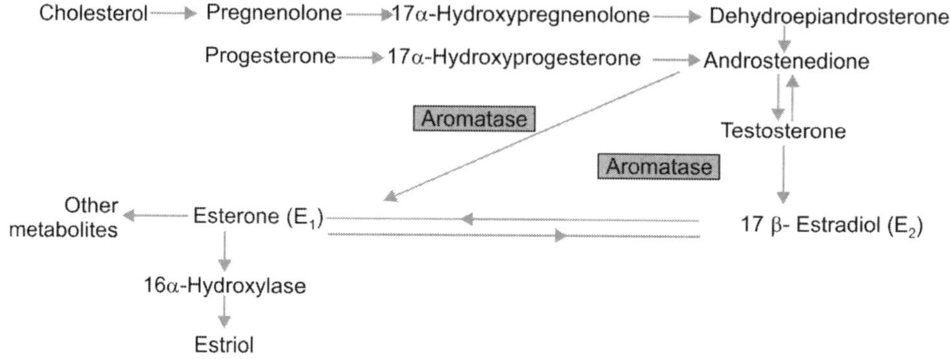

Fig. 21.1 Biosynthesis of progesterone and estrogens

Transport and Metabolism

- The female sex steroids are transported bound to the plasma albumin and sex hormone binding globulin in loose combination such that it readily is released to target tissues. It has a half-life approximately 30 minutes.
- Estrogens are metabolized at the liver by glucuronidation and sulfation to be eliminated with bile in feces and urine.
- Progesterone is rapidly metabolized to other nonprogestational steroids within few minutes.
- Liver degrades the progesterone to pregnendiol—Major end-product of progesterone metabolizm and is excreted in urine.

Regulation of Secretion

- The regulation of secretion of the female sex steroids is under the hypothalamo – pituitary hormonal axis control.
- The hypothalamic hormone GnRH stimulates the anterior pituitary to secrete FSH and LH which in turn stimulate the ovaries to secrete the estrogens and progesterone.

Functions of Female Sex hormones

Effects of Estrogens

- Estrogens cause the uterus to develop and increase in size at puberty.
- Estrogens cause the breast tissue to proliferate (stroma and ductal) and increase fat deposition at puberty causing development of breasts.
- Estrogens inhibit osteoclastic activity of bones, increase bone deposition causing rapid growth but also cause epiphyseal union so the height is not very much.
- Estrogens cause increased subcutaneous fat deposition.
- Estrogens make the skin soft and smooth.
- Estrogens are similar to aldosterone in action that it causes retention of Na and water at kidneys.
- Estrogens make the fallopian tube more glandular and ciliary to propel the fertilized ovum towards the uterus.

Effect of Progesterone

- It enhances the development of the uterine endometrium—Makes it more secretory to make it suitable for implantation of the fertilized ovum.
- It makes the fallopian tubes more secretory to nourish the fertilized ovum.
- It causes alveolar development in breasts such that they become secretory.

The GnRH, FSH and LH along with the female sex steroids regulate the female monthly sexual cycle that includes ovulation and menstrual cycle.

Pathophysiology

- *Primary hypogonadism:* The ovaries are defective so there is decreased ovulation and ovarian hormones secretion.
- *Secondary hypogonadism:* There is loss of pituitary gonadotropins function.
- *Turner's syndrome:* The individuals are with a karyotype XO so are females with delayed puberty.
- *Polycystic ovary disease:* In this case there is an over-production of androgens causing obesity, irregular menses, hirustism, etc.

A Quick Look at the Hormones of Gonads

- Gonads are the male and female sex organs secreting male and female sex hormones.
- The most important male sex hormones are testosterone, androstenedione, DHEA.
- The hormone testosterone secretion is under the regulation of GnRH from hypothalamus which in turn through LH and FSH regulates the synthesis and secretion of testosterone and spermatogenesis.
- Testosterone is responsible for the development of secondary sexual characteristics at puberty in males.
- It is transported bound to a SHBG to target tissues and unused testosterone is conjugated at the liver and is excreted.
- Female sex hormones are secreted by the ovaries.
- Estrogen, estriol, estradiol and progesterone are the principal female sex hormones.
- The secretion of female sex hormones is regulated by GnRH from hypothalamus and then LH and FSH from anterior pituitary.
- Estrogens are responsible for the female secondary sexual characteristics.
- GnRH, FSH, LH and female sex hormones regulate the female sexual cycle—Menstrual cycle.
- Male and female hypogonadism is characterized by reduced secretion of their sex hormones.

Section – 5

Genetics

- DNA Replication and Repair
- Transcription—RNA Synthesis
- Genelic code, Mutation and Translation of mRNA
- Regulation of Gene Expression
- Recomdinant DNA Technology

CHAPTER

22

DNA Replication and Repair

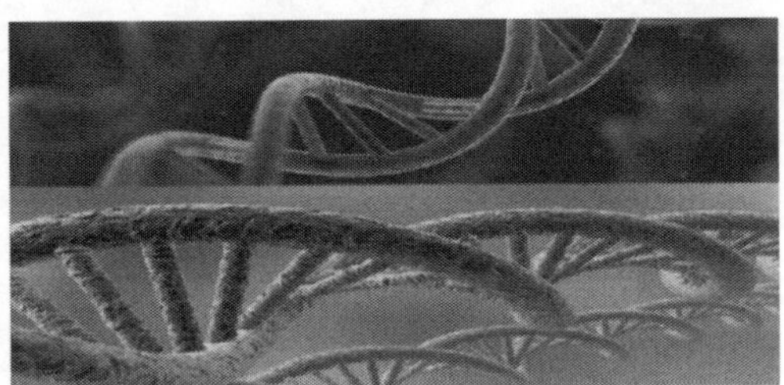

Chapter Framework

Introduction

- Every living organism in order to perpetuate needs to multiply and produce its progeny that is a copy of its parent cell or multicellular organism.
- The genetic information of the organism has to be completely and correctly replicated for the exact copy of the parent to be formed.
- The complete genetic information of an organism is present in the form of genes in its genome.
- *Genes* are defined as the region of DNA that contains the information for determining the primary structure of proteins or noncoding RNA.
- *Genome* is defined as the overall DNA contained in one cell. In eukaryotic somatic cells there are two sets of genes thus these are diploid cells whereas their germ cells have only one set of genes and are haploid in nature.
- Certain regions of the genome in the eukaryotes are repetitive and do not code for any proteins, these are known as the *introns (noncoding sequences of DNA).*
- Only a small portion of the complete genome is responsible for coding the entire organism these are the *exons (coding sequences of DNA).*
- The DNA is replicated in a highly specific, organized and semiconservative manner, such that an exact copy of the parent organism is produced.
- In multicellular organisms, the DNA is organized as chromosomes.
- The DNA combines with basic nucleoproteins—Histones (H_1, H_2A, H_2B, H_3 and H_4) which are rich in arginine and lysine.
- A single strand of DNA wounds around a core histone octamer (H_2A,H_2B, H_3, H_4) with two such octamers linked up by a linker DNA (30 base pairs) and H_1.
- A single histone octamer with DNA wound around it in 1.75 super helical turns is termed as a nucleosome.

- A chain of nucleosomes is chromatin fibril (10 nm in diameter), which is further condensed sequentially to 30nm (solenoid form—6 nucleosomes per turn) then 300 nm (50 turns per loop of the chromatin on chromosomal matrix) then 700 nm (18 loops condensed together in a minibands) finally to a 1400 nm chromatid (several minibands stacked together) [Figure 22.1].
- Two such chromatids form a complete chromosome. Thus, a single chromatid has haploid information and a chromosome has diploid genetic information.

Cell Cycle

- The complete life span of a cell is divided into different phases gap 1 (G_1), synthetic (S), gap 2 (G_2) and mitosis (M) phase which is termed as the cell cycle.
- The G_1 and G_2 phases are the non synthetic phases of the cell. The cell is in interphase in the G_1 phase.
- During the S phase there is the synthesis of the proteins necessary for the new cell and the replication of the DNA molecule.
- This process of cell cycle is regulated by a group of proteins—Cyclins.
- The cyclins are a family of proteins whose concentration increases and decreases throughout the cell cycle.
- There are specific kinases—Cyclin-dependent kinases that are activated by the cyclins and which phosphorylate specific cellular proteins essential for progression through different stages of cell cycle (Fig. 22.2).
- Cyclin D increases during G_1 phase that activates the kinases Cdk 4 and 6. These kinases phosphorylate cellular proteins such that the cell moves through the restriction point to S phase. One such substrate is retinoblastoma gene product—Rb protein which inhibits the transcription factor E2F and thus inhibits cell division acting as cell cycle regulator. Rb on phosphorylation is inhibited; E2F is relieved of Rb and cell cycle proceeds from G_1 to S phase which is otherwise inhibited by Rb.
- Other cyclins are Cyclin E, A and B which respectively help in transition from G_1 to S, S to G_2 and G_2 to M.

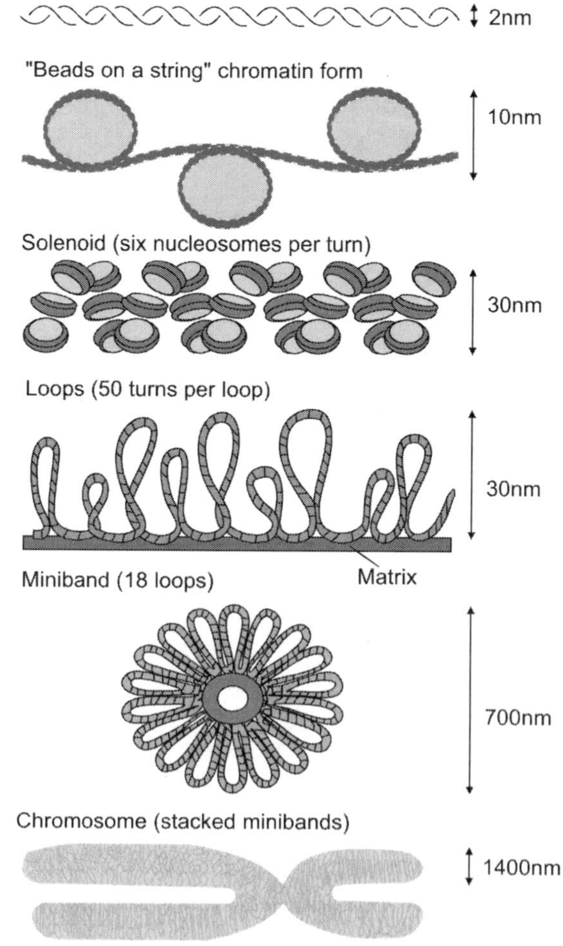

Fig. 22.1 Organization of chromosome

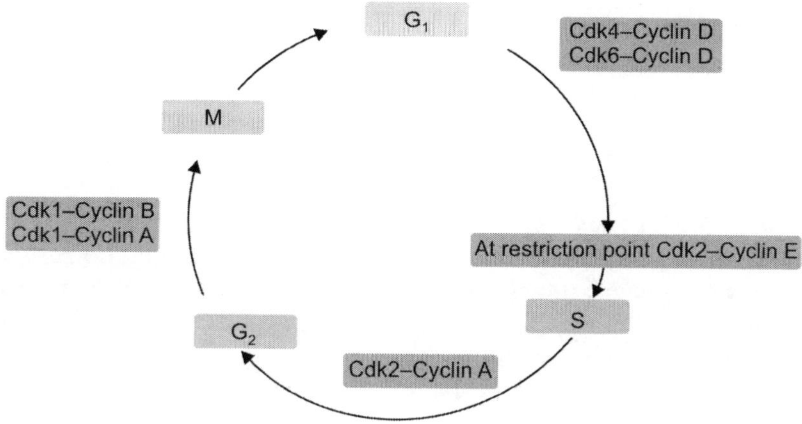

Fig. 22.2 Cell cycle regulation

DNA Replication

- DNA replication occurs during the S – phase of cell cycle just before the cell is about to divide.
- The process of DNA replication occurs in a semi-conservative manner, i.e. the two parent strands separate and act as a template on which two new daughter DNA molecules are synthesized. Thus, each new DNA molecule has one strand from the parent, i.e. the parent DNA is half conserved in the daughter DNA—Semiconservative replication (Fig. 22.3).
- The process of DNA replication in the prokaryotes occurs in the cytosol as they do not have a nucleus; however in the eukaryotes the DNA is well-organized as chromosomes in the nucleus and thus replication occurs in the nucleus of eukaryotes.

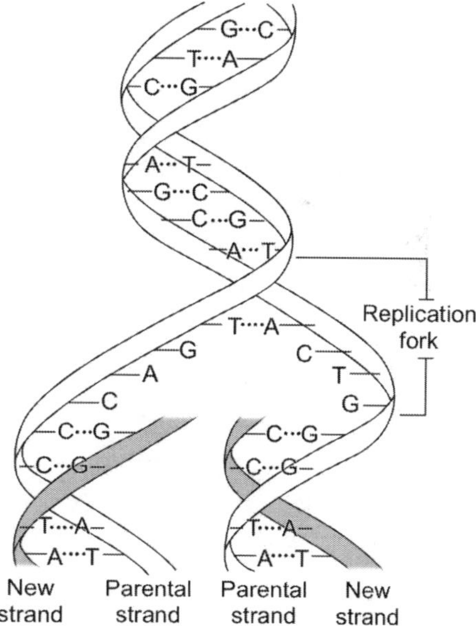

Fig. 22.3 Semiconservative DNA replication

Process of Replication

- DNA replication was studied by Kornberg in *E. Coli*.
- The process of DNA replication is highly complex, yet organized and involves a number of enzymes and cellular proteins that are important for ensuring the specificity and fidelity of replication.
- The process of replication involves following steps:
  - Recognition of origin of replication (ORI) and separation of the two complementary DNA strands.
  - Formation of replication fork.
  - RNA primer formation and initiation of replication.
  - Chain elongation.
  - Proof reading of the newly synthesized DNA.

Recognition of Origin of Replication (ORI) and Separation of two Complementary DNA Strands

- Prokaryotes have one site of origin (Ori) on each chromosome (Fig. 22.4A).
- Eukaryotes have multiple ori considering the large genome size (Fig. 22.4B).
- Initiation of DNA replication requires the recognition of the origin of replication by a group of proteins that form the prepriming complex. These proteins include DNA A protein, Single strand binding (SSB) proteins, DNA helicases (DNA B).
- In the eukaryotes the origin of replication is termed as the ARS (Autonomously Replicating Sequences) which contain 11bp sequence ORE (Origin Replication Element) the ORE binds a set of proteins like DNA A, Helicase, SSB etc. to form a ORC (Origin Replication Complex).
- *DNA A protein* has 20-50 monomers that bind to specific nucleotide at origin of replication, particularly region rich in A and T base pairs. It causes the separation of the ds DNA forming localized ss DNA. This process requires ATP.
- *SSB proteins* (Helix-destabilizing proteins) then bind cooperatively to ssDNA i.e. binding of one molecule makes it easier for additional molecules of SSB tightly to the single DNA strand thus DNA A and SSB protein stabilize the ssDNA and also protects it from nucleases.

Formation of Replication Fork

- The process of replication is bidirectional, i.e. the ss DNA thus separated and stabilized by the SSB proteins now is further separated in both the directions like the unzipping of a zip by a DNA helicase enzyme (Fig. 22.5).
- *DNA Helicases* cause the unwinding of the DNA double helix. They require ATP for the process. These enzymes bind to ssDNA and cause the separation of the double-stranded helix forming a replication fork.

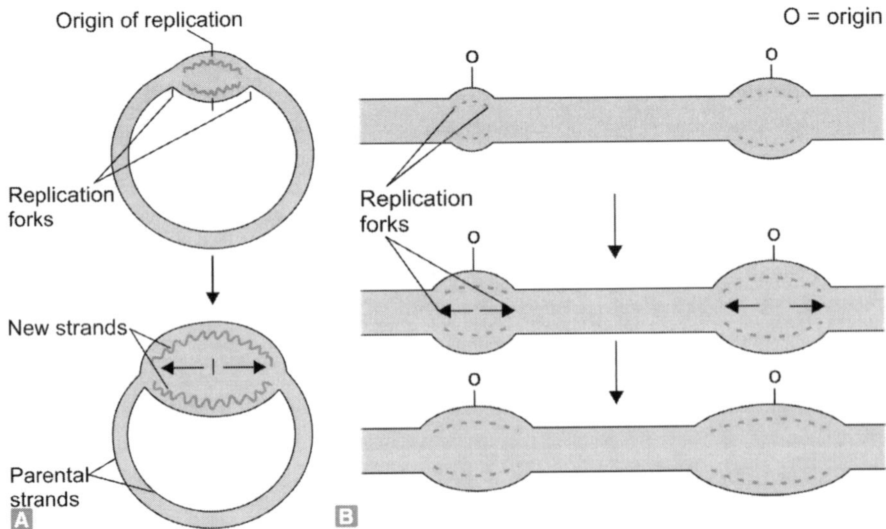

Fig. 22.4 ORI in (A) Prokaryotes (B) Eukaryotes

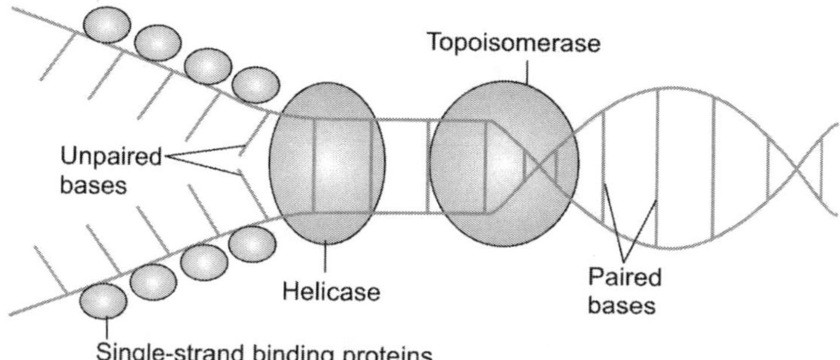

Fig. 22.5 Replication fork

- Synthesis of new DNA strand begins at the origin and occurs at two replication forks that move away from the origin bi-directionally.
- As the 2 strands of the double helix are separated it causes accumulation of the positive supercoils which are removed by DNA topoisomerases. They are of 2 types:
  - *Type I Topoisomerases:* Cut a single–strand of DNA (nuclease activity) and causes the removal of both positive (those that contain more turns of the helix than relaxed DNA) and negative (those that contain fewer turns of the helix than relaxed DNA) super coiling in eukaryotes. They have ligase activity by which they ligate the DNA strand back after removal of the supercoiling and does not require ATP but use the energy of the phosphodiester bond. In prokaryotes type I topoisomerases cause the removal of negative super coiling.
  - *Type II Topoisomerases:* They cause transient breaks in both the strands of the DNA. Both negative and positive super coils are removed but it requires ATP for the process of ligating the DNA strands again.

RNA Primer Synthesis and Initiation of Replication

- DNA polymerase (DNA synthesizing enzyme) cannot initiate the synthesis of new DNA strand all by itself; it needs a RNA primer for initiating the synthesis catalyzed by a primase.
- *There are three prokaryotic DNA polymerases (Pol I, II and III) and five eukaryotic DNA polymerases* (pol α, β, γ, δ and ε) (Table 22.1).
- Recent studies have shown the eukaryotes to have 4 more DNA polymerases that are primarily 'bypass polymerases' i.e. they bypass the DNA fragments that have errors and thus avoid replication of such sequences.
- The DNA polymerases read the parental nucleotide sequences in 3' 5' direction and synthesize new DNA strand in the 5' 3' direction (Fig. 22.6).

Table 22.1 Prokaryotic DNA polymerases

Polymerases	*Functions*	*Exonuclease Activity*
Pol I	Filling of gap after removal of RNA primer DNA repair removal of RNA primer in conjunction with RNAse H	5' to 3' and 3' to 5'
Pol II	DNA repair	3' to 5'
Pol III	Replication—synthesis of DNA	3' to 5'

Table 22.2 Eukaryotic DNA polymerases

Polymerase	*Functions*	*Exonuclease Activity*
Pol α	Replication (in a complex with primase and aids in starting the primer) DNA repair	None
Pol β	DNA repair exclusively	None
Pol γ	DNA replication in mitochondria	3' to 5'
Pol δ	Replication (processive DNA synthesis on leading and lagging strands) DNA repair	3' to 5'
Pol ε	Replication (in some tissues takes the place of Pol d) DNA repair	3' to 5'

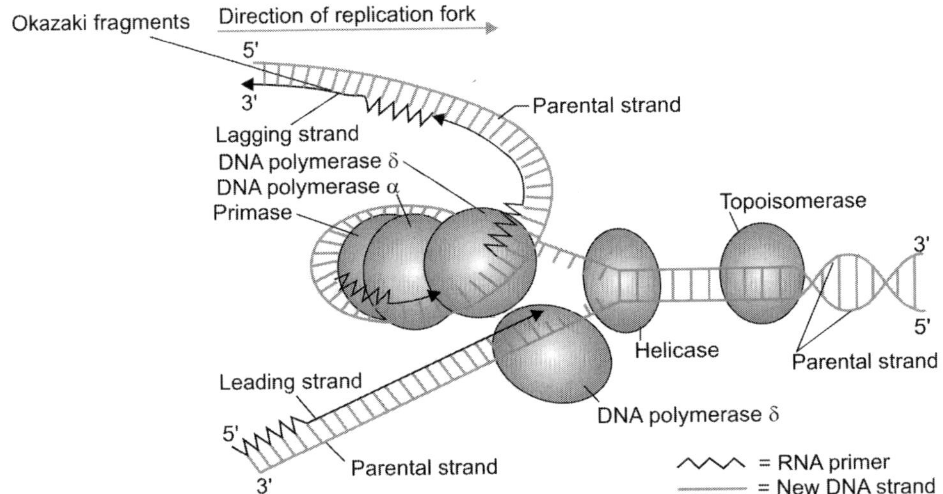

Fig. 22.6 Replication fork formation and movement of DNA polymerase on leading and lagging strands of DNA.

- One strand of the DNA is copied in the direction of progressing replication fork continuously. This is the leading strand.
- The other strand is copied in direction opposite to the advancing replication fork and it is replicated discontinuously lagging strand. On the lagging strand DNA is copied as short stretches termed as Okazaki fragments. Okazaki fragments are joined by DNA ligase.
- The complete unit of helicase and primase is known as the Primosome.

Chain Elongation

- DNA polymerases can only copy a DNA template in the 3' to 5' direction and produce the newly synthesized strand in the 3' to 5' direction.
- The new incoming nucleotides are complimentary to the sequence of nucleotides on the template parent strand.
- The new nucleotide enters as a high energy phosphate—ATP/GTP/CTP/TTP according to base pairing rule and links up with the phosphodiester backbone with hydrolysis of 2 high energy bonds and incorporation of the nucleotide occurs as a mononucleotide one after the other as per base pairing rule.

Proof Reading

- It is highly important for the survival of the organism that the newly synthesized DNA is replicated correctly with minimum errors. However if there is some mistake in the incorporation of the nucleotides, then the DNA polymerases III carries out a 3' $\rightarrow$ 5' exonuclease activity, this is termed as proof reading (eukaryotic analog pol is pol ε,β).

Excision of RNA Primer

- DNA polymerase III continues to add up new nucleotides until it comes close to a RNA primer. Then a DNA polymerase I excises the RNA primer and gap left is filled by the same DNA polymerase I and a DNA ligase join the pieces of DNA synthesized by DNA polymerase I and III.
- Eukaryotic DNA then combines with new histone proteins to form nucleosomes and is reorganized into chromatin. Even during the process of replication, the nucleosomes are not totally dislodged from the parent strand rather they are slightly loosely bound to one of the parent strand and after replication they are properly bound again to reorganize into chromatids.

Telomerase

- Telomeres are the ends of linear DNA that the DNA polymerase cannot replicate and thus are shortened after each replication cycle, contributing to the process of ageing.
- However, germ cells, embryonic cells and cancer cells have an enzyme telomerase which has a RNA primer and a reverse transcriptase activity that maintains the telomeric ends preventing ageing and giving the immortality to the cancer cells.

DNA Repairs

- DNA is constantly is exposed to a number of environmental and physiological stresses which can cause an alteration in the structure of the DNA by altering the base sequences.
- Since DNA is the carrier of the genetic information of an organism, its sequence of bases should be replicated with great fidelity as has been discussed in process of replication. However if any alterations in this base sequences occur after the replication process they must be removed and corrected in order to avoid permanent changes in these base sequences that may otherwise lead to mutations which may or may not be viable for the organism.
- Thus a number of DNA repair and proof reading mechanisms have evolved in the cells which help remove the errors of DNA replication or alteration in base sequences incurred later on due to various reasons (Table 22.3).

Types of DNA Repairs

Mismatch Repair

- It repairs the copying errors made during DNA replication like an adenine may pair up with cytosine or the DNA polymerase may slip and incorporate extra bases.

Mechanism of Repair

- Specific proteins scan the new DNA for an error.
- Methylation of adenine of a GATC sequence (on either sides of the error) occurs on template strand and is taken as reference point.

Table 22.3 Types of DNA damages

I.	Single-base alteration
	A. Depurination
	B. Deamination of cytosine to uracil
	C. Deamination of adenine to hypoxanthine
	D. Alkylation of base
	E. Insertion or deletion of nucleotide
	F. Base-analog incorporation
II.	Two-base alteration
	A. UV light-induced thymine-thymine-thymine (pyrimidine) dimer
	B. Bifunctional alkylating agent cross-linkage
III.	Chain breaks
	A. Ionizing radiation
	B. Radioactive disintegration of backbone element
	C. Oxidative free radical formation
IV.	Cross-linkage
	A. Between bases in same or opposite strands
	B. Between DNA and protein molecules (e.g. histones)

- Now a GATC endonuclease cuts the strand with the error taking methylated adenine of GATC as reference point.
- The defect is then removed by an exonuclease.
- The defect is repaired by a DNA polymerase.
- A DNA ligase then seals the nick.
- Thus, mismatch repair corrects problem caused due to copying errors (single base / 2 to 5 base unpaired loop are corrected).

Base Excision Repair

- Spontaneous depurination of DNA occurs due to the thermal lability of the purine N- glycosidic bond, at a rate of 5000 to 10000 bases/cell/day at 37°C.
  - Cytosine → uracil
  - Adenine → hypoxanthine
  - Guanine → xanthine
- The depurinated site can be recognized by specific cellular enzymes and it is replaced by an appropriate purine directly without breakage of the phosphodiester backbone of the DNA strand.
- These enzymes are N – glycosylases which recognise the defect and remove the basic sugar with the help of an apurinic or apyrimidinic endonucleases. A proper base is then ligated by the DNA polymerase and ligase.

Nucleotide Excision Repair

- This mechanism removes and replaces damaged DNA regions up to 30 bases in length, e.g. damage caused by UV light which induces formation of cyclo butane Pyrimidine-pyrimidine dimers or damage caused by smoking (benzo[a] pyrene – guanine adducts), ionizing radiations, cross linkages between bases on opposing strands or cross linkages between DNA and proteins.

Mechanism of Repair

- An exinuclease (16 subunits in eukaryotes) cuts between 3rd to 5th phosphodiester bond from the 3′ end of the lesion and between 21st and 25th bond from 5′ end.
- The strand is removed and new strand synthesized by DNA polymerase and ligated by DNA ligase.
- Thus removing about 27 to 29 nucleotides at a time.
- Xeroderma pigmentosa (AR) occurs in subjects having low activity of nucleotide – excision repair the subjects show marked sensitivity to sunlight which leads to multiple skin cancers.

Double–strand Break Repair

- This repair mechanism is important for repairing DNA damaged as a result of ionizing radiations, oxidative free radical generation, chemotherapeutic agents, etc. that cause double-strand DNA breakages.
- The repair mechanism involves heterodimeric protein – *Ku* protein that binds to the free ends of the DNA and recruits another DNA-dependent protein kinase *(DNA-PK)* just inside the free ends of the DNA.
- The Ku protein has an ATP, dependent helicase activity so it unwinds the DNA free ends whereas the DNA-PK in association with the *Ku* protein causes activation of the kinase activity and phosphorylates the *Ku* and other DNA-PK molecules activating the *Ku* helicase activity and bringing the free ends in close approximation.
- This causes base pairing between unpaired bases and extra nucleotide tails are removed by the exonuclease, gap filled by DNA ligases.
- This mechanism also has physiological significance as during gene rearrangement during immunoglobulin synthesis.

A Quick Look at the DNA Replication and Repair

- The genes are specific sequences of DNA that code for proteins and non-coding RNA.
- DNA is replicated with high degree of specificity and fidelity to conserve the genetic information of the parent in the progeny and to avoid mutations that may be fatal.
- DNA replication occurs at specific time during the cell cycle (S-phase).
- Cell cycle (G_1, S, G_2 and M phases) is regulated by specific proteins—Cyclins.
- DNA replication occurs in a semiconservative way.
- DNA replication involves the stages of:
  - Recognition of ori
  - Formation of replication fork
  - Formation of RNA primer
  - Chain elongation
  - Gap filling
  - DNA proof reading
  - Reorganization of chromatid.
- Errors of DNA copying or any other DNA damage is recognized by specific cellular proteins and corrected using different mechanisms like—
  - Mismatch repair
  - Base excision repair
  - Nucleotide excision repair
  - Double-strand break repair.

CHAPTER

23

Transcription—RNA Synthesis

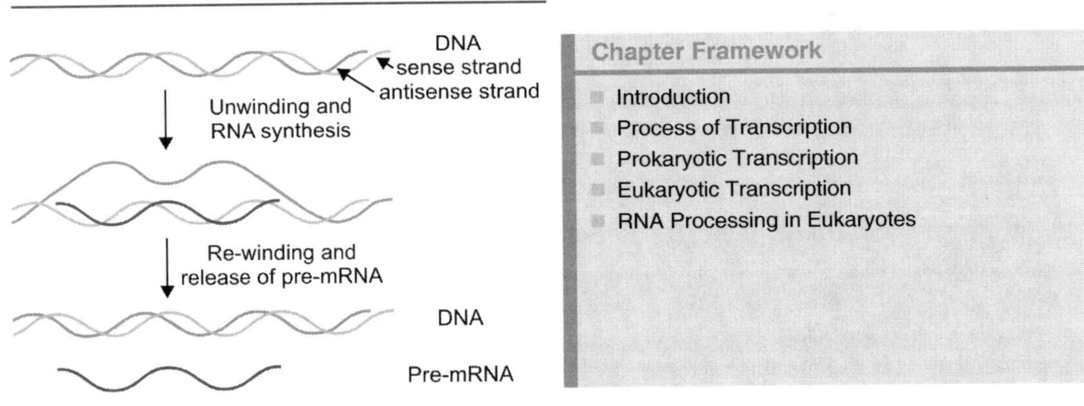

Introduction

- The genetic information of an organism is present as a sequence of nucleotides in the DNA; however, this genetic information achieves its expression through the RNA.
- The sequence of nucleotides on the DNA is copied into the complimentary copy of nucleotides on RNA by the process of transcription.
- During transcription one of the strand of DNA acts as a template strand complimentary to which the nucleotides are polymerized to form RNA molecule with an exception of inclusion of a U base complimentary to T instead of A.
- Also the sugar involved in the phosphodiester linkage is ribose in place of deoxy ribose.
- Not all the genetic sequences present in the genome are transcribed to RNA; certain regions of the genome are actively transcribed these are the *euchromatin regions* and others that are inactive during transcription are *heterochromatin.*
- Some regions of the chromatin are activated for transcription when required at other times they are condensed inactive heterochromatin, these are termed as *facultative heterochromatin*, e.g. One out of two X chromosomes of females is a facultative heterochromatin and becomes active only during gametogenesis.
- Certain regions are transcriptionally inactive at all times—*Constitutive heterochromatin* — e.g. Regions of chromosome near telomeres and centromeres.

Process of Transcription

An Overview (Fig. 23.1)

- The process of transcription of DNA to RNA requires the DNA to open up and provide single-strand to act as a template on which the RNA is transcribed. Thus, the DNA opens up at the site of initiation of transcription (Promoter region) with the binding of a DNA-dependent RNA polymerase.
- The strand of the DNA to which the RNA is complimentary is the template strand and the strand of DNA that is exact copy of the RNA (with exception of U for A) is termed as the coding strand.
- Not all genes are present on the same DNA strand and thus the same DNA strand can act as template strand for some genes and coding strand of other genes.
- The new nucleotides are added one after the other as per the base pairing rule during the elongation of the RNA.
- The process of elongation continues till a termination signal comes across the RNA polymerase and releases the RNA molecule.
- The process of transcription is slightly different in prokaryotes and eukaryotes.

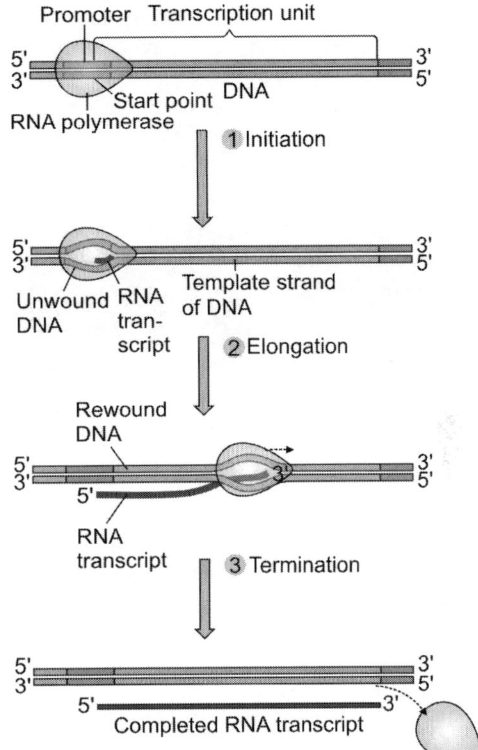

Fig. 23.1 Process of transcription

- The process of transcription begins from specific genetic sequences—Promoter region, then elongates and terminates at the terminating sequences. The complete genetic sequences from the promoter to the termination region are termed as single transcription unit.
- The DNA is transcribed into RNA by a DNA-dependent RNA polymerase. This enzyme reads the DNA molecule from 3′→5′ end and the new RNA molecule is synthesized from 5′→ 3′ end.
- The position from where transcription begins is +1. Any bp sequence before this point is upstream (-1) and after it is downstream (+2, +3, and so on).
- Multiple RNA polymerases can transcribe a single template DNA strand simultaneously but at different positions at least 20 bp apart.
- The same DNA strand can act as a coding or template strand for one gene and may be the noncoding strand for other genes, i.e. the same strand may be coding for one gene and noncoding for the other one.

Prokaryotic Transcription

Bacterial RNA Polymerase

- RNA polymerase in *E. coli* contains five subunits that combine to form a holo enzyme designated $\alpha 2\beta\beta'\sigma$. The $\alpha 2\beta\beta'$ make up the core enzyme and the σ subunit gets dissociated from the core enzyme after its purpose is served, i.e. to help find the promoter region and initiate the RNA synthesis.

- The σ subunit binds rather strongly to the promoter region. A number of σ subunits are present each designed to recognize a different promoter site.

Initiation of Transcription

- The holo-enzyme slides across the DNA template strand and recognizes the promoter region.
- The DNA dependent RNA polymerase causes the melting (unwinding) of the DNA-double helix of about 20 bp length.
- *Bacterial Promoters:* These are approximately 40 nucleotides in length and contain two consensus sequences *TATA Box at—8 to—10 positions* (Pribnow box) and at position*—35 is a GACA box*. These promoter consensus sequences help in the regulation of the transcription process.
- The first nucleotide incorporated is almost always a purine.
- Once the transcription is initiated, the process continues till about 11 nucleotides have been added, then the σ subunit is separated from the core enzyme.

Chain Elongation

- Successive residues are added to the 3′-OH terminus of the nascent RNA molecule according to the base pairing rule.

Chain Termination and Release

- Chain termination of the prokaryotes is regulated by two mechanisms:
  - *Rho* (ρ) *dependent:* A set of consensus sequences that are rich in C nucleotides about 40 nucleotides long are identified by a protein—rho (ρ) factor. Rho (ρ) is an ATP-dependent RNA-stimulated helicase that disrupts the nascent RNA-DNA complex.
    - The termination signals are followed by AT series.
    - When the RNA polymerase reaches the termination sequences, the ρ–factor recognises and reads through the AT region and the RNA terminal end folds upon itself in a hairpin loop such that the RNAP cannot move downstream anymore, thus terminating the transcription process.
    - The completed RNA chain and RNAP are released from the template.
  - *Rho* (ρ) *independent:* Some genes have the rho (ρ) independent transcription termination characterized by presence of:
    - *Palindrome sequences:* A palindrome is a region of double-stranded DNA in which each of the two strands contain stretches that have the same nucleotide sequence when read in the opposite direction e.g. GAATTC. These sequences in the template DNA strand would cause the transcription of a RNA strand that fold upon itself to from a hairpin loop at termination of transcription.
    - *Polyadenylate residues:* Beyond the hairpin turn, the RNA transcript contains a string of U's. The bonding of U's to the corresponding DNA template A's is weak and causes the dissociation of the RNA transcript.

Eukaryotic Transcription

Eukaryotic RNA Polymerase

- The eukaryotic cells have three RNA polymerases—Pol I, Pol II and Pol III respectively transcribing rRNA (28 S, 18 S and 5.8 S), mRNA and tRNA/5 S rRNA.
- These RNAP are sensitive to one peptide toxin—Amanitin produced by a mushroom *Amanita phalloides.*

RNAP	*Sensitivity to Amanitin*
Pol I	Insensitive
Pol II	High sensitivity
Pol III	Intermediate sensitivity

Initiation of Transcription

- Initiation of transcription occurs as in the bacterial cells, in coordinated regulation for frequency and fidelity by eukaryotic promoters.
- The eukaryotic promoters are more complex than the prokaryotic ones.
- There are:
  - *TATA box/Hogness box:* TATAAA consensus sequences at 25 to 30 bp upstream the mammalian gene to be transcribed. TATA box binds to TATA box binding proteins (TBP) and TBP associated factors (TAFs) during the formation of the transcription initiation complex. This determines the fidelity of transcription process.
  - *Initiator sequences (Inr) and Downstream Promoter elements (DPE):* These are present downstream the TATA box sequences. These are also responsible for the fidelity of transcription. Certain genes may lack a TATA box such genes fidelity is regulated by these sequences—Inr and DPE.

    In a survey of over 200 eukaryotic genes, roughly 30% contained a TATA box and Inr, 25% contained Inr and DPE, and 15% contained all three elements, while ~ 30% contained just the Inr.
  - *CAAT/GC box:* The CAAT box sequences are present further upstream the TATA box sequences and are responsible for the regulation of the frequency of transcription. Several other elements are also involved in some genes for determining the frequency of transcription like – Sp1, NF1, AP1, etc.
  - *Enhancers and silencers:* These are responsible for regulated gene expression. Enhancers enhance the expression of a gene and are independent of orientation, i.e. can act in either $5' \rightarrow 3'$ orientation or $3' \rightarrow 5'$ orientation. Silencers act in vice versa fashion to enhancers, i.e. they repress the expression of a gene and are also independent of orientation. Both these sequences can be either upstream or downstream the transcription start site.
  - *Hormone response elements:* These are present for the regulation of genes specifically expressed in response to hormones and they act in conjunction with the enhancers and repressors.

- The RNAP and its transcription factors bind to the promoter sequences in a stepwise manner to form the transcription basal complex.
- The basal complex of Pol II has TF II—A, B, D, E and F that extends from – 30 to + 30 bp corresponding to the transcription initiation site.

Chain Elongation

- The process of chain elongation occurs as in the prokaryotes with the sequential addition of the polynucleotides according to the base pairing rule with an exception of uracil pairing up with adenine instead of thymine.

Chain Termination

- The process of transcription termination is not very clearly understood in the eukaryotes. However it does not have a rho (ρ) factor as in the prokaryotes ,i.e. it is rho (ρ) independent termination.

RNA Processing in Eukaryotes

- The eukaryotic RNA when it is synthesized is the heteronuclear RNA which needs further processing to be converted to mature and functional RNA molecules.
- RNA processing of the eukaryotic RNAs involves:
  - mRNA processing by—Splicing of exons and alternative promoter ligation.
  - mRNA processing by—Poly A tailing and 5′ capping.
  - rRNA processing by—Trimming the large preribosomal RNA by ribonucleases to mature rRNA.
  - tRNA processing by—Trimming the large pre-tRNA by ribonucleases to mature tRNA and adding – CCA end and modification of bases to form specific unusual bases.

mRNA Processing

- The heteronuclear RNA synthesized during transcription process is further post-transcriptionally modified to form the mature mRNA by removing the noncoding nucleotide sequences (introns) using spliceosomes.
- Spliceosomes are organelles that have small nuclear RNAs (snRNPs) with some proteins. These bind to either sides of an intron and clip it off to be removed and the exons are spliced together as shown in Figure 23.2 autoimmune disorders with auto antibodies against the snRNPs and other host proteins is seen in an inflammatory disorder—*Systemic Lupus Erythematous*.
- Another mechanism for the mRNA processing is alternative splicing, i.e. one particular gene has a number of alternative sites of splicing the introns thus there is generation of alternative or variants of an mRNA leading to the production of different variants of proteins, e.g. Hb variants.
- Faulty splicing can cause diseases like β-thalassemia where the β-globin gene of hemoglobin is severely under expressed due to some alteration in the nucleotides at the intronexon junction causing faulty splicing.
- Variants of RNA can also be generated by using alternative promoters as are seen in the tissue specific expression of certain genes.

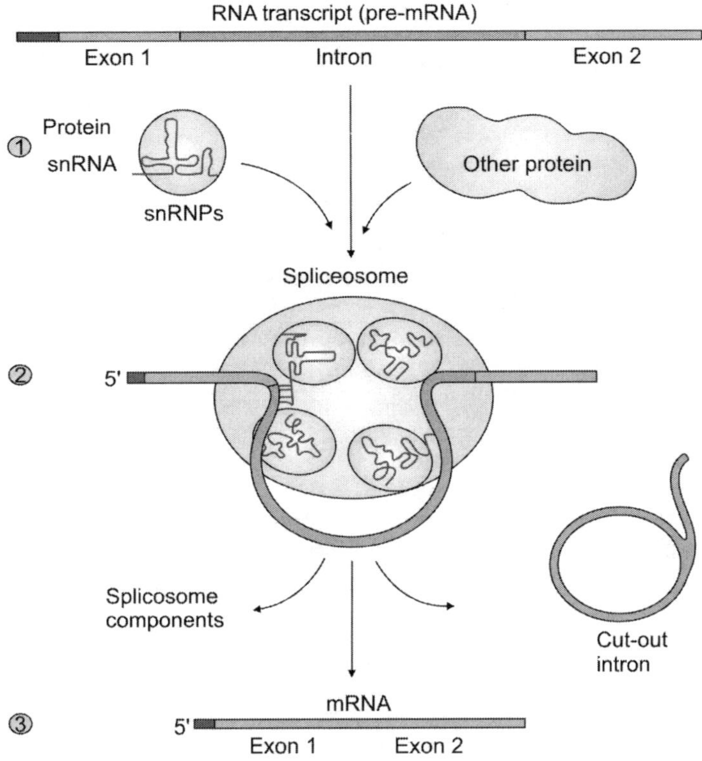

Fig. 23.2 mRNA processing by spliceosomes

- mRNA is modified at its 5′ end and its 3′ end. There is an addition of a poly adenylate tail *(Poly A tail)* at the 5′ end that protects against the 5′→3′ exonuclease activity. It may be about 200 nucleotides long. However not all cytoplasmic mRNAs have a poly tail. Histones mRNAs are an exception.
- Similarly the 3′ end has a 7-methyl guanosine cap added posttranscriptionally that also serves as a protective shield against the 3′ exonuclease activity.
- *RNA editing* is another method for mRNA processing. A very significant example for it is the tissue specific expression of apo-B as apo-B_{100} at liver and apo-B_{48} at the intestines. This RNA editing occurs posttranscriptionally at intestinal cells when the codon of glutamine (CAA) is deaminated by *cytidine deaminase* such that it is converted to a stop codon UAA. Thus the intestinal apoprotein translation gets terminated to give a shorter apo-B_{48}. But there is no RNA editing at the hepatocytes and a complete apo-B_{100} is produced.

tRNA Processing

- The processing of the tRNA primary transcript includes the:
  - Removal of introns as in mRNA processing.
  - Addition of a – CCA end at the acceptor arm by a nucleotidyl transferase at the 3′ end.
  - Modification of bases at specific positions to produce modified bases.

rRNA Processing

- The 28S, 18S, and 5.8S rRNAs of eukaryotes are synthesized form a single large precursor molecule. Eukaryotic rRNA is synthesized by RNA polymerase I and is modified separately. The preribosomal RNAs are cleaved by ribonucleases yield intermediate-sized pieces of r RNA, which are further trimmed.
- The 5 S r RNA is synthesized from a separate precursor molecule and processed separately.

A Quick Look at the Transcription—RNA synthesis

- The genetic information of an organism is present in the DNA which is transcribed to RNA using the DNA as template and a DNA-dependent RNA polymerase.
- The process involves initiation, elongation and termination.
- DNA acts as a template on which RNA is synthesized in 5′ to 3′ direction.
- The prokaryotic transcription promoters are at –8 to – 10 (TATA box) and –35 (CAAT box).
- The termination of prokaryotic transcription occurs by rho (ρ) dependent and rho independent mechanism.
- Eukaryotes have three different types of RNA polymerases Pol I, II and III.
- Eukaryotic transcription is regulated by TATAA box at – 25 to – 35 bp, Inr sequences, DPE, CAAT box, enhancers, silencers, HREs.
- Eukaryotic RNA when synthesized is heteronuclear RNA and needs processing to form mature RNA.
- RNA processing occurs by—splicing of exons, alternative promoter splicing, RNA editing, poly tailing, 5′ capping, 3′ capping (mRNA processing) addition of CCA terminal end (tRNA) and rRNA processing.

CHAPTER

24

Genetic Code, Mutations and Translation of mRNA

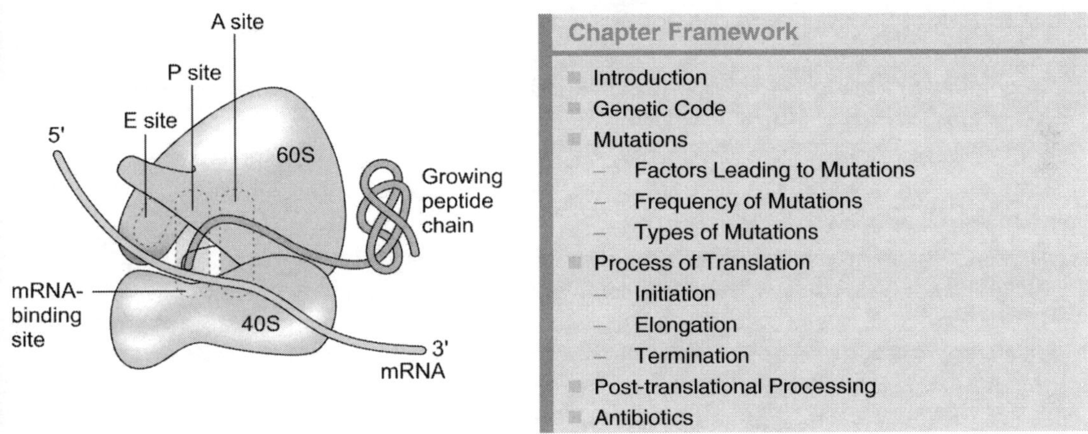

Chapter Framework

Introduction

The genetic information of an organism is organized in the form of genes. A gene is a piece of DNA that determines the amino acid sequence of a protein, and the synthesis of a protein based on genetic information is called translation. The genetic information on the DNA is transcribed into the RNA (transcription) and the RNA then acts as a template on which the protein is synthesized—*Central dogma* (Fig. 24.1).

Genetic Code

The genes that carry the genetic information are organized as a set of 3 nucleotides termed as '*triplet codon*'. The triplet codon format for the genetic code was given by *Kornberg*. Each codon codes for a particular amino acid.

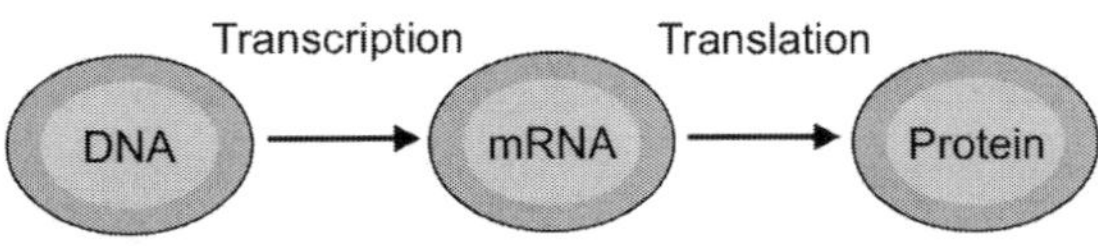

Fig. 24.1 Central dogma

Salient features of the triplet codon (Fig. 24.2)

- There are 64 codons in the genetic code. Out of 64 three are noncoding and do not code for any amino acid. These are also termed as *stop codons/nonsense codons*. They are amber (UAA), ochre (UAG) and opal (UGA).
- The genetic code is *unambiguous,* i.e. a given triplet codon shall code for only one specific amino acid and not for any other amino acid.
- The genetic code although is unambiguous however it also shows *degeneracy,* i.e. one amino acid can be coded for by multiple codons that are specific for it. There are many amino acids coded by multiple codons like—Ser, Val, Arg, Thr, etc. Serine has 6 codons coding for it. These six codons of Ser shall code only for Ser and not any other amino acid, i.e. *genetic codes are unambiguous as well as degenerate at the same time.*
- Degeneracy of the genetic code is explained by the phenomenon of *Wobble* at the third nucleotide i.e. the third nucleotide of the triplet codon is not stringently conserved for a codon, it can wobble. Amino acids like—Ser, Thr, Val, Arg etc. which have multiple codons show the phenomenon of wobble at the third nucleotide for e.g. "2 codons of Arg, AGA and AGG bind to the same anticodon UCU".
- The genetic code is *nonpunctuated and continuous,* i.e. the codons are read by the translation machinery continuously without any punctuation till a stop codon comes across.
- The genetic code is *universal,* i.e. same genetic code is valid for all living organisms prokaryotes or eukaryotes with exception of mitochondrial codons have AUA instead of AUG as the initiation codon coding for methionine. Another exception is in mitochondria UGA codes for tryptophan instead of acting as termination codon and the termination codons in mitochondria are AGA and AGG (which in normal eukaryotic translation codes for arginine).

First letter	Second letter: U	Second letter: C	Second letter: A	Second letter: G	Third letter
U	UUU Phe UUC Phe UUA Leu UUG Leu	UCU Ser UCC Ser UCA Ser UCG Ser	UAU Tyr UAC Tyr UAA Stop UAG Stop	UGU Cys UGC Cys UGA Stop UGG Trp	U C A G
C	CUU Leu CUC Leu CUA Leu CUG Leu	CCU Pro CCC Pro CCA Pro CCG Pro	CAU His CAC His CAA Gln CAG Gln	CGU Arg CGC Arg CGA Arg CGG Arg	U C A G
A	AUU Ile AUC Ile AUA Ile AUG Met	ACU Thr ACC Thr ACA Thr ACG Thr	AAU Asn AAC Asn AAA Lys AAG Lys	AGU Ser AGC Ser AGA Arg AGG Arg	U C A G
G	GUU Val GUC Val GUA Val GUG Val	GCU Ala GCC Ala GCA Ala GCG Ala	GAU Asp GAC Asp GAA Glu GAG Glu	GGU Gly GGC Gly GGA Gly GGG Gly	U C A G

Fig. 24.2 Genetic code

Mutations

- A mutation is any heritable change in DNA sequence. This may, or may not, affect the phenotype of the organism. Such a change may occur either spontaneously or be induced as a consequence of treatment with a DNA damaging agent (X-rays, ultraviolet light, chemicals, etc.). Mutations may affect the cell growth regulation and lead to an uncontrolled cellular growth, i.e. cancer. However, mutations have had a very positive effect on the process of biologic evolution as different species have evolved as a result of mutations that were viable for better survival.

Factors Leading to Mutations

Changes in the Environment or Mutagens

- Ultraviolet radiation
- Pollutants and chemicals
- Tar from tobacco.

Errors During Replication, Transcription, or Translation

Frequency of Mutations—is it good; is it bad?

- Mutations are not very frequent, they are rare events. Humans inherit 3×10^9 base pairs of DNA from each parent. No process is 100% accurate. So it is with DNA replication. Like a conscientious typist, the cell does proofread the accuracy of its copy. But, even so, errors slip through. It has been estimated that in humans and other mammals, uncorrected errors (= mutations) occur at the rate of about 1 in every 50 million (5×10^7) nucleotides added to the chain. But with 6×10^9 base pairs in a human cell, that means that each new cell contains some 120 new mutations.
- Only 1.2% of our DNA encodes the exons of our proteome, and for a long time it was thought that much of the rest was "junk" DNA. Mutations in it would most likely be harmless and even in coding regions the existence of synonymous codons could result in the altered (mutated) gene still encoding the same amino acid in the protein.
- But it now appears that as much as 80% of our DNA seems to participate in regulating genes which are expressed, in response to the signals (nutrients, hormones, etc.) they receive. Mutations in these regions might well have harmful, if subtle, effects.
- Mutations also help in evolutionary process as it has been observed that certain genetic sequences in the genomes of vertebrates are highly conserved even though they do not encode any protein, suggesting their importance in the organisms survival and certain genes although mutated do not code for a nonviable protein.
- Recent advances have enabled the coding portions of the genome of single cells to be sequenced. Preliminary results indicate that each normal cell in an adult has accumulated ~20 somatic mutations, and that its collection of mutations differs from cell to cell (Cancer cells accumulate many more mutations [often in the hundreds].

Types of Mutations

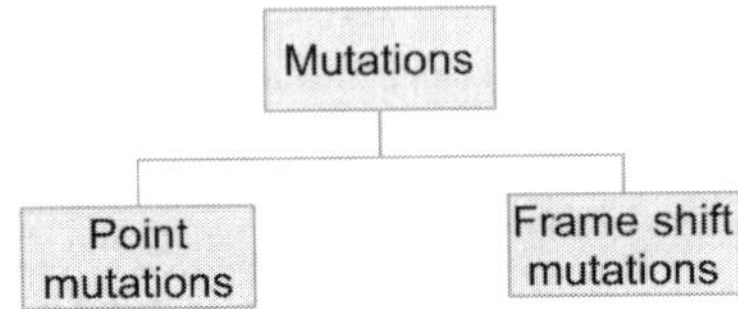

Point Mutations

Point mutations occur due to change in a single nucleotide of the DNA. It may be either transition or transversion type.

Transition: When a purine is replaced by a purine and a pyrimidine by a pyrimidine.

Transversion: When a purine is replaced by a pyrimidine and vice-versa.

Effects of Point Mutations

Due to point mutation there occurs an alteration in the nucleotide sequence of DNA which changes the genetic code on mRNA and the protein translated may or may not be altered depending upon the alternation of amino acid.

- Silent Mutation.
  - This occurs when the point mutation of the DNA alters the genetic code on mRNA in such a way that the codon formed due to mutation is a synonym of the original codon so the amino acid translated is not altered, e.g. Arg has 2 codons AGG and AGA; silent point mutation would be such that one of the codons would change to the 2nd codon (AGG-AGA) (G-A, i.e. a transition of mutation).
- Missense Mutation.
  - Missense point mutation occurs when the point mutation causes an altered genetic code on mRNA that is translated into a protein with variable viability of the mutation. Depending upon the viability of the mutation it is of further 3 types:
    - *Acceptable Missense Mutation:*
      This occurs when the point mutation leads to an altered mRNA being translated into a protein with altered amino acid sequence. However, the new mutated protein formed is physiologically functional just like the original protein, e.g. Hb Hikari has β61 Asn instead of Lys. This Hb functions like normal Hb and there is no alternation in functional capacity of Hb. The individuals with Hb Hikari, no disease is observed.
    - *Partially Acceptable Missense Mutation:*
      This occurs when the point mutation leads to an altered mRNA being translated into a protein with altered amino acid sequence such that the mutated protein is abnormal and has reduced or compromised physiological function, e.g. HbS–β6 glutamic acid is replaced by valine. Such HbS is normal in the oxygenated state but on losing its oxygen to the tissues, it develops a sticky patch causing HbS to precipitate out. This causes the HbS to form crystals that deshape RBC to "Sickle" shape leading to hemolysis and sickle cell anemia.

- *Unacceptable Missense Mutation:*
  This occurs when the point mutation leads to an altered genetic code on mRNA being translated into a protein that is not viable and not suitable for survival. This protein does not carry out its assigned function, e.g. HbM is formed when HbA α58 His is replaced by Tyr. This methemoglobin cannot transport O_2.

- Nonsense mutations:
  - In this type of point mutations, the alteration of a single nucleotide suddenly generates nonsense codon, terminating the translational process abnormally and producing a protein molecule abnormally small.

Frame Shift Mutations

- As discussed earlier the translation machinery reads the genetic code on mRNA in a continuous nonpunctuated manner till it reaches a termination codon. If there occur a sudden mutation due to either insertion or deletion of a nucleotide in the genetic sequence, it will alter the reading frame (garbled reading frame) and the protein translated will be different. Such mutations are called frame shift mutations. They are further classified as:
  - Insertional mutagenesis
  - Deletional mutagenesis

  Frame shifts often create new STOP codons and thus generate nonsense mutations. Perhaps that is just as well as the protein would probably be too garbled anyway to be useful to the cell.

Process of Translation

- The process of translation involves the sequential polymerization of amino acids one after the other according to the genetic code on the mRNA. The translation machinery comprising the tRNA and the ribosomes scan and read the genetic codes on the mRNA. The tRNA carrying specific amino acids recognise their specific codons (complimentary to their anticodon loop) which then polymerize to form specific protein.
- The amino acid carrying tRNA is activated to amino acyl tRNA by specific amino acyl tRNA synthetases. There are 20 different amino acids and for each there is a tRNA. Some of the amino acids have more than one tRNA. Thus in all there are 31 tRNAs. Mitochondria have separate translation machinery and have 22 tRNAs.

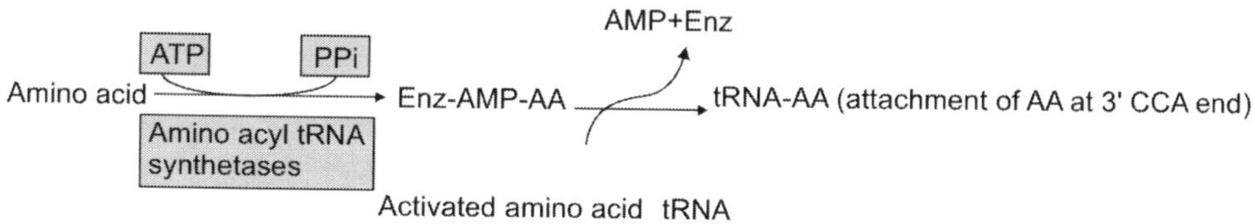

- The D arm of tRNA helps in the proper recognition of a given tRNA by its amino acyl tRNA synthetases.
- The TψC arm helps the tRNA bind to the ribosome.

Initiation

- Initiation of translation requires that an mRNA molecule be selected and bound to a ribosome. Once the mRNA binds to ribosome, the ribosome finds the correct reading frame on the mRNA and translation begins.
- In prokaryotic mRNA there is a consensus sequence—Shine-dalgarno sequence which is complementary to a sequence of nucleotides on the 30s ribosomal RNA and indicate initiation site.
- In eukaryotes initiation involves—
  - *Dissociation of 80s ribosome:* The eukaryotic initiation factors 3 and 1A bind to the 80s ribosome dissociating it into 60s subunit and a 40s subunit bound to eIF3 and eIF1A preventing the re-association of 40s and 60s.
  - *Formation of 43s Pre-initiation complex*: For this first a GTP binds to eIF2 to form a binary complex. Binary complex then binds met-tRNA^{i} to form ternary complex. 40s ribosome + ternary complex gives the pre-initiation complex 43s.
  - *Formation of 43s Initiation complex (pre-initiation complex + mRNA)*: The 7-methyl GTP cap at 5′ end helps in binding the mRNA to the 43s pre-initiation complex to give initiation complex. This complex formation needs a few initiation factors like eIF 4F, 4E and 4G. This complex now scans the mRNA for the initiation codon AUG. Its position in eukaryotes is determined by a consensus sequence termed KOZAK consensus sequences as they surround AUG. These sequences are like Shine-Dalgarno sequences of prokaryotes.
  - *Formation of 80s initiation complex*: The 60s ribosomal subunit binds to the initiation complex with the help of eIF2 and hydrolysis of GTP and all the initiation factors bound are now released since 80s initiation complex is formed. These initiation factors are recycled to be used in another translation process.

Elongation

- The ribosomes elongate the polypeptide chain by sequential addition of amino acids. The ribosomes have 2 sites:
  - A-site → acceptor site where incoming amino acid enters.
  - P-site → peptidyl site where the new polypeptide chain is present.
- Both these sites cover at least 2 neighbouring codons. The tRNA charged with amino acid recognizes a proper codon as the ribosome moves down, via its anticodon loop and a new amino acid enters 'A' site. This is assisted by elongation factor EEF-1 α and GTP hydrolysis. Once the amino acid has entered, elongation factor and GDP and Pi are released.
- Now the new amino acid tRNA in A site carries out a nucleophilic attack on the peptidyl tRNA of 'P' site. The reaction is catalyzed by enzymatic activity peptidyl transferase of 28s ribosomal RNA (of 60s).
- So now the growing chain is on 'A' site. It translocates back to 'P' site and 'A' site is again free to take up new amino acid according to the codon on mRNA.

  Thus energy requirements for formation of 1 peptide bond:

  → Activation of amino acid → 2 ATP
  → Entry of aminoacyl tRNA into A-site → 1 GTP → GDP
  → Translocation A → P-site → 1 GTP → GDP
  4 ~ Pi

Termination

- After multiple cycles of elongation, when a nonsense codon is read by the ribosomal machinery at A-site, then instead of a new amino acid tRNA entering, a molecule of water is added up.
- The eukaryotic releasing factors (eRFs) recognize the termination signal.
- These eRF along with GTP and peptidyl Transferase cause the hydrolysis of bond between new peptide chain and tRNA at P-site and release a new polypeptide chain, tRNA and a free P-site.
- Many ribosomes can translate the same mRNA molecule simultaneously. The ribosomes should be at least 80 nucleotides apart. Such an assembly of multiple ribosomes on single mRNA is termed as polysome/polyribosome.
- In prokaryotes, a single mRNA codes for multiple proteins thus are polycistronic.
- In eukaryotes, a single mRNA codes for single polypeptide thus are monocistronic.
- The rate of incorporation of amino acid in eukaryotes is 6/sec in prokaryotes 18/sec.

Post-translational Processing

- In animal cells many proteins are synthesized from the mRNA template as a precursor molecule, which then must be modified to obtain an active protein, e.g. Insulin, blood clotting factors (II, VII, IX and X), collagen, etc.

Insulin

- It is a low molecular weight protein synthesized as a prohormone having 2 polypeptide chains connected by a connecting peptide or C-peptide.
- It folds in a specific way to allow formation of inter and intra chain disulfide bonds necessary in mature insulin molecule. A specific protease then clips out the C- peptide to form functional insulin.

Collagen

- It is an abundant protein in the extracellular spaces of higher eukaryotes. It is synthesized as procollagen.
- Three procollagen polypeptide molecules align themselves in a specific way guided by their amino terminal sequences and twist around themselves in a left-handed helix. The left-handed triple helix then undergoes post-translational modification.
- Now specific enzymes carry out the hydroxylation of proline and Lys residues.
- Oxidations of hydroxy proline and hydroxy lysine side chains within the procollagen to aldehyde groups provide sites for cross-links between these amino acid residues. The cross-links give strength to the molecule.
- Next the amino terminal sequences are removed to give the mature, strong, insoluble collagen molecule.

Maturation of Clotting Factors II, VII, IX and X

- The blood clotting factors are synthesized as inactive precursors for, preventing in vivo, spontaneous and haphazard coagulation. These factors, particularly factors II, VII, IX and X are converted to their active forms at liver via a vitamin K-dependent γ-carboxylation of glutamic acid residues.

- Besides these there are many other post-translations modifications of proteins like covalent modification by acetylating, phosphorylation and glycosylation.

Antibiotics

- Many antibiotics work because they selectively inhibit protein synthesis in bacteria this is so because of the difference in the ribosomes of prokaryotes and eukaryotes.
- The antibiotics interact with the bacterial ribosomes and inhibit protein synthesis thus arresting growth of the bacteria and death of the bacteria.

Antibiotics Acting in Only Prokaryotes

- Tetracyclin—It prevents binding of amino acyl tRNA to A-site.
- Chloromycetin—It binds to 23s RNA (which plays role in peptide bond format). Clinically not useful but helps in research.

Antibiotics Acting in Both Prokaryotes and Eukaryotes

- Puromycin—It inhibits protein synthesis in both *pro and eukaryotes.* It is structural analog of tyrosinyl tRNA, so gets incorporated in its place inhibiting further translation.

Antibiotics Acting in Eukaryotes Only

- Cycloheximide—It is active in eukaryotes only. It inhibits the peptidyl transferase activity of 60s ribosome.
- Ricin—It is active in eukaryotes only. It inactivates 28s ribosomal RNA.
- Diphtheria toxin—It is active in eukaryotes only since it inactivates eukaryotic elongation factor.

Protein Turnover/Degradation

- Proteins are constantly being synthesized and degraded. Degradation of proteins is a selective process. Cell can distinguish of proteins that are to be degraded because such proteins are tagged with ubiquitin (a 76 a.a. protein).
- The carboxy terminal glycine of ubiquitin makes linkage with ε amino groups of the several Lys residues of the protein to be degraded.
- Regulation of protein degradation is important since inappropriate tagging by ubiquitin of regulatory protein for degradation can lead to tumor formation, e.g. Human papilloma Virus (HPV) encodes a protein that activates the enzyme necessary for ubiquitin tagging of proteins. This causes tagging and degradation of tumor suppressor protein like p53 and other proteins necessary in DNA repair.

A Quick Look at the Genetic Code, Mutations and Translation of mRNA

- Genes are a sequence of nucleotides that code for an amino acid.
- Genetic code is collection of codons coding for different amino acids.
- Translation is the process of translating the genetic information on an mRNA into a sequence of amino acids—Proteins.
- There are 61 codons coding 20 different amino acids and 3 nonsense or stop codons that stop the process of translation.
- The genetic code is unambiguous, degenerate, shows wobble, universal (with exceptions of AUA, AGG, AGA and UGA), nonpunctuated, nonoverlapping.
- Mutations area change in the genetic sequence of nucleotides on the DNA that causes an altered reading frame on the mRNA for the translation machinery giving rise to a protein that may be or may not be viable.
- Mutations may be point mutations or frame shift mutations.
- Point mutations will be—Silent, missense (acceptable, partially acceptable and unacceptable) and nonsense mutations.
- Frame shift mutations will be—Insertional or deletional.
- Translation in eukaryotes requires various protein factors:
  - Initiation—eIF3, eIF1A, eIF4E, F, G.
  - Elongation—eEF1α
  - Termination—eRF
- Four high-energy phosphates are required for the formation of a single peptide bond.
- Posttranslational processing is required for Insulin, clotting factors II, VII, IX, and X, collagen.
- Ubiquitin is used for tagging the proteins for degradation.
- Antibiotics act by the inhibition of various components of the translation machinery like 23S ribosomal RNA (tetracyclin), 28S ribosomal RNA (Ricin), 60S ribosomal RNA (Cycloheximide), etc.

CHAPTER

25

Regulation of Gene Expression

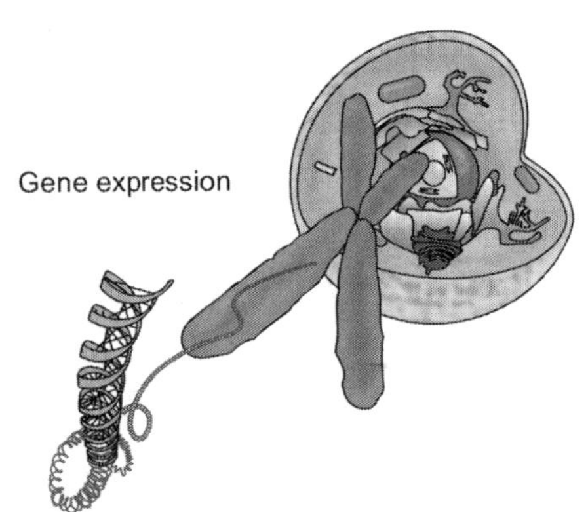

Chapter Framework

- Introduction
- Prokaryotic Gene Expression—Lac Operon Concept
  - The Lac Operon of *E. coli*
  - Bacteriophage Lambda—Switch Between Lysogenic and Lytic Phase
- Eukaryotic Gene Expression Regulation
  - Chromatin Structure and Gene Regulation
  - Transcriptional Control in Eukaryotic Eells
  - Gene Control through Messenger RNA Processing
  - Gene Control through RNA Stability
  - Gene Amplification
  - Gene Rearrengemet
  - Translational and Post-translational Control

Introduction

- The complete organization of an organism is bestowed upon the millions of genes that are present in each cell of that organism. In other words each cell has the complete genetic information for the formation of the whole organism. However, different cells have difference in structure, physiological function, biochemical properties and lifespan.
- All this is due to the differential expression of the genes in different cells such that a cell of pancreas is specialized to specifically produce the proteolytic enzymes and another set of cells in pancreas would act like an endocrine gland secreting hormones insulin, glucagon and somatostatin each from different islet cells. Similarly the cells of thyroid would produce their specific thyroid hormones and so on. This tissue specific expression of the genes is the basis of the organization of multicellular organisms. This occurs due to the genes switching on and off in a particular tissue.
- The fundamental unit of gene expression is a *cistron*. A cistron is a sequence of nucleotides that code for a polypeptide chain. The prokaryotic genes are poly-cistronic genes, i.e. a single mRNA codes for more than one separately translated protein.
- Bacterial genes that have related functions are clustered and are under the control of a single promoter. These genes are often transcribed together into a single mRNA.
- However, the eukaryotic genes are mono-cistronic, i.e. each mRNA encodes for a specific polypeptide chain.

Prokaryotic Gene Expression—*Lac Operon Concept*

- The prokaryotic gene expression and its regulation are best explained by the operon concept proposed by *Jacob and Monod (1961)*. They proposed the Lac Operon model (Fig. 25.1A nd B) of gene expression in the *E. coli* bacteria.
- Bacterial genomes usually contain several thousand different genes.
- Some of the gene products are required by the cell under all growth conditions and are called *housekeeping genes.* Housekeeping genes must be expressed at some level all of the time. These include the genes that encode such proteins as DNA polymerase, RNA polymerase and DNA gyrase.
- Some of the gene products are required under certain circumstances in response to a metabolite or a substrate; these are called the *inducible genes* and the substrate or metabolite is the inducer.
- An operon comprises a group of structural genes that are transcribed together under the influence of a single promoter and additional sequences that regulate transcription.
- A typical example of operon is the lac operon model which comprises the three structural genes – (Fig. 25.1)
  - Lac Z—It encoding the β–galactosidase enzyme that hydrolyses the β1-4 glycosidic linkage of lactose.
  - Lac Y—It encoding permease that helps lactose to permeate the bacterial cell wall.
  - Lac A—It encoding detoxifying enzyme β–galactoside transacetylase.

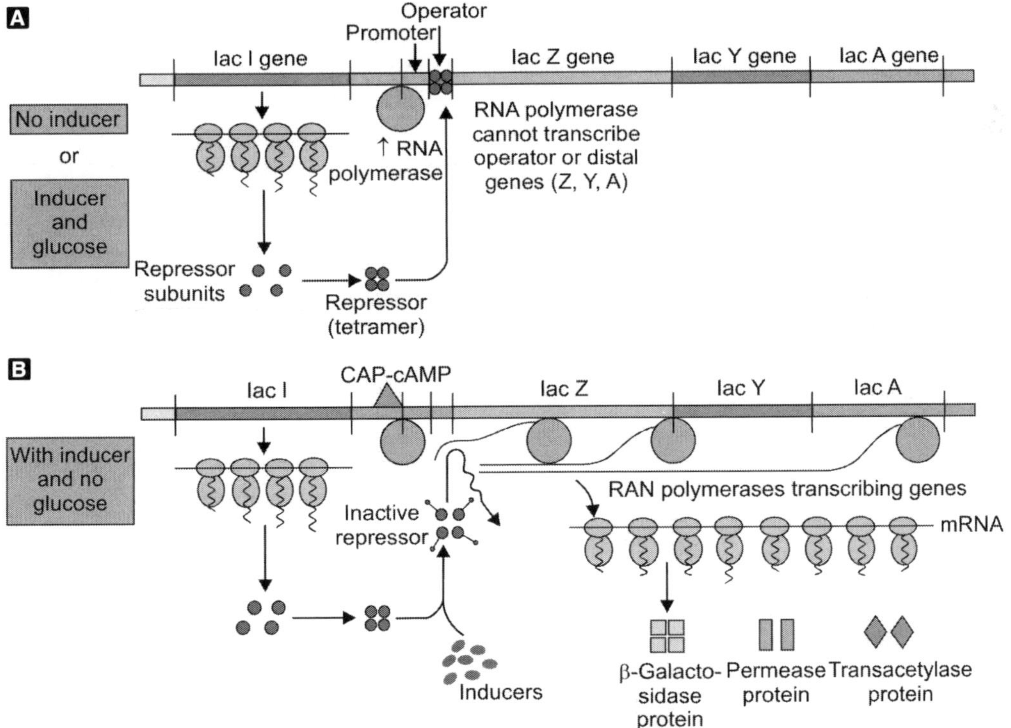

Figs 25.1A and B Lac Operon concept

- The structural enzymes of lac operon are inducible genes that are expressed only in the presence of inducer lactose. Whereas the regulatory gene lac I is constitutively expressing (housekeeping gene) producing the lac repressor.
- When the *E. coli* is in a medium rich in glucose, it specifically utilizes glucose as a source of energy and the lac operon is inhibited. This is because the lac I gene product—Lac repressor is expressed constitutively and binds on to the operator region, inhibiting the downstream movement of the RNA polymerase.
- During this phase of glucose utilization, the *E. coli* also accumulates cAMP and a cAMP binding protein (CAP).
- In glucose deficiency and presence of the inducer lactose, the repressor molecules are bound to the inducer which inhibits the aggregation of former on the operator region. Thus the operator region is now free to bind to the RNA polymerase which then transcribes and translates all the downstream structural genes of the lac operon.
- This expression is also enhanced by the binding of the CAP protein on the operator region.
- The expression of lac operon genes helps in the utilization of lactose as a source of energy.
- In this case, lactose is a positive regulator of lac operon that increases its expression and glucose acts as its negative regulator of lac operon.

Bacteriophage Lambda—Switch between Lysogenic and Lytic Phase

- Certain bacteriophages show the next higher level of gene expression regulation by switching on and off the structural genes, e.g. Lambda bacteriophage.
- The lambda bacteriophage may follow a lysogenic (integrated into host DNA) pathway or a lytic pathway (where there is synthesis of multiple copies of bacteriophages ultimately killing the host cell) (Fig. 25.2A and B).
- The choice whether the lysogenic or the lytic phase shall be followed is dependent upon the binding of the regulatory protein Croprotein and repressor protein on an operator region that has three distinct parts O_R1, O_R2 and O_R3.
- The binding of the repressor protein to the operator region in an order O_R1, O_R2 and O_R3 (cooperatively) blocks the DNA dependent RNA polymerase to transcribe the Cro gene and thus the bacteriophage is lysogenic as the lytic genes downstream cro are not transcribed. Here the repressor is switching off the cro gene since the cro promoter overlaps with the OR1.
- Conversely in presence of stimuli like UV rays/other DNA damaging agent, the repressor protein is degraded and the operator region is now free such that cro protein is translated.
- The cro protein binds to the O_R3 and then sequentially to O_R2, O_R1 thus switching off the translation of the repressor gene permanently and all the genes of the lytic phase are translated causing lysis of the host cell. This is because the repressor promoter is overlapped by the O_R3.

Eukaryotic Gene Expression Regulation

- The eukaryotic gene expression is regulated in a much more complex manner than the prokaryotes since the eukaryotes have a highly organized genome, which is monocistronic in nature. This control requires a number of different types of proteins and regulatory elements.

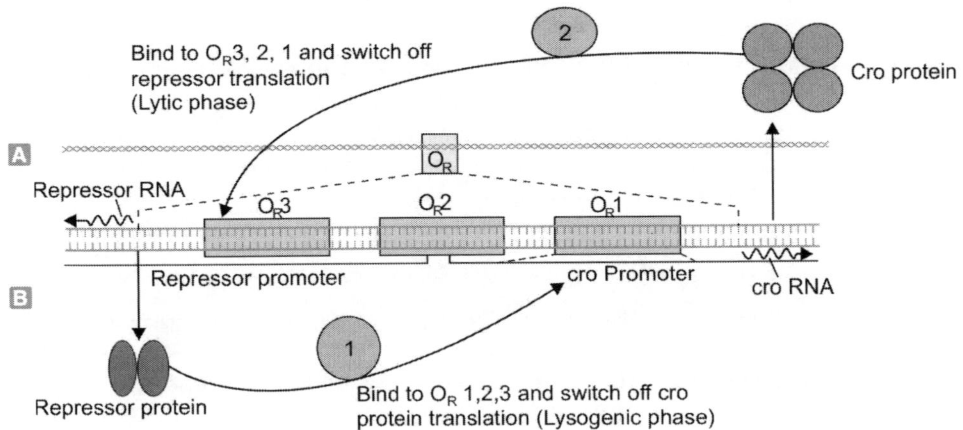

Figs 25.2A and B Lambda bacteriophage switch between lysogenic and lytic phase

- The regulation of gene expression in the eukaryotes can occur in several ways at any step of the information pathway from DNA ⟶ RNA ⟶ Protein.
- The different ways of regulating gene expression in eukaryotic ells are:
  - Chromatin structure and gene expression regulation
  - Transcriptional control in eukaryotic cells by Cis-acting DNA sequences
  - Gene control through messenger RNA processing
  - Gene control through RNA stability
  - Gene amplification
  - Gene rearrangement
  - Translational and post-translational control
  - Protein interactions.

Chromatin Structure Remodelling and Gene Expression Regulation

- The eukaryotic DNA is organized into chromosomes (as shown in chapter 22). The chromatin provides yet another level of regulation of gene expression since not all the chromatin is transcriptionally active. As already mentioned in Chapter 22 the transcriptionally active chromatin is euchromatin and inactive is heterochromatin.
- The regulation at the chromatin level is assisted by the presence of nucleosomes. These nucleosomes do not allow a ready access to the DNA by various transcription factors.
- Furthermore the nucleoproteins—Histones present in the nucleosomes are modified covalently such that an additional level of gene expression is achieved.
- Histones may be *acetylated* at the lysine residues on amino terminal ends. Such acetylated histones have a reduced affinity for a negatively charged DNA, thus the histones are dissociated form the DNA which is then easily accessible to the various transcription factors.
- De-acetylated histones would have reverse affect.
- Another feature is the methylation of deoxycytidine residues. It has been reported that methylation of deoxycytidine residues can cause inactivation of the DNA transcriptionally. However, this is not a rule.

Transcriptional Control by Cis acting DNA Sequences

- The transcriptional regulation of frequency of the gene expression is under the control of Cis-acting DNA sequences—*Enhancers and repressors (or silencers)* that respectively increase or decrease the rate of expression of a gene respectively.
- These DNA sequences can act when present hundreds of base pairs apart from the gene and in either orientation upstream or downstream.

Regulation through mRNA Processing

- The eukaryotic mRNA is transcribed first as a large precursor molecule—Heteronuclear RNA that has multiple coding and noncoding sequences. However, the functional mRNA that reaches the cytoplasm is much shorter and has only the coding sequences. This splicing of the exons occurs during mRNA processing (*see* Chapter 23).
- The RNA processing involves several methods like—Alternative splicing of exons, use of alternative promoters.
- Thus genes are expressed differentially depending on the type of mRNA processing.

Gene Control through RNA Stability

- The mRNA molecules stability is directly proportional to their rate of translation; greater the stability higher the amount of protein being translated and vice – versa.
- The stability of the mRNA molecule is determined by 5′poly A tails and the 3′ 7-methyl GTP cap that protect against the action of 3′and5′exonuclease activity.
- Besides the caps at the two ends, the mRNA molecules have also been reported to have stem loop structures at 3′noncoding sequences especially in the histones mRNAs which lack the poly A cap.

Gene Amplification

- Gene expression in eukaryotes may be enhanced in response to drugs, e.g. the anticancer drug methotrexate causes the amplification of genes of folate reductase leading to drug resistance.
- Another example is the amplification of genes of egg shell proteins in Drosophila during oogenesis only, i.e. gene expression is so regulated that the number and frequency of expression is raised when needed.

Gene Rearrangement

- The expression of certain genes like the genes of the antibody producing cells is regulated at level of post-transcriptional where the variety of genes of the light and heavy chains of immunoglobulins rearrange themselves in multiple combinations giving rise to a large number of different antibodies. It is because of this gene rearrangement that millions of different antigens are recognized by rearrangement of 1000s of different genes of light and heavy chains in the plasma cells.
- A faulty gene rearrangement can cause cancer.

Translational and Post-translational Control of Gene Expression

- The different genes of the eukaryotes are regulated at the level of translational and post-translational control.
- Ribosomes, amino acyl tRNAs, initiation factors, and elongation factors are all required for the translation of mRNA molecules. The availability of these components affects the rate of translation and therefore influences gene expression.
- Many eukaryotic proteins are extensively modified after translation by the selective cleavage and trimming of amino acids from the ends, by acetylation, or by the addition of phosphates, carboxyl groups, methyl groups, and carbohydrates to the protein. These modifications affect the transport, function, and activity of the proteins and have the capacity to affect gene expression.

Protein Interactions

- Much of gene regulation is accomplished by proteins that bind to DNA sequences and influence their expression. These regulatory proteins generally have discrete functional parts—Called domains, typically consisting of 60 to 90 amino acids—That are responsible for binding to DNA.

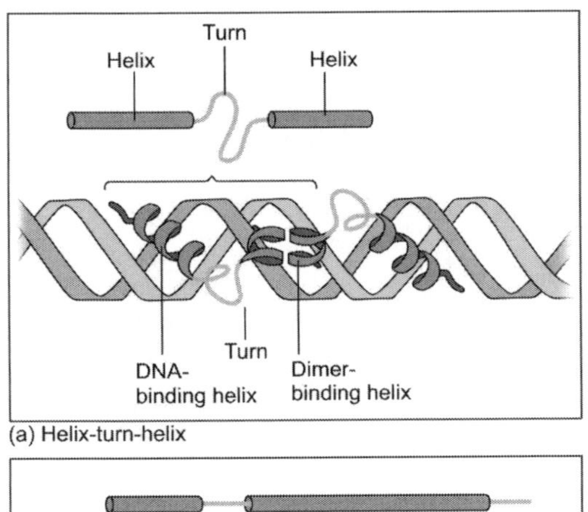

(a) Helix-turn-helix

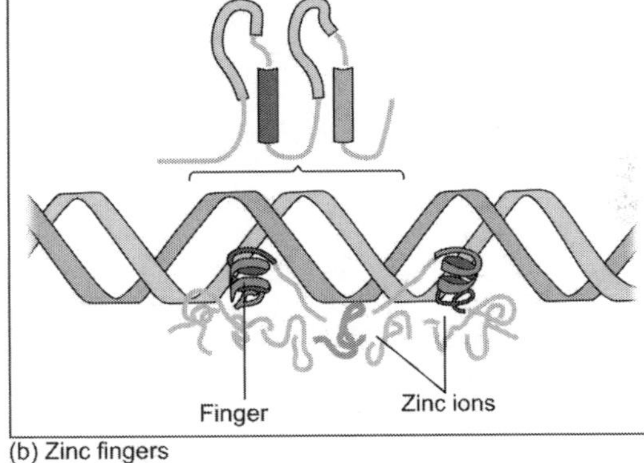

(b) Zinc fingers

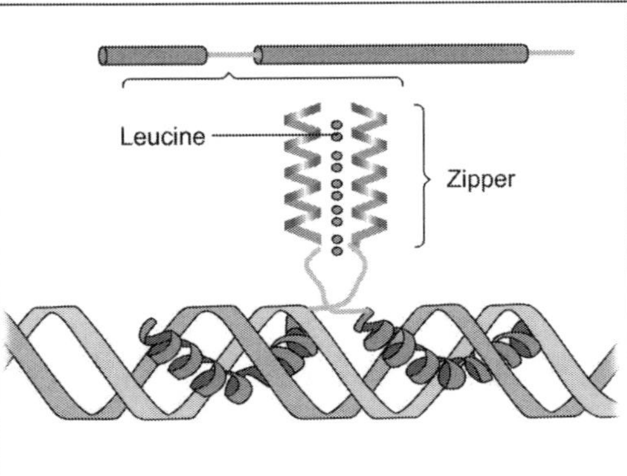

(c) Leucine zipper

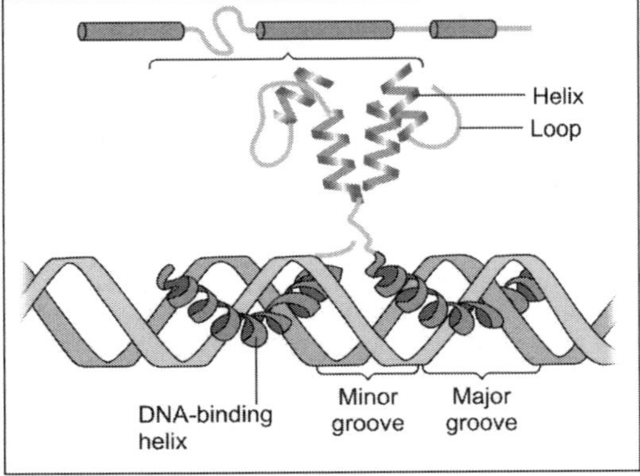

(d) Helix loop helix

Fig. 25.3A to D DNA-binding motifs

- Within a domain, only a few amino acids actually make contact with the DNA (most commonly asparagine, glutamine, glycine, lysine, and arginine).
- Many regulatory proteins have additional domains that can bind other molecules such as other regulatory proteins.
- DNA-binding proteins can be grouped into several distinct types on the basis of a characteristic structure, called a motif, found within the binding domain. Motifs are specific simple structures like α-helix which easily fits into the DNA major grooves.
- Some common DNA-binding protein motifs in eukaryotic gene expression are:
  - Helix turn helix—It has two α-helices and binds at DNA major groove.
  - Zinc finger motif—It has loop of amino acids with Zn at its base and binds at DNA major groove.
  - Leucine zipper motif—It has two leucine arms interdigitate or helix of Leucine residues with a basic arm. It binds two adjacent major grooves.
  - Helix – loop – helix—It has two α-helices separated by a loop of amino acids and it binds DNA major groove (Fig. 25.3A to D).

A Quick Look at the Gene Expression

- Gene expression is responsible for the organization of a complete organism as the complete genetic information of the organism is expressed selectively and specifically giving rise to the different tissues and organs.
- In prokaryotes the genes are polycistornic, i.e. a single mRNA is translated into different proteins.
- In eukaryotes the mRNA is mono-cistronic, i.e. each mRNA encodes for a specific protein.
- The prokaryotic gene expression is explained by the lac operon model.
- An operon is a collection of structural genes clustered together on an mRNA such that their expression is regulated by a single promoter.
- Bacteriophage lambda has a genetic switch, i.e. the structural genes are regulated by two proteins repressor and cro protein which respectively switch on either the lysogenic or the lytic phase.
- Eukaryotic gene expression is exerted at various levels:
  - Chromatin structure remodelling
  - Cis acting DNA sequences—Enhancers and silencers
  - mRNA processing
  - Gene rearrangement
  - Gene amplification
  - mRNA stability
  - Translational and post-translational modification
  - Protein interaction.

CHAPTER

26

Recombinant DNA Technology

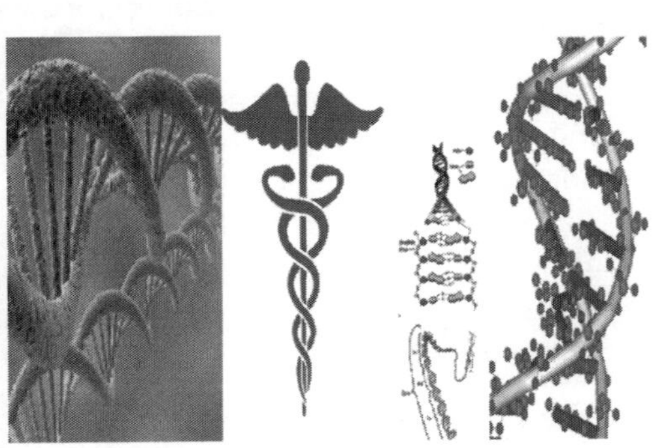

Chapter Framework

- Introduction
- What is rDNA?
- Restriction Endonucleases
- Cloning Vectors
- Steps for Synthesis of rDNA
- PCR—Artificial Cloning Technique
- Various Techniques of rDNA
  - Southern Blotting
  - Western Blotting
  - FISH
  - RFLP
- Significance of rDNA
- Future of rDNA Technology in Medicine—Gene Therapy

Introduction

- The early 1970s saw the birth of what is today the epitome of molecular biology success—recombinant DNA (rDNA) technology.
- Two scientists—Kathleen Danna and Daniel Nathans published a paper in 1971 on the isolation of a bacterial enzyme that was used to cleave viral DNA at specific sites; today we call them as the restriction endonucleases. These enzymes are one of the basic tools needed for the synthesis of rDNA.
- This marks the birth of the rDNA era.
- The synthesis of an rDNA involves the separation, cleavage and the splicing together of DNAs from two different sources. The rDNA thus formed can be manipulated in a variety of ways like for studying the expression of specific genetic sequences or in vitro synthesis of specific proteins or hormones, etc.
- This technique unravels the mystery of the genetic information contained in the DNA sequences.

What is rDNA?

- Naturally the process of recombination between homologous chromosomes is seen during the process of cell division. The word 'recombinant DNA' comes from the fact that DNA from two different sources might be combined together. Genes from two different bacteria might be joined, for example, a human gene might be inserted into a viral chromosome.

- The prerequisite for this rDNA is thus the separation of DNA from different sources and their splicing together.
- Molecular biologists have been able to:
  - Isolate DNA from cells and viruses.
  - Cleave their DNA at specific sites using enzyme—Restriction endonucleases.
  - Splice together the DNA from two different sources and the products of these innovations are the rDNA molecules.
- Thus rDNA technology is the set of methods used to locate, analyse, alter, study, and recombine DNA sequences.
- It is used to probe the structure and function of genes, address questions in many areas of biology, create commercial products, and diagnose and treat diseases.
- The two fundamental units required for the rDNA technology are the enzymes that cleave the DNA from the two sources site specifically, i.e. Restriction endonucleases and a source for the cloning of the rDNA, i.e. A cloning vector.

Restriction Endonucleases

- The key development that made rDNA technology possible was the discovery in the late 1960s of restriction enzymes (also called restriction endonucleases) that recognize and make double-stranded cuts in the sugar–phosphate backbone of DNA molecules at specific nucleotide sequences.
- Restriction enzymes are produced by bacteria as a defence mechanism against infection by viruses. They restrict or prevent viral infection by degrading the DNA of invading viruses.
- More than 3500 restriction enzymes have been identified, and over 250 are commercially produced and available for use by researchers (Table 26.1).
- The site where the restriction enzymes act is termed as restriction site.
- Each restriction enzyme is referred to by a short abbreviation that signifies its bacterial origin.
- The sequences recognized by restriction enzymes are usually from 4 bp to 8 bp long; most enzymes recognize a sequence of 4 bp or 6 bp long. Most recognition sequences are palindromic—Sequences that read the same forward and backward.
- Some of the enzymes make staggered cuts in the DNA. For example, Hind III recognizes the sequence as shown in Figure 26.1.
  - Hind III cuts the sugar–phosphate backbone of each strand at the point indicated by the arrow, generating fragments with short, single-stranded overhanging ends. Such ends are termed as cohesive/sticky ends as they have a tendency to readily anneal.
- Some restriction enzymes like Hae III produce blunt ends, i.e. they cut the DNA sequences such that there is no overhanging unpaired DNA left (Fig. 26.2).

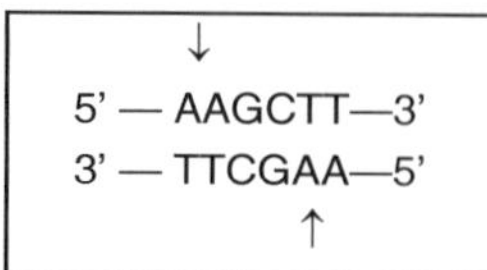

Fig. 26.1 Restriction site of Hind III

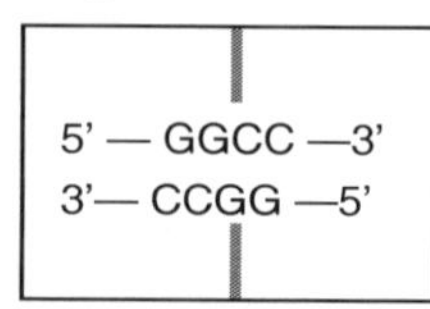

Fig. 26.2 Restriction site of Hae III

Table 26.1 Characteristics of some common restriction endonucleases

Enzyme	*Microorganism from which Enzyme is isolated*	*Recognition Sequence*	*Type of Fragment End Produced*
BamHI	*Bacillus amyloliquefaciens*	↓ 5' — CGATCC—3' 3' — CCTAGG—3' ↑	Cohesive
CofI	*Clostridium formicoaceticum*	↓ 5' — CCGC—3' 3' — CCCG—5' ↑	Cohesive
DraI	*Deinococcus radiophilus*	↓ 5' — TTTAAA—3' 3' — AAATTT—5' ↑	Blunt
EcoRI	*Escherichia coli*	↓ 5' — CAATTC—3' 3' — CTTAAC—5' ↑	Cohesive
EcoRII	*Escherichia coli*	↓ 5' — CCACG—3' 3' — GGTCC—5' ↑	Cohesive
Hae III	*Haemophilus aegyptius*	↓ 5' — CGCC—3' 3' — CCGG—5' ↑	Blunt
Hind III	*Haemophilus influenzae*	↓ 5' — AACCTT—3' 3' — TTCCAA—5' ↑	Cohesive
Hpa II	*Haemophilus parainfluenzae*	↓ 5' — CCGG—3' 3' — GGCC—5' ↑	Cohesive

Cloning Vectors

- Vectors are DNA molecules that accept DNA fragments and replicate inserted DNA fragments when vectors are placed into host cells.
- A vector should fulfil following criteria to be used as a cloning tool:
  - A vector should contain several restriction sites that allow insertion of the DNA fragments to be cloned.
  - Vectors must be introduced into host cells to allow for independent replication of the vector DNA and any DNA fragment it carries.

- To distinguish host cells that have taken up vectors from host cells that have not, the vector should carry a selectable marker gene (usually an antibiotic resistance gene or the gene for an enzyme absent from the host cell).
- The vector and its inserted DNA fragment should be easy to isolate from the host cell to recover cloned DNA for different applications.
  - Four types of cloning vectors are commonly used for cloning genes in bacteria: plasmids, bacteriophages, cosmids and yeast artificial chromosome (YAC).
    Plasmids carry 6 kilo to 10 kilo bp genetic information.
    Bacteriophages carry 10 kilo to 20 kilo bp genetic information.
    Cosmids carry 20 kilo to 50 kilo bp genetic information.
    Yeast Artificial Chromosome (YAC) carry more than 1 mega bp (0.5 mbp – 3 mbp)

Plasmids (Fig. 26.3)

- The most commonly used cloning vector is bacterial plasmid. These were the first vectors to be used and still are a preferred choice.
- Plasmids are extra chromosomal, double-stranded DNA molecules that replicate independently from the chromosomes within bacterial cells.
- The pUC19 plasmid is a typical cloning vector. It has an origin of replication and two selectable markers—An ampicillin-resistance gene and a lac Z gene.
- Ampicillin is an antibiotic that normally kills bacterial cells, but any bacterium that contains a pUC19 plasmid will be resistant to this antibiotic.
- The lac Z gene encodes the enzyme β-galactosidase, which normally cleaves lactose to produce glucose and galactose.
- The enzyme will also cleave a chemical called X-gal, producing a blue substance; when X-gal is placed in the medium, any bacterial colonies that contain intact pUC19 plasmids will turn blue and can be easily identified—Serving as a reporter or marker gene.

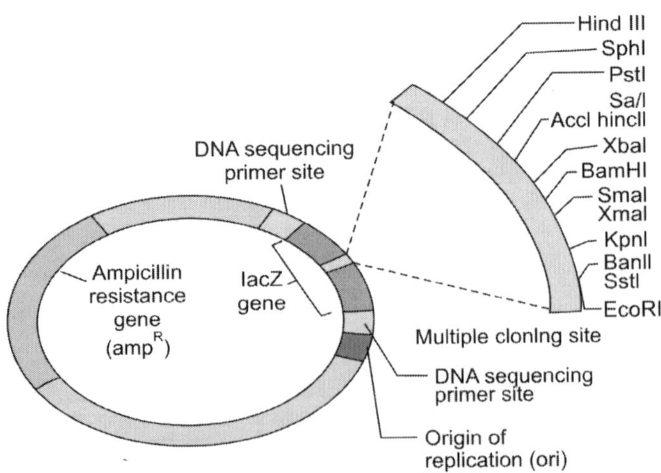

Fig. 26.3 A typical plasmid isolated from *E. coli* (pUC19)

Limitations of Plasmids

- Plasmids are still the workhorses for many applications of rDNA technology, but they have one limitation: because they are small, they can only accept inserted pieces of DNA upto about 10 kilo bases (kb) in size and most plasmids can often only accept substantially smaller pieces. Therefore as rDNA technology has developed and it has become desirable to clone large pieces of DNA, other vectors have been developed primarily for their ability to accept larger pieces of DNA and because they can be used with other types of host cells beside bacteria.
- Another limitation of the plasmids is that they can become virulent and damage the host.

Cosmids

- Cosmid is a hybrid DNA formed by the joining of a plasmid and L (lambda) phage DNA carrying a "cos site". In brief cosmid is a plasmid carrying the cos site of a Lambda phage DNA. The cosmid is not naturally found in living cells. It is a "constructed vector".
- The cosmid DNA does not code for the synthesis of viral proteins. The cosmid does not participate in the multiplication of phage particles.
- They can carry larger DNA fragment.

Expression Vectors

Sometimes just the cloning of a gene is not the only target of synthesizing an rDNA rather the purpose is to synthesize a particular protein within the host bacterial cell (for commercial use, e.g. The rDNA may be synthesized with the human insulin gene inserted into a vector that also has specific promoter sequences of the insulin gene leading to an expression of the insulin gene within the bacterial cell. Such vectors which contain additional promoter sites for the expression of the foreign gene are called expression vectors.

Some eukaryotic cloning vectors are—Yeast artificial chromosome (YAC) and Bacterial artificial chromosome (BAC).

Steps for the Synthesis of rDNA

The synthesis of rDNA is done as per the following protocol (Figs 26.4 and 26.5):

Isolation of the desired gene of interest from the human genome

- The gene of interest is selected from the mRNA of the host. Since, mRNA has just the coding sequences for a particular protein, it is chosen and a cDNA is synthesized on it by reverse transcriptase (RNA-dependent DNA polymerase). This cDNA is then exposed to a restriction enzyme which will cleave it on specific restriction sites.

Choosing the Vector

- The vector is chosen – plasmids mostly are used. The plasmids are then exposed to the same restriction enzyme as that of the human gene such that both the human and the plasmid DNA have cut ends complimentary to each other.

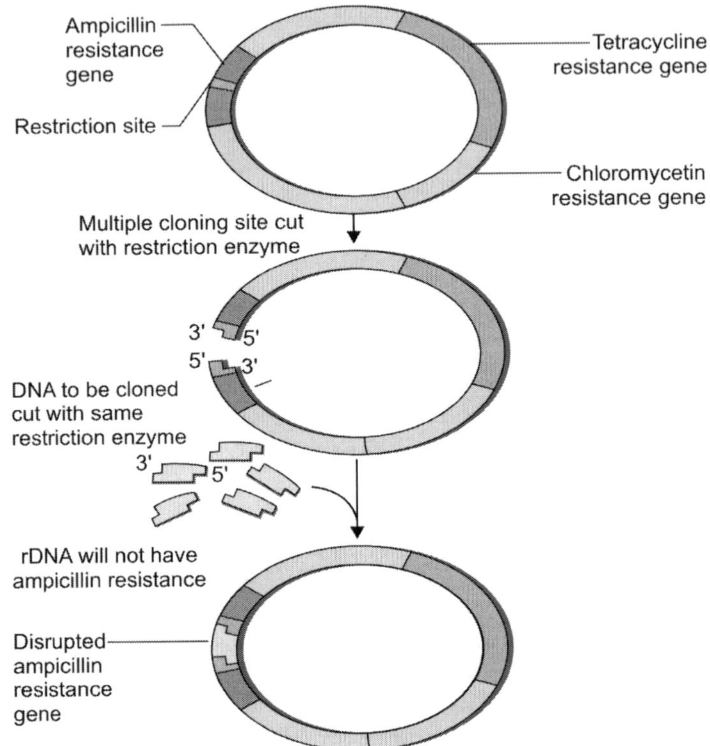

Fig. 26.4 Synthesis of r – DNA

Mixing the Vector and Human Gene

- The cut DNA from two different sources is joined together covalently by using DNA ligase such that the two DNAs fuse together and give rDNA.

Transfection of rDNA into Host Cells

- The rDNA is transfected into host bacteria and the host cells are then incubated in an environment conducive for multiplication. Transfection may be carried out by various methods like—Electroporation or using liposomes etc. (Discussion of these methods is beyond the scope of this book).

Amplification of the Vector

- The host cells multiply rapidly and increase the number of copies of the rDNA. The increased number of rDNA molecules can be isolated from the host cells. If the human gene is inserted along with a sequence for its expression, it will cause the expression of this gene and the respective protein can then be harvested from the bacterial colony.

Selection of Transfected Cells

- The rate of transfection is not very high, i.e. not all the bacterial cells are able to take up the rDNA molecules therefore the transfected cells have to be selected from all the host cells.

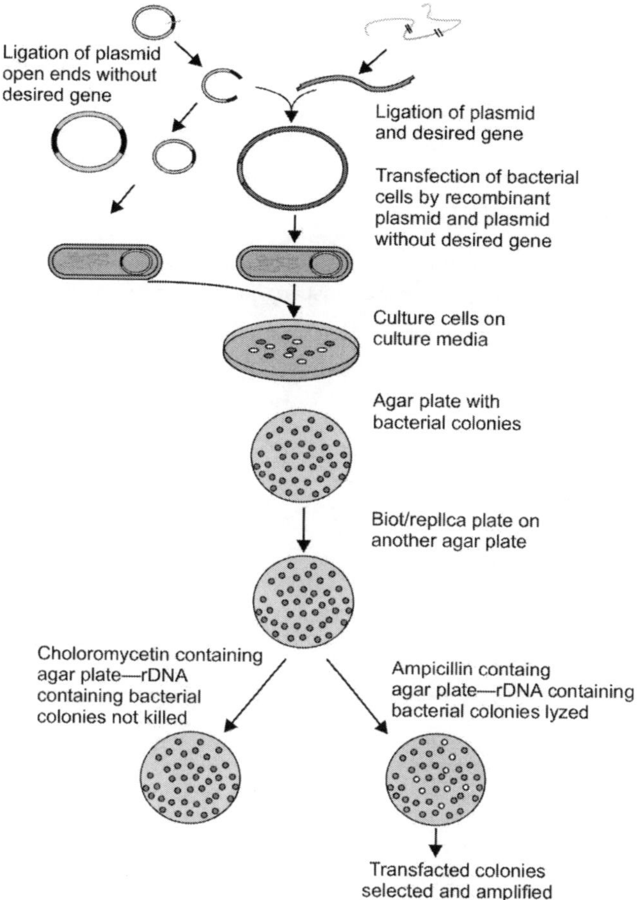

Fig. 26.5 Transfection, cloning and selection of rDNA

- This is done using the marker gene. The plasmid antibiotic resistance can be used as a marker gene. For example, a plasmid resistant to ampicillin, chloromycetin and tetracycline is fused with a human gene such that the human gene disrupts the ampicillin gene. Such a plasmid when transfected into a bacterial host, the transfected cells shall be resistant to tetracycline and Chloromycetin but not to ampicillin.
- The bacterial colonies cultured on the culture plate are replica-plated on to two more culture plates containing respectively ampicillin and tetracycline. The transfected colonies will be killed in the ampicillin plate and their corresponding colonies can now be selected from the original plates.

Polymerase Chain Reaction (PCR)—Artificial DNA Cloning Technique

In 1983, Kary Mullis of the Cetus Corporation conceptualized a new technique for amplifying DNA in a test tube—Polymerase chain reaction (PCR) (Fig. 26.6). PCR is a technique for artificially cloning DNA without a cloning vector. It allows DNA fragments to be amplified a billion fold within just a few hours. It can be used with extremely small amounts of original DNA, even a single molecule. The polymerase chain reaction has revolutionized molecular biology and is now one of the most widely used of all molecular techniques. The basis of PCR is replication catalyzed by a DNA polymerase enzyme, which has two essential requirements:

- A single-stranded DNA template from which a new DNA strand can be copied and
- A primer with a 3′-OH group to which new nucleotides can be added.

DNA Libraries

- DNA libraries are the set of all genes of an organism form where a particular gene can be isolated just as books can be taken from a library. Different types of DNA libraries are:

Genomic Library

- The mammalian genome contains 106 kbp genes approximately. To isolate a single gene of 10 kbp would be a task similar to searching a needle in a haystack. Thus the complete genome is split via restriction enzymes and cloned into different vectors such that at least one of the clones would have a part of the intended gene.

cDNA Library

- Complimentary DNA (cDNA) is prepared on a template of mRNA. A cDNA library comprises of cDNAs constructed on the cellular mRNA which is particularly important in eukaryotes as they have a lot of noncoding DNA sequences in their genome and mRNA has particularly the exons.

Techniques for Identifying the DNA Sequences

- Detection of specific DNA sequences—Southern blotting, northern blotting and western blotting.
- Chromosomal mapping of genes—In–situ hybridization.
- Gene mapping—Restriction fragment length polymorphism (RFLP).

Detection of Specific DNA Sequences—Southern Blotting, Northern Blotting and Western Blotting

- Detection of specific DNA sequences is done using the blotting techniques (Fig. 26.7).
- DNA is usually transferred to a solid support, such as a sheet of nitrocellulose paper.
- After bands of DNA are transferred to nitrocellulose paper, the paper is treated with an alkaline solution. Alkaline solutions denature DNA (that is, separate the two strands of each double helix).
- The single-stranded DNA is then hybridized with a probe, and the regions on the nitrocellulose blot containing DNA that base-pairs with the probe are identified. [*Probe*—It is a single-stranded polynucleotide (DNA or RNA) that is used to identify a complementary sequence on a larger single-stranded DNA or RNA molecule. A probe contains a radioactive P^{32} in it so as to be identified autoradiographically.]

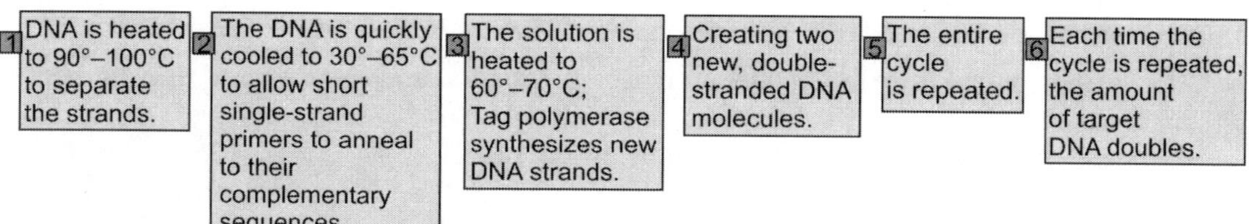

Fig. 26.6 PCR mechanism

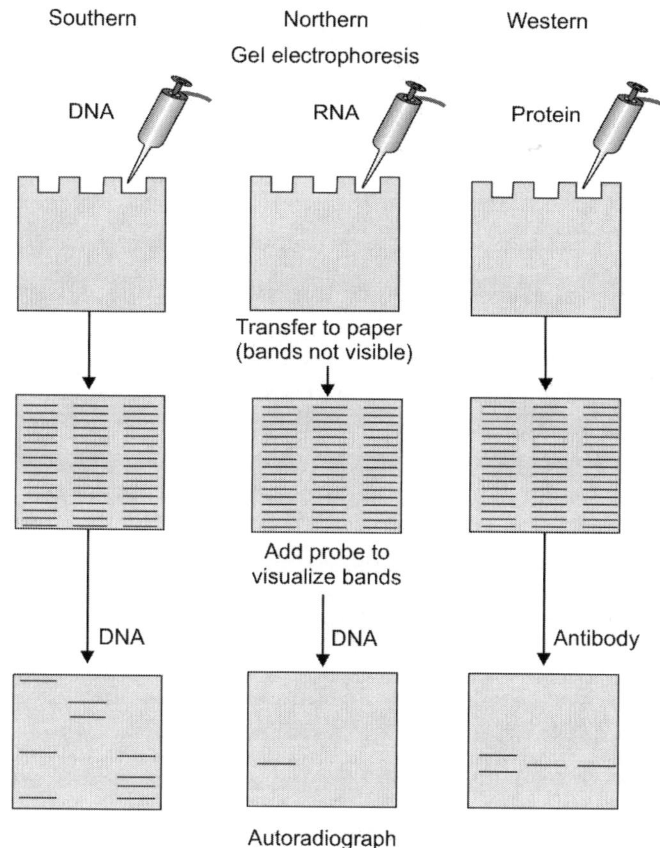

Fig. 26.7 Comparative blotting techniques

- Southern blots are produced when DNA on a nitrocellulose blot of an electrophoretic gel is hybridized with a DNA probe i.e. it helps identify specific nucleotide sequences on DNA molecule.
- Northern blots are produced when RNA on a nitrocellulose blot is hybridized with a DNA probe, i.e. it helps identify specific nucleotide sequences on RNA.
- Western blot is similar to these techniques with a modification that the probe used is a labelled antibody to a particular protein that has been electrophoresed and blotted on to a nitrocellulose blot.

Chromosomal Mapping of Genes—In-situ Hybridization

- DNA probes can be used for locating genes on a chromosome and the process is termed as in-situ hybridization.
- The technique can also be used for locating cellular mRNA.
- It is termed as 'insitu' since the DNA or RNA is not isolated form the cell for locating rather it is present in-situ, i.e. within the cell.
- The technique involves the preparation of a slide of the tissue concerned, fixing it and denaturing the cellular DNA using high pH. Then a labelled probe is added, excess probe washed and bound probe indicating the position of specific DNA sequences is detected autoradiographically.
- *If the probe is labelled with a fluorescent reagent, it is termed as fluorescent—in-situ hybridization (FISH).*
- Cellular mRNA can also be detected by same method, except that denaturation is not required.

Gene Mapping —*Restriction Fragment Length Polymorphism (RFLP)*

- Polymorphisms are variations among individuals of a species in DNA sequences of the genome.
- Each restriction enzyme has specific sites on the human genome. If there is any alteration in nucleotide of a restriction site it will cause a variation in the length of the restriction fragment length causing restriction fragment length polymorphism.
- A mutation can also generate a new restriction site which would be absent in normal individuals but will be present in mutated persons.
- Some polymorphisms occur within the coding region of genes. Others are found in noncoding regions closely linked to genes involved in the cause of inherited disease, in which case they can be used as a marker for the disease.
- Many of the RFLPs although present in the exons but are tightly linked with certain coding sequences and will serve as biologic markers of genetic diseases.
- RFLPs of no two individuals are identical thus the mapping of RFLPs can also be termed as *DNA finger printing.*

Significance of rDNA Technology in Medicine

The rapid development of techniques in the field of molecular biology is revolutionizing the practice of medicine. The potential uses of these techniques for the diagnosis and treatment of disease are vast. Some of the important uses of rDNA technology in modern day medicine are:

Production of Pharmaceuticals

- rDNA technology has revolutionized todays' pharmaceutical industries. The first pharmaceutical product to be synthesized using the rDNA technology was human insulin. Today all of the insulin being used is produced commercially by rDNA technology. This is highly advantageous since the earlier insulin used by diabetics was extracted from farm animals which caused allergic reactions in some individuals. However, the human insulin derived by rDNA technology is safe.

Oligonucleotide Drugs

- Oligonucleotide drugs are short pieces of DNA or RNA that prevent the expression of particular genes. Such oligonucleotide drugs are nowadays used for treatment of AIDS and cancer. The ss – oligonucleotide DNA binds to the ds – DNA of host cell or to viral RNA and inhibits the transcription and translation respectively thus killing the cell and the virus.

Preparation of Vaccines

- Vaccines like hepatitis B vaccines are today prepared using the rDNA technology. Earlier the hepatitis vaccines were prepared from pooled serum of hepatitis patients. This posed a risk of contamination of the vaccines by virus particles. However, the rDNA hepatitis vaccines are highly advantageous over the earlier vaccines since there is no risk of contamination.

Forensic Use

- The use of rDNA technology has proved be of tremendous use in forensics as even a trace of DNA from a crime scene can be amplified using the PCR technique and then be matched with the DNA of the accused person using the DNA finger printing technique.

Prenatal Diagnosis of Genetic Diseases

- There are a number of inherited disorders that are not compatible with a healthy living. Such disorders if diagnosed prenatally can be useful and fetus not compatible with a healthy life be terminated. This prenatal diagnosis of genetic diseases has become possible due to r – DNA technology where the fetal cells and cells from amniotic fluid can be drawn and their DNA isolated and mapped for the presence of an abnormal gene or absence of a normal gene.

Gene Therapy

Gene therapy was considered a fantasy which actualized on 15th September 1990 when a young girl was treated for severe immunodeficiency (SCID) due to lack of adenosine deaminase by injecting correct gene.

Steps of Gene Therapy

- Isolate cells from patient.
- Isolate and form rDNA with correct gene.
- Transfect the rDNA into a vector like retroviruses.
- Infect the isolated patient cells with retroviruses containing rDNA.
- Retrovirus DNA incorporates into patients DNA with the correct gene.
- Introduce the patient cells with correct gene back into patient. Gene Therapy has cured—(1) SCID (2) Duchene muscular dystrophy (3) Cystic fibrosis. Gene therapy conducted to date has targeted only non-reproductive, somatic cells. Correcting a genetic defect in these cells (termed somatic gene therapy) may provide positive benefits to patients but will not affect the genes of future generations. Gene therapy that alters reproductive, or germ-line, cells (termed germ-line gene therapy) is technically possible but raises a number of significant ethical issues, because it has the capacity to alter the gene pool of future generations.

A Quick Look at the Recombinant DNA Technology

- rDNA technology is the epitome of molecular diagnosis and therapy in modern medicine.
- rDNA is the synthesis of a rDNA by fusing DNA fragments from two different sources like—Human gene with a bacterial or viral or plasmid DNA.
- rDNA preparation requires:
  - Isolation of desired gene
  - Exposure of desired gene to restriction endonucleases (RE)
  - Selection of vector and exposure of vector to same RE
  - Fusion of the two DNA fragments
  - Transfection of the rDNA into a host
  - Selection of transfected host
  - Cloning/Amplification of rDNA
  - Harvesting the product of the rDNA
- Amplification of DNA can also be carried out by PCR, i.e. artificial cloning of a DNA fragment.
- A gene can be selected from genomic library or cDNA library.
- Isolation of a DNA fragment can be done using Southern Blotting.
- Isolation of a gene can also be done using Northern Blotting (mRNA).
- Proteins of interest can be identified by using Western Blotting technique.
- The advantages of rDNA technology are:
  - In pharmaceutical industry
  - Preparation of vaccines
  - Preparation of oligonucleotide drugs
  - Forensic use
  - Prenatal diagnosis of genetic diseases
  - Gene therapy.

Section – 6

Miscellaneous

- Cancer and Oncogenes
- Immunology
- AIDS
- Xenobiotics Metabolism
- Free Radicals and Antioxidants in Health and Disease
- Regulation of Acid-Base Balance
- Biochemistry of Saliva and Dental Caries
- Biochemistry of Connective Tissue and Bones
- Current Topics in Biochemistry

CHAPTER

27

Cancer and Oncogenes

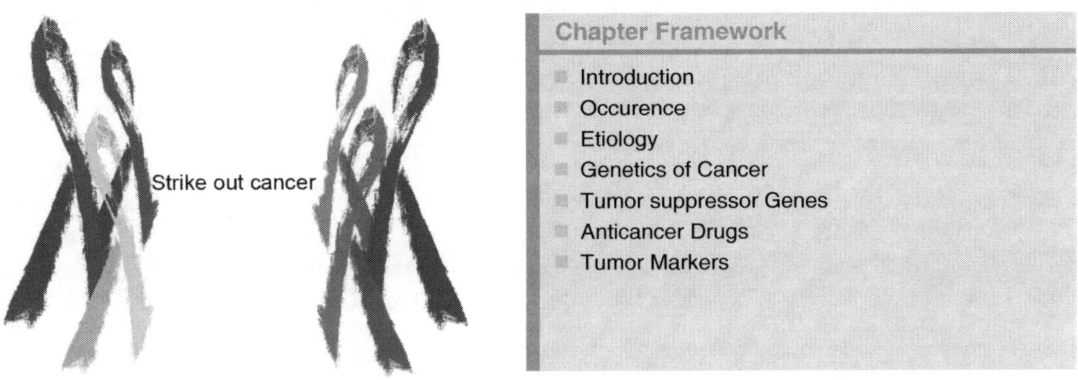

Introduction

Under normal circumstances, the proliferation of body cells is under strict control. The cells proliferate, differentiate and die in a highly regulated manner. However, cancer is a phenomenon where a group of cells defies all rules of cell division and divides uncontrollably leading to the development of a mass of cells—'Tumor'. The term "Cancer" is derived from Latin word 'cancrum' that means crab. The disease is so called because of the swollen veins around the area, resembles a crabs limb. Thus cancer is characterized by loss of control of cellular growth and development leading to excessive proliferation and spread of cells or metastasis (spread of cancer to other tissues) and invasion of local tissues.

Tumors are of 2 types:

- *Benign Tumors:* They show diminished control of growth but do not invade local tissue by metastasis.
- *Malignant Tumors:* They are cancerous and show uncontrolled cellular proliferation, invade local tissue and metastasize.

Occurrence

- Cancer is the 2nd most common cause of human death in developed countries, second only to cardiovascular diseases. The incidence of cancer increases with an increase in life expectancy. More than 70% of the new cancer cases occur in persons over 60 years of age. Prevalence of

Cancer in India as per a representative survey is constantly increasing and ICMR projects the number to increase to 11.61 lakhs by the year 2015.

Etiology

- All cancers are multifactorial in origin. They include genetic, physical, chemical and environmental factors. Most human cancers are spontaneous. However, some of the common causes of carcinogenesis are:

Genetic/Hereditary

- Hereditary plays an important role in carcinogenesis some of the cancers are inherited, e.g. Xeroderma pigmentosa, childhood retinoblastomas (AD).

Environmental Factors

- Many of the human cancers are caused by environmental factors, mainly chemicals/ carcinogenic agents. The entry of the carcinogenic chemicals into the body may occur by:
  - *Occupation:* Asbestos, benzene, etc. various industries.
  - *Dietary:* Aflatoxin B_1—A carcinogenic agent produced by *Aspergillus* infecting the foodstuffs like groundnut.
  - *Lifestyle:* Smoking, tobacco chewing.
  - *Drugs:* Some drugs can be carcinogenic.

Physical Carcinogenic Agents

Physical carcinogenic agents cause carcinogenesis by radiations by 2 ways:

- *Direct effect:* X-Rays, γ-Rays or UV-rays cause damage to DNA thus can be mutagenic and carcinogenic.
- *Indirect effect:* In addition to direct effect, the radiations cause generation of free radicals that lead to DNA damage and carcinogenesis.

Chemical Carcinogens

- A large number of chemicals are carcinogenic in nature some of them act directly, however, a majority of them are present as procarcinogens and are converted to ultimate carcinogenic chemicals in the body (Fig. 27.1 and Table 27.1).
- The procarcinogens are not chemically reactive but in the body after metabolism they are converted to ultimate carcinogens which are highly carcinogenic.
- The metabolic activity involves one or more enzymes, e.g.—Cytochrome P450 or a monoxygenase.
- Some of the chemicals require promoters/promoting agents for their carcinogenic activity e.g. Croton oil and benzo (a) pyrene individually are not carcinogenic but when benzo (a) pyrene

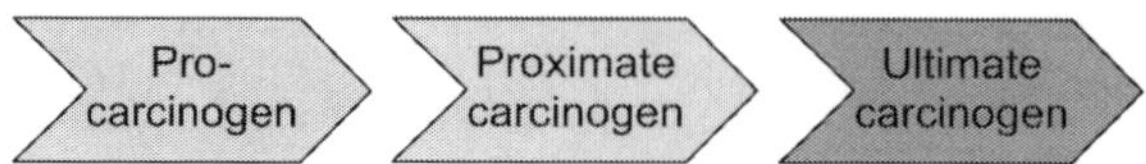

Fig. 27.1 Activation of procarcinogen to ultimate carcinogen

Table 27.1 Chemical carcinogenic agents and cancer caused

	Chemical Carcinogens	*Cancer caused*
1.	Aromatic hydrocarbons (e.g. Benzpyrene A)	Present in cigarette smoke and cause lung cancer
2.	Aniline azodyes	Used in rubber industry and cause bladder cancer
3.	Nitrosamines	Generated from nitrates in GIT and can cause gastric cancer
4.	Aflatoxin B1	Produced by *Aspergillus flavus* and causes liver cancer (hepatoma)

is applied on the skin of rat followed by application of croton oil, tumor develops. Thus croton oil is the promoting agent.

Oncogenic Viruses (Table 27.2)

- Animals contain proto-oncogenes in their genome (which are inactive and do not cause cancer unless activated).
- Oncogenic viruses are virus particles that picked up oncogenes from their animal hosts.
- Oncogenic virus in the etiology of cancer was first reported by Rous (1911). The study of Rous showed that cell free filtrates of chicken sarcomas (tumors of connective tissue) causes new sarcomas in chicken. This was due to the oncogenic virus Rous sarcoma virus.
- The oncogenic viruses can be either DNA/RNA viruses.

DNA Viruses

These viruses have DNA as their genetic material. For e.g:

- Epstein–Barr virus causes Burkitt's lymphoma.
- Hepatitis – B virus causes liver carcinoma.
- Human Papilloma virus causes multiple warts and cervical cancer.

Mechanism of Action of DNA Viruses

- The DNA viruses form stable associations with human genome. The viral genes integrated into the human genome produce specific proteins which act and derange the normal growth regulation.

RNA Viruses

- RNA viruses have RNA as their genetic material and all oncogenic RNA viruses are retro viruses, i.e. they use reverse transcriptase as the key enzyme during their infection and multiplication in the host. Reverse transcriptase is an RNA-dependent DNA polymerase that synthesizes DNA using RNA as a template.

Mechanism of Action of RNA Viruses

Taking Rous sarcoma virus as an example—The genome of this retrovirus contains 4 genes.

Gag: Codes for group specific antigens of the virus.

Table 27.2 RNA viruses and their oncogenic products

	Type of RNA virus	*Oncogenic product*	*Cancer caused*
1.	Rous sarcoma	(src) Tyrosine kinase	No human cancer
2.	Avian myelocytoma virus	(myc) DNA-binding protein	Burkitt's lymphoma, Neuroblastoma, Lung cancer
3.	Murine sarcoma virus	(sis) GTP-binding protein	Bladder cancer, colon cancer, leukemia

Pol: Codes for reverse transcriptase.

Env: Codes for envelop protein.

Src: Codes for tyrosine kinase.

- The product of src gene causes abnormal phosphorylation of several cellular proteins that could cause carcinogenesis. The different proteins that undergo modification are:
  - *Vinculin* – It is a protein, found in focal adhesion plates of cells. This causes the cells to be transformed. Such transformed cells loose the sense of contact inhibition and grow over the surrounding, cells growing uncontrollably as a mass of cells—tumor.
  - *The process of cell change in which a cell loses its ability to control its rate of division, and thus becomes a tumor cell, is called cell transformation.*
- Transformed cells apparently, undergo a change in the property of their cell membranes which become less adhesive. This change enables the cells to dissociate from neighboring cells and to infiltrate other organs (metastasis) where they form metastatic tumors. Cancer cells apparently lack proper recognition and communication.
- *Loss of anchorage dependence:* Most normal cells must be attached to a rigid substratum (i.e. they must be anchored) in order to grow. Transformed cells can grow even when they are not attached to the substratum and even in multi-layers as opposed to mono – layer in normal cells.
- *Glycolytic enzymes*: The glycolytic enzyme proteins are so modified that the rate of glycolysis is increased in transformed cells.

Tyr kinase could cause abnormal phosphorylation of phosphatidyl inositol to inositol mono and bis PO_4 which in-turn increases the production of IP_3 and DAG. The IP_3 increases intracellular Ca^{++}. This raised Ca^{++} concentration further is responsible for the activation of various cell membrane channels that may promote cell division.

Genetics of Cancer

- With the advancement in our knowledge of molecular biology we have learnt a great deal about the genetic basis of cancer.
- All cells have a controlling center *nucleus* that contains genes—which are the precise controlling feature of all cellular functions right from metabolism to cell division.
- There are three major types of genes involved in tumor genesis—*proto-oncogenes, tumor suppressor genes and genes involved in mutations of DNA repair.*

Proto-oncogenes

These are normal genes that can become oncogenic due to:

Mutations in DNA Mismatch Repair Genes

- This is seen in hereditary nonpolyposis cancer. DNA repair genes normally eliminate any error in DNA replication that may cause a mutant transformation of the cells into cancerous cells. Any mutations of these repair genes will cause cancers due to accumulation of lethal mutations and HNPCC.

Chromosomal Abnormalities

- There are a number of chromosomal abnormalities seen in different leukemias.

Chromosomal Translocation

- It is seen in 8 and 14 chromosomes; leading to activation of *Myc* proto – oncogene which Burkitt's lymphoma. Other examples are—Acute myeloid leukemia and acute lymphocytic leukemias.

Point Mutations

- A point mutation in a proto-oncogene can activate it to an oncogene for e.g. K-ras point mutation cause cancer of colon, lung and pancreatic melanoma.

Tumor Suppressor Genes

- These are genes that supress normally the formation of tumors but on mutation can lead to tumor genesis.
- These genes protect an individual from cancer. These are also called anti -oncogenes and are written in capital letters e.g.:

RB Gene—Retinoblastoma Gene

When there is homozygous deletion of RB gene-retinoblastoma results. This gene produces protein p105 which suppresses cell proliferation and prevents activity of various viral oncogenes by forming inactive complexes with them.

P53 Gene

- It produces p53 protein which acts like a regulator of transcription and regulator of cell cycle.
- The level of p53 increases when cells are exposed to DNA damaging agents. This causes increased G1 Phase so that cell gets time for repair.
- P53 also triggers apoptosis (programmed cell death) of damaged cells. Thus acts like a Molecular Policeman.
- P53 binds various viral oncogenes to form inactive complexes thus suppressing carcinogenesis.

Telomeres and their Role in Cancer

- Telomeres are the terminal ends of the chromosomes where there are number of DNA repeats, e.g. In human chromosomes there are about 1500 bp of sequences TTAGGG.
- The telomeres are maintained with the help of an enzyme telomerase/telomere terminal transferase.

- This enzyme is unique in that it is composed of proteins as well as RNA molecules.
- The activity of telomerase helps maintain the terminal ends of the DNA which otherwise gradually are lost (especially on the lagging strand) causing cell senescence/cell death.
- Cancer cells multiply uncontrollably probably because of a very active telomerase enzyme.
- Thus telomerase has become a very potent site of cancer therapeutic research.

Anticancer Drugs

- Since the cancer cells multiply rapidly the major target for cancer therapy has been inhibition of DNA replication.
- The anticancer drugs are classified as:
  - Cell cycle specific—Acting at a particular stage of cell cycle – G_1, or S and effect rapidly dividing cells.
  - Cell cycle nonspecific—Acting on all cells irrespective of cell cycle stage and thus affect a wide variety of cancerous as well as noncancerous cells.
- Important anticancer drugs are listed in Table 27.3.

Tumor Markers

- These are factors/biochemical indicators that help to detect the presence of cancers.
- They are useful for:
  - Follow-up of cancer and monitor the effectiveness of therapy.
  - Detecting recurrence of tumor.
  - Diagnosis of cancer.
    - These can be tumor cell surface antigens, enzymes, cytoplasmic proteins, hormones, fetal antigens (produced normally in fetuses but may be abnormally expressed in certain types of cancers).
    - They may be detected in blood and body fluids.

Table 27.3 Important anticancer drugs

Class of compound	*Action*	*Treatment of*
Alkylating agents like Melphalan	Alkylates DNA	Myeloma
Antimetabolites like Purine antagonists (Mercaptopurine) or Folate antagonists (Methotrexate)	A faulty purine gets incorporated during DNA replication and inhibits it. Or Folate reductase is inhibited (*see* Chapter 6)	Colorectal caner Choriocarcinoma
Antitumor antibiotics like Doxorubicin	Intercalates with DNA strand stabilizing DNA topoisomerase –II complex.	Hodgkin's disease
Corticosteroids like Prednisone	Inhibits lymphocyte proliferation	Myeloma
Sex hormones like Estrogens	Block effect of androgens	Prostate cancer
Plant compounds like Vinblastine	Inhibits microtubule formation by binding to them	Kaposi sarcoma
Others like Cisplatin or hydroxyurea	Cause DNA strand breakage or inhibit ribonucleotides reductase	Lung cancer and chronic myelocytic leukemia

Characteristic Features

- Should have high sensitivity.
- Should have high specificity.
- Method should be simple and economically viable.
- Should be disease-sensitive with no false results.

Some common examples of tumor markers are:

- Bence Jones proteins—Multiple myeloma.
- β-HCG, PTH, GH, ACTH, etc. hormonal.
- LDH isoenzymes
- PSA } Prostate cancer
- Acid phosphatase } Prostate cancer
- ALP — Bone cancer
- Carb Ag, e.g. CA- 125—Ovarian Cancer
- Oncofetal Products α-Fetoproteins—Hepatoma, germ cells cancer
- Carcinoembryonic Ag Colorectal, lung cancer and GIT cancer.

A Quick Look at the Cancer and Oncogenes

- Cancer is a phenomenon where a group of cells defies all rules of cell division and divides uncontrollably leading to the development of a mass of cells – 'tumor'.
- Tumors are of 2 types i.e. benign and malignant.
- Cancer is caused by:
  - Hereditary
  - Lifestyle
  - Physical carcinogens
  - Chemical carcinogens
  - Oncogenic viruses—DNA viruses and RNA viruses
- Tumor suppressor genes that supress normally inhibit formation of tumor like RB gene, P53 gene.
- Cancer cells multiply uncontrollably probably because of a very active telomerase enzyme.
- The anticancer drugs are classified as:
  - Cell cycle specific—Acting at a particular stage of cell cycle—G_1, or S and effect rapidly dividing cells.
  - Cell cycle nonspecific—Acting on all cells irrespective of cell cycle stage and thus affect a wide variety of cancerous as well as non cancerous cells.

CHAPTER

28

Immunology

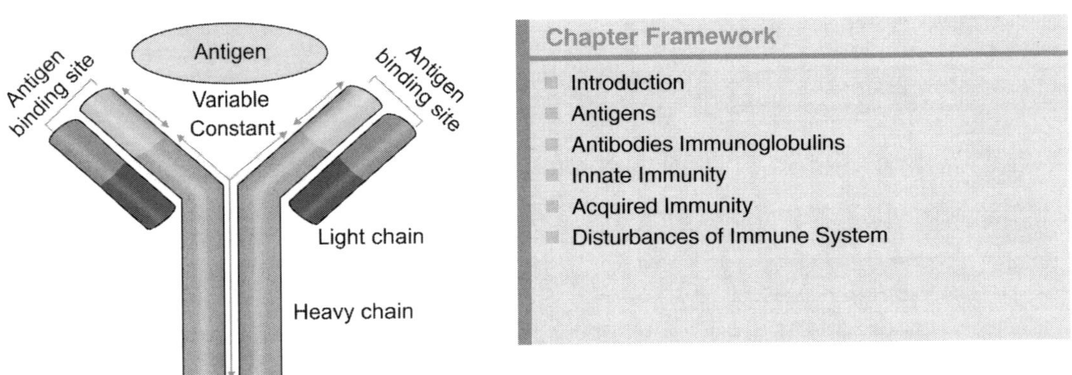

Chapter Framework

- Introduction
- Antigens
- Antibodies Immunoglobulins
- Innate Immunity
- Acquired Immunity
- Disturbances of Immune System

Introduction

The human body is constantly exposed to a large variety of foreign agents (antigens) like microorganisms or chemicals that pose threat of diseases which may be severe and even fatal at times. However, we are equipped with a highly effective and sensitive defence mechanism—Immune system. The immune system confers two types of immunities—*Innate (we are born with) and acquired (we acquire during our lifetime).*

The immune response to different antigens involves the innate and acquired immunities. Immune response may be either humoral or cell mediated.

Antigens

- Antigens are defined as foreign chemicals or groups that are present either on a microbe (bacteria/virus) or free which when enters our body evokes an immune response.
- An antigen is chemically a polysaccharide or a protein of high molecular weight that occurs as repeating units on the bacteria/viruses and can evoke an immune response.
- Only a little portion of the antigen is responsible for evoking the immune response—Epitope.
- A hapten is a small molecule that is antigenic but cannot evoke an immune response all by itself but becomes immunogenic on combining with some larger molecule.

Antibodies/Immunoglobulins

- Immunoglobulins are proteins synthesized by the immune system in response to the antigenic stimulus.
- They are capable of binding to the antigen. Structurally antibodies comprise of 4 polypeptide chains (2 heavy and 2 light chains). Thus they are heterodimeric proteins.
- There are two light chain types (lambda and kappa) about 25,000 in molecular weight and 5 heavy chain types molecular weight >50,000 (gamma (γ), alpha (α), mu (μ), delta (δ) and eta (ε). Depending upon the heavy chains types there are 5 types of immunoglobulins:
  IgG, IgA, IgM, IgD and IgE (Table 28.1).
- The immunoglobulins are synthesized in response to the immunogenic stimulus of an antigen.
- Each light chain is bound to a heavy chain by a disulfide bond, and by such noncovalent interactions as salt linkages, hydrogen bonds, and hydrophobic bonds, to form a heterodimer (H-L) (Fig. 28.1).
- Similar noncovalent interactions and disulfide bridges link the two identical heavy and light (H-L) chain combinations to each other to form the basic four-chain (H-L)2 antibody structure.
- Each of the heavy and light chain have at their—NH_2 terminal ends a variable region (V_L and V_H) which identifies and binds to the different antigens at their epitopes. The portion of variable region binding to epitope is termed as paratope.
- A small number of antibodies are capable of identifying large spectra of antigens due to the variation in the type and sequence of amino acids at the variable region.
- On this variable region there are specific regions which are responsible for the variation; these are the complementarity determining regions (CDRs) or hyper variable regions. There are 3 such regions in V_L and V_H each.
- The regions of relatively constant sequence beyond the variable regions have been dubbed C regions, C_L on the light chain and C_H on the heavy chain.
- Antibodies are glycoproteins; with few exceptions, the sites of attachment for carbohydrates are restricted to the constant region.
- F_{ab} is a region on the V_H that participates in binding the antigen.
- F_c is the region on the C_H carboxy terminal end that does not participate in antigen binding but it helps the Ig to bind on to specific B-lymphocytes.
- These variable and constant regions are joined by a hinge like Joining region (J chain).
- We are capable of synthesizing millions of different antibodies each specific for an antigen due to the gene rearrangement of the genes of heavy and light chains.
- Different effector functions of Ig include (Table 28.2):

Table 28.1 Immunoglobulin types

Class	*Heavy chain*	*Subclasses*	*Light chain*
IgG	γ	γ1, γ2, γ3, γ4,	K or λ
IgM	μ	None	K or λ
IgA	α	α1, α2,	K or λ
IgE	ε	None	K or λ
IgD	δ	None	K or λ

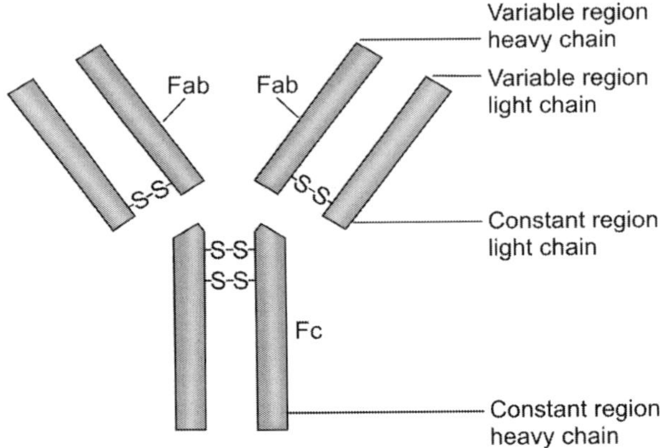

Fig. 28.1 Structure of immunoglobulin

- Neutralization—Antibodies coat the antigens on the surface of pathogens and prevent their entry in host cells.
- Opsonization—Antibodies coat the surface of pathogens and facilitate phagocytosis by attracting phagocytes and natural killer cells.
- Complement activation—It consists of a group of proteins present in plasma that act in concert with Igs. Complement proteins are pro-enzymes which are converted into enzymes by a cascade of reactions similar to blood coagulation cascade. There are two complement pathways finally leading to cell lysis (bacteriolysis)—Classic complement cascade and alternate complement pathway.

Innate/Passive Immunity

- It is the immunity a person is born with.
- Innate immunity can be seen to comprise four types of defensive barriers—anatomic, physiologic, phagocytic, and inflammatory (Table 28.3).

Table 28.2 Types of immunoglobulins and their effector functions

Class	*Half-life*	*Activity against*	*Unique features*
IgG	23 days	Bacteria and viruses	Cross placenta and activate complement system
IgA	5 – 6 days	Strong antiviral and moderate antibacterial	Secretory IgA in secretions like tear, saliva etc.
IgM	5 – 6 days	Strong antiviral and moderate antibacterial	Ist Ig to be synthesized. Activate complement system
IgE	2 – 3 days	Parasites	Mediate allergic reactions
IgD	2 – 3 days	Unknown function	

Table 28.3 Modes of innate immunity

Defensive barrier of innate immunity	*Mechanism of action*
Anatomic barrier Skin Mucous membranes	Mechanical barrier Check the entry of microbes, acidic environment (pH 3-5) impedes growth of microbes Normal flora competes with microbes, mucus traps the microbes and cilia propel the microbes out of body
Temperature	Normal body temperature inhibits growth of some pathogens. Fever response inhibits growth of some pathogens
Low pH	Acidity of stomach contents kills most ingested microorganisms
Chemical mediators	Lysozyme cleaves bacterial cell wall; Interferon induces antiviral state in uninfected cells; Complement lyses microorganisms or facilitates phagocytosis.
Phagocytic/endocytic barriers (lymphocytes, monocytes, macrophages, etc.)	Various cells internalize (endocytose) and break down foreign macromolecules
Inflammatory barriers	Tissue damage and infection induce leakage of vascular fluid, containing serum proteins with antibacterial activity, and influx of phagocytic cells into the affected area

Acquired/Adaptive immunity

- It is acquired during the lifetime by a person on exposure to a variety of antigens and involves:
  - Humoral immunity—Production of antibodies against specific Ags by B-lymphocytes (produced in bone marrow).
  - Cell mediated immunity—Operates through activated T-lymphocytes (produced by thymus) that differentiate into helper T-cells, cytotoxic T-cells/natural killer cells, suppressor T-cells and memory cells.
- Adaptive immunity displays four characteristic attributes:
  - Antigenic specificity
  - Diversity
  - Immunologic memory
  - Self/nonself—Recognition
- Adaptive immunity is capable of recognizing and selectively eliminating specific foreign microorganisms and molecules. It varies in different individuals depending upon the exposure different antigens during their lifetime.
- It requires a concerted action of the T-lymphocytes and the B-lymphocytes with the antigen processing cells.
- The different antigens that encounter the immune system are processed by antigen processing cells (APCs)—Macrophages, B-lymphocytes, dendritic cells which engulf and degrade the antigen to present it on their surface with a major histocompatibility complex (MHC).

- MHC proteins are present on cells of all individuals specific to each individual. The antigen processing cells present the antigen on their surface in association with its MHC proteins. It is this combination that is recognized by the helper T-cells.
- The helper T-cells then release specific lymphokines that carry out the effect of cell mediated immunity by increasing the titer of helper T-cells, B-cells, attract macrophages and mediate inflammatory response.
- If the Ags are not presented with MHC proteins the T-cells cannot recognise them. In case of graft rejection it is the MHC proteins of the donor that are destroyed as foreign Ags unless immunosuppressive drugs are used.
- The cytotoxic T-cells destroy the APC along with the Ag. Some of the T-cells become memory T-cells to evoke immune response on subsequent infections. Suppressor T-cells are responsible for preventing an exaggerated immune response.

Disturbances of Immune System

Autoimmunity

- It is the development of immune response against self-antigens that either do not reach the thymus and bone marrow in fetal life or are not synthesized during fetal life or become immunogenic on combining with a foreign antigen. Such self-antigens are then destroyed by the immune system. Some important autoimmune diseases are—Type-I diabetes mellitus, Hashimoto's Thyroiditis, systemic lupus erythematous, rheumatoid arthritis, etc.

Immunodeficiency

- Immunodeficiency is caused due to inherited or acquired defect in the humoral and/ or cell mediated immunity. Few example of inherited immunodeficiency are—Congenital agammaglobulinemia (humoral immunity defect), Di George syndrome (Cell mediated immunity defect), Severe combined immunodeficiency (both humoral and cell mediated immunity defective). AIDS is an important acquired immunodeficiency disease.

Hypersensitivity/Allergy

- It is an exaggerated immune response to an allergen and is mediated by mast cells and basophils that have on their surface IgE antibodies. The binding of the allergen to the IgE antibodies on mast cells and basophils causes the release of a number of chemical like histamine, heparin, slow reacting substance of anaphylaxis, etc. that cause allergic reaction. Common features of allergic reactions are—Vasodilation, increased capillary permeability, edema, itching, rashes, allergic rhinitis, sneezing, bronchospasm, etc. and sometimes in severe cases anaphylactic shock that may be fatal.

A Quick Look at the Immunology

- Antigen is a foreign chemicals or groups that are present either on a microbe (bacteria/ virus) or free which when enters our body evokes an immune response.
- Immunoglobulins are proteins synthesized by the immune system in response to the antigenic stimulus. Each Ig made of 2 heavy and 2 light chains.
- Different classes of Ig – IgG, IgA, IgM, IgD and IgE based on 4 types of heavy chains γ, α, μ, δ, ε.
- Innate or inborn due to physical barriers and physiologic barriers.
- Acquired immunity is acquired due to exposure to different antigens during lifetime of an individual.
- Acquired immunity involves a concerted action of B-lymphocytes and T-lymphocytes.
- This may either humoral or cell mediated.
- Humoral immunity is antibody mediated and involves the B-lymphocytes.
- Cell mediated immunity involves T-lymphocytes.
- The T-cells recognize antigens presented by APCs in association with MHC.
- Graft rejection occurs when T-cells do not recognize the donor MHC complex.
- Autoimmunity is development of immune response against self-antigens as in Type-I DM, systemic lupus erythematous, rheumatoid arthritis, Hashimoto's thyroiditis.
- Immunodeficiency is defect in either humoral and or cell mediated immunity as in Digeorge's syndrome (inherited) and AIDS (acquired).
- Allergic reaction is exaggerated immune response to an allergen and is IgE mediated.

CHAPTER

29

AIDS

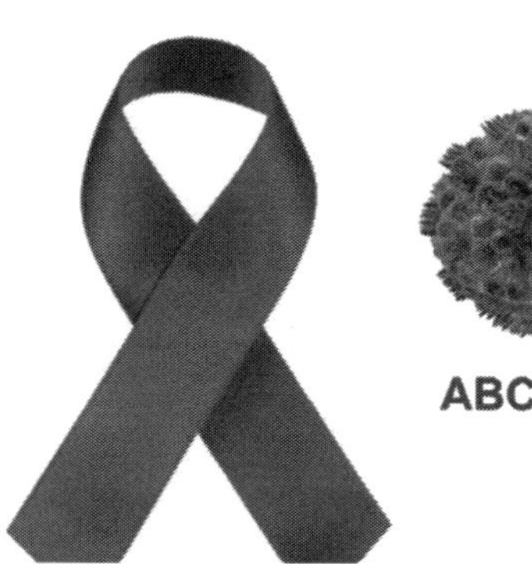

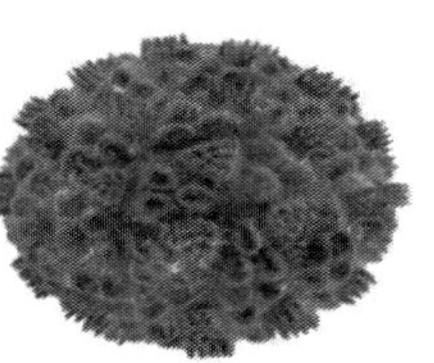

ABC of AIDS

Chapter Framework

- Introduction
- AIDS Virus
- Immunology and Infection by AIDS Virus
- Modes of Infection and Prevention
- Diagnostic Tests for AIDS

Introduction

AIDS is an acquired immunodeficiency syndrome of humans. It is caused by a retrovirus-HIV (Human Immunodeficiency Virus). This virus was first discovered in the year 1981 when there was a sudden increase in opportunistic infections like Pneumonia *(Pneumocystis carinii)* and Kaposi sarcoma in the United States of America. Earlier reports were that it is similar to the Human T-cell Lymphotropic viruses-I and II (HTLV-I and II). However, it was soon realised that it was different from these two retro viruses and was termed as HIV. This was reported independently by Robert Gallo and Luc Montagnier (1983). Today, it has reached pandemic proportions with maximum numbers in Africa—The continent that has been proven genetically to be the site of origin of HIV. India's first known HIV infection was diagnosed in a female sex worker in Chennai in February 1986. It is highly probable that HIV had been circulating for some years before that, since screening during 1986 to 87 found as many as 3% to 4% of sex workers infected in Vellore and Madurai. According to National Family and Health Survey (NFHS-II) figures, India had an estimated 2.5 million people (range 2 and 3.1 million) between the ages of 15 and 49 years living with HIV in 2006.

AIDS Virus

- It is around 120 nm in diameter.
- It is a retro virus, i.e. its genetic material is an RNA molecule which when enters the host cell, copies its genetic information into a DNA molecule via a RNA-dependent DNA polymerase—Reverse transcriptase.

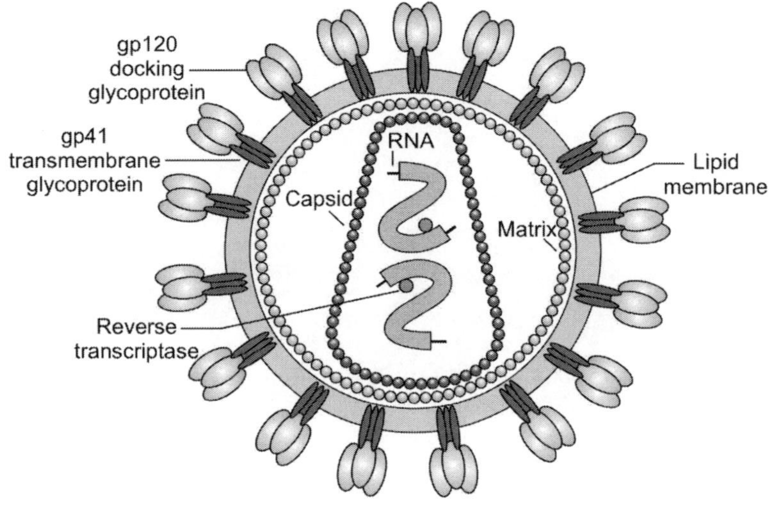

Fig. 29.1 HIV structure

- The new viral DNA molecule then integrates with the host cell genome and uses the host's cellular machinery for synthesizing new virus particles (Fig. 29.1).
- There are two copies of the genomic RNA in each virion encapsulated in capsid protein.
- The different viral proteins are named based on their molecular weights. Certain significant proteins are:
  - p66 and p55 that have reverse transcriptase activity.
  - p32 which is an endonuclease.
  - p9 a nucleocapsid.
  - p10 which is a protease.
  - p24 which is the major capsid.
  - p17 which is the membrane antigen.
- The important genes are (Fig. 29.2)
  - gag—coding for p55 .
  - pol—coding for p160.
  - env—coding for gp160.
- Besides these are some other accessory genes—vif, vpr, vpu, vpt and tev/tnr.
- The regulatory genes are tat, rev and nef.
- All these structural genes are flanked on either side by long terminal repeats (LTRs).

Immunology and Infection by AIDS Virus

- HIV infects cells in the immune system and the central nervous system. The main type of cell that HIV infects is the T helper lymphocyte. These cells play a crucial role in the immune system, by coordinating the actions of other immune system cells. A large reduction in the number of T helper cells seriously weakens the immune system.

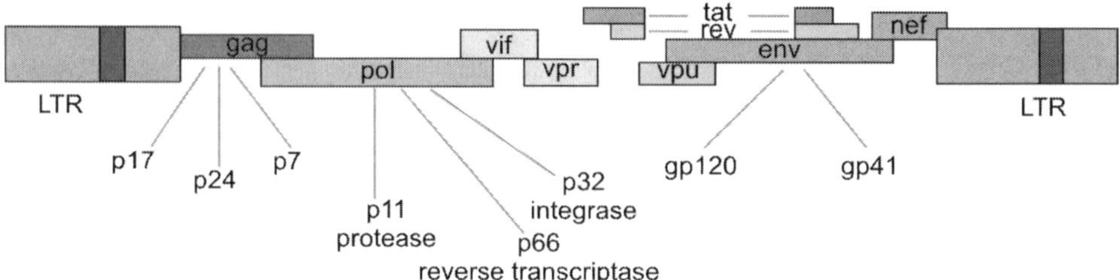

Fig. 29.2 HIV genes

- HIV infects the T helper cell via the CD4 protein on its surface, which HIV uses to attach itself to the cell before gaining entry. (This is why the T helper cell is sometimes referred to as a CD4+ lymphocyte.)
- Once it has found its way into a cell, HIV produces new copies of itself, which can then go on to infect other cells.
- HIV infection leads to low levels of CD4+ T cells through three main mechanisms—
  - First, direct viral killing of infected cells.
  - Second, increased rates of apoptosis in infected cells and
  - Third, killing of infected CD4+ T cells by CD8 cytotoxic lymphocytes that recognize infected cells.
  - When CD4+ T cell numbers decline below a critical level, cell-mediated immunity is lost, and the body becomes progressively more susceptible to opportunistic infections.
- The process usually takes several years.
- HIV infection can generally be broken down into four distinct stages: primary infection, clinically asymptomatic stage, symptomatic HIV infection, and progression from HIV to AIDS.

Primary Infection/Window Period

- This stage of infection lasts for a few weeks and is often accompanied by a short flu-like illness.
- Upto about 20% of people the HIV symptoms are serious enough to consult a doctor, but the diagnosis of HIV infection is frequently missed.
- During this stage there is a large amount of HIV in the peripheral blood and the immune system begins to respond to the virus by producing HIV antibodies and cytotoxic lymphocytes.
- This process is known as seroconversion. If an HIV antibody test is done before seroconversion is complete then it may not be positive.
- This is also termed as the *Window Period* and the viral capsid protein p24 can be detected during this time.

Clinically Asymptomatic HIV Infection/Seropositive Stage

- Antibodies can be detected in blood—Seropositive.
- HIV levels drop low but the patients are infectious and carriers of the virus.

- They remain normal without any symptoms.
- 10% go to next stage of AIDS within 5 years, 50% within 10 years and 90% within 15 years.

Symptomatic HIV Infection and Progression to AIDS

- The immune system is depressed or is 'burnt out' due to years of activity.
- HIV mutates and becomes more pathogenic.
- Antiretroviral therapy is started in this stage when CD4 count depletes severely. For e.g. – Reverse transcriptase inhibitors that may be nucleoside analogues like zidovudine or Nonnucleoside inhibitors like nevirapine or nucleotide inhibitor like Adefovir; Protease inhibitors like saquinavir, ritonavir, etc.
- Body becomes host to a number of commensal microbes resulting in multiple infectious diseases and the patient dies in two years.
- Clinically the AIDS patients show symptoms of:
  - Lymphadenopathy
  - Fever
  - Lesions of skin, GIT, lungs, urinary tract and brain.

Modes of Infection and Prevention

- Sexual transmission of the disease is a major contributor making up 80% of the total load.
- About 15% of the patients get the disease by infected blood or infected syringes as in case of drug addicts or in healthcare workers exposed to the virus during their work due to negligence of proper safety procedures.
- Rest 5% of the cases are of transmission from infected mother to fetus.
- Prevention is the best cure for AIDS. The major steps for prevention are:
  - Avoid unsafe sexual contact.
  - Dispose-off the syringes properly and do not reuse syringes unless autoclaved or boiled for more than 10 minutes.
  - Use of gloves and safety glasses by the laboratory and health care workers while dealing with AIDS patients and their blood samples.
  - Properly sterilize instruments and gloves. Blood spills to be decontaminated by 1% hypochlorite solution.
  - Checking the expecting mothers for the presence of the virus and medical termination of the pregnancy in case found seropositive.

Diagnostic Tests for AIDS

- Antibodies are detected using ELISA technique.
- Western blot is performed for further confirmation.
- T-helper cell count is checked.
- Real time PCR is done to count the number of HIV particles.

A Quick Look at the AIDS

- It is a retro virus, i.e. its genetic material is an RNA molecule which when enters the host cell, copies its genetic information into a DNA molecule via a RNA-dependent DNA polymerase—Reverse transcriptase.
- The important genes are:
  - gag – coding for p55 .
  - pol – coding for p160.
  - env – coding for gp160
- HIV infection leads to low levels of CD4+ T cells through three main mechanisms—
  - First, direct viral killing of infected cells.
  - Second, increased rates of apoptosis in infected cells
  - Third, killing of infected CD4+ T cells by CD8 cytotoxic lymphocytes that recognize infected cells.
  - When CD4+ T cell numbers decline below a critical level, cell-mediated immunity is lost, and the body becomes progressively more susceptible to opportunistic infections.
- HIV infection can generally be broken down into four distinct stages: primary infection, clinically asymptomatic stage, symptomatic HIV infection, and progression from HIV to AIDS.
- Diagnostic tests for AIDS:
  - Antibodies are detected using ELISA technique.
  - Western blot is performed for further confirmation.
  - T-helper cell count is checked.
  - Real time PCR is done to count the number of HIV particles.

CHAPTER

30

Xenobiotics Metabolism

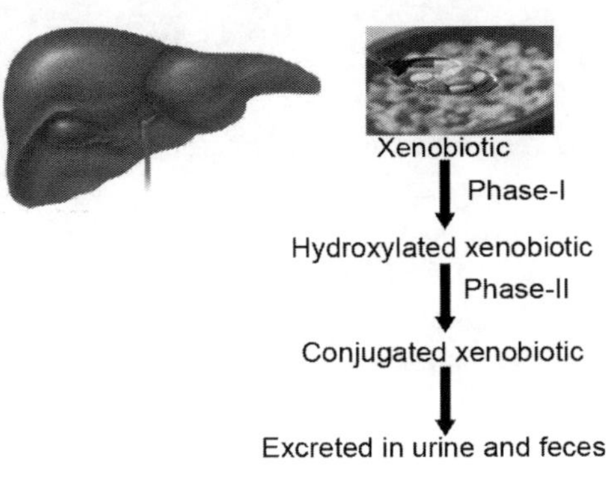

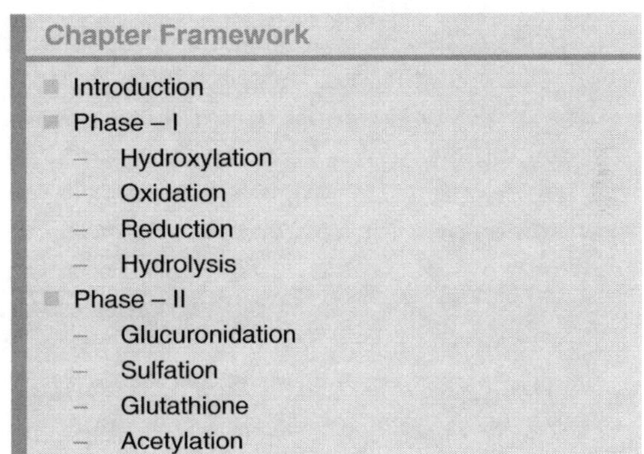

Chapter Framework

- Introduction
- Phase – I
  - Hydroxylation
  - Oxidation
  - Reduction
  - Hydrolysis
- Phase – II
  - Glucuronidation
  - Sulfation
  - Glutathione
  - Acetylation

Introduction

Human body is a bundle of miracles. It has all the necessary mechanisms not only for sustaining life but also various means to protect against harmful pathogens, viruses and chemicals.

Since time immemorial humans have been exposed to various chemicals, both endogenously produced and environmental. With the advancements in the human knowledge of drugs/ pharmacology and industrial chemistry there has been a barrage of chemicals to which the humans are exposed. Most of these chemicals are harmful either directly or on metabolism in body and must be removed; such compounds are called xenobiotics.

The enzymes machinery of human body has also evolved and devised techniques that help in detoxifying and removing these harmful drugs and chemicals. Xenobiotics metabolism involves 2 phases:

1. Phase—I-Where the xenobiotic is hydroxylated/oxidized/hydrolyzed/reduced.
2. Phase—II-Where the hydroxylated xenobiotic is conjugated with polar metabolites making them more water-soluble and easily excreted.

Phase – I

Hydroxylation of Xenobiotics Using CytP450

Site: Microsomes

- Cytochrome P450 is considered as one of the most versatile biocatalyst known.
- It is present in the microsomal fractions of the cell. The phase – I hydroxylation reaction occurs as shown in the reaction below by involving NADPH-CytP450 reductase, CytP450 and molecular oxygen.
- The substrate gets hydroxylated in the process by one atom of O2 and the second atom forms water. Due to this dual fate of oxygen they are also call the "*mixed function oxidases*".
- This is one of the most important enzymes of drug metabolism that is responsible for metabolizing 50% of drugs that humans ingest.
- There are about 150 different isoforms of CytP450, belonging to a single large super family.
- The different isoforms have been given a systemic nomenclature with CYP depicting CytP450, followed by an Arabic numeral, an alphabet and finally an Arabic numeral, each depicting family, sub family and individual number in that sub family respectively.
- CytP450 are widely distributed among tissues but highest concentration is present in liver and small intestine, in their microsomal fraction.
- However, in the adrenal gland, mitochondrial CytP450 is alone present which is involved in steroid hormones biosynthesis.
- Most CytP450 isoforms are inducible, for example administration of phenobarbital causes hypertrophy of ER. This has importance in drug interaction. This can be explained as follows:
  - If a patient is on warfarin to prevent blood clotting (metabolized by CYP2CP) and is administered phenobarbital, to treat epilepsy, the dosage of warfarin will have to be increased. This is because phenobarbital will induce CytP450 causing rapid metabolism of warfarin. Conversely, on discontinuing Phenobarbital, the dosage of warfarin will have to be reduced as there will be a decline in number of CytP450.
  - Not all CytP450 hydroxylation reactions cause drug detoxication, there are some which cause the hydroxylation of polycyclic aromatic hydrocarbons (PAHs) and make them carcinogenic and thus promote carcinogenesis.
  - Polymorphism shown by CtyP450 isoforms is responsible for the varied response of individuals to same drug.

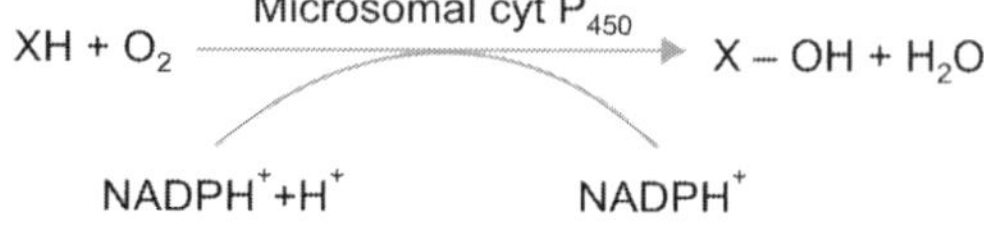

Oxidation

Oxidation of Alcohols and Aldehydes to Acids

- Alcohols and aldehydes are converted to corresponding acids by oxidation. For example:

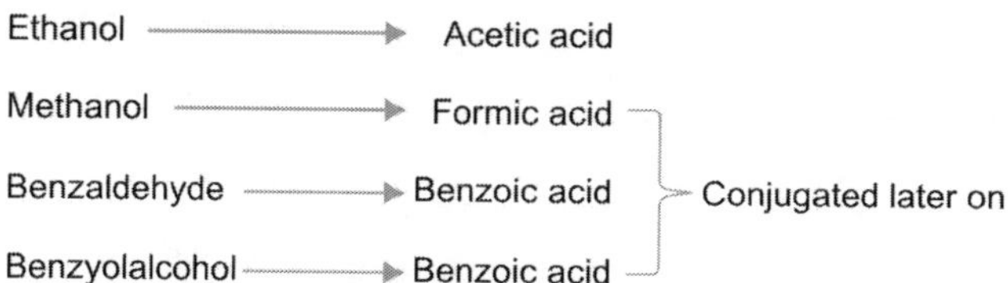

- Oxidation of methanol results in the production of formic acid, a more toxic compound then methanol which may be removed by phase II conjugation reaction.

Oxidation of Aromatic Hydrocarbons

Aromatic hydrocarbons are oxidized to phenols. Phenols may be removed by conjugation reaction. For e.g.

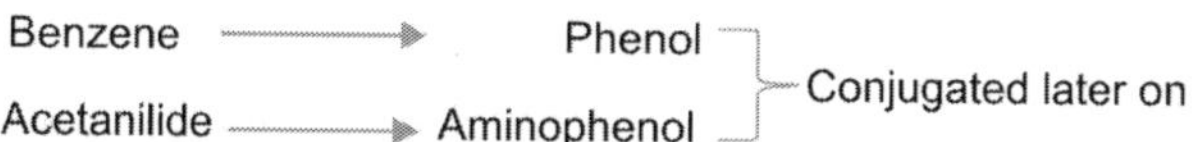

Oxidative Deamination of Amines

Aliphatic amines undergo oxidative deamination to the corresponding acids and nitrogen is converted to urea. For example—

Butylamine ⟶ Phenol
Benzylamine ⟶ Aminophenol

Oxidative Dealkylation of Hydrocarbons

Aromatic hydrocarbons containing alkyl group is oxidized to acids. For example—

Toluene ⟶ Benzoic acid

Reduction

Reduction is less common than oxidation. The major group of compounds, which are reduced and detoxified by the liver are azo-compounds and nitro-compounds. Some important reactions are:

- Aldehydes may be reduced to alcohol, e.g.

  Chloral ⟶ Trichloroethanol
- Aromatic nitro-compounds are reduced to amines, e.g.

  Picric acid ⟶ Picramic acid
- Compounds with S-S bonds reduced to –SH, e.g.

  Disulfiram ⟶ Dithiocarbamic acid (Used in the treatment of alcoholism)

Hydrolysis

Foreign compounds that are esters, amides or glycosides are subject to hydrolysis by esterases, amidases and glycosidases.

Phase – II

It involves 5 different types of conjugation reactions with polar entities, making the xenobiotics water-soluble and easily excretable.

Glucuronidation (Addition of Glucuronic Acid)

Molecules like aniline, benzoic acid, phenol, many steroids, bilirubin and 2-acetyl aminofluorine (carcinogen) are glucuronidated and excreted as glucuronides. UDP-glucuronic acid is the glucuronate donor.

Sulfation

- The sulfur donor is phospho adenosyl phospho sulfate (PAPS) also called active sulfate. Compounds which get sulfated are phenols, cresols, indole, skatole, steroids and aliphatic and aromatic amines.

Glutathione

- It is a tripeptide γ-glutamyl cysteinyl glycine. It is abbreviated as GSH depicting the thiol group present in it.
- Glutathione conjugates with various potentially toxic xenobiotics, renders them less toxic and finally the glutamyl and glycinyl groups are removed and an acetyl group (donated by acetyl CoA) is added producing mercapturic acid which is excreted.
- The compounds removed by glutathione are aromatic nitro-compounds, halogenated compounds, aliphatic halides, epoxides formed during phase-I reactions.
- The reaction is as follows:

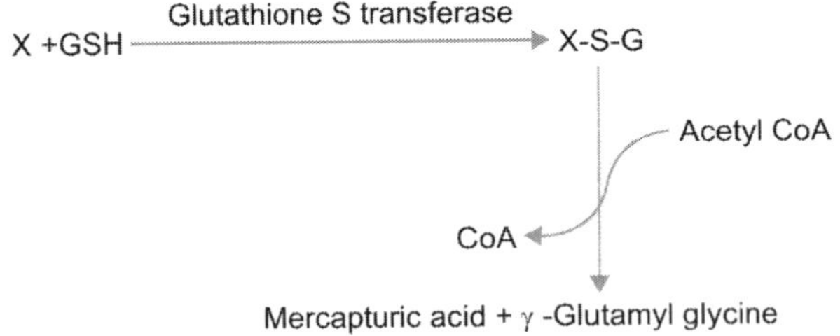

- This occurs in liver cells.

Acetylation

- Acetylation is addition of acetyl group to a xenobiotic in presence of transferases.
- This enzyme is present in the cytosol of liver cells, though is widely distributed.
- Drugs like—Isoniazid (anti-tubercular drug) is detoxified by this method.
- Some individuals are fast acetylators and some are slow acetylators, depending upon the polymorphic form of acetyl transferases present in them.

- Slow acetylators are prone to the toxic effects of isonazid, as the slow clearance causes the drug to persist in the body for a longer duration.
- There are several other conjugating agents used in drug detoxification like—Methylation (by S-adenosyl methionine), thiosulfate, cysteine, glycine (bile salts), british anti lewsite (BAL) detoxified by heavy metals, glutamine conjugates phenyl acetyl glutamine.
- Responses to xenobiotics on metabolism varies with age, gender and also individual to individual these responses may be pharmacologic, i.e. the xenobiotic maybe metabolized to form the biologically active form of drug.
- The xenobiotic in some cases converts to a more toxic form, e.g. Pro-carcinogen gets activated to carcinogen which exerts the toxic effect by binding to cellular proteins, DNA, RNA or enzymes and become cytotoxic or exert carcinogenic effect.
- Some xenobiotics may bind to a cellular protein and become antigenic, exerting immunologic effect.
- With advancements in our knowledge regarding xenobiotic metabolism, it is hoped we will be able to devise drugs that have fewer side effects and avoid undesirable drug interactions.

A Quick Look at the Xenobiotics

- Xenobiotics are the various chemicals and drugs to which the human body is exposed and are harmful either directly or on metabolism.
- Xenobiotic metabolism occurs in two stages:
  - Phase-I, where the xenobiotic is hydroxylated/ oxidized/ hydrolyzed/ reduced.
  - Phase-II, where the hydroxylated xenobiotic is conjugated with polar metabolites making them more water-soluble and easily excreted.

CHAPTER

31

Free Radicals and Antioxidants in Health and Disease

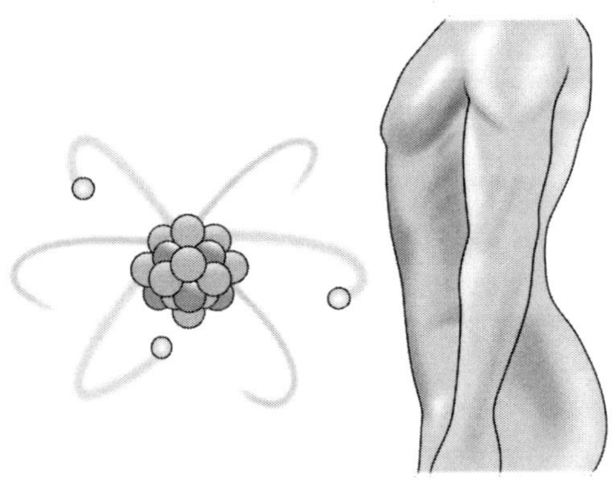

Chapter Framework

- Introduction
- What are Free Radicals?
- Generation of Free Radicals
- Free Radicals in Diseases
- Antioxidants

Introduction

- Over the last 20 years scientists have been able to demonstrate a common link among the various chronic diseases that currently plague people all over the world for example, conditions such as cancer, Alzheimer's disease, rheumatoid arthritis, cardiovascular disease, and cataracts as well as the actual aging process itself all may be, in part, caused by a phenomenon known as oxidative or free radical damage. The term oxidative is used because oxygen is frequently involved.
- Antioxidants, on the other hand, are chemical compounds that can prevent, stop, or reduce oxidative damage.
- It is the balance between the free radicals that are produced and the amount of antioxidants available to prevent or reduce the free radicals that actually determines the amount of tissue damage.

What are Free Radicals?

- Normal atoms have a central nucleus containing positive protons and neutral neutrons with electrons revolving in fixed orbits around the nucleus.
- The electrons in atoms are paired. However, if these atoms loose an electron leaving an unpaired electron, it now becomes the free radical.
- Free radicals are highly reactive molecules that are generated by the process of oxidation and invariably involve an oxygen molecule too. Thus these are also termed as the reactive oxygen species (ROS).

- Types of ROS include the hydroxyl radical, the superoxide anion radical, hydrogen peroxide, singlet oxygen, nitric oxide radical, hypochlorite radical, and various lipid peroxides.

Generation of Free Radicals

- Many compounds of our body are capable of being converted to free radicals by natural events that remove one of their electrons, or by radiation. Radiation, for example, dissociates water into the hydrogen atom and the hydroxyl radical.

$$H_2O \longrightarrow OH^{\cdot} + H^{\cdot}$$

- Transition metal ions like Cu^+, Co^{++}, Ni^{++} and Fe^{++} can react non enzymatically with oxygen or H_2O_2 leading to formation of hydroxyl free radicals.
- Free radicals are also generated during the defence mechanism by the macrophages which engulf bacteria and by respiratory burst generate a superoxide anion in the presence of respiratory burst oxidase and NADPH+ H^+.
- Another source of free radicals is the mitochondrial and microsomal electron transport chains. Although their end-products are not radicals; however considerable radicals leak through.
- 3% to 5% of the daily consumption of 30 mols of oxygen by an adult human being is converted to singlet oxygen, hydrogen peroxide, and superoxide, perhydroxyl and hydroxyl radicals, rather than undergoing complete reduction to water.
- The most damaging radicals in biological systems are oxygen radicals especially superoxide (O_2), hydroxyl (OH), and perhydroxyl (O_2H). Tissue damage caused by oxygen radicals is often called oxidative damage.
- Free radicals are self-perpetuating by chain reaction.

Free Radical in Diseases

- Free radicals cause damage to the biochemical integrity of the cells by interacting with DNA, lipids and proteins. Free radical damage in germ cells DNA causes heritable mutations that may be extremely harmful.
- Free radicals cause single strand breakage of DNA strand which causes somatic mutations and even cancer.
- The ROS cause peroxidation of the PUFA of the biological membranes. This causes the loss of membrane integrity and cell damage.
- The peroxidation of PUFA can further cause chemical modification in the amino acids constituting body proteins. Such proteins are considered as immunogenic to the immune system generating antibodies.
- Free radicals also cause the depolymerization of the mucopolysaccharides leading to the degradation of the ground cementing substance of the tissues and tissue necrosis.
- Oxidative damage to DNA, proteins, and other macromolecules has been implicated in the pathogenesis of a wide variety of diseases.
- Most important diseases that are caused by free radical damage are—Cancer, heart diseases, pulmonary disorders, cataracts, etc. Some other important diseases caused by oxidative damage are shown in Table 31.1.

Table 31.1 Diseases related to oxidative stress

• Atherosclerosis	• Multiple Sclerosis
• Cancer	• Pancreatitis
• Pulmonary dysfunction	• Inflammatory bowel disease and colitis
• Cataracts	• Parkinsons's disease
• Arthritis and inflammatory diseases	• Neonatal lipoprotein oxidation
• Diabetes	• Drug reactions
• Shock, trauma and ischemia	• Skin lesions
• Renal disease and hemodialysis	• Aging

Antioxidants

- Mother nature has armed the human body with a variety of antioxidants that give protection against the free radical damage.
- The antioxidants are mainly categorized as:
  - Endogenous antioxidants
  - Exogenous antioxidants.

Endogenous Antioxidants

- The human body is armed with a number of enzyme systems and proteins that act as antioxidants and give protection against the free radical damage.
- The most significant of these endogenous antioxidant systems are:
  - Glutathione peroxidase (Se-dependent) (Discussed under Selenium)
  - Superoxide dismutase (Cu and Zn-dependent) (Discussed under Copper)
  - Catalase (Fe-dependent) (Discussed under Iron)
  - Other antioxidants are—Bilirubin, uric acid, CoQ10, metal binding proteins like—ceruloplasmin, transferrin, ferritin, myoglobin, metallothionin, etc.

Exogenous Antioxidants

- The endogenous antioxidants are further strengthened by a host of exogenous/dietary antioxidants. Most of these exogenous antioxidants are plant products hence also termed as phytochemicals.
- These dietary antioxidants are further classified as water-soluble and fat-soluble antioxidants.
- The water-soluble antioxidants include:
  - *Vitamin C*—Well over 100 studies have reported that reduction in cancer risk is associated with a diet high in vitamin C.
  - *Polyphenols like* flavonoids—Flavonoids have been demonstrated to have anti-inflammatory, antiallergenic, antiviral, anti-aging, and anticarcinogenic activity.
- The fat-soluble antioxidants include:
  - *β-carotene*—Carotenoids, especially β-carotenes have been implicated in reducing the risk of lung cancer and an increased incidence of lung cancer in populations consuming

diet low in β-carotenes have been reported. Other carotenoids are: Lycopene found in tomatoes, watermelon etc. Lutein found in corn and egg yolk, zeaxanthin and anthocyanin all of which have been reported to have antioxidant properties.

- *Resveratrol*—It found in grapes, peanuts and red wine. It maintains the telomeric ends, thus has anti-ageing effect proven in experimental animals.
- *Tocopherols (Vitamin—E)* It is the first line of defence against peroxidation of PUFA by ROS (details discussed in Chapter 6).

The various endogenous and exogenous antioxidants together work as a team and protect the cellular machinery against the harmful effects of the ROS. As shown in the Figure 31.1, the various antioxidants are focused at different cellular sites like:

- Peroxisomes—It contain catalase.
- Mitochondria—It contain superoxide dismutase (Mn-dependent)
- Nucleus and ER are protected by Vitamin E and β-carotene.
- Cytoplasmic SOD (Cu and Zn-dependent) is a strong antioxidant protecting against the cytoplasmic ROS.
- The various ROS are neutralized by the antioxidants as shown in Table 31.2.

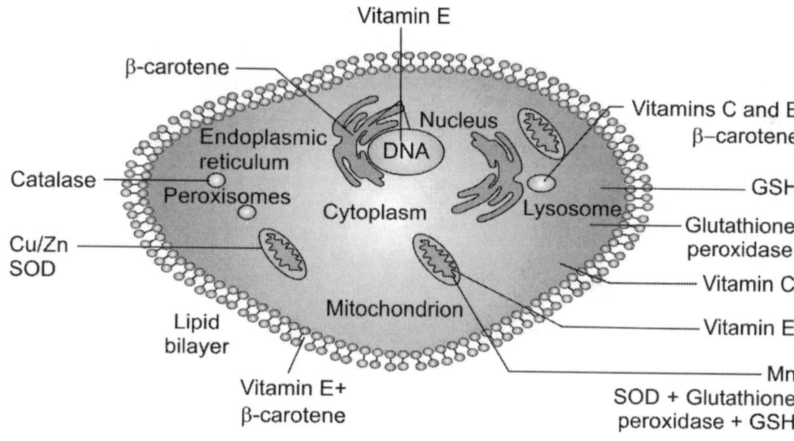

Fig. 31.1 Cellular sites of various antioxidants

Table 31.2 ROS and their neutralizing antioxidants

Reactive oxygen species	*Neutralizing antioxidants*
Hydroxy radical	Vitamin C, GSH, flavanoids
Superoxide anion	Vitamin C, GSH, flavonoids, SOD
H_2O_2	Vitamin C, GSH, β-carotene, vitamin E, CoQ_{10}, flavonoids
Lipid peroxides	β–carotene, tocopherols, ubiquinone, flavonoids, GSH peroxidase

A Quick Look at the Free Radicals and Antioxidants

- Free radicals are reactive oxygen species with an unpaired electron in their valence shell.
- Important free radicals are—Hydroxy, peroxy, alkoxy, lipid peroxides and superoxide anion.
- The free radicals are generated by oxidative mechanisms during metabolic reactions.
- These are produced in a chain reaction and continue to produce more and more free radicals thus posing great health risk.
- The free radicals cause damage to the:
  - DNA by causing single strand DNA breakage leading to somatic mutations.
  - Cell membrane by causing disturbance in membrane integrity due to peroxidation of membrane PUFA.
  - Tissues as they cause depolymerization MPS of ground substance of tissues.
- A number of diseases are caused by free radical damage like cancer, Alzheimer's, diabetes, cardiovascular diseases, parkinson's disease, etc.
- Free radicals are scavenged by antioxidants.
- Antioxidants can be endogenous and exogenous.
- Endogenous antioxidants are certain enzymes present in the body like GSH peroxidase, catalse, SOD, etc.
- Exogenous antioxidants are derived from the diet we consume as vitamins and minerals like Vitamin E, β-carotene, selenium, etc.

CHAPTER

32

Regulation of Acid-Base Balance

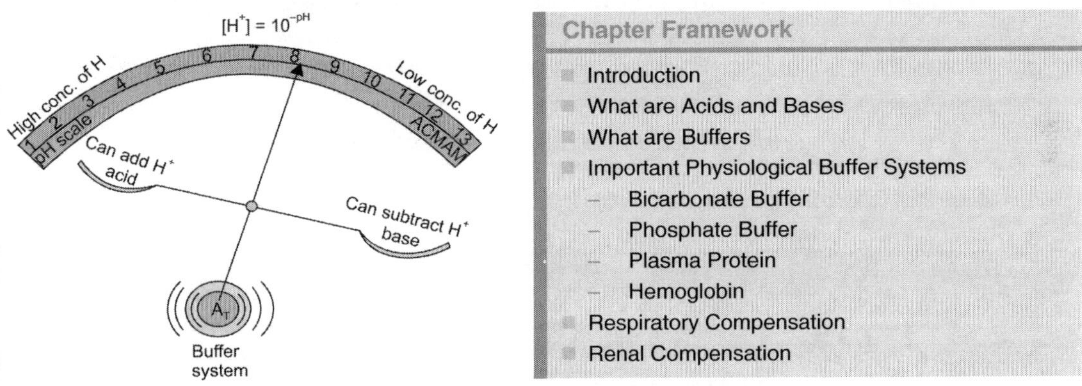

Chapter Framework

Introduction

- The regulation of a normal pH/ acid–base balance in the human body is of pronounced significance for the maintenance of normal cellular function.
- pH is a number ranging from 0 to 14, defining the acidity or alkalinity of a medium. pH 7 is neutral, below 7 is acidic and above 7 is alkaline. The normal physiological pH ranges from 7.35 to 7.45.
- pH is negative log of H^+ concentration and according to the *Henderson – Hasselbalch equation* it is dependent upon pKa and concentration of weak acid and its corresponding base.

$$\frac{pH = pKa + \log[A^-]}{[HA]}$$

- This balance is controlled by the lungs, kidneys, and serum buffers, interacting and responding to physiologic changes.
- Physiologic insults such as vomiting, diarrhea, respiratory failure, kidney dysfunction, diabetes, toxic ingestions, among others can result in life-threatening acid–base crises.

What are Acids and Bases?

Acids

- Acids are defined as substances that release H^+ on dissolving in water causing a rise in the $[H^+]$ and dropping the pH.

- A number of organic acids are generated during metabolic processes in the human body like lactic acid, citric acid, oxalic acid, ketone bodies, carbonic, acid etc. Carbonic acid is volatile acid since it dissociates to give water and CO_2 which is expired and the other metabolic acids are nonvolatile acids (N-V acids)
- Some acids are added through the diet or drugs we consume like organic acids—Citric acid or phosphoric acid or mandelic acid, etc.

Bases

Bases are defined as substances that pick up free H^+ from their surrounding medium causing a drop in $[H^+]$ concentration and raising pH.

- Physiologically, pH of blood rises not due to addition of alkali but more so due to the drop of H^+ concentration raising the blood pH.
- The different lines of defence against the alteration in blood pH are:
  - Physiological buffers
  - Respiratory compensation
  - Renal compensation.

What are Buffers?

- Buffers may be defined as solution of a weak acid and its corresponding salt with its strong base.

$$H^+ + \text{buffer-Na} \longrightarrow \text{buffer-}H^+ + Na^+$$

- A buffer is a substance that prevents a drastic change of pH by acting as an acid (donating H^+) when the medium turns alkaline sharply or as a base (accepting extra H^+) when the medium turns acidic sharply. Thus extreme changes of pH are prevented in presence of buffers.
- *Henderson-Hasselbalch equation* for buffers can be represented as

$$\frac{pH = pKa + \log [base]}{[acid]}$$

- The maintenance of a normal physiological pH is achieved by certain important blood buffers like—$NaHCO_3/H_2CO_3$, plasma proteins.

Important Physiological Buffer Systems (1st line of defence) (Table 32.1)

Physiological buffers are the first line of defence against any change in the acid–balance of our body.

Bicarbonate Buffer

- $NaHCO_3/H_2CO_3$ 20/1
- It is the most significant buffer of ECF.
- The concentration of bicarbonate in plasma is fairly high (26 mmol – 28 mmol/L). The concentration of H_2CO_3 is calculated by the product of arterial PCO_2 (40 mm of Hg) and solubility constant of $CO_2 = 0.03$.
- Thus HCO^-_3 concentration comes to be 1.2 mmol/L which is much lower than plasma bicarbonate concentration.

Table 32.1 Important physiologic buffers

ECF buffers	*ICF buffers*	*RBCs buffers*
$NaHCO_3/H_2CO_3$	$KHCO_3/H_2CO_3$	$KHCO_3/H_2CO_3$
Na_2HPO_4/NaH_2PO_4	K_2HPO_4/ KH_2PO_4	K_2HPO_4/KH_2PO_4
Na^+/H^+ Albumin	K^+/Protein/H^+/Protein	K^+-Hb/H^+-Hb

- This is the most important physiological buffer as it is present in high concentration 26 mEq to 28 mEq/L.
- This system provides the *alkali reserve.*
- Alkali reserve is the concentration of $NaHCO_3$ which has not yet combined with a non- volatile acid.
- The system is open-ended; continuous removal of organic acid is made possible by the exhalation of carbon dioxide (CO_2). In equilibrium, the equation is as follows:

$$H^+ + HCO_3 - Na \longrightarrow H_2CO_3 \longrightarrow H_2O + CO_2$$

$$\text{Nonvolatile acid} + NaHCO_3 \longrightarrow H_2CO_3 + \text{Na salt of N-V acid}$$

$$\downarrow$$

$$H_2O + CO_2\uparrow$$

- This system is directly linked to the lungs and a normal respiratory mechanism is must.

Phosphate Buffer

- Na_2HPO_4/NaH_2PO_4::4/1
- It is mainly linked to the kidney and is not a very good physiological buffer as it is present in low concentration (1mmol/lit).
- This is mostly intracellular.

Plasma Proteins

- Proteins being amphoteric in nature act as physiological buffers i.e. they prevent the change in blood pH from normal physiological range. The prime plasma protein to act as a buffer is albumin.
- NaPr/HPr

Na Pr	+	HL ⟶	NaL	+	Pr H
Sodium salt of Protein		N-V acid	Sodium salt of N-V acid		Weak acid of plasma protein

Hemoglobin

- Hb is also a very important buffer system.
- It acts as a buffer due to the presence of multiple -NH2 group, -COOH group and most importantly imidazole group of histidine in its globin part.
- The imidazole group of histidine is attached with Fe^{++} of heme and also has an -NH group that is dissociated when required for buffering action.
- During oxygenation of heme, the imidazole NH releases H^+ at lungs such that it combines to HCO_3 to form $H_2CO_3 \longrightarrow CO_2 + H_2O$.

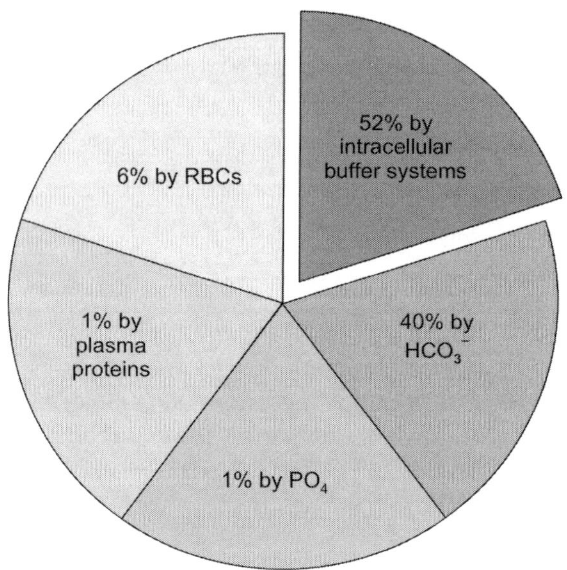

Fig. 32.2 Blood buffers

- Conversely during deoxygenation or release of O_2 at tissues it acts as a base picking up H^+ present at the tissues along with CO_2.
- If hemoglobin did not exist, venous blood would be 800 times more acidic than arterial blood, circulating at a pH of 4.5 instead of the normal venous pH of 7.37.
- Of the total buffering by the blood buffers:
  - Intracellular buffers are similar to the extracellular ones, i.e. bicarbonate buffer ($KHCO_3$/H_2CO_3), phosphate buffer ($KHPO_4$/H_2PO_4) except that they have K salts rather than Na salts since K is the major intracellular cation.

Respiratory Compensation (2nd line of Defense)

- Respiratory compensation is a rapid compensation, helping maintain the acid – base balance in acute conditions.
- The respiratory compensation is the secondary mode of managing the acid – base balance. It involves the peripheral and central chemoreceptors located at the carotid arteries and medulla oblongata respectively. An alteration in PCO_2 alters the blood pH.

$$CO_2 + H_2O \longrightarrow H_2CO_3 \longrightarrow H^+ + HCO^-_3$$

- An increased H^+ concentration owing to the metabolic activities producing CO_2 stimulates the respiratory centers for hyperventilation, flushing out excessive CO_2 thus reducing the concentration of H_2CO_3 and the ratio of $H_2CO_3/HCO_3 < 20$ thus the normal pH is maintained.
- Alternately if the blood pH is raised, the respiratory centers at medulla and the carotid chemoreceptors shall be inhibited thus causing hypoventilation, retention of CO_2 so that the concentration of H_2CO_3 is raised and the ratio of H_2CO_3/HCO_3 is >20.
- For respiratory compensation a healthy respiratory system is a must.

Renal Compensation (3rd line of Defense)

- Kidneys are another significant mode of compensation for an alteration in the acid – base balance and come next in the line to the respiratory compensation.
- However, kidneys respond slow and not to acute changes in acid – base imbalances but give a permanent solution to acid – base imbalances by secreting H^+ ions. Thus the pH of normal urine is slightly acidic (approximately 6.0).
- Kidneys maintain the acid – base balance by primarily secreting H + and reabsorbing the HCO_3 at the renal tubules.
- There are three different mechanisms for secretion of H+ ions at the renal tubules:
  - Bicarbonate method (at PCT)
  - Phosphate method (PCT and DCT) } *Contribute to titrable acidity of urine*
  - Ammonia method (PCT)

Bicarbonate Method

Site—Proximal Convoluted Tubules

- At the PCT of kidneys, the tubular cells synthesize carbonic acid from metabolic CO_2 or CO_2 which diffuses into tubular cells (Fig. 32.3).
- Carbonic acid in presence of carbonic anhydrase dissociates into H^+ and HCO_3^-.
- The tubular cells then secrete H^+ actively into the tubular lumen in exchange for a Na^+ into the tubular cell.
- The bicarbonate ions passively follow the Na^+ ions thus maintaining the alkali reserve of blood. The normal urine is thus free of HCO_3^-.
- Thus, each time an H^+ is formed in the tubular epithelial cells, an HCO_3^- is also formed and released back into the blood.
- The HCO_3^- reabsorbed is not the one that is filtered at glomerulus because the filtered HCO_3^- combines with secreted H^+ to form carbonic acid and is excreted. The reabsorbed bicarbonate is the one formed during metabolic activities.

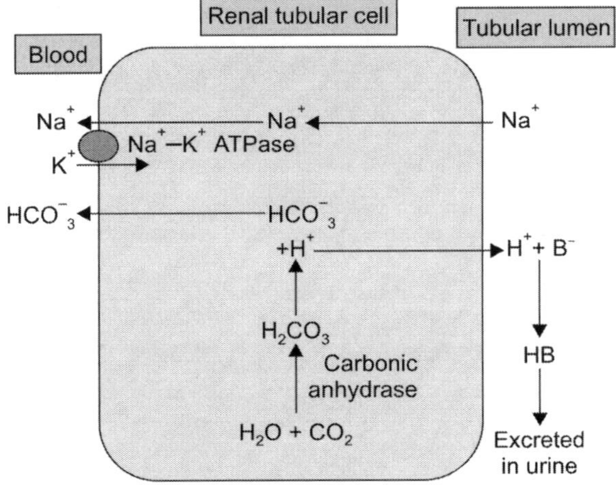

Fig. 32.3 Bicarbonate method of renal acid – base regulations

Phosphate Method

Site—Complete Renal Tubules

- The titrable acidity of urine is contributed by this method.
- The plasma phosphate exists as monohydrogen phosphate (80%) and dihydrogen phosphate (20%).
- At the PCT and DCT the H^+ are secreted with an anti – port of Na^+ as shown in Figure 32.4.

Ammonia Method

Site—PCT, Loop of Henle and DCT

- The ammonia buffer is yet another important renal tubular buffer system that is quantitatively more than phosphate buffer.

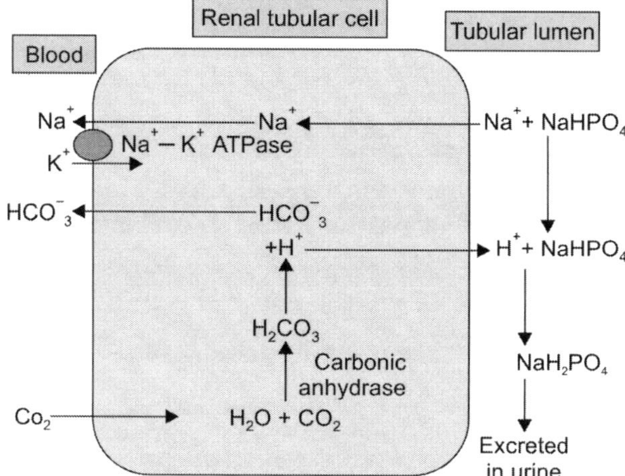

Fig. 32.4 Titrable acidity of urine added by phosphate method

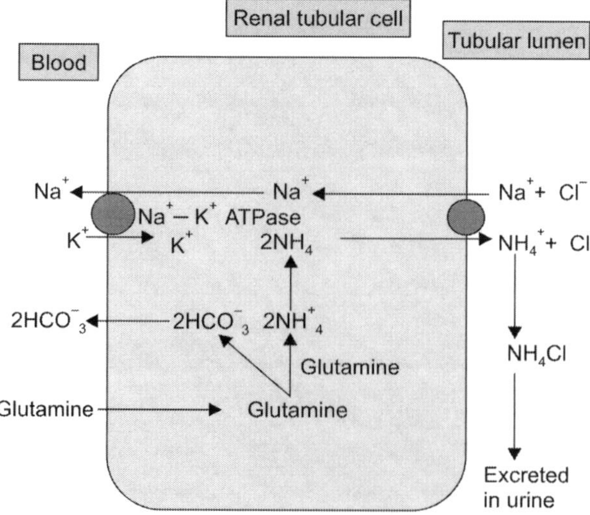

Fig. 32.5 Ammonia method of urine acidification

- The glutamine synthesized as a result of amino acid metabolism at liver is transported to the renal tubules where in the presence of glutaminase it splits into 2 NH_4^+ and HCO_3^- (Figure 32.5).
- NH_4^+ ions are secreted into the renal tubules as titrable acidity. For every glutamine metabolized at kidneys, two moles of bicarbonate ions are reabsorbed into blood and 2 H^+ secreted into renal tubules as NH_4^+ ions adding up to acidity of urine.

Imbalances of Acid – Base and Their Compensatory Mechanisms

Table 32.2 Comparison of Acidosis and Alkalosis

	Respiratory acidosis	*Metabolic acidosis*	*Respiratory alkalosis*	*Metabolic alkalosis*
pH (7.35 – 7.45)	decreases (↓)	decreases (↓)	increases (↑)	increases (↑)
Pco_2 (40 mm of Hg)	increases (↑↑)	decreases (↓)	decreases (↓↓)	increases (↑)
HCO_3^- (22 mmol–26mmol/L)	increase (↑) disproportionate increase in HCO_3/ H_2CO_3	decrease (↓↓) disproportionate decrease in HCO_3/ H_2CO_3	decrease (↓)	increases (↑↑)
Compensation	1^0 Renal 2^0 Respiratory	1^0 – Respiratory (hyperventilation) 2^0 – Renal	1^0 Renal 2^0 Respiratory	1^0 – Respiratory (hypoventilation) 2^0 – Renal
Urine acidity	Increased titrable acidity	Increased titrable acidity	Reduced titrable acidity	Reduced titrable acidity
Causes	Hypoventilation due to inhibition of respiratory centers, Air way obstruction – asthma, reduced elasticity of lungs as in emphysema	Diabetic and starvation ketoacidosis, severe exercise lactic acidosis, severe diarrhea, ingestion of acidic drugs like mandelic acid or ammonium salts.	Hyperventilation due to excessive stimulation of respiratory centers as in CNS diseases, meningitis, salicylate poisoning, hyperpyrexia.	Excessive loss of HCl as in high intestinal obstruction, pylorospasm, due to alkali ingestion, excessive loss of K^+, X-ray therapy or uv radiation therapy.

Anion gap

- *Plasma anion gap: It is the gap between positively and negatively charged ions: $(Na^+ + K^+) - (Cl^- + HCO_3^-)$*
- *Normal range: 8 mmol to 16 mmol/l. The net negative charge on albumin accounts for most of the normal anion gap.*
- *The ionic charges of other cations (Mg^{2+} Ca^{2+}) and anions (HPO_4^- and urate-) tend to balance each other.*
- *Urinary anion gap: $(Na^+ + K^+)U - (Cl^-)U$.*
- *Normal range: minus 20 mmol to 50 mmol.*
- *It helps in differential diagnosis of metabolic acidosis.*

A Quick Look at the Regulation of Acid – Base Balance

- The normal physiological pH ranges from 7.35 – 7.45.
- This balance is controlled by the lungs, kidneys, and serum buffers, interacting and responding to physiologic changes.
- Acids are defined as substances that release H^+ on dissolving in water causing a rise in the $[H^+]$ and dropping the pH.
- Bases are defined as substances that pick up free H^+ from their surrounding medium causing a drop in $[H^+]$ concentration and raising pH.
- Buffers may be defined as solution of a weak acid and its corresponding salt with its strong base.
- Physiological buffers first line of defence.
- Bicarbonate buffer—$NaHCO_3$/ H_2CO_3 :: 20/1.
- Alkali reserve is the concentration of NaHCO3 which has not yet combined with a nonvolatile acid.
- Phosphate buffer—Na_2HPO_4 / NaH_2PO_4 :: 4/1
- Hb acts as buffer due to multiple NH_2 and -COOH groups and imidazole group.
- Respiratory mechanism is the second line of defence.
- Respiratory compensation is a rapid compensation, helping maintain the acid – base balance in acute conditions.
- Kidneys are the third line of defence.
- Kidneys respond slow and not to acute changes in acid – base imbalances but give a permanent solution to acid – base imbalances by secreting H^+ ions.

CHAPTER

33

Biochemistry of Saliva and Dental Caries

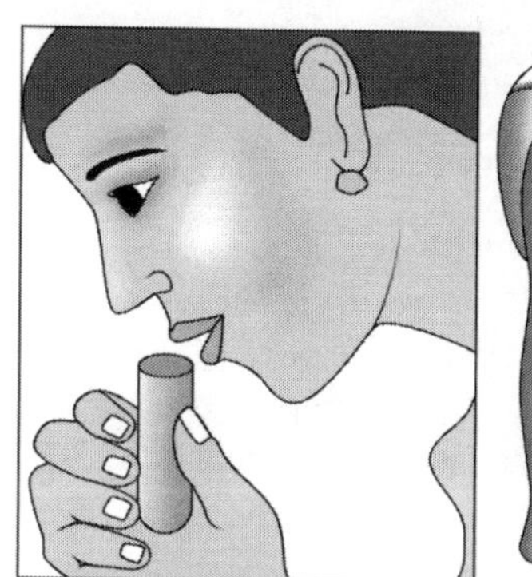

Saliva collection

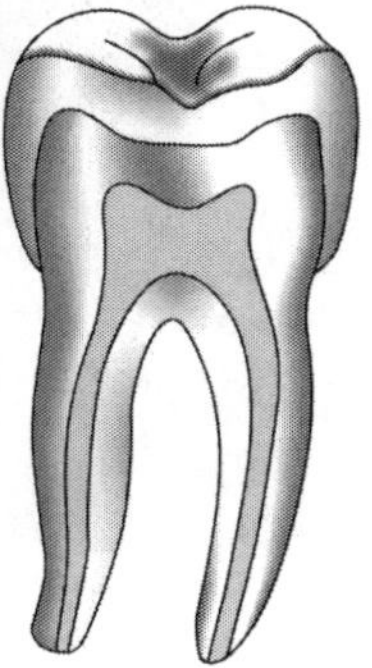

Chapter Framework

- Introduction
- Saliva Composition and Functions
- Saliva Analysis and its Clinical Significance
- Dental Caries

Introduction

Saliva is the watery secretion of the salivary glands. It is secreted in response to both sympathetic and parasympathetic stimulation. Adequate saliva is essential in maintaining oral health. It is a complex body fluid that has both digestive as well as protective functions. The ancient Greeks were among the first to recognize the medicinal value of saliva over 2000 years ago when they placed nonvenomous snake saliva on wounds to aid in healing. Today salivary analysis is proving to be an important noninvasive mode of diagnostics and shows promise for the future. Saliva has been attributed one very important role that of oral clearance or flushing and thus help prevent dental caries—A very important and frequently encountered dental problem.

Saliva Composition and Functions

Composition of Saliva

- The human salivary gland system can be divided into two distinct exocrine groups. The major salivary glands include the paired parotid, submandibular, and sublingual glands.
- Additionally, the mucosa of the upper aero-digestive tract is lined by hundreds of small, minor salivary glands.
- A healthy person's mean daily saliva production ranges from 1–1.5 to 4L. The salivary flow (SF) index is a parameter allowing stimulated and unstimulated saliva flow to be classified as normal, low, or very low (hyposalivation).
- Individuals should be analyzed for both stimulated and unstimulated SF index since there are biologic variations in the stimulated and unstimulated saliva.

- Human saliva is composed of 99.5% water, while the other 0.5% consists of electrolytes, mucus, glycoproteins, enzymes, and antibacterial compounds such as secretory IgA and lysozyme.
- The major electrolytes of saliva are NaCl and Na_2CO_3.
- Mucin provides for the viscosity of saliva. Besides mucin the other major proteins of saliva are α-amylase and proline-rich proteins.
- Total salivary proteins in an individual maintaining good oral hygiene is 1.6mg/ml (approximately) which is much lower than plasma concentration of proteins. Half of these proteins are as amylase, proline-rich proteins (40%–45%) and 5%–10% is mucin.
- Stimulated saliva has 20% less protein than unstimulated.
- Salivary glands also secrete urea which is converted to ammonia and carbon dioxide by urease enzyme. Ammonia in the oral cavity helps buffer acids and gives protection from caries.
- Calcium and phosphorous are also present in the saliva in supersaturating state but their precipitation is avoided by the proteins chelation.
- Whole saliva also contains several other proteins in small concentrations like–Proteases, protease inhibitors, lysozyme, carbonic anhydrase, immunoglobulin A and salivary agglutinins.
- Total or whole saliva refers to the complex mixture of fluids from the salivary glands, the gingival fold, oral mucosa transudate, in addition to mucus of the nasal cavity and pharynx, nonadherent oral bacterial, food remainders, desquamated epithelial and blood cells, as well as traces of medications or chemical products.

Functions of Saliva

- The important functions of saliva are:

Lubrication and Digestion

Mucin and water together help in lubrication. Lubrication of oral cavity helps in proper speech. Lubrication of food bolus and to hold together food bolus. This property of lubrication has a dual role of both assistance in chewing and digestion of food. Salivary amylase helps digest boiled starch and lingual lipase hydrolyses emulsified fats.

Protection Against Bacterial Acid

Carbonic anhydrase helps protect teeth from bacterial acid dissolution.

Immune Function

Innate immunity of saliva mediated by peroxidase, lactoferrin and lysozyme and various other proteins like salivary agglutinins and proline-rich proteins protects against bacterial infections.

Oral Health

One of the important functions of saliva is maintenance of oral hard tissue integrity by providing mechanical cleansing, buffering effect, antimicrobial actions and maintaining saturation with respect to hydroxyapatite (calcium and phosphate) in the saliva.

Oral Clearance

Saliva dilutes and eliminates dietary sugars and acids as well as oral micro-organisms from the mouth by a process referred to as oral clearance which depends upon SF index. Reduce the adherence of bacteria to teeth by the washing out/ clearance of oral cavity.

Buffering Action

Another important function of saliva is its ability to buffer acids, which is essential for maintaining pH values in the oral environment above the critical pH for hydroxyapatite. The saliva buffer capacity includes the bicarbonate, phosphate and protein systems.

Saliva Analysis and its Clinical Significance *(Biochemical Analysis of Saliva in Practical Biochemistry Section)*

- As we approach the threshold of genomic medicine, the increasing use of salivary diagnostics will help catalyze a shift from disease diagnosis to health surveillance. With new techniques for detecting small quantities of salivary components, including proteins and messenger RNA (mRNA), the field of salivary diagnostics has emerged as one of dentistry's most promising areas of research.
- Because collecting saliva is noninvasive, it is becoming the popular way diagnostic field today.
- With the establishment of the saliva research base, dental and biomedical researchers now have the scientific foundation upon which it can develop clinical tools that accurately screen salivary samples for the presence or absence of disease-specific biomarkers.
- Today a number of diseases can be diagnosed using salivary analysis in a clinical laboratory. A number of analytical kits have been developed for the purpose and found to be useful in diagnosis of a number of diseases like:
  - Salivary hormone levels *(Cortisol in Cushing's syndrome)*.
  - Salivary viral particles have been found to be reliable in HIV1 and 2 diagnosis.
  - Salivary proteomic analysis in *Prediabetes*.
  - Salivary TC, TG, LDLc and VLDL have been found to be high in patients of *Ischemic stroke*.
  - Researchers have found that panels of salivary mRNA (messenger ribonucleic acid) and protein markers can serve as biomarkers for *Oral cancer* detection.

Implications of Salivary Diagnostic Research for the Dental Profession

- Saliva-based tests also offer the following advantages for patients and providers:
  - Ease of collection.
  - Lower costs for sample collection.
  - Elimination of the common fear of needle.
  - Reduced risks of percutaneous injury.
- Salivary diagnostics could dramatically change the clinical practice by introducing point-of-care testing and real-time disease surveillance. Dentistry can help this vision become a reality, because many patients see their dentists more often than their physicians.

Dental Caries

- The tooth surface is unique among all body surfaces in two ways. First, it is a nonshedding hard surface, and, second, this surface is introduced into the human mouth during the first years of life.
- Dental caries is an infectious microbiologic disease of the calcified tissues of teeth, characterized by demineralization of the inorganic portion and destruction of the organic substance of the tooth.

- It is common disease that spreads across all age groups with frequency of incidence more among children than adults.
- The disease begins from the surface of the tooth and if left untreated can progress through the dentin to the pulp cavity leading to pain, infection and even tooth loss.

Etiology

- The lubricating and antimicrobial functions of saliva are maintained mainly by resting saliva. Stimulation of saliva results in a flushing effect and the clearance of oral debris and noxious agents.
- The demineralization of dental caries is caused by acids produced by bacteria, particularly *Mutans Streptococci* and possibly *Lactobacilli* that ferment dietary carbohydrates. This occurs within a bacteria-laden gelatinous material called *dental plaque* that adheres to tooth surfaces and becomes colonized by bacteria. Thus, caries results from the interplay of three main factors over time:
  - Dietary carbohydrates.
  - Cariogenic bacteria within dental plaque.
  - Susceptible hard tooth surfaces.
- Children who develop colonization of *mutans streptococci* in early life are difficult to manage and suffer from caries than those who get the bacteria later since it is difficult to completely eliminate them.

Prevention of Dental Caries

- Probably the most important caries-preventive functions of saliva are the flushing and neutralizing effects, commonly referred to as "salivary clearance" or "oral clearance capacity". In general, the higher the flow rate, the faster the clearance and the higher the buffer capacity and lesser the incidence of caries.
- Another very significant modus operandi for prevention is to encourage healthy eating habits with low sweets, refined foods, fast foods, etc. with maintenance of good oral hygiene with use of fluoride toothpaste at least twice a day (morning and bedtime).

A Quick Look at the Saliva and Dental caries

- Saliva is a complex watery body fluid.
- It is composed of 99% water and 1% solids including—Mucin, digestive enzymes, proline-rich proteins, lysozyme and electrolytes.
- Its prime function is lubrication for helping in chewing, bolus formation, swallowing and speech.
- It also has antibacterial activity due to lysozyme and innate immunity given by salivary agglutinins and IgA antibodies.
- It buffers the acid formed in oral cavity by bacterial activity.
- Saliva secretion has an oral clearance effect/flushing effect that helps prevent formation of dental caries.
- Dental caries are infectious microbiological diseases of oral cavity characterized by demineraliszation of the hard surface of tooth due to plaque formation and bacterial colonization of the plaque.
- The caries start from the tooth surface and erode gradually right through the dentin upto the pulp cavity of tooth leading to sensitivity and pain in tooth and if not treated even tooth loss.
- Dental caries can be prevented by the maintenance of good oral hygiene, making healthy food choices and using fluoridated tooth paste twice a day.

CHAPTER

34

Biochemistry of Connective Tissue and Bones

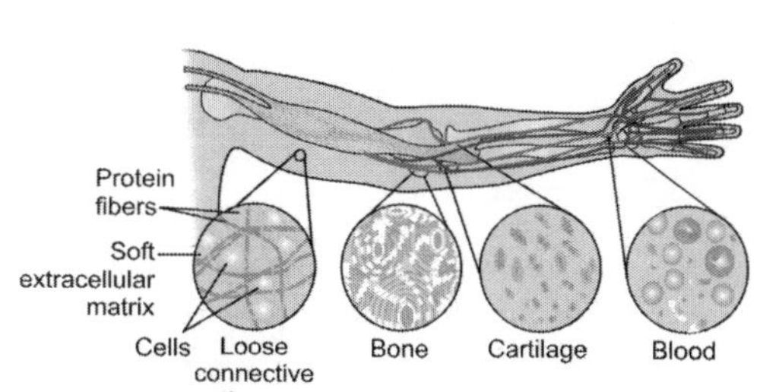

Chapter Framework

Introduction

The human body is composed of approximately 100 trillion cells, located in different tissues. The tissues are surrounded by what we call the extracellular matrix/connective tissue. This extracellular matrix fills the spaces between the cells and binds together tissue giving it a shape and also separating it from other surrounding tissues. Basic components of the extracellular matrix include:

1. The structural proteins, collagen and elastin.
2. Certain specialized proteins, such as fibrillin, fibronectin, and lamilin, which have specific functions in the ECM.
3. Proteoglycans, which consist of long chains of repeating disaccharides (glycosaminoglycans, GAGs, formerly called mucopolysaccharides) attached to specific core proteins.

Types and Functions of Connective Tissue

Different types of connective tissue include:

- Ordinary/Special
- Loose/Dense
- Regular/Irregular
- Other—Fibrous, elastic, adipose, lymphoid, areolar, blood, bone and cartilage.

Functions of connective tissue are:

- Transport
- Immunological defence
- Mechanical support
- Growth and repair

- Energy economics
- Hemopoiesis

Components of Connective Tissue

- Connective tissue consists of cells embedded in an extracellular matrix. (Fig. 34.1) The matrix, in turn, consists of fibers and ground substance. As a result of this basic topology, other tissues are either supported upon connective tissue (epithelial surfaces), invaginated into connective tissue (glandular epithelium), or embedded within the connective tissue (blood vessels, muscles, and nerves).

Collagen

- It is the most abundant protein in animals constituting approximately 25% of the total proteins in mammals.
- It is a family of fibrous proteins, is produced by a variety of cell types but principally by fibroblasts (cells found in interstitial connective tissue), muscle cells, and epithelial cells.
- At least 19 distinct types of collagen made up of 30 distinct polypeptide chains (each encoded by a separate gene) have been identified in human tissues. Although several of these are present only in small proportions, they may play important roles in determining the physical properties of the tissues. (Table 34.1)
- Newly synthesized collagen undergoes extensive posttranslational modification before becoming part of a mature, extracellular collagen fiber. Like most secreted proteins, collagen is synthesized on ribosomes in a precursor form, preprocollagen, which contains a leader or signal sequence that directs the polypeptide chain into the vesicular space of the endoplasmic reticulum. As it enters the endoplasmic reticulum, this leader sequence is enzymatically removed to give procollagen.

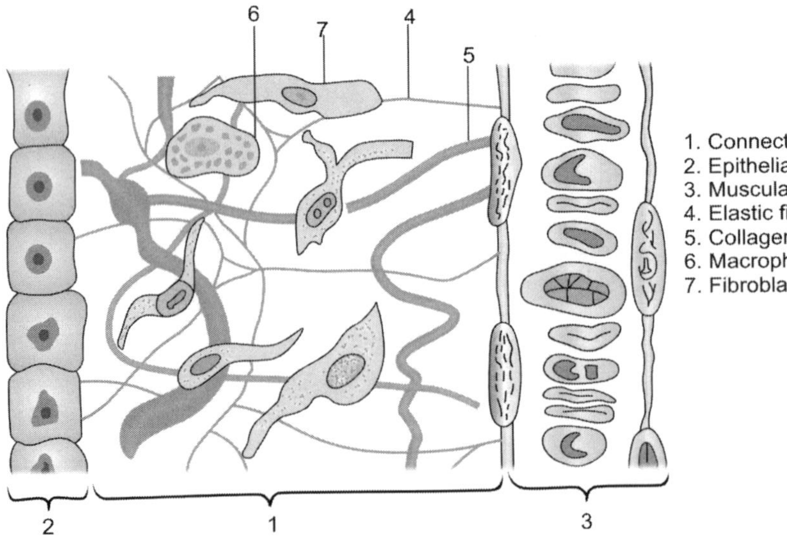

Fig. 34.1 Components of a typical connective tissue

Table 34.1 Types and Functions of Collagen

Collagen Type	*Structural Details*	*Localization*
I	Fibrils	Skin, tendon, bone, cornea
II	Fibrils	Cartilage, vitreous humor
III	Fibrils	Skin, muscle associates with type I collagen
IV	Nonfibrillar, mesh collagen	All basal laminae (basement membranes)
V	Small fibers, N-terminal globular domains	Associated with type I collagen in most interstitial tissues
VI	Microfibrils, with both N and C-terminal globular domains	Associated with type I collagen in most interstitial tissues
VII	An anchoring collagen	Epithelial cells, dermal-epidermal junction
VIII	Nonfibrillar, mesh collagen	Cornea, some endothelial cells
IX	Fibril-associated collagens with interrupted triple helices (FACIT) N-terminal globular domain	Associated with type II collagen in cartilage and vitreous humor
X	Nonfibrillar, mesh collagen, with C-terminal globular domain	Growth plate, hypertrophic and mineralizing cartilage
XI	Small fibers	Cartilage, vitreous humor
XII	FACIT	Interacts with types I and II collagen in soft tissues
XIII	Transmembrance collagen	Cell surfaces, epithelial cells
XIV	FACIT	Soft tissue
XV	Endostatin—Forming collagen	Endothelial cells
XVI	Other	Ubiquitous
XVII	Transmembrane collagen	Epidermal cell surface
XVIII	Endostatin-forming	Endothelial cells
XIX	Other	Ubiquitous

- Procollagen the precursor of collagen is a triple helix composed of three polypeptide chains that are twisted around each other, forming a rope-like structure (Fig. 34.2).
- All collagen types have a triple helical structure. Each polypeptide subunit or α-chain is twisted into a left-handed helix of 3 residues per turn. Three of these α-chains are then wound into a right-handed super-helix, forming a rod-like molecule 1.4 nm in diameter and about 300 nm long.
- A striking characteristic of collagen is the occurrence of glycine residues at every third position of the triple helical portion of the α-chain. This is necessary because glycine is the only amino acid small enough to be accommodated in the limited space available down the central core of the triple helix.
- Other amino acids with conspicuous repetitions in collagen are proline and lysine. Both proline and lysine are hydroxylated in the presence of vitamin C-dependent hydroxylase enzyme and are converted to hydroxy proline and hydroxy lysine during the post-translational modification of procollagen to collagen.
- These hydroxy proline and hydroxy lysine give strength to the mature collagen fibers.

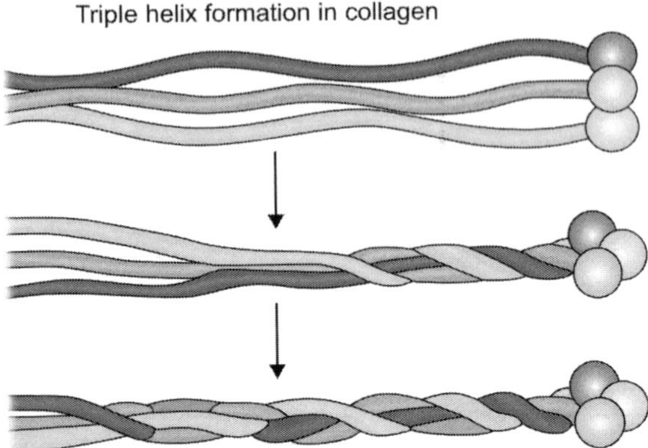

Fig. 34.2 Collagen triple helix

Fibronectin

- The same cells that secrete collagen also secrete fibronectin, a large glycoprotein present on cell surfaces, in the extracellular matrix, and in blood.
- Fibronectin binds to aggregating procollagen fibres and alters the kinetics of fibre formation in the pericellular matrix.
- Associated with fibronectin and procollagen in this matrix are the proteoglycans heparan sulfate and chondroitin sulfate.
- In fact, type IX collagen, a minor collagen type from cartilage, contains attached proteoglycan chains. Such interactions may serve to regulate the formation of collagen fibers and to determine their orientation in tissues.

Elastin

- Elastin is a connective tissue protein that is responsible for properties of extensibility and elastic recoil in tissues. Although not as widespread as collagen, elastin is present in large amounts, particularly in tissues that require these physical properties, e.g. lung, large arterial blood vessels, and some elastic ligaments. Smaller quantities of elastin are also found in skin, ear cartilage, and several other tissues.
- In contrast to collagen, there appears to be only one genetic type of elastin, although variants arise by differential processing of the hnRNA for elastin.
- Elastin is synthesized as a soluble monomer of 70,000 MW called tropo-elastin. Some of the prolines of tropo-elastin are hydroxylated to hydroxy-proline by prolyl hydroxylase, although hydroxy-lysine and glycosylated hydroxy-lysine are not present.
- Unlike collagen, tropo-elastin is not synthesized in a pro- form with extension peptides. Furthermore, elastin does not contain repeat Gly-X-Y sequences, triple helical structure, or carbohydrate moieties.

Proteoglycans

- Proteoglycans are proteins that contain covalently linked glycosaminoglycan (GAGs).
- The proteins bound covalently to GAGs are called core proteins; they have proved difficult to isolate and characterize.

- The amount of carbohydrate in a proteoglycan is usually much greater than is found in a glycoprotein and may comprise up to 95% of its weight
- There are at least 7 GAGs: hyaluronic acid, chondroitin sulfate I and II, heparin, heparan sulfate, and dermatan sulfate. A GAG is an unbranched polysaccharide made up of repeating disaccharides, one component of which is always an amino sugar (hence the name GAG), either D-glucosamine or D-galactoseamine. *(Discussed in detail in chapter 1).*
- The GAGs present in the proteoglycans are poly-anions and hence bind poly-cations and cations such as Na and K.
- Proteoglycans are found in every tissue of the body, mainly in the extracellular matrix. There they are associated with each other and some of them—with collagen, another—with elastin. These interactions are important in determining the structural organization of the matrix. In addition, some of them interact with certain adhesive proteins, such as fibronectin and laminin.
- The glycosaminoglycan chains of proteoglycans are degraded by lysosomal enzymes that cleave one sugar at a time from the nonreducing end of the chain. An inability to degrade proteoglycans leads to a set of diseases known as the mucopolysaccharidoses *(Discussed in chapter 1).*
- Proteoglycans, collagen and fibrin have distinct binding domains for adhesion proteins, such as fibronectin and laminin. These domains allow these adhesion proteins to bind the various components of the extracellular matrix. They also contain specific binding domains for specific cell surface receptors known as the integrins.

Bones

- Bone is a very dense form of connective tissue and its matrix is predominantly a mixture of:
  - Tough fibers (mainly type I collagen fibrils).
  - Solid particles (calcium phosphate formed as hydroxyapatite crystals).
- There are two main types of living cells in the bone matrix:
  - Osteoclasts, which eats up old bone matrix.
  - Osteoblasts, which deposits new bone matrix.

Bone Formation/Osteogenesis

- Bone formation and resorption (remodeling) occurs on bone surfaces of microscopic units called osteons. Formation is carried out by active osteoblasts that secrete collagen into the extracellular space.
- The bone matrix is deposited as layers. This uncalcified bone matrix (consisting chiefly of type I collagen) is called osteoid.
- The next step in osteogenesis is calcification of the matrix.
- Calcification involves the formation of numerous crystallites of hydroxyapatite [$Ca_{10}(PO_4)_6(OH)_2$] within the matrix.
- Osteoblasts initiate the calcification process by releasing matrix vesicles (MVs) that contain apatite crystals.
- These vesicles also contain alkaline phosphatase and other enzymes. The loaded matrix vesicles rupture, causing an increase in the local concentration of minerals initiating mineralization

and formation of hydroxyapatite crystals, which are deposited within and at the surfaces of these vesicles.

- The small centers of mineralization grow and eventually fuse with each other (Fig. 34.3).
- Ground substance (collagens and proteoglycans) surrounds and stabilizes these crystals. The interaction of hydroxyapatite with collagenous fibers and proteoglycans brings about the hardness and rigidity of bone.
- Surface osteoblasts mature into osteocytes as they become surrounded by mineralized bone but they remain in contact with the bone surface and help maintain the bone structure.
- The bone is in a dynamic state of deposition and reabsorption. The osteoclasts excavate through the bony matrix demineralizing and digesting the organic matrix until they reach the haversian canals capillary branch where they transform into the pre – osteoblasts and then finally osteoblasts to deposit the new bone once again.

Inherited Disorders of Connective Tissue

- Inherited disorders associated with Collagen—*Ehler's-Danlos syndrome and osteogenesis imperfecta*. Both the disorders occur due to the mutations that cause formation of abnormal collagen. Ehler's-Danlos syndrome is characterized by hyperextensibility of skin and fragility of tissue; whereas osteogenesis imperfecta is characterized by fragility of bones.
- Inherited disorder associated with Elastin—*Williams syndrome* is characterized by impaired synthesis of elastin and adversely affects CNS and connective tissue.
- Inherited disorder associated with Fibrillin—*Marfan's syndrome* characterized by hyperextensibility of joints and skeletal system thus the patients have long digits and are tall. Besides cardiovascular problems are observed.

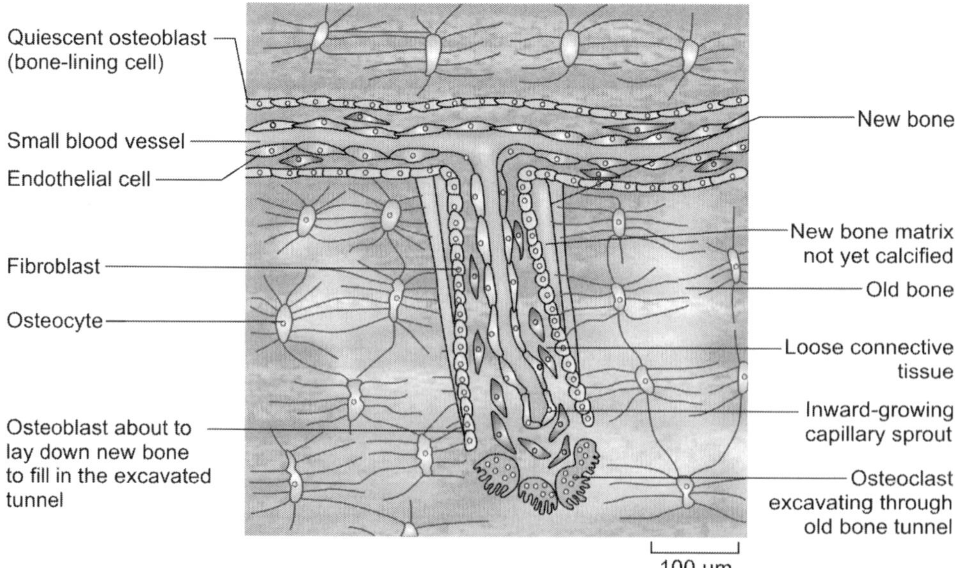

Fig. 34.3 Bone remodeling

A Quick Look at the Biochemistry of Connective Tissues and Bones

- Connective tissue/extracellular matrix are present in between the tissues filling the spaces between them.
- The major components of connective tissue are—Collagen, elastin, fibrillin, proteoglycans.
- Collagen is the most abundant human protein comprising 25% of total proteins.
- There are 19 types of collagen.
- Each molecule of collagen is made of a triple helix with an abundance of hydroxy proline, hydroxy lysine and glycine.
- Elastin is a connective tissue protein that is responsible for properties of extensibility and elastic recoil in tissues.
- Proteoglycans are proteins that contain covalently linked glycosaminoglycan (GAGs).
- Proteoglycans are found in every tissue of the body, mainly in the extracellular matrix.
- Bone is a very dense form of connective tissue and its matrix is predominantly a mixture of:
  - Tough fibers (mainly type I collagen fibrils).
  - Solid particles (calcium phosphate formed as hydroxyapatite crystals).
- There are two main types of living cells in the bone matrix:
  - Osteoclasts, which eats up old bone matrix.
  - Osteoblasts, which deposits new bone matrix.
- Inherited disorders of
  - Collagen—Ehler's-Danlos syndrome and osteogenesis imperfecta
  - Elastin—William's syndrome
  - Fibrillin—Marfan syndrome

CHAPTER

35

Current Topics in Biochemistry

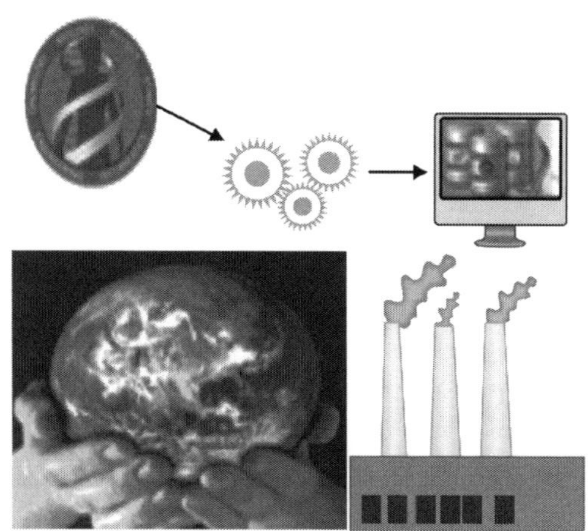

Chapter Framework

- Human Genome Project
- Bioinformatics
- Environmental Biochemistry

Human Genome Project (HGP)

- Modern day medicine is rapidly advancing with the progress of one of the latest branches of genetics – *Human Genomics*.
- It is the study of the complete human genome, i.e. 3×10^9 base pairs of genetic information.
- In earlier days we knew the causative organism of most of the diseases but with progression of the medical science today we have come across diseases that are *multifactorial* in origin rather than being dependent on a single organism, e.g. Cancer, diabetes, Alzheimer's, etc.
- For the better diagnosis and prognosis of such diseases a sound knowledge of the complete human genome is a must so that all the proteins coded by it and their interactions may be understood.
- For this purpose in the year 1990 the Human Genome Project was launched in USA.
- This culminated in July 2000, when leaders of the two groups involved in this effort (the International Human Genome Sequencing Consortium and Celera Genomics, a private company) announced that over 90% of the genome had been sequenced.
- Draft versions of the sequence were published in early 2001. With the exception of a few gaps, the sequence of the entire human genome was completed in 2003, 50 years after the description of the double-helical nature of DNA by Watson and Crick.

Method for Sequencing the Human Genome

- The mapping of the human genome is what was desired for when the HGP was initiated. The mapping of human genome can be done by:
  - Cytogenetic mapping (mapping the active genes by chemical dyes).
  - Gene linkage map (prepared by RFLPs, VNTRs, Small nucleotide repeats).
  - Physical mapping (high resolution base sequence mapping active genes).
- The various techniques used for mapping in HGP are:
  - DNA sequencing
  - Using DNA probes
  - Fluorescent in-situ hybridization (FISH)
  - Cloning vectors
  - PCR
  - Chromosome walking
  - Data base utility.

Impact of Human Genome Project

- The HGP has had a tremendous impact on modern day medicine and has rather helped in evolving newer areas better for diagnosis of different diseases like proteomics, metabolomics, lipidomics, pharmacogenomics, molecular diagnosis, Nutrigenomics, glycomics, stem cell biology, bioinformatics, biotechnology, gene therapy, etc.
- All these fields have sprung up only because the HGP has equipped us with the complete information of all the genetic sequences in the human genome and how these sequences express and interact with other genes and proteins to cause disease process.

The Salient Features of HGP are

- The human genome contains 3.2 billion chemical nucleotide base pairs (A, C, T, and G).
- The average gene consists of 3,000 base pairs, but sizes vary greatly, with the largest known human gene being dystrophin at 2.4 million base pairs.
- Functions are unknown for more than 50% of discovered genes.
- The human genome sequence is almost exactly the same (99.9%) in all people.
- About 2% of the genome encodes instructions for the synthesis of proteins.
- Repeat sequences that do not code for proteins make up at least 50% of the human genome. Repeat sequences are thought to have no direct functions, but they shed light on chromosome structure and dynamics. Over time, these repeats reshape the genome by rearranging it, thereby creating entirely new genes or modifying and reshuffling existing genes.
- Human DNA show 98% similarity with the chimpanzee genome.
- Genes appear to be concentrated in random areas along the genome, with vast expanses of noncoding DNA between them.
- Chromosome 1 (the largest human chromosome) has the most genes (3,168), and Y chromosome has the fewest (344).
- Particular gene sequences have been associated with numerous diseases and disorders including breast cancer, muscle disease, deafness, and blindness.

- Scientists have identified millions of locations where single-base DNA differences (Single nucleotide polymorphism—SNPs) occur in humans. This information promises to revolutionize the processes of finding DNA sequences associated with such common diseases as cardiovascular disease, diabetes, arthritis, and cancers.

Protein Coding Regions of Human Genome

- It was earlier known that the human genome contains some 80,000 to 100,000 base pairs since that are the number of cellular proteins; considering the one gene one protein hypothesis. However with the completion of HGP it was found that the complete human genome contains 3.2 billion base pairs which are much larger than the number of proteins being encoded. But out of the total genetic information present in the genome, it is just 30,000 to 40,000 genes that code for proteins. This variation in number of genes and proteins is due to the process of RNA editing enabling a single gene to code for more than one protein.
- The total genes (noncoding genes have been excluded) in the human genome can be categorized as:
  - Genome maintenance and gene expression—23%
  - Signal transduction—21%
  - General biochemical functions of cells—17.5%
  - Synthesis of structural, transport proteins, Immunoglobulins, etc.—38%.

Bioinformatics

- Biological data are being produced at a phenomenal rate with the advancement of human genomics and the huge barrage of information gathered after the completion of HGP. Thus the advanced computational tools and interdisciplinary experts are needed to capture, represent, store, integrate, distribute, and analyze the data.
- Bioinformatics is the youngest branch to come up in the field of science, the term first tracing its use in the 1990s.
- It is the combination of biology and information technology where the flood of biological data being obtained is stored, analyzed, integrated and correlated for unravelling the mysteries of science.
- It is the application of computational techniques to analyze the information associated with biomolecules on a large-scale that has now firmly established itself as a discipline in molecular biology, and encompasses a wide range of subject areas from structural biology, genomics to gene expression studies.
- This unexpected union between the two subjects is largely attributed to the fact that life itself is an information technology; an organism's physiology is largely determined by its genes, which at its most basic can be viewed as digital information.

Aims of Bioinformatics

- The aims of bioinformatics are threefold.
  - At its simplest bioinformatics organizes data in a way that allows researchers to access existing information and to submit new entries as they are produced.

- The information stored in these databases is essentially useless until analyzed. Thus the purpose of bioinformatics extends much further. The second aim is thus to develop tools and resources that aid in the analysis of data.
- The third aim is to use these tools to analyze the data and interpret the results in a biologically meaningful manner. Traditionally, biological studies examined individual systems in detail, and frequently compared those with a few that are related. However, with the birth of bioinformatics, we can now conduct global analyses of all the available data (Table 35.1) with the aim of uncovering common principles that apply across many systems and highlight novel features.

- The biological database is the set of/collection of biological data on a computer that can be manipulated in a variety of ways to appear in a number of varied arrangements and subsets. Some important databases used in bioinformatics have been listed in Table 35.2.

Table 35.1 Type of data being used in bioinformatics and the bioinformatics subject area utilizing the data

Data source and size	*Bioinformatics topics*
Raw DNA sequences—8.2 million sequences	Separation of introns and exons, their identification, predicting gene product and forensic use.
Protein sequences—300,000 sequences	Preparing and comparing sequence algorithms, multiple sequence algorithms alignment and identifying conserved motifs
Macromolecular structure	Protein geometry measurements, secondary (2°), tertiary (3°) organizsation prediction, intermolecular interactions analysis, molecular simulations
Genomes—40 complete genomes (1.6 billion – 3.2 billion base pairs)	Characterization of repeats, Structural assignments to genes, Phylogenetic analysis, characterization of protein content, metabolic pathways, linkage analysis for relating specific genes to diseases
Gene expression	Correlating expression patterns, mapping expression data to sequence, structural and biochemical data
Literature—11 million citations	Digital libraries for automated bibliographic searches and knowledge database of data from literature

Table 35.2 Important biological databases being used in bioinformatics

Database	*Salient features*
Primary nucleotide sequence databases (www.ncbi.nih.gov/Genebank)	Provides nucleotide sequence databases and is maintained by National Centre for Biotechnology Information (NCBI)
Protein sequence databases SWISS-PROT (www.expasy.ch/sport)	Provides the description of the structure of a protein, its domains, posttranslational modifications, variants.
Protein sequence motif databases (www.expasy.ch/prosite)	Provides information on protein families and domains, and also has patterns and profiles for sequences and biological functions
Others Unigene (www.ncbi.nih.gov/Unigene) Genome biology (www.ncbi.nlm.nih.gov/genomes)	Nucleotide sequences of Gene bank in the form of clusters is available Information about complete genomes is available

Applications of Bioinformatics

Applications of data mining to bioinformatics include:

- Gene finding
- Protein functional domain detection
- Functional motif detection
- Protein function inference
- Disease diagnosis
- Disease prognosis
- Disease treatment optimization
- Protein and gene interaction network reconstruction
- Data cleansing
- Protein sub-cellular location prediction.

Environmental Biochemistry

Environmental biochemistry is the scientific study of the chemical and biochemical phenomena that occur in environment. It can be defined as the study of the sources, reactions, transport, effects, and fates of chemical species in the air, soil, and water environments; the effect of human activity on these and their effect on human health.

The major components of environment are shown in Fig. 35.1.

- The interaction of the atmosphere, lithosphere, hydrosphere and biosphere is continuing for years together. On account of the various activities of man, the composition and complex nature of environment gets changed.

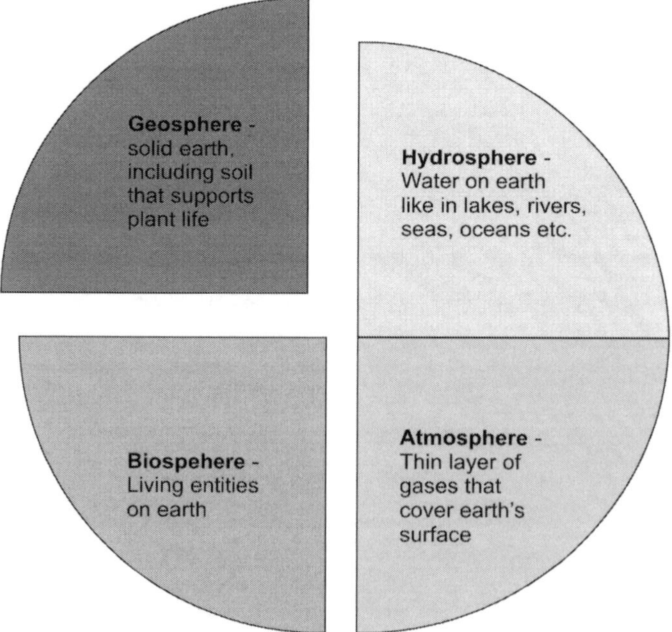

Fig. 35.1 Components of environment

- These activities include industrialization, construction, and transportation. Such activities, although desirable for human development and welfare, lead to generation and release of objectionable materials into the environment thus turning it foul, and rendering our life miserable.
- The natural environment is clean, but due to multifarious activities of man it gets polluted resulting in what is called as environmental pollution.
- Environment pollution is a wide-reaching problem and it is likely to influence the health of human populations greatly. A brief insight view about the causes and effects of environment pollution (in the perspective of air pollution, water and/soil waste pollution) on human by diseases and problems is discussed here.

Environmental pollution is classified into various types like:

- Pollution of air is termed as the atmospheric pollution.
- The pollution of hydrosphere or water is termed as water pollution.
- In addition to these major sources of pollution we have pollution of lithosphere called soil pollution.
- Urban areas are blessed with the menace of noise, which at times becomes intolerable. It is called noise pollution.

Air/Atmospheric Pollution (Fig. 35.2)

- Air is the name given to the Earth's atmosphere used in breathing and photosynthesis. It is composed of 78.1% N_2, 21% O_2 and 0.03% CO_2 alongwith water vapor and suspended particles.
- Amongst the various types of pollution, air pollution is of greatest importance. It can be readily noticed as it causes immediate health problems. The hazardous gases that lead to pollution are oxides of carbon, nitrogen and sulfur. Particulate matter also causes air pollution. The emission due to auto-exhaust causes serious pollution of air due to formation of oxides of nitrogen and benzopyrene.

Important Air Pollutants and their Effects on Humans

Sulfur Dioxide

- It is emitted by the burning of coal and oil. It affects the respiratory system the worse in humans by destroying the lung surfactant causing respiratory distress, air way obstruction and even lung cancer in certain cases.

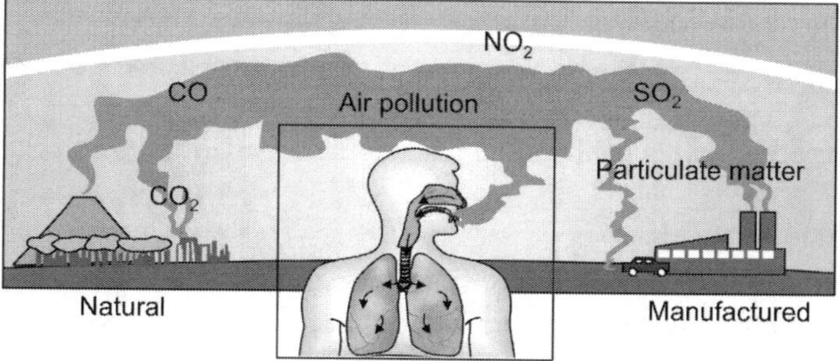

Fig. 35.2 Air pollution

Carbon Monoxide

It is produced by the incomplete combustion of carbon-rich fuel in automobiles, rails, aeroplanes, or in industries. CO has a high affinity to Hb (600 times that of CO_2). It combines with Hb to form carboxy Hb and in high concentration causes impaired mental function, dizziness, loss of consciousness and death occurs at a concentration 750ppm.

Carbon Dioxide

This gas is normally present in the atmosphere but at a lower concentration and is responsible for maintaining the temperature in our atmosphere, which in its absence would be extremely cold. Thus it is the green-house gas. However, higher concentrations of this gas would cause soaring temperatures as is seen nowadays and is termed as global warming. CO_2 is used by the green plants for photosynthesis and thus plantation of more trees can prevent the green-house effect.

Nitrogen Dioxide

It is also harmful to humans and combines with Hb reducing its oxygen carrying capacity. It along with SO_2 combines to water vapor and causes acid rain.

Particulate Matter

Solid particles of dust and soot from exhaust fumes, grinding, spraying, etc. are important source of particulate matter as pollutants. These particles adversely affect the respiratory system in humans by lodging in airways and causing coughing, sneezing, aggravate asthma and may have even toxic effect.

Indoor Pollutants

Poor ventilation is one of the prime causes of indoor pollution. Major indoor pollutants are the volatile organic compounds released by paints, varnishes, disinfectants, fumigation, carpets or spores in hospital air etc. These pose severe hazard to the human health and can cause acute respiratory problems which include running nose, cough, sore throat, lung infection, asthma, difficulty in breathing, noisy respiration and wheezing.

- Chlorofluorocarbons (CFC)
  - These are used in perfumes, sprays, referigerators, air conditioners, foams, etc. These on leaking into the air are photodissociated on reaching the stratosphere releasing the chlorine atoms which destroy the ozone layer (protective layer against UV rays of sun).

The consistent increase in the air pollution is adding up to the global heating and temperatures of earth have shown extremes in either side, i.e. summers have been hotter and winters chillier in last few decades phenomenally. The rising temperatures can cause heat stress causing heat stroke (failure of thermoregulation). Similarly, exposure to extremely cold temperatures can cause cold stress leading to shivering and nonshivering thermogenesis and in severe conditions hypothermia.

Water Pollution

- Water pollution is the contamination of water bodies (e.g. lakes, rivers, oceans, aquifers and groundwater). Water pollution occurs when pollutants are discharged directly or indirectly into water bodies without adequate treatment to remove harmful compounds.
- The important water pollutants and their effects on human health are shown in Tables 35.3 to 35.5.

Table 35.3 Classification of water pollutants

Inorganic pollutants	*Organic pollutants*
Heavy metals (As, Cd, Pb, Hg, etc.)	Organic acids
Cyanides, Thiocyanides	Bio-medical waste
Dyes, Bleaches, Pigments, etc.	Oil, grease, pesticides
Sulfides, Ammonia	Bacteria, viruses, algae, worms
Minerals (Zn, Se, F, Cl, Cu, Fe, Ba, etc.)	
Detergent solvents	

Table 35.4 Effects of water pollutants on human health

Water Pollutant	*Effect on Human health*
Cadmium (Cd)	Cd is very toxic, 50 mg may cause vomiting, diarrhea, abdominal pains, loss of consciousness.
Mercury (Hg)	Mercury is very toxic. More than 100 mg may cause headache, abdominal pain, diarrhea, destruction of Hb, tremors, very bad effects on cerebral functions and CNS, paralysis, inactivates functional proteins, nephrotoxic, hyper coagulability of blood, minamata disease, and even death.
Lead (Pb)	More than 400 mg of Pb in human body can cause brain damage, vomiting, loss of appetite, convulsions, and uncoordinated body movements. It is retained in liver, kidney, brain, muscle, soft tissues, bones. Leads to high rate of miscarriages, affects skin, and respiratory system, liver, brain cells, and nephrotoxic. Disturbs endocrine system, causes anemia, and long-term exposure may cause even death.
Arsenic (As)	Greater than 25 mg of arsenic causes vomiting, diarrhea, nausea, irritation of nose and throat, abdominal pain, skin eruptions, inflammations and even death. It binds Hb in erythrocytes. May cause cancer of skin, lungs and liver, chromosomal aberration and damage, gangrene, loss of hearing, injury to nerve tissue, liver and kidney damage. Minor symptoms of As poisoning, weight loss, hair loss, nausea, depression, fatigue, white lines across toe nails and finger nails.
Radioactive materials/ metals/ substances	These generally cause 'Gene' mutation, ionization of body fluids, chromosomal mutations and cancers. Destroy body cell tissue, adversely effects reproductive system. When mother is exposed to radiation during pregnancy, it causes severe mental retardation and leukemia in infants. Radioactive metals like heavy metals are nephrotoxic.
Fluoride	Excess fluoride intake in body results in progressive crippling scourge (sponging)/fluorosis of bones, teeth.
Selenium (Se)	Signs of Se poisoning (more than 4 mg) are fever, nervousness, vomiting, falling of blood pressure, causes damage to liver, kidney and spleen, loss of nails and hair. It can cause growth inhibition, skin discoloration, bad teeth, psychological problem, and gastrointestinal problems.
Oil/Grease/Oil Sludge	Many constituents of oily sludge are even carcinogenic and potent immunotoxicants.
Surfactants and detergents	They are toxic and harmful for aquatic life, animals and humans. Inhibit self-purification of water.
Cyanides	Apart from acute toxicity and chronic toxicity, it leads to development of iodine deficiency disorders.
Pesticides/ Insecticides	Plays a role in development of Parkinson's disease, destruction of nerve cells in certain regions of brain resulting in loss of dopamine which is used by nerve cells to communicate with brain. Some act as protoplasmic, nerve or respiratory poisons

Table 35.5 Diseases due to water pollution and their causative organisms

Waterborne diseases *Bacterial* Typhoid Cholera Paratyphoid Gastroenteritis bacterial dysentery	 *Salmonella typhi,* *Vibrio cholera* *Salmonella paratyphi* Enterotoxigenic *Escherichia coli*, Variety of *Escherichia coli*
Viral Infectious hepatitis Poliomyelitis Diarrhea	 Hepatitis—A virus Poliovirus Rotavirus, other virus like *Echono-virus*, *Coxsackie-virus*
Water-washed diseases Sabies Trachoma Bacillary dysentery	 Various skin fungus species Trachoma infecting eyes *E. coli*
Water-based diseases Schistosomiasis Guinea worm	 Schistosoma sp. Guinea worm
Infection through water related insect vectors Sleeping sickness Malaria	 *Trypanosoma* through Tsetse fly *Plasmodium* through Anaphelis
Infections due to defective sanitation/ polluted water Hookworms	 Hookworms, Ascaris

Soil Pollution

- Soil is the thin layer of organic and inorganic materials that covers the earth's rocky surface. The organic portion, which is derived from the decayed remains of plants and animals, is concentrated in the dark uppermost topsoil. The inorganic portion made up of rock fragments, was formed over thousands of years by physical and chemical weathering of bedrock. Productive soils are necessary for agriculture to supply the world with sufficient food.
- Soil pollution is defined as the build-up in soils of persistent toxic compounds, chemicals, salts, radioactive materials, or disease-causing agents, which have adverse effects on plant growth, animal and human health.

Causes of Soil Pollution

- Soil properties are affected by past land use, current activities on the site, and nearness to pollution sources.
- Human activities have intentionally added substances such as pesticides, fertilizers and other amendments to soils.
- Accidental spills and leaks of chemicals used for commercial or industrial purposes have also been sources of contamination. Some contaminants are moved through the air and deposited as dust or by precipitation.
- Once contaminants are in soils, where they go and how quickly they travel depends on many factors like:

- Soil mineralogy and clay content (soil texture)
- pH (acidity) of the soil
- Amount of organic matter in the soil
- Moisture levels
- Temperature
- Presence of other chemicals.

- The soil contaminants then end up into:
  - End up in water held in the soil or in the underlying groundwater (by leaching through the soil).
  - Volatilize (evaporate) into the air; or
  - Bind tightly to the soil.

  Important soil pollutants are as shown in Table 35.6

  Effects of soil pollution on human health is shown in Table 35.7
- Besides the effects on human health, soil pollution has some other effects like:
  - Pollution runs off into rivers and kills the fish, plants and other aquatic life.
  - Crops and fodder grown on polluted soil may pass the pollutants on to the consumers.

Table 35.6 Important soil pollutants

Inorganic	*Organic*
Heavy metals like Cd, Hg, Pb, As, Cr, Zn, Cu, cyanides, radioactive minerals, nuclear war fare etc.	Herbicides, pesticides, oils, hydrocarbons, tars, dioxins

Table 35.7 Effect of soil pollution on human health

Pollutant	*Source*	*Effect on human health*
As	Naturally occurring	Chronic poisoning causes loss of appetite, GI disturbances like diarrhea alternating with constipation, peripheral neuritis, conjunctivitis, sometimes skin cancer
Cd	Mining, metallurgy, chemical industry, electro-plating	Leads to chronic poisoning and affects the proximal tubules of the kidney, causing formation of kidney stones
Pb	Lead smelters, Pb batteries	Pb poisoning can cause severe mental retardation and even death
Hg	Industrial waste	Neurological problems and shows nephrotoxicity
Cyanides	Wastes from heat treatment of metals, dismantling of electroplating shops etc.	Apart from acute toxicity and chronic toxicity, it leads to development of iodine deficiency disorders
Dioxin	Herbicide use in farms	Skin cancer and infertility
Plastic bags	They are nonbiodegradable and burning them releases into air toxic gases like CO_2, CO, Phosgene, and poisonous chlorinated compounds	See harmful effects of air pollution
Oil spills	Spills from gas stations, fuel tanks, etc. release toxic compounds like toluene, benzene and xylene in high levels	Can cause cancer

- Polluted soil may no longer grow crops and fodder.
- Soil structure is damaged (clay ionic structure impaired).
- Blockage of pipelines in urban areas and corrosion of foundations and pipelines.
- Impairs soil stability and causes deforestation.
- May release vapors and hydrocarbon into buildings and cellars.
- May create toxic dusts.

Noise Pollution

Noise Pollution is when humans make and produce high levels of noise, which are beyond the regular levels. Important sources are traffic; concerts; airplanes; industrial machinery; construction or demolition. The human being can tolerate on an average 45 dB to 60 dB without much discomfort however, beyond this limit it causes mental fatigue, irritation and other health hazards.

A Quick Look at the Current Topics in Biochemistry

- It is the study of the complete human genome, i.e. 3×10^9 base pairs of genetic information.
- The various techniques used for mapping in HGP are:
  - DNA sequencing
  - Using DNA probes
  - Fluorescent in-situ hybridization (FISH)
  - Cloning vectors
  - PCR
  - Chromosome walking
  - Database utility
- The total genes (noncoding genes have been excluded) in the human genome can be categorized as:
  - Genome maintenance and gene expression—23%
  - Signal transduction—21%
  - General biochemical functions of cells—17.5%
  - Synthesis of structural, transport proteins, Immunoglobulins, etc—38%.
- Bioinformatics is the application of computational techniques to analyze the information associated with biomolecules on a large-scale.
- Applications of data mining to bioinformatics include:
  - Gene finding
  - Protein functional domain detection
  - Functional motif detection
  - Protein function inference
  - Disease diagnosis
  - Disease prognosis
  - Disease treatment optimization
  - Protein and gene interaction network reconstruction
  - Data cleansing
  - Protein subcellular location prediction.
- Environmental biochemistry is the study of the sources, reactions, transport, effects, and fates of chemical species in the air, soil, and water environments; the effect of human activity on these and their effect on human health.

Section – 7

Practical Biochemistry

- Part A: Introduction to Practical Biochemistry
- Part B: Qualitative Exercises
- Part C: Quantitative Exercises
- Part D: Urine Analysis
- Part E: Applications of Clinical Biochemistry
- Part F: Demonstrations

Part A

Introduction to Practical Biochemistry

- Practical Biochemistry in Dentistry and Allied Health Sciences
- A Peep into the Biochemistry Laboratory
- Quality Control and Precision of Results
- How to work in a Biochemistry Laboratory

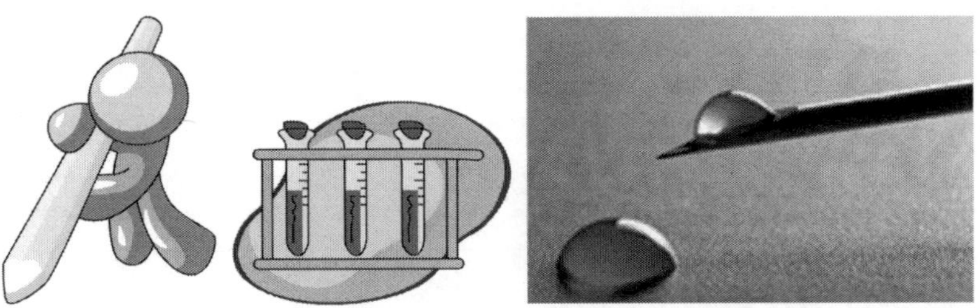

Practical biochemistry has become an essential part of the undergraduate teaching of all students of health sciences including dentistry. The undergraduate teaching of practical biochemistry aims at imparting to the student the basic skills of working in a biochemistry laboratory safely and to achieve accurate results with minimum errors. Thus, in this introductory section, the students are introduced to the Practical Biochemistry Laboratory, the instruments present in the laboratory, procedures to work safely and to get results with accuracy and precision.

CHAPTER

36

Practical Biochemistry in Dentistry and Allied Health Sciences

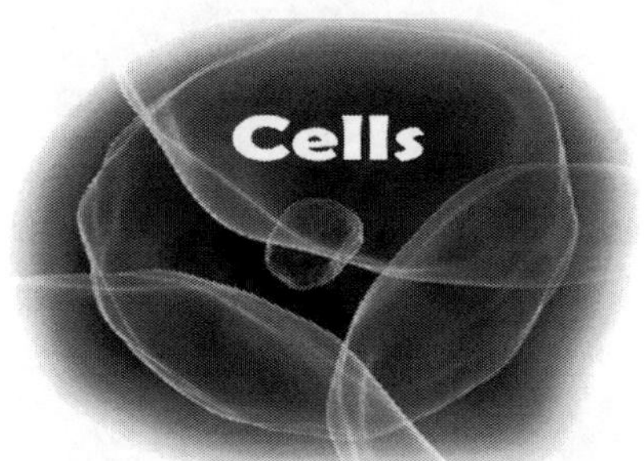

The Chemistry of life

Biochemistry is a science concerned with the chemical constituents of living cells and the various reactions or processes they undergo. Biochemists study the chemical reactions going on in the human cells. Remarkable advances in the biochemical techniques have helped to study the cell's molecular biology, DNA and taken today's researchers to the threshold of understanding the regulation of cellular functions. Thus, help in the better understanding of the basis of health and disease.

Biochemistry can therefore be better defined as a science concerned with the chemical basis of life (Greek word *'bios'* means life).

A sound knowledge of biochemistry is essential to medicine and its allied branches including dentistry.

The dental profession has a primary responsibility for the oral health care of the community. A dentist's role is not just merely to treat and manage diseases related to the oral cavity, but he/she has to treat the patient as a whole. For this a dentist should be well-versed with other aspects of health and disease. The dentists have to be well-trained in managing patients with medical diseases that may affect the dental treatment. Therefore, they should have a sound foundation for basic sciences of medicine like Biochemistry.

A dentist is traditionally taught to perform a complete oral examination of the patient and to develop a treatment plan from the examination findings. Before making the diagnosis and developing a treatment plan, the dentist should evaluate the facts properly as there may be some underlying pathology.

A sound knowledge of biochemistry would help in investigation of the etiology of the oral disease as well as the underlying pathologic condition, which otherwise could complicate the dental treatment.

Therefore, a sound knowledge of clinical biochemistry is of paramount importance to the dental students.

CHAPTER

37

A Peep into the Biochemistry Laboratory

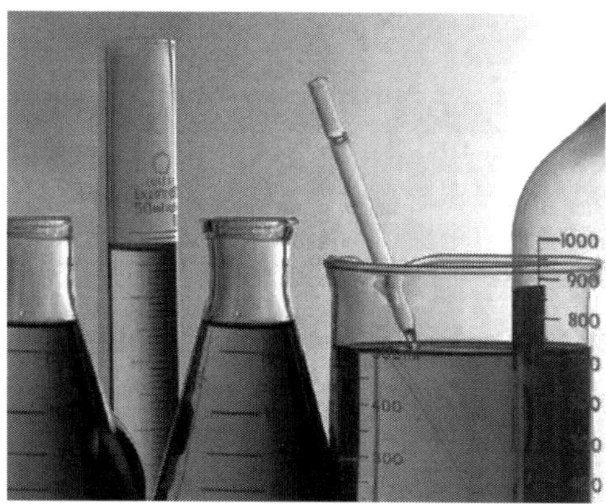

Chapter Framework

Common Lab Equipment and Instruments

The various types of equipment and instruments used in an undergraduate biochemistry laboratory are:

a. Balances
b. Centrifuges
c. Hot air ovens
d. Incubators
e. Water baths
f. Photometers and Spectrophotometers
g. pH meters
h. Semiautomated analyzers
i. Fully automated analyzers
j. Distillation plants

Balances

- Accurately weighing balances are of great significance in a biochemistry laboratory for proper reagent preparation. There are two types of balances used commonly in a biochemistry laboratory—

- Double pan chemical balance
- Monopan electronic balance.

The former is very accurate when standardized weights are used and can weigh from 100 mg to a few gm. The latter is highly sensitive, easy to operate and very accurate but is not economically priced.

Centrifuges

- Centrifuges are designed to accelerate the sedimentation process by using centrifugal forces. Two commonly used centrifuges in biochemistry laboratory are:
  - Swingout head type (Horizontal rotor)—This type has a maximum speed of 5000 rpm (revolutions per minute) due to the heat generated by the rotors on friction with air.
  - Angle head type (Fixed angle rotor)—This can have a maximum speed of 100,000 rpm due to the reduced friction of rotors fixed at an angle.

Hot Air Ovens

Hot air ovens are used for:

- Dry sterilization of syringes and needles (140°C–160°C)
- Drying glassware
- Heating chemicals used for preparation of standards.

  Hot air ovens comprise of double-walled, heavy gauge aluminium chamber logged with insulating material and fitted with heating element. The electricity passing through the heating element/coil generates heat. It is fitted with a thermostat and ventilator to regulate temperature. (Temperature range—40°C–300°C).

Incubators

They are used for incubating various samples at an optimal temperature, which can be regulated using a thermostat. (Temperature ranges between 30°C–80°C).

Water Bath

The water bath is used to provide optimum temperature to carry out various chemical reactions which occur at specific temperature. It comprises of a nickel plated tank (20–30 liter capacity) fitted with a strip heater under the tank. Temperature is controlled by a thermostat. They also are fitted with specific slots to put test tubes.

Spectrophotometer/colorimeter

It is an instrument used to measure the pH of a given solution. It works on the principle of measuring the electromotive force (EMF) generated between two electrodes due to their difference in the H^+ concentration.

pH meter

They are the most commonly used photometric instruments and are indispensible for clinical biochemistry laboratory. They will be discussed in detail separately in clinical biochemistry section.

Semiauto Analyzers

These are an improved version of the colorimeters and spectrophotometers. They are fitted with digital read outs and printing devices, making the work simpler to a great degree. They are used for kinetic assays and end – point assays.

Fully Automated Analyzers

These analyzers use robotics for repetitive pipetting and mixing of samples and reagents and for taking observations in large samples. They are very costly and used in large laboratories.

Distillation Plants

It is used to prepare distilled water free from all impurities and interfering ions (that may be present in the tap water and may interfere with reagents preparation). It is made up of stainless steel or heavy gauge brass sheet, fitted with steam condenser tube and heating coils. It works on the principle of distillation, i.e. boiling of water and condensation of it by cooling it and the distilled water is free from all impurities.

Common Lab Glassware

The laboratory glassware is usually manufactured from borosilicate glass. It is resistant to action of chemicals (except HCl). Such glassware is resistant to breakage due to sudden changes of temperature. Commonly used glassware in the undergraduate biochemistry laboratory are:

a. Beakers
b. Flasks (conical/volumetric)
c. Measuring cylinders
d. Reagent bottles (plane/amber colored)
e. Dropping bottles
f. Burettes
g. Pipettes (various volumes)
h. Test tubes (broad/narrow bore)
i. Funnels
j. Centrifuge tubes
k. Cuvettes
l. Wash bottles.

Samples

Commonly used samples in the clinical biochemistry laboratory include:

- Whole blood—For analysis of sugar, urea, blood gases.
- Plasma—For analysis of sugar, enzymes, electrolytes, metabolites like creatinine, uric acid, cholesterol, etc.
- Serum—For analysis of sugar, enzymes, electrolytes, metabolites like creatinine, uric acid, cholesterol, etc.

- CSF—For analysis of sugar, protein, chloride.
- Gastric Juice—For analysis of HCl, blood.
- Sweat—For analysis of chloride.

Blood is the most commonly used specimen. Venous blood is obtained from antequbital vein by venepuncture. Arterial blood is required for blood O_2 evaluation. It is obtained from radial and femoral artery.

Anticoagulants

For various biochemical parameters requiring plasma, different anticoagulants are used like:

- Heparin—Prevents thrombin formation.
- Oxalate salts of Na^+, K^+ and NH_4^+ — Ca^{++} precipitation.
- Sodium citrate—It forms calcium complex.
- EDTA—Causes of Ca^{++} chelation.

Other samples that may be analyzed in the clinical biochemistry laboratory are—Pleural fluid, ascetic fluid, urinary stones, gallstones, amniotic fluid, gastric and duodenal aspirations.

CHAPTER

38

Quality Control and Precision of Results

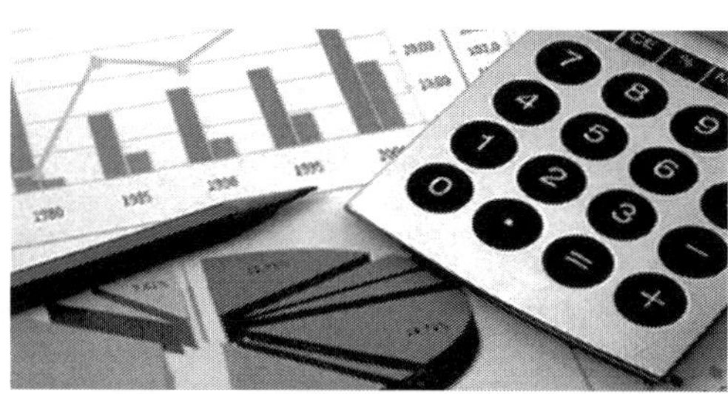

Chapter Framework

- Importance of Quality Control in Clinical Practice
  - Precision
  - Sensitivity and Specificity
  - Internal Quality control
  - External Quality control
  - Importance of Quality Control in Clinical Biochemistry

Introduction

The results of a clinical biochemistry laboratory are of great help and significance to a practicing Physician. The correct results would help in accurate diagnosis and management of the patient's clinical condition, however, erroneous results may even lead to a false diagnosis. Thus there has to be a high level of quality control, precision and accuracy in the laboratory.

Laboratory quality control is designed to detect, reduce, and correct deficiencies in a laboratory's internal analytical processes prior to the release of patient results and improve the quality of the results reported by the laboratory.

Quality control can be defined as the study of those errors that are the responsibility of the laboratory and the procedures used to recognize them and minimize them.

It is the analytical phase of quality assurance which is monitored in terms of:

- *Accuracy:* It refers to the reliability of the method in determining the real or true value of the analyte. It shows how close the measured value is to the actual value.
- *Precision:* It is the reproducibility of an analytical method. Besides abiding by these two terms, a high degree of quality control is achieved by:
  - Cleanliness of glassware
  - Proper reagents preparation
  - Proper sample collection, handling, storage, etc.
  - Proper data collection.

Few definitions necessary for discussing quality control are:

- *Standard:* It is a substance with constant composition with sufficient purity to be used for standardization.
- *Control:* It is the sample which is chemically and physically similar to the unknown specimen. In a clinical laboratory often a high and a low control are run along with the normal.

- *Standard deviation:* It is the statistical expression of the scatter or dispersion of values around a central average (mean) value.
- *Specificity and sensitivity:* Specificity is how good the assay is at discriminating between the analyte under study and a potentially interfering substance.
  Sensitivity of an assay is a measure of the lowest quantity of the analyte that can be detected by the method used.

Quality control in clinical biochemistry laboratory can be conducted by:

1. Internal Quality Control
   Internal quality control includes:
   - Use of standardized glassware, reagents and equipment.
   - Employment of conscientious and well-trained staff.
   - Maintenance of:
     a. Proper analytical skill from start to finish.
     b. Required quality of reagents.
     c. Desired performance of the instruments.
   - Selection of accurate and precise methods.
2. External Quality Control
   External quality control includes comparison of the results of the laboratory with those of some standardized external laboratory for authentication of the results of the laboratory. Quality control charts are used for inter laboratory comparison. Various charts used for this purpose include:
   a. The Levey-Jennings control charts:
      In this chart the control values are plotted on the Y-axis and time on the X-axis. The chart shows the expected mean value in the center and indicates the control limits or range of acceptable values. The run is considered to be normal when the control values fall within control limits (± 2 SD).
   b. CUSUM (Cumulative sum) chart:
      In order to check the accuracy of analyses and quality control values, a CUSUM chart is prepared. Systematic errors can be checked by such charts. When systematic errors (all low or high values) are present, CUSUM values will rise steadily. At a certain stage the error will be too large to be accepted and the method will be considered out of control. CUSUM technique provides better determination of systemic errors than can be obtained by Levey-Jennings charts.

Importance of Quality Control in Clinical Practice

Today's physicians rely heavily on the clinical biochemistry laboratory reports for the diagnosis, follow-up and planning the therapeutic dosage for their patients. In accuracy and erroneous results may cost the patients dearly.

Thus, a good quality control practice helps to attain correct reports enhancing the laboratory performance and contribute to the satisfaction of the physicians and patients alike. Further this would contribute to better patient care and management in an efficient way.

CHAPTER

39

How to Work in a Biochemistry Laboratory

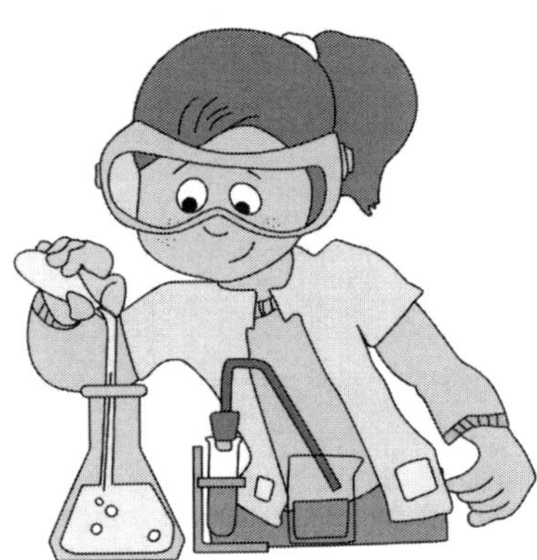

Chapter Framework

- Instructions for Working in a Biochemistry Laboratory

This course is intended to introduce you to some of the most widely used experimental procedures in biochemistry.

The biochemistry laboratory course, like all laboratory courses, is an exploration of procedures. This means that, in order to get full benefit from the course, you will need to read the manual, and you should participate as much as possible in the discussions. You should ask questions in or out of the class. You should participate in the actual lab work (and not simply allow your lab partners to do things for you). The more effort you put into the course work, the more you will learn. The class is an opportunity to learn valuable skills; take full advantage of it !

Instructions for Working in a Biochemistry Laboratory

Laboratories contain hazards of various kinds. Therefore, students should follow these instructions for their own safety and the safety of their colleagues.

1. The students should use aprons (laboratory coats) to protect themselves from chemical splashes and infectious agents.
2. All chemicals should be considered as potentially dangerous and should avoid contact with skin or clothing.
3. The gas burners should be turned off when not in use.
4. The reagent bottles should be covered with their lid/stopper after use.
5. The glassware and reagents should be replaced on their appropriate place after use.
6. The students should keep their work stations clean.

7. The students should work systematically during practical classes:
   - They should not talk during the practical work.
   - They should wear their aprons.
   - They should carry their practical journals and writing material before entering the laboratory.
   - They should record their observations for the practical in practical journal directly.
   - They should take down their practical data in their practical journal with proper description of—Aim, principle of method, procedure of method, normal range, clinical significance if any of the test, observations and result.
   - Do not say—"Well, I will remember what this means"; instead, write it down!
   - Do not say—"I will remember what I was thinking while I did this experiment"; instead, write it down! If you use your lab notebook properly, you will find that writing your practical results is much easier, and you will be developing good habits for the future.

Part B

Qualitative Exercises

- Carbohydrate Analysis
- Lipid Analysis
- Protein Analysis

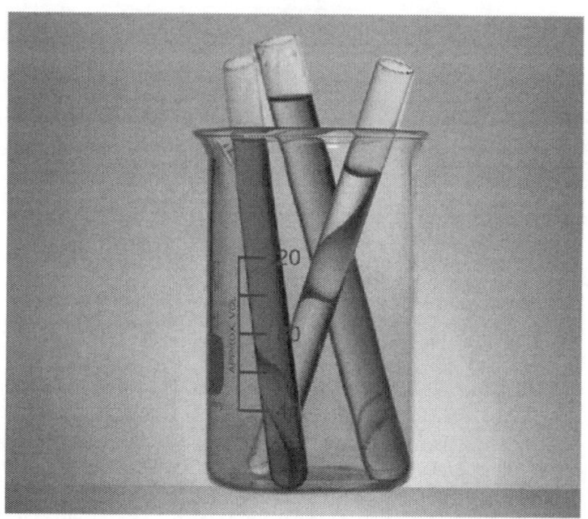

The qualitative exercises form an important section in practical biochemistry for the learners of biochemistry. Biochemistry is the study of biomolecules like carbohydrates, lipids, proteins, amino acids, vitamins, enzymes, etc. To study these biomolecules in laboratory we should be able to identify their presence or absence in a sample by chemical analysis. Qualitative analysis basically is concerned with this procedure of identification of the presence of a particular biomolecule in a given sample along with the analysis of the basic chemical nature of that biomolecule.

CHAPTER

40

Carbohydrate Analysis

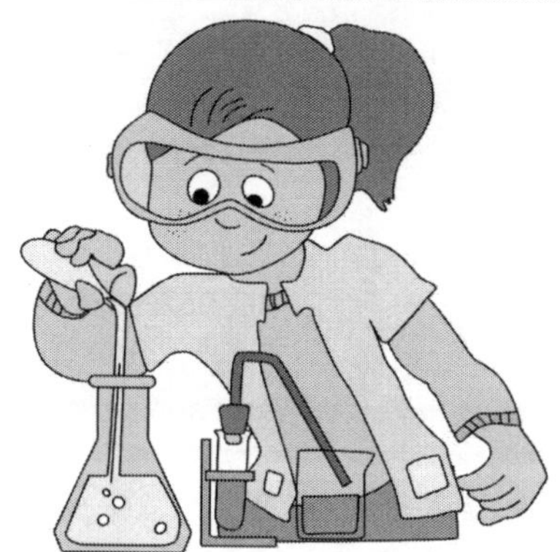

Chapter Framework

- Definition
- Classification
- Tests for Analysis of Carbohydrates
  - Molisch's Test
  - Reduction Tests
  - Fehling's Test
  - Benedict's Test
  - Test for Detecting Monosaccharides
  - Test for Keto-Sugars
  - Tests for Disaccharides
  - Osazone Test
  - Glacial Acetic Acid
- Tests for Polysaccharides
  - Iodine Test
  - Half and Full Saturation Test
- Identification of Unknown Carbohydrate

Definition

Carbohydrates can be defined as aldehyde or ketone derivatives of polyhydroxyl alcohols and compounds which yield these on hydrolysis.

Classification

Carbohydrates can be classified as follows:

1. *Monosaccharides:* These are the simplest sugars which cannot be hydrolyzed further, e.g. Glucose, fructose. These can be further classified on the basis of number of functional group into aldoses and ketoses.
   a. *Aldoses:* Those monosaccharides which contain an aldehyde group, e.g. Glucose, galactose, ribose, etc.
   b. *Ketoses:* Those monosaccharides which contain a ketone group e. g. Fructose, ribulose, erythrulose, etc.
   Furthermore the aldoses and ketoses are classified on the basis of number of carbon atoms into:
2. *Disaccharides:* Those carbohydrates which can be hydrolyzed further to produce 2 monosaccharide units are called disaccharides, e.g. lactose, maltose.

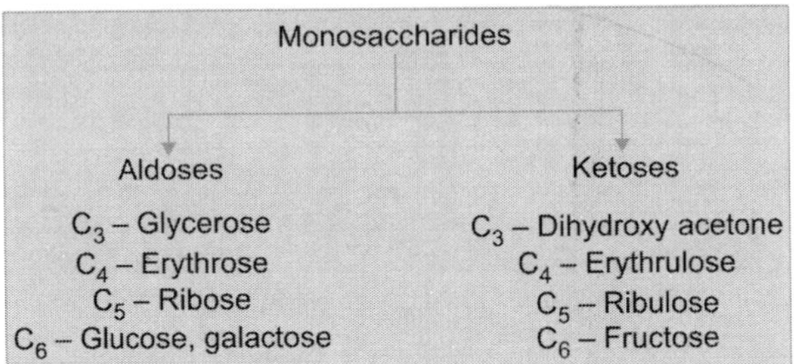

3. *Oligosaccharides:* Those carbohydrates which can be further hydrolyzed into 3 to 9 monosaccharide units are called oligosaccharides, e.g. raffinose.
4. *Polysaccharides:* Those carbohydrates which are made up of more than 10, i.e. 100s and 1000s of monosaccharide units are called as polysaccharides.

Polysaccharides can be further classified as:

a. Homopolysaccharides: Those polysaccharides which are made up of similar monosaccharide units, e.g. Starch, dextrin, glycogen, etc.
b. Heteropolysaccharides: Those polysaccharides which are made up of repeating units of [–amino sugar + uronic acid –] derivatives, e.g. Chondroitin, hyaluronic acid, etc.

The common carbohydrates used for analysis in the undergraduate laboratory are such that they include monosaccharides (glucose and fructose), disaccharides (nonreducing—sucrose, reducing—lactose and maltose) and polysaccharides (homopolysaccharides—starch and dextrin).

Tests for Analysis of Carbohydrates

Molisch's Test

This test is given by all soluble carbohydrates and similar color is developed at the surface of insoluble carbohydrates under appropriate conditions. Thus, it is the group specific test for carbohydrates.

Reagents

- Molisch reagent—5% α-naphthol in 95% ethyl alcohol
- Concentrated sulfuric acid (conc. H_2SO_4).

Principle

Strong acids like sulfuric acid, hydrolyze polysaccharides and disaccharides into monosaccharides. The monosaccharides then are dehydrated to corresponding furfural derivatives. The reaction is due to the formation of furfural and hydroxyl methyl furfural by the action of concentrated acid on pentoses and hexoses. The furfural derivatives then condense with a naphthol to give the violet colored ring at the junction of the two liquids.

Procedure

Add 2 drops of Molisch reagent (5% solution of a - naphthol in 95% ethyl alcohol) to 2 ml dilute sugar solution (1%) in a narrow bore test tube. Mix thoroughly, incline the test tube and add about 3 ml of concentrated sulfuric acid down the side of the test tube, forming a layer beneath the sugar solution. Be sure that the acid does not mix to a large extent with the solution. A purple violet color at the interface of the two liquids is an indication of positive test.

Precautions

- Always use a narrow test tube for obtaining a good ring at the junction.
- Do not confuse brown ring as a positive test.
- Do not add the acid too rapidly else the sugar would get charred and give a false-negative result.

Reduction Tests

Many sugars have the property of readily reducing the alkaline solution of the ions of certain metals such as copper, bismuth, iron and silver. The alkali in all these reagents brings about a considerable decomposition of the sugar molecule into reactive fragments (the enediols) which may also reduce the metal ions. This, while the total reduction for a given concentration of sugar may be constant under carefully defined conditions and is, therefore, utilizable for quantitative purposes.

Fehling's Test

Reagents

Fehling's solution A: 34.65 gram copper sulfate dissolved in water and made up to 500 mL.

Fehling's solution B: 125 gram potassium hydroxide and 174 gram Rochelle salt dissolved in water and made up to 500 mL.

These solutions are prepared separately. The Rochelle salt helps to prevent the precipitation of cupric hydroxide.

Procedure

Take 1 mL each of Fehling's solution A and B in a test tube and boil for 2 minutes. Now add 1 mL of sugar solution and boil for about a minute. Reducing sugars will give a precipitate of Cu_2O with the oxidation of sugars to their respective aldonic acids.

Drawbacks

- The reagent has low stability, therefore has to be prepared and stored separately.
- The procedure is cumbersome since it involves two steps.
- The alkali used, i.e. potassium hydroxide is strong and causes destruction of the sugar.

Benedict's Test

Reagents

Copper sulfate—17.3 g
Sodium citrate—173 g
Sodium carbonate—100 g
Distilled water (to make)—1 liter.

Dissolve sodium citrate and sodium carbonate in about 800 ml distilled water by application of heat. Dissolve copper sulfate in about 100 ml distilled water. Now add copper sulfate slowly to the carbonate citrate mixture with constant stirring. Make the volume up to 1 liter.

Principle

Both Fehling's test and Benedict's test are based upon the principle of reduction of cupric ions in hot alkaline medium (KOH in Fehling's test and Na_2CO_3 in Benedict's test) by reducing carbohydrates having a potentially free aldehyde or ketone group to Cu_2O and the carbohydrate gets oxidized to corresponding aldonic acid.

Procedure

Heat 5 ml Benedict's reagent with 8 drops of sugar solution. Boil the solution to then allow it to cool. There is a formation of red/yellow/green precipitate indicating a positive test.

Advantages of Benedict's Test

- The reagent is stable, i.e. has a longer shelf life.
- The procedure is single step procedure.
- The alkali used is a weak alkali therefore the sugar does not get charred/destroyed.

Clinical Importance of the Benedict's Test

The test is a semiquantitative test when performed in a standard way and gives an idea of the percentage of sugar in urine sample.

Standard Way to Perform the Benedict's Test with Urine Sample

Take 5 mL of the Benedict's reagent in a test tube. Add 8 drops of urine sample to it and boil for one and half minute. If sugar is present in urine sample yellow/green/orange/brick red colored precipitate is observed. The color of the precipitate formed gives idea of the percentage of sugar in the given urine sample. (0.5%—yellow, 1%—green, 2%—orange, >2%—brick red).

Test for Detecting Monosaccharides

Barfoed's Test

Reagents

Dissolve 12.3 gram of neutral crystalline copper acetate in 200 mL water, filter if necessary and add 1.8 mL of glacial acetic acid.

Principle

Strongly reducing carbohydrates like the monosaccharides will cause reduction even in a mildly acidic medium (provided by glacial acetic acid) and form the brick red precipitate of Cu_2O.

Disaccharides do not give this test positive on heating for 30 seconds. However, on boiling for 15 to 20 minutes, the disaccharides are hydrolyzed to their constituent monosaccharides and will give a false positive test.

Procedure

Take 3 mL of Barfoed's reagent in a test tube and add 1 ml of reducing sugar to it. On boiling this solution for 30 seconds exactly, a brick red colored precipitate is obtained at the bottom of the test tube, indicating the presence of reducing monosaccharides.

Precautions

Do not boil the solution for a longer duration else the disaccharides would give a false positive test.

Test for Keto-Sugars

Seliwanoff's Test

Reagents

Dissolve 0.05 gm of resorcinol in 100 mL of dilute HCl to form Seliwanoff's reagent.

Principle

The keto sugars react with dilute HCl form hydroxylmethylfurfural derivatives which, then condense with resorcinol to give a pink-red colored complex.

Procedure

Take 3 mL of Seliwanoff's reagent in a test tube and add 1 ml of keto sugar solution to it. Boil for 2 minutes. A pink-red colored complex is formed indicating the presence of keto sugar.

Tests for Disaccharides

Inversion Test for Sucrose

Reagents

- Concentrated HCl
- Solid sodium carbonate
- Benedict's reagent
- Seliwanoff's reagent.

Procedure

Boil 3 mL of the sucrose solution with few drops of conc. HCl. Now cool this solution and add solid sodium carbonate to it for neutralizing the solution. Keep adding Na_2CO_3 till effervescence ceases. This is now termed as the hydrolysis mixture/hydrolysate. Divide the hydrolysate into 2 parts and perform the Benedict's test with one part and Seliwanoff's test with the second portion. A positive test indicates the that sucrose is now hydrolyzed into reducing sugars glucose and fructose which give the positive test respectively Benedict's test and Seliwanoff's test.

Osazone Test

Reagents

Osazone Mixture

It is prepared by mixing 1 part phenyl hydrazine and 2 parts sodium acetate by weight.

Glacial Acetic Acid

Principle

When reducing carbohydrates are heated with osazone mixture, they undergo specific chemical reactions giving rise to crystals of characteristic shape on cooling.

Procedure

Take 5 mL of reducing carbohydrate solution, i.e. glucose, fructose, maltose, lactose in separate test tubes and label them. Now Osazone mixture is added. Add 5 drops of glacial acetic acid into each test tube and warm gently to dissolve the solids. Keep the test tubes in boiling water bath for the following time period:

Glucose and fructose—2 to 5 min

Lactose and maltose—45 min

Then cool it gradually, pore precipitate on slide and observe under microscope for different types of crystals.

Glucose and fructose—Needle-shaped/Hay stack like crystals.

Lactose—Cotton puff-shaped crystals.

Maltose—Sunflower-shaped crystals (Fig. 40.1).

Tests for Polysaccharides

Iodine Test

Reagents—I_2 Solution

Principle

Polysaccharide being macromolecules have affinity to adsorb I_2 giving characteristically colored complexes.

Explanation

The test depends on the property of adsorption of I_2 by large polysaccharide molecules.

The small I_2 molecules adsorbed on the surface, form complex of lose physical combination. On heating the I_2-polysaccharide complex dissociates and therefore disappears on cooling the

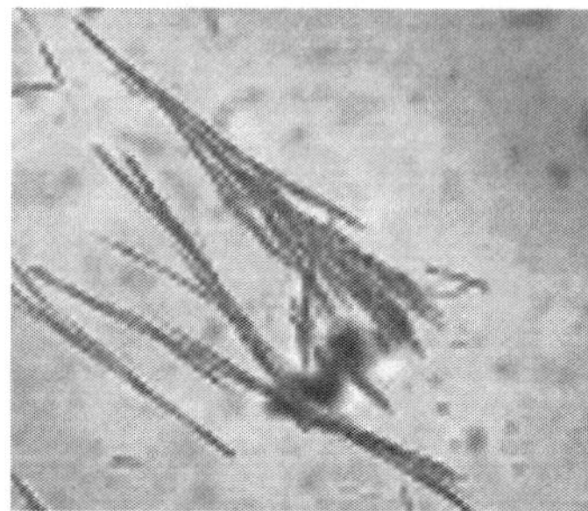

Glucose/Fructose

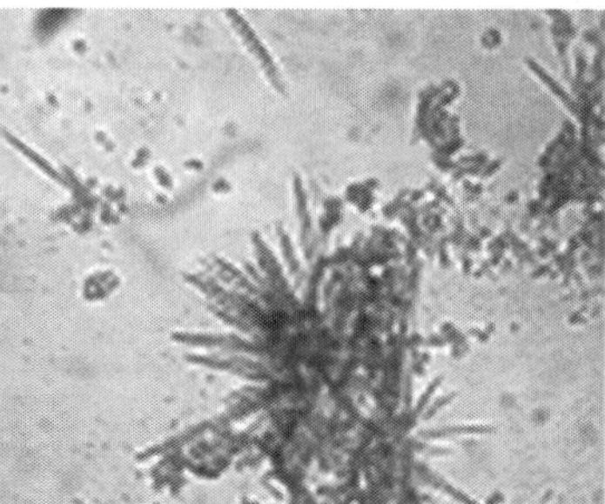

Lactose

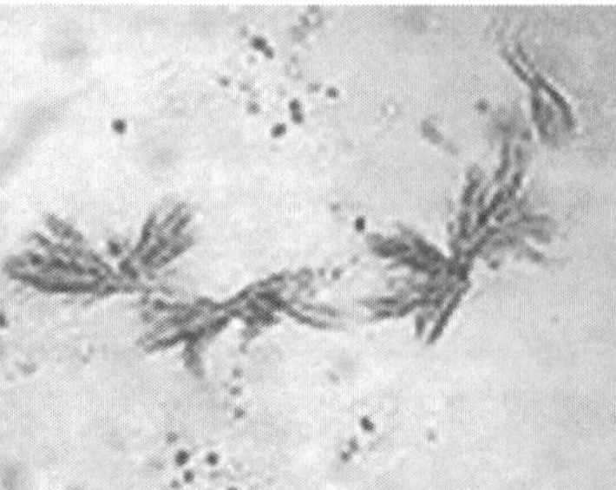

Maltose

Fig. 40.1: Osazone crystals

complex is reformed and the color reappears, except in the case of dextrin. Heating produces change on the surface of dextrin as the result of which they lose the property of adsorption.

Precaution

Excess of I_2 should not be added. It will give black color.

Procedure

Take 3 mL of carbohydrate solution and add few drops of I_2 solution, mix and observe the color. Starch gives a blue color which disappears on heating and reappears on cooling.

Dextrin gives a reddish purple color on addition of I_2, which disappears on heating and does not reappears on cooling.

Half and Full Saturation Test

Reagents

Solid Ammonium Sulfate

Saturated solution ammonium sulfate in water.

Principle

Polysaccharides form colloidal solution in water. Colloids are kept in solution by two factors:

- Electric charges: Similarly charged particles repel each other and therefore their coalescence is prevented.
- Shell of hydration: Each molecule is surrounded by shell of water known as shell of hydration; this prevents the coalescence of particle.

Starch is a bigger molecule and easily precipitated by half saturation in ammonium sulfate while dextrin is smaller molecule so it is precipitated by full saturation.

Procedure

Half Saturation

Take 2 mL of carbohydrate solution and add equal volume of saturated solution of ammonium sulfate shake vigorously and allow standing. A white precipitate indicates that the carbohydrate under test is precipitated by half saturation. The test is given positive by starch.

Full Saturation

Take 2 ml of carbohydrate solution and shake and allow standing. A white precipitate indicates that the carbohydrate under test is precipitated on full saturation with solid $(NH_4)_2SO_4$. This test is given by both starch and dextrin.

Identification of Unknown Carbohydrate

Identification of unknown carbohydrate can be done as shown in the Flow chart 40.1.

Flow chart 40.1 Identification of unknown carbohydrate

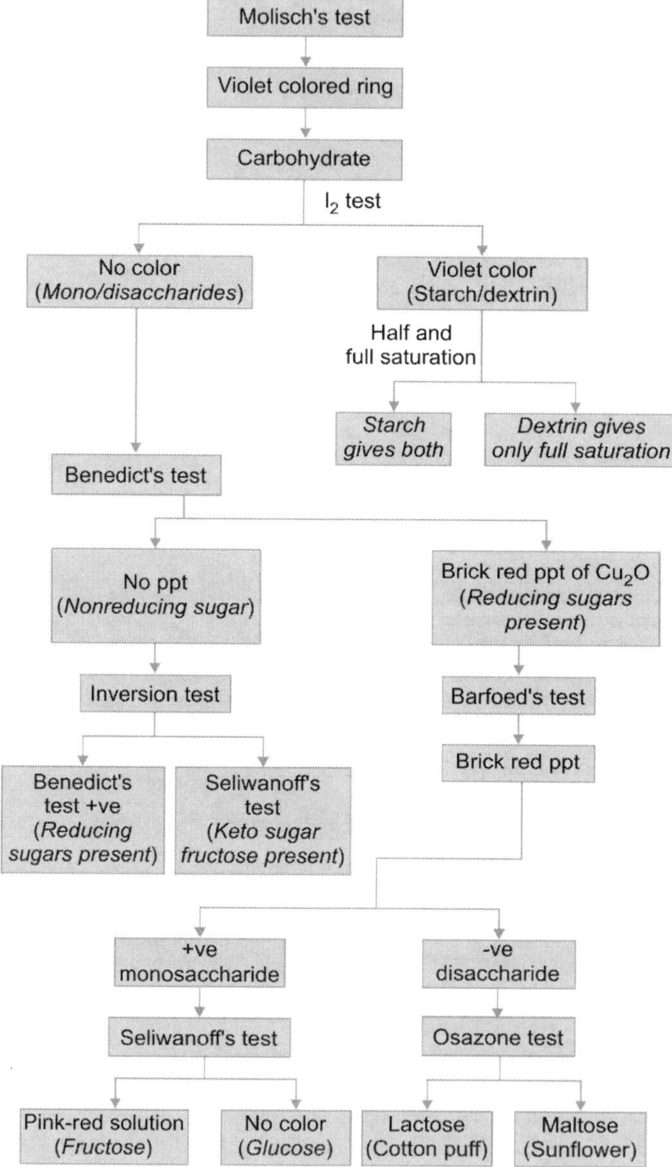

Viva Voce

Q1. What does the green fluorescence in Molisch's test indicate?

Q2. Why is Benedict's test preferred over Fehling's test?

Q3. Why is the Barfoed's test given by only monosaccharides and not by reducing disaccharides?

Q4. Can sucrose give a direct positive Seliwanoff's test?

Q5. Why do glucose and fructose have identical osazone crystals?

Q6. Why does starch give both half and full saturation tests whereas dextrin gives only full saturation test?

CHAPTER

41

Lipid Analysis

Chapter Framework

Definition

Lipids are heterogeneous group of organic component, which are characterized by solubility in nonpolar solvent and insolubility in polar solvent. Chemically, they are esters of fatty acid with certain alcohol.

Classification

Lipids are classified into three classes:

Simple Lipids

These are esters of fatty acid with alcohol. They are subdivided into two groups:

- Fats and oils—they are fatty acids esterified with glycerol.
- Fats are solid and oils are liquid at room temperature. Waxes—these are esters of fatty acid with high molecular weight alcohol like cetyl alcohol.

Compound Lipids

They contain some substances in addition to fatty acids and alcohol. They can be subdivided into:

- *Phospholipids*—They contain fatty acids and alcohol which may or may not be glycerol; besides this they contain phosphoric acid and nitrogenous base, e.g. Lecithin, cephalin, sphingomyelin, plasmalogens, etc.
- *Glycolipids*—They contain fatty acid, carbohydrate and sphingosine, an amino alcohol. They can be subdivided into:
  - *Cerebrosides*—These contain fatty acid, carbohydrate (glucose or galactose) and sphingosine, e.g. Kerasin, nervon, oxynervon and cerebron.

- *Gangliosides*—These are similar, to cerebrosides except that they contain fatty acid, sphingosine, N-acetyl neuraminic acid and hexoses—glucose and galactose.
- *Lipoproteins*—These are lipids conjugated with a protein as prosthetic group, e.g. Chylomicrons, VLDL, IDL, LDL, HDL. They help in transport of nonpolar lipids in aqueous medium of plasma.
- *Sulfolipids*— These are sulfated glycolipids

Derived Lipids

These can be derived by the hydrolysis of the simple and compound lipids, e.g. Cholesterol, fatty acids, glycerol, etc.

Analysis of Lipids Based on Physical Properties

Lipids show typical physical properties like insolubility in polar solvents, lighter than water and greasy nature. All these properties can be demonstrated by performing the following tests:

Solubility Test

Reagents

- Chloroform
- Ether
- CCl_4.

Principle

The test is based on the property of solubility of lipids in organic solvents and its insolubility in lipids in organic solvents and its insolubility in water.

Procedure

Take 3 mL each of water and chloroform, CCl_4, ether in separate test tubes. Now add 5 drops of oil into each test tube. Shake vigorously and allow to stand the oil and water separate quickly whereas clear solutions are formed in case of organic solvents showing that oils are insoluble in water and soluble in organic solvents.

Grease Spot Test

Reagents

Ether.

Principle

Lipids are greasy in nature therefore they leave a greasy spot on filter paper. This test may be taken as a group test for lipids.

Procedure

Take 3 mL of ether in a test tube dissolve 5 drops of oil in it. Put a drop of this solution on a filter paper and let it dry by ether evaporation leaving a translucent spot on filter paper indicating lipids are greasy in nature.

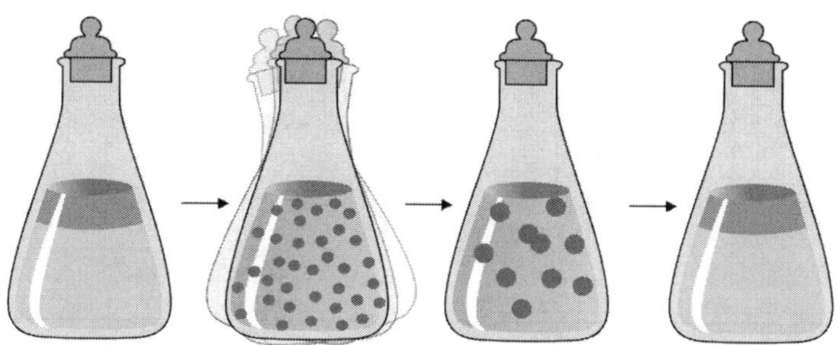

Fig. 41.1 Emulsification of lipids

Emulsification Test (Fig. 41.1)

Reagents

- 0.5% Na_2CO_3 solution in water
- Soap solution
- Bile salt solution 0.5% in water.

Principle

When oil and water are shaken together oil in broken up into very tiny droplets which are dispersed in water. This is known as oil in water emulsion. Water molecules due to their high surface tension have a tendency to come together and form a separate layer, this is why oil in water emulsion is unstable in the presence of substances that lower the surface tension of water, for example—Na_2CO_3, soap solution, bile salts, etc. decrease the tendency of water molecule to coalesce together. Thus, the emulsion gets stabilized. Since bile salts cause greatest decrease in surface tension, they are the best emulsifying agent.

Procedure

Take 5 ml of water, Na_2CO_3, soap solution with bile salt solution in separate test tube add 5 drops of oil into each test tube, shake vigorously and allow standing. The oil-water emulsion is least stable for the Na_2CO_3 solution, slightly more stable with the soap solution and maximum stable with the bile salts solution. Thus the oil takes minimum time to form separate layer with the Na_2CO_3 solution and maximum with the bile salts solution.

Analysis of Derived Lipids

Test for Glycerol

Dunstan's Test (with Dilute Glycerol)

Reagents

- 0.5% solution of sodium borate
- Phenolphthalein indicator.

Principle

Borax hydrolyses into NaOH and Boric acid. As NaOH is strong alkali and boric acid is a relatively weak acid, the medium becomes alkaline, indicated by the pink color of phenolphthalein.

On adding glycerol, a strong glyceroboric acid is formed and its medium becomes acidic indicated by the disappearance of the pink color.

On heating the glyceroboric acid dissociates into glycerol and boric acid and the medium becomes alkaline again, so that the pink color of phenolphthalein reappears.

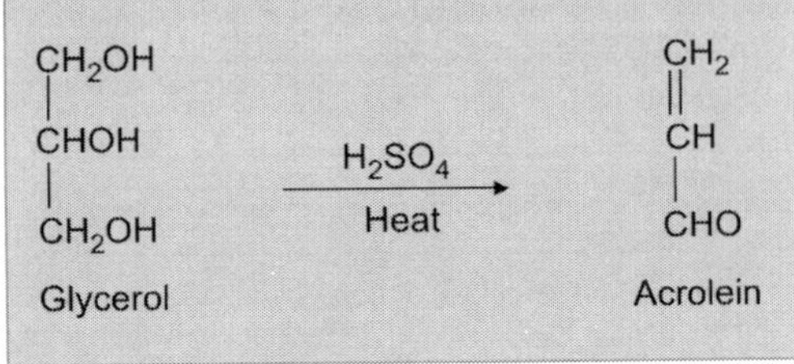

Procedure

Take 3 mL of borax solution in a test tube add a drop of phenolphthalein indicator. A pink color is produced indicated that the medium is alkaline. Now add 20% glycerol drop by drop until the pink color disappears indicating that the medium has become acidic. Heat the solution until the pink color reappears indicating that the medium has become alkaline again.

Acrolein Test (with Concentrated Glycerol)

Reagents

- Conc. H_2SO_4.

Principle

On heating with H_2SO_4, glycerol gets dehydrated and forms unsaturated aldehyde termed as acrolein.

Procedure

In an absolutely dry test tube pour a few drops of conc. glycerol add and drop of concentrated H_2SO_4. Heat the test over a small flame a typical pungent odor is present.

Tests for Cholesterol

Salkowski's Test

Reagents:

- Conc. H_2SO_4.
- 0.5% solution of cholesterol in $CHCl_3$.

Principle

Cholesterol in presence in conc. H_2SO_4 get dehydrated into 3, 5-cholestadiene. Two molecules of 3, 5-cholestadiene 1-one react with H_2SO_4 to form monosulfonic acid which is green in color or form disulfonic acid which give cherry-red color.

Procedure

Take 2 mL of cholesterol in a dry test tube. Add 2 mL conc. H_2SO_4, shake and allow standing. $CHCl_3$ and H_2SO_4 layer separates. On standing the $CHCl_3$ layer is cherry-red and acid layer shows a green fluorescence.

Liebermann-Burchard's Test

Reagents

- Conc. H_2SO_4
- Acetic anhydride.

Principle

The exact chemical reactions involved in Liebermann-Burchard's test and Salkowski's test is not known. It is presumed that cholesterol is dehydrated by conc. H_2SO_4 and acetic anhydride to form 3, 5-cholestadiene and 2, 4-cholestadiene. The cholestadiene then combine to form their dimer or trimer, which react with H_2SO_4 to form their sulfonic acid derivatives. Various colors appear at different stages.

Procedure

Take 3 mL cholesterol salt in dry test tube. Add 10 drops of acetic anhydride and 2 drops of conc. H_2SO_4. A red color develops at first followed by blue, finally the whole solution becomes green.

Viva Voce

Q1. The hydrophobic nature of lipids is explained by which test?
Q2. Washing powder and bile salts work on the same principle named as ....
Q3. Glycerol (concentrated) on heating with strong acid gives pungent fumes of ....
Q4. The dilute glycerol is detected by .... test.
Q5. Liebermann-Burchard and Salkowski test are clinically significant. Why?
Q6. Name the colored products formed during the tests of cholesterol Liebermann-Burchard and Salkowski's.

CHAPTER

42

Protein Analysis

Chapter Framework

- Definition
  - Classification
- Group Specific Test of Proteins
  - Biuret Test
  - Ninhydrin Test (for α-amino Acids)
- Color Reactions for Identification of Various Amino Acids
  - Xanthoproteic Test (for Aromatic Amino Acids)
  - Millon Nasse's Test (for Tyrosine)
  - Lead Sulfide Test (for Sulfur Releasing amino acids—Cystine and Cysteine)
  - Aldehyde Test (for Tryptophan)
- Precipitation of Proteins
  - Heat Coagulation Test
  - Heller's Nitric Acid Test
  - Half and Full Saturation Test
  - Precipitation by Heavy Metals Test
  - Precipitation by Alkaloidal Reagent (Sulfo-salicylic Acid)
  - Precipitation at Isoelectric pH
  - Neumann's Test
- Identification of Unknown Protein

Definition

Proteins are complex nitrogenous compounds which yield amino acids hydrolysis.

Chemically, they are macromolecules made up of amino acids linked by peptide linkage.

Classification

Proteins can be classified into three classes based upon their solubility.

Simple Proteins

Simple proteins are made up of only amino acid. They can be subdivided on the basis of their solubility and heat coagulability into albumin, glutelins, protamines, prolamines, histones and albuminoids.

Conjugated Proteins

They are made up of amino acids and a nonprotein part which is known as the prosthetic group. Depending on the nature of prosthetic group the conjugated proteins are of the following types.

Mucoproteins, lipoproteins, nucleoproteins, phosphoproteins, chromoproteins and metalloproteins.

Derived Proteins

They are derived by denaturation or hydrolysis of native proteins. They are further of two types:

Primary derived
These are formed by intramolecular changes not involving hydrolysis, e.g. protein, metaproteins, denatured proteins and coagulated proteins.

Secondary derived
These are formed by the hydrolysis of native proteins, e.g. Primary proteoses, secondary proteoses and peptones.

The major proteins given for analysis in an undergraduate laboratory are albumin (simple protein), casein (conjugated protein) and gelatin and peptone (derived proteins). Analysis of these proteins is done as this would help understand the chemical nature of the proteins and also to identify the proteins which contain essential amino acids like aromatic amino acids— Phe, Trp, Sulfur releasing amino acid—Met. Thus, emphasizing the dietary importance of good quality proteins like milk protein or egg protein.

Group Specific Test of Proteins

Proteins are polymers of amino acids and group specific tests are given by compounds having peptide linkage (Biuret) or those containing a-amino acids (Ninhydrin). Thus, these tests are given by all proteins.

Biuret Test

Reagents

- 10% NaOH
- 5% $CuSO_4$.

Principle

Proteins and compounds with 2 or more peptide linkage gives violet color with Cu^{++} ions in presence of NaOH.

Note: Whenever urea is heated it is converted into biurets and these biurets give a violet color when treated with NaOH and $CuSO_4$. Hence it is known as biuret test.

Procedure

Take 2 mL of protein solution and 1 mL of NaOH solution. Then add $CuSO_4$ slowly drop by drop, mixing constantly till a violet color is seen. In the 2nd test tube, take 2 mL of water add 1 mL NaOH and 2 drops of $CuSO_4$ and compare it with the test.

Ninhydrin Test (for α-Amino Acids)

Reagents

- Ninhydrin reagent (1, 2, 3-trihydro hydantene hydrate).

Principle

When an a-amino acid is heated with ninhydrin a violet color compound is formed. CO_2, NH_3 are also formed during the reaction, which are evolved as effervescence.

Explanation

When Ninhydrin, which is a powerful oxidizing agent is heated is α-amino acid decarboxylation and oxidation takes place, releasing CO_2 and producing an aldehyde with one carbon atom less. Ninhydrin itself is reduced. The reduced ninhydrin then reacts with NH_3 and one molecule of nonreduced ninhydrin forming bluish violet color complex.

Practical Importance

This test forms the basis of several different types of quantitative methods for determination of amino acids in biological fluids by techniques like electrophoresis or chromatography.

Procedure

Take 3 mL of protein solution. Add few drop of ninhydrin solution. Mix the solution and heat for about 1 to 2 minute. Now allow the test Cube to cool. Development of bluish violet purple color indicates the presence of α-amino acid. This is a group specific test given positive by all α-amino acids.

Color Reactions for Identification of Various Amino Acids

The color reactions of the proteins include those tests which help in the detection of specific amino acids by development of unique colors unique to that particular amino acid or group of amino acids.

Xanthoproteic Test (for Aromatic Amino Acids)

Reagents

- Conc. HNO_3
- 40% NaOH.

Principle

When the protein containing aromatic amino acids is heated with HNO_3, there is nitration of benzene group of amino acids. Nitrophenyl group impacts yellow color to the solution. On adding NaOH, the nitrophenyl group ionizes to give orange color.

Procedure

Take 3 ml of protein solution. Add 1 mL of HNO_3 to it. White ppt may develop. Heat the solution for some times, it turns yellow. Now add 40% of NaOH (2 mL). Mix it, orange color appears which shows presence of aromatic amino acids.

Millon Nasse's Test (for Tyrosine)

Reagents

- 15% $HgSO_4$ in 6 NH_2SO_4
- 1% $NaNO_2$ fresh solution.

Principle

There occurs mercuration and nitration of phenolic group of tyrosine resulting in formation of red-colored complex.

Note:

a. *The test is carried out in strong acidic medium as Hg is precipitated in alkaline medium.*
b. *The $NaNO_2$ reacts with H_2SO_4 to form (HNO_2) nitrous acid.*

Procedure

Take 3 mL of protein solution and 1 mL of Millon Nasse's reagent. Boil it than cool. After cooling add 1 mL of freshly prepared $NaNO_2$ solution. The solution and precipitate turns pink showing the presence of tyrosine.

Lead Sulfide Test (for Sulfur-releasing Amino Acids—Cystine and Cysteine)

Reagents

- 40% NaOH
- 2% Lead acetate.

Principle

On boiling with NaOH the sulfur present in protein is liberated as sodium sulfide. This reacts with lead acetate to form a black brown precipitate or brown color of lead sulfide.

Explanation

Cysteine and cystine respond to this test but the sulfur present in methionine is not released by the above treatment. Casein and gelatin which contain methionine but practically negligible amount of cystine and cysteine give a negative test.

Procedure

Take 2 mL of protein solution and add 2 mL of 40% NaOH. Boil, then, cool and add few drops of lead acetate. The brown or black precipitate shows the presence of sulfur-releasing amino acids.

Aldehyde Test (for Tryptophan)

Reagents

- Dilute formaldehyde
- Conc. H_2SO_4.

Principle

Tryptophan contains an indole ring which combines with formaldehyde in the presence of conc. sulfuric acid to from a violet-colored compound.

Procedure

Take 2 mL of protein solution and add 4–5 drops of formalin and shake well. Now add 2 mL of sulfuric acid by the sides of test tubes slowly. A violet-colored ring at the junction of 2 liquids shows positive test.

Precipitation of Proteins

Proteins form colloidal solutions in water. These can be precipitated out by various reagents. Depending upon the chemical nature of the proteins, different proteins get precipitated under different condition and by different reagents. Thus, the precipitation reactions are performed to determine whether the proteins are simple/conjugated/derived.

Heat Coagulation Test

Principle

Certain physical agents (heat, cold, etc.) disrupts the secondary, tertiary and quaternary level of structural integrity of natural protein molecule by breaking H_2 bond and removal of physical forces like van der Waals and electrostatic forces thereby denaturing the protein molecule and polypeptide chain get uncoiled, i.e. irregularly shaped.

The denatured protein of albumin and globulin is less soluble at isoelectric pH so is thrown out as white coagulum.

Procedure

Fill 2/3 rd of test tube with protein solution. Hold test tube at its bottom and incline slightly and warm the upper part of solution. A dense coagulum is formed in upper part of solution. This may be compared with the lower part of test tube. The test is given by heat coaguable protein like albumin and globulin.

Heller's Nitric Acid Test

Reagents

- Conc. HNO_3.

Principle

Simple and conjugated proteins react with conc. nitric acid to form acid metaprotein that turn yellow due to nitration.

Procedure

Take 3 mL of conc. HNO_3 in test tube. Incline the test tube and add 3 mL of protein solution along the wall of test tube. A yellow white precipitate appears at the junction of the two liquids indicating that protein is precipitated by conc. HNO_3.

Half and Full Saturation Test

Reagents

- Saturated solution of $(NH_4)_2$ SO_4 in H_2O
- Solid $(NH_4)_2$ SO_4.

Principle

Protein solutions are colloidal nature and are stabilized by 2 factors:

- Electrical charges
- Shell of hydration.

Some charges (depending on pH of the solution) are present on surface of protein molecules. Similarly charged molecules repel each other preventing coalescence. Each molecule is surrounded by a film of water known as shell of hydration. This also prevents coalescence of particles. If both these factors are removed then the particles will coalesce. This can be done by adding $(NH_4)_2SO_4$, which neutralizes electrical charges and removes the shell of hydration as it has greater affinity for water. Smaller the molecule greater will be the number of charges to be neutralized and greater will be the surface area with larger shell of hydration requiring large amount of ammonium sulfate for neutralization. Therefore, peptone is of very small size thus it does not give half as well as full saturation test. Larger the molecule smaller will be the surface are of the molecule smaller will be the shell of hydration to be removed. Thus, gelatin a bigger molecule gives both the tests.

Procedure

Half Saturation Test

Take 3 mL of protein solution in a test tube and add 3 mL of saturated solution of $(NH_4)_2SO_4$ solution. Shake vigorously and allow standing. A white precipitate is seen in case of casein and gelatin.

Full Saturation Test

Take 3 mL of protein solution add solid $(NH_4)_2SO_4$ and shake vigorously and allow standing. A white precipitate is seen in case of albumin, casein and gelatin.

Precipitation by Heavy Metals Test

Reagents

- $AgNO_3$ solution or $HgSO_4$ or lead acetate.

Principle

Metals being heavily charged when added to protein solution (negatively charged) in alkaline medium result in precipitation. The insoluble precipitate is a metal proteinate. Thus with $AgNO_3$ it forms silver proteinate with lead acetate it from lead proteinate, with mercuric sulfate it forms mercuric proteinate, etc.

Practical Importance

In heavy metal poisoning egg white is used as an antidote due to the capability of protein to precipitate with heavy metals and to prevent the heavy metal from absorption by GIT and exerting their toxic effect.

Procedure

Take 3 mL of protein solution in a test tube and add heavy metal salts solution drop by drop till precipitate appears.

Precipitation by Alkaloidal Reagent (Sulfosalicylic Acid)

Reagents

- Sulfosalicylic acid

Principle

Proteins are amphoteric in nature, i.e. they behave as acids in alkaline medium and as bases in acidic medium. In the presence of sulfosalicylic acid they act as bases and react with the acid to form an insoluble salt, i.e. protein salicylate.

Clinical Importance

The test is used for the detection of protein in urine.

Procedure

Take 3 ml of protein solution in a test tube. Add sulfosalicylic acid drop by drop mixing after each addition. White turbidity appears.

Precipitation at Isoelectric pH

Reagents

- 1% acetic acid.

Principle

The solubility of proteins at their isoelectric pH is minimum casein (casein is precipitated at its isoelectric pH, i.e. 4.6 at room temperature) is milk protein and is stable only in alkaline medium above IEP. In milk, it is kept soluble by various factors. On addition of acid the medium becomes acidic and various factors are removed precipitating casein.

Procedure

Take 3 mL of casein solution add 1% acetic acid drop by drop till casein is precipitated.

Neumann's Test

Reagents

- Ammonium molybdate
- Conc HNO_3

Principle

Casein when reacts with ammonium molybdate, in presence of HNO_3 it forms canary yellow color solution or precipitate of phosphoammonium molybdate.

Note: This test is given by phosphoproteins and thus casein is phosphoprotein.

Procedure

Take 3 mL of casein solution add 1% acetic acid slowly drop by drop till casein is precipitated.

Explanation

Casein is digested by the conc HNO_3 to release phosphoric acid group, which reacts with ammonium molybdate to give a canary yellow colored solution or precipitate.

Identification of Unknown Protein

Identification of unknown protein sample can be done as shown in the Flow chart 42.1.

Flow chart 42.1 Identification of unknown protein

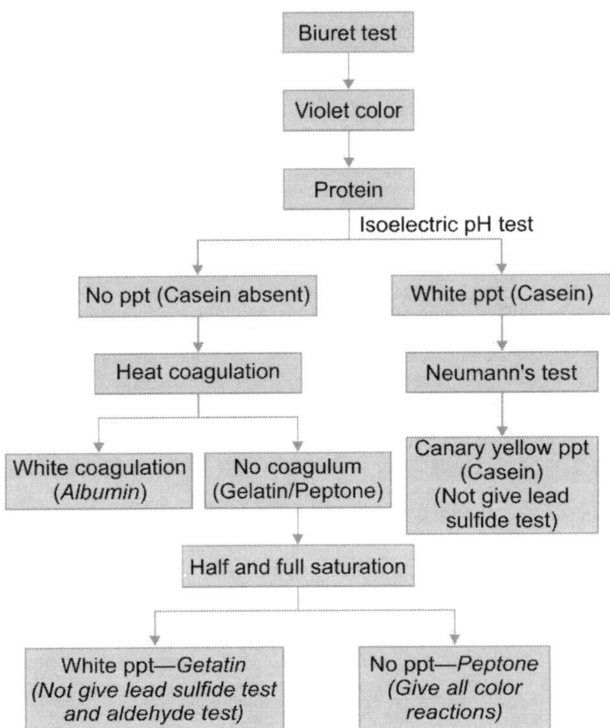

Viva Voce

Q1. Why is the Biuret test given positive by all proteins?
Q2. Why is the Biuret test named so?
Q3. What is the clinical importance of Ninhydrin test?
Q4. Name the color reaction specific for aromatic amino acids?
Q5. Name the color reaction specific for sulfur-releasing amino acids?
Q6. Why is the lead sulfide test not given by casein?
Q7. Faint pink color of Millon Nasse's test by Gelatin indicates what?
Q8. Which protein gives all the color reactions positive and what does that show?
Q9. Name a precipitation test given exclusively by casein.
Q10. What is the clinical importance of the Sulfosalicylic acid test?
Q11. During the heat coagulation test which bonds are broken in the albumin molecule?
Q12. What is the clinical importance of heavy metal test?

Part C

Quantitative Exercises

- Gastric Juice Analysis
- Colorimetry
- Blood Sugar
- Total Protein and A: G ratio
- Serum Urea
- Serum Creatinine
- Serum Lipid Profile
- Estimation of Sugar in urine (Benedict's Quantitative Method)

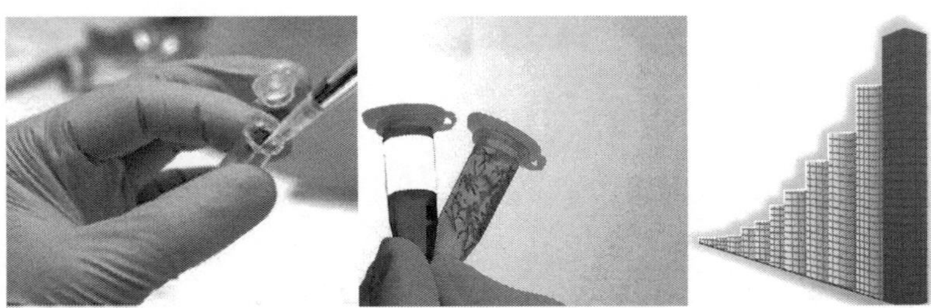

Quantitative Exercises

Quantitative estimations are the most important applications of a clinical biochemistry laboratory. These include the estimations of various biochemical parameters in body fluids like blood, serum, plasma, urine or secretions like gastric juice, etc.

The quantitative analyses may be done manually like the estimations of free and total acidity of a gastric juice sample or they may be performed using clinical laboratory instruments like colorimeters or semiautomated analyzers or fully automated analyzers for various serum and plasma investigations (blood sugar, urea, creatinine, lipid profile, etc.).

The quantitative exercises to be performed by the undergraduate students include mainly the analysis of gastric juice for its free and total acidity and the analysis of blood and serum parameters like sugar, urea, creatinine, cholesterol, etc.

CHAPTER

43

Gastric Juice Analysis

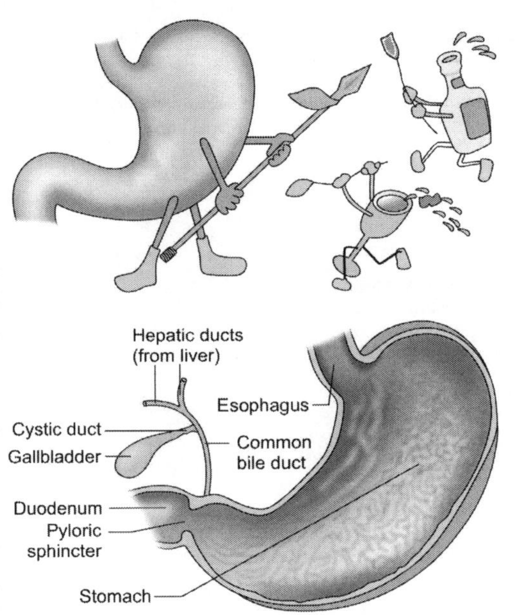

Chapter Framework

Gastric juice is a combined secretion of 3 different types of cells of the gastric mucosa. The chief cells secrete pepsinogen, the parietal cells secrete HCl and the mucous cells secrete mucus. The gastric juice is a clear, pale yellow, odorless fluid, having a pH around 1 to 2 and specific gravity around 1.007.

Analysis of Gastric Juice

It includes analysis of acid fraction and enzyme concentration. The various tests performed with gastric juice are related with detection of disorders of secretory activity of gastric glands.

For determining gastric function, gastric juice is analyzed for free and total acidity. The free acidity of gastric juice is due to free HCl secreted by oxyntic cell of gastric glands. The combined acidity is due to acid-protein complex—protein hydrochloride and traces of weakly ionized agents like citric acid, lactic acid, pyruvic acid, etc. which may be present as remnants of food digestion. The free and combined acidity together constitute total acidity.

Method of Collection of Gastric Juice

The patient is asked to come after an overnight fast. Ryle's tube (diameter—4 mm) is lubricated with wax or liquid paraffin which is passed through nasogastric route. The position of the lower end of the tube in judged by the marking on the Ryle's tube. The fasting juice sample is collected as first sample as shown in Figures 43.1A and B.

Test sample is collected after 100 mL of 7% alcohol or cup of tea (without milk) with toast is given to the patient. After 15 min the first sample after the test meal is withdrawn. Nearly 10–12 mL of gastric juice is withdrawn each time at 30 minutes interval and such total of 6 samples are collected. The gastric juice is then examined quantitatively and qualitatively. Readings are than plotted on graph paper taking time and concentration as the 2 axis. This procedure is called fractional test meal (FTM).

The FTM curve shows the complete course of gastric juice secretion as shown in Figure 43.2.

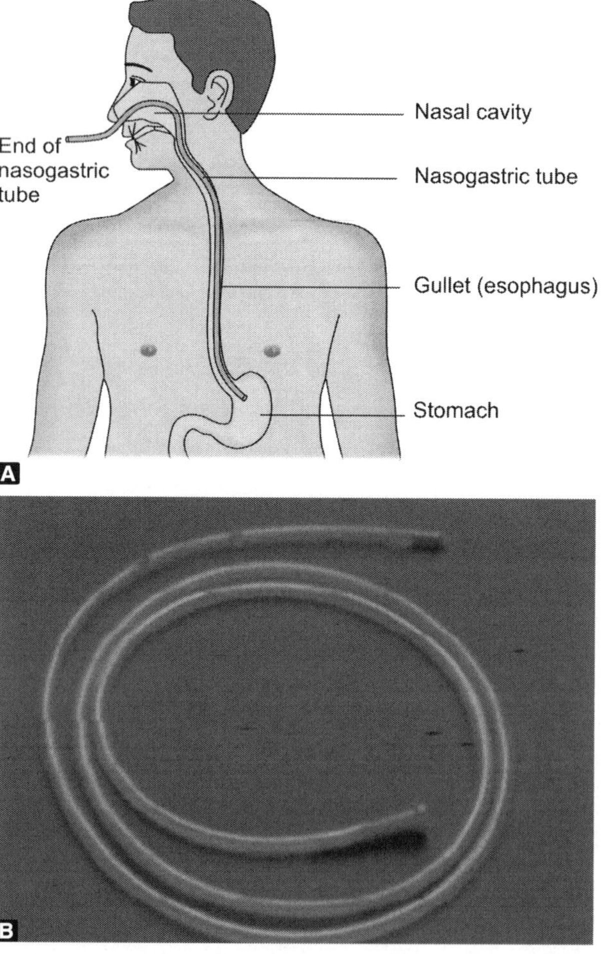

Fig. 43.1A and B (A) Route of Ryle's tube insertion (B) Ryle's tube

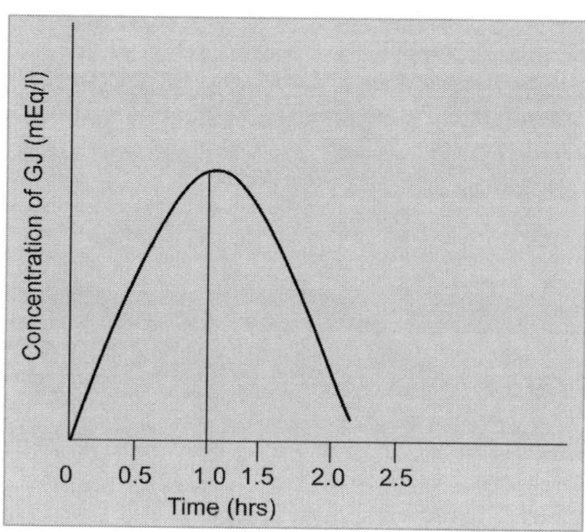

Fig. 43.2 FTM curve

Determination of Free and Total Acidity

Reagents

- NaOH—N/10
- Toffer's indicator—Dimethyl amino azobenzene
- Phenolphthalein indicator.

Principle

A fixed volume of gastric juice is titrated with standard NaOH first to pH 3.6 when free acidity is neutralized and then upto pH 8.5 when all acids in gastric juice is neutralized.

Procedure

Take 10 mL of gastric juice into a conical flask and add 4 to 5 drops of toffer's indicator so that solution turns red. Now take N/10 NaOH in a burette and add dropwise to the gastric juice with regular shaking. The red color of solution in flask is gradually replaced by orangish yellow color also called salmon pink. This is recorded as first-end point indicating amount of free acid present in gastric juice. Now add 1 drop of phenolphthalein indicator, further addition of alkali leads to change in color from orangish yellow to lemon yellow which is followed by appearance of stable pink color. This is the second end point which denotes total acidity of gastric juice.

Observation Table

S.No.	Initial burette reading (x mL)	Ist-end point (y mL)	IInd-end point (z mL)	Free acidity (y–x)	Total acidity (z–x)
1.					

Calculation

N_1 = X (normality of gastric juice)
V_1 = 10 mL (volume of gastric juice taken)
N_2 = Normality of NaOH – N/10
V_2 = A (average of reading)
$N_1 V_1 = N_2 V_2$
$N_1 \times 10 = 1/10 \times A$
N_1 = A/100 Eq/L
N_1 = 10 A mEq/L

Normal Values

Free acidity—15–40 mEq/L
Total acidity—25–55 mEq/L

Interpretation

Hyperchlorhydria—It is excessive secretion of HCl. In this condition, free acidity exceeds 60 mEq/L. It shows a high FTM curve.

General Causes

- Excessive alcohol intake.
- Excessive tea and coffee intake with poor food.
- Chain smoking for emotional stress. All these stimulate secretion of gastric juice. This leads to gastric and peptic ulcer.
- Zollinger-Ellison syndrome—It is a genetic or inherited cause of excessive HCl secretion. In this condition, a gastrin secreting tumor causes excessive secretion of gastric juice.
- Hypochlorhydria—It is less secretion of HCl and a low FTM curve is obtained.
- Bile regurgitation due to reverse peristalsis.
- Chronic gastritis.
- Achlorhydria—A flat curve is obtained. It means no HCl secretion.
- Pernicious anemia—There is autoimmune destruction of oxyntic cells which secrete HCl.

Viva voce

Q1. The gastric juice is secreted by which cells of the gastric mucosa?
Q2. The normal pH of gastric juice ranges from 1 to 2, however, the mucosal wall is not digested by the strong acid. Why?
Q3. The first-end point indicated by Toffer's shows the neutralization of .... acid.
Q4. The second-end point indicated by phenolphthalein shows the neutralization of .... acid.
Q5. The fractional test meal includes tea without milk. Why?
Q6. A high FTM curve indicates ....
Q7. A flat FTM curve is seen in pernicious anemia. Why?
Q8. A genetic condition showing a high FTM curve is ....
Q9. What are the common causes for hypochlorhydria?
Q10. Hyperchlorhydria leads to .... and .... ulcers.

CHAPTER

44

Colorimetry

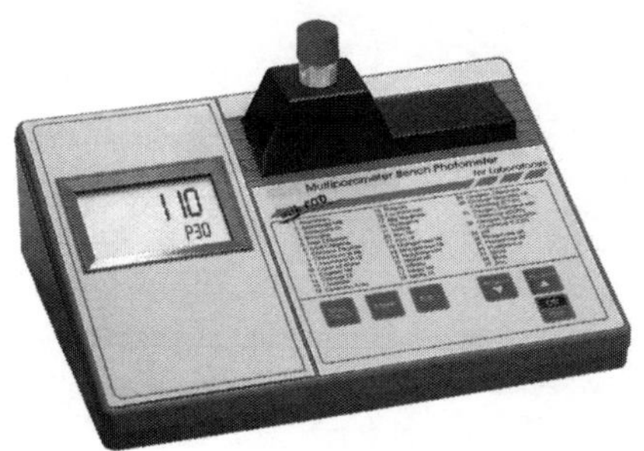

Chapter Framework

- Photometry
  - Theory of Colorimetry
  - Photoelectric Colorimeter
  - Significance of Blank Solution
  - Choice of Filters
  - Spectrum
  - Instruction of Operating of Instrument

Colorimetry means *measurement of color*. Biochemical analyses are mostly done by colorimetric methods. In these methods the substance to be determined is treated in the final step of the test procedure with a reagent which forms a colored product and the intensity of the color is measured by the instrument called—Photoelectric colorimeter or spectrophotometer.

Nowadays, the principle of color matching used in older technique has been replaced by the measurements of light and therefore, it is now called photometry.

Photometry

It is an instrument technique used for determining the concentration of a substance by measuring the amount of light transmitted or absorbed by the substance present in the solution.

Theory of Colorimetry

When monochromatic light passes through a colored solution a certain percentage of light is absorbed and rest is transmitted. Two laws of photochemistry explain the theory of colorimetry. These are:

- Law of Lambert
- Law of Beer

Together these laws are termed as the Lambert – Beer's Law.

According to this law, the optical density (OD) or absorbance of a colored solution is proportional to the concentration of the colored substance and also to the distance through which light has to pass.

The OD can be defined as log of the ratio of the intensity of incident to transmitted light.

$OD = Log\ I_o/T$

I_o = Intensity of incident light

T = Intensity of transmitted light

Where incident light intensity is taken as 100% and T-refers to the percentage of light transmitted.

Hence,

$$OD = \log 100/T$$
$$= \log 100 - \log T$$
$$= 2 - \log T$$

If transmittance is 100%, then

OD = 2 – log 100

i.e. OD = 0

It follows that the ratio of OD of unknown to that of standard is equal to ratio of concentration of unknown to that of standard.

$$\frac{\text{OD of unknown}}{\text{OD of standard}} = \frac{\text{conc. of unknown}}{\text{conc. of standard}}$$

$$\text{conc. of unknown} = \frac{\text{OD of unknown}}{\text{OD of standard}} \times \text{conc. of standard}$$

Photoelectric Colorimeter

In photoelectric colorimeter the wavelength of incident light and thickness of solution through which the light passes are kept constant. The emergent light enters a photocell which converts light energy into electrical energy. This can be measured by a sensitive galvanometer and is directly proportional to intensity of emergent light. Intensity of light emerging from unknown and standard solution is measured. Thus the concentration of the unknown sample can be determined.

The basic components of a photoelectric colorimeter are:

- Source of light
- Filters
- Cuvettes
- Photocell
- Galvanometer.

Individual photoelectric colorimeter differs with respect to mode of calibration of colorimeter. Most of them display calibration in both of OD and percent transmission scale. If the readings are taken in percent transmission than for calculation purpose it has to be converted into OD by adapting the formula.

OD = 2 – log T

Significance of Blank Solution

In all the colorimetric analyzes preparation of blank becomes necessary. This is because of the fact that some color comes from reagent, in addition to the color that is developed due to the unknown substance. Hence, if a blank solution is prepared using all the reagents except the substance which is being measured and its OD value subtracted from the OD of unknown or standard the remaining values represent only the true optical density.

Choice of Filters

This is another key feature in colorimetric estimation. If conc. v/s OD relationship is to be linear monochromatic light is necessary. In every case the precise wavelength to be selected is that of light which is most strongly absorbed by the colored solution. This is usually a color which is complementary to the color of solution, e.g.

For blue solution—Red
for red solution—Green
for yellow solution—Blue.

Spectrum

Light consist of electromagnetic radiation. These EM waves are measured in terms of wavelengths represented by symbol λ. A wavelength is distance between 2 peaks of wave and is expressed in μm or nm. The analysis of EM-radiation in terms of bands of wavelength is called spectrum. There are 3 main spectra:

1. Ultravoilet (UV)
2. Visible (V)
3. Infrared (IR).
   - Ultravoilet (Invisible)
     - This covers the wavelength between 190–400 nm.
     - These wavelengths are not associated with colors, hence colorless solutions are measured in this region.
   - Visible spectrum (V)
     - This covers wavelength between 400 nm to 760 nm.
     - These wavelengths are associated with colors.
     - Each color is associated with a band of wavelength.

Some of which are:

Violet—400 nm to 450 nm
Blue—450 nm to 500 nm
Green—500 nm to 570 nm
Yellow—570 nm to 590 nm
Orange—590 nm to 620 nm
Red—620 nm to 760 nm

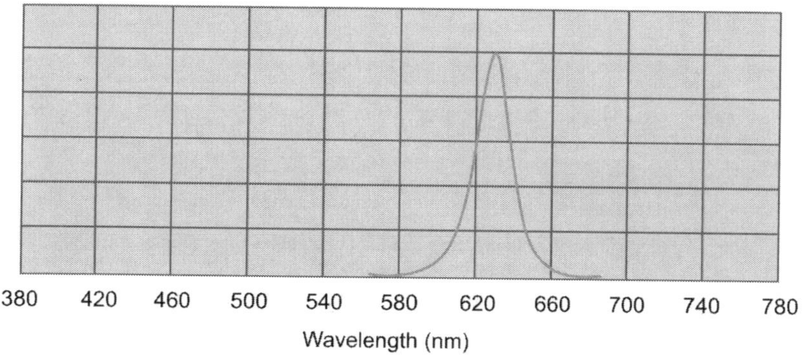

- Infrared (Invisible)
  This is beyond the wavelength 760 nm. The wavelength of this spectrum is not used in photometry.

Instruction of Operating of Instrument

- Switch the instrument on and leave it to warm up for about 7 min to 10 min.
- Insert the correct filter in the slot provided.
- Take blank or distil water in a cuvette and adjust the instrument in such a manner that needle shows 100% transmission, i.e. zero OD
- Now fill another cuvette with test and standard solution in succession and put them in place of blank and read their absorbance in succession.
- After taking the OD reading switch off colorimeter and disconnect from the mains.
- Clean the cuvette thoroughly with distil water.
- Make sure you do not cause scratches on the cuvette and then calculate the concentration of the substance present in given sample.

Viva voce

Q1. What is the principle of colorimetry?
Q2. What are different parts of a spectrum?
Q3. What is the significance of a reagent blank?
Q4. Why should the colorimeter be switched on 10 minutes to 15 minutes before use?
Q5. What is optical density?
Q6. What are the contents of reagent blank?
Q7. Which solutions are measured in UV region?
Q8. Why complementary colored filters are used?
Q9. Which part of spectrum is not used in photometry?
Q10. Name the different components of photoelectric colorimeter.

CHAPTER

45

Blood Sugar

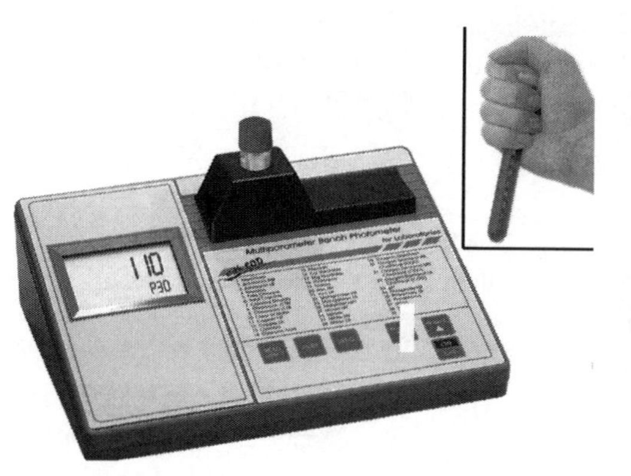

Chapter Framework

- Estimation of Blood Glucose by Ortho-toluidine Method of Dubowski, (1962)
  - Principle
  - Reaction
  - Reagents
  - Procedure
  - Calculation
- Estimation of Blood Glucose by Glucose Oxidase or Peroxidase
  - Reagent
  - Principle
  - Procedure
  - Calculation
  - Normal Value and Clinical Significance

Glucose is the principle sugar of the blood. It is used as a fuel source by the cells and it is the exclusive fuel source for the RBCs, brain, CNS. Any fall of blood sugar below the fasting level causes headache, nausea and if not treated brain dysfunction, coma and finally death. Similarly the high blood sugar levels are harmful as in case of diabetes mellitus. Therefore, estimation of blood sugar is of prime importance.

Estimation of blood sugar was done initially by the O-toluidine method and is performed nowadays by the enzymatic method.

Estimation of Blood Glucose by Orthotoluidine Method of Dubowski, (1962)

Principle

O-toluidine reacts with aldehyde group of glucose at 100°C in glacial acetic acid solution to form a Schiff's base which is blue green in color. The intensity of color developed is proportional to the amount of glucose present in solution and can be determined colorimetrically at 635 nm.

Reaction

$$\text{Glucose} + \text{O-toluidine} \rightarrow \text{N-glucosyl amine} + H_2O + \text{Schiff's Base}$$

Reagents

1. Orthotoluidine reagent—1.5 g thiourea is dissolved in 940 mL of analytical grade glacial acetic acid and 66 mL rthotoluidine is added to it and mixed.
2. Standard glucose solution—100 mg of glucose dissolved in 100 mL water.

Procedure

A set of three tubes is prepared, marked as blank, standard and test. Take 0.1 mL serum or plasma in test tube labeled as test, 0.1 mL glucose standard in test tube labeled as standard and 0.1 mL water in test tube labeled as blank. Pipette 5 mL O-toluidine reagent into all the tubes and mix well by shaking the tubes. Place all the tubes in a boiling water bath for 10 min to 12 min. Read color intensity of unknown and standard against blank at 635 nm (red filter).

Calculation

$$\text{mg of glucose per 100 mL serum} = \frac{\text{OD of unknown} \times \text{Standard glucose} \times 100}{\text{OD of standard} \times \text{volume of serum}}$$

$$= \frac{\text{OD for unknown} \times 0.1 \times 100 \text{ mg / dL}}{\text{OD of standard} \times 0.1}$$

This method is not used now days because:

1. The method requires larger amount of serum as compared to the enzymatic method.
2. O-toluidine used as a reagent is carcinogenic in nature, thus the method has been discarded.

Estimation of Blood Glucose by Glucose Oxidase or Peroxidase

Reagent

Working reagent: It contains glucose oxidase, peroxidase, phenol and 4-amino antipyrine [Chromogen] and buffer.

Principle

Glucose in acted upon by an enzyme glucose oxidase and oxidised to gluconic acid and H_2O_2 is released. H_2O_2 reacts with phenol and 4-amino antipyrine in presence of peroxidase enzyme to give a pink color dye quinonemine. The intensity of the color developed is measured colorimetrically at 635 nm (red filter).

Procedure

Reagent	*Blank*	*Standard*	*Test*
Working reagent	1 mL	1 mL	1 mL
Standard solution	-	0.01 mL	-
Plasma/serum	-	-	0.01 mL

Calculation

$$\text{Blood glucose (mg/dL)} = \frac{\text{OD for unknown}}{\text{OD of standard}} \times 100$$

Normal Value and Clinical Significance

The normal value of blood glucose in a healthy adult during fasting conditions (6 – 9 hours after the last meal) varies from 70 mg to 110 mg per 100 mL of blood. This level rises after meal. The renal threshold value of glucose is 180 mg/dL, beyond which glucose starts appearing in urine.

There are many clinical conditions leading to a state of hyperglycemia, the most important and common amongst them being diabetes mellitus. Estimation of blood sugar is an important investigation to detect and diagnose cases of borderline and frank diabetes. It also serves, as a guideline for prescribing and adjusting the doses of antidiabetic drugs used to treat cases of diabetes mellitus.

Fasting blood sugar level may be within normal range but postprandial level may be on the higher side in borderline cases of diabetes. In general blood sugar is estimated as:

1. Fasting blood sugar.
2. Postprandial blood sugar (one and half hour after meal).
3. One hour after administration of 100 gm of glucose orally (depending upon body weight).
4. Glucose tolerance test (GTT) (Figs 45.1 and 45.2).

In GTT blood samples are collected at zero hours (fasting) and half hour intervals after administration of 100 gm of glucose orally (1 gm glucose/kg body weight) and analyzed for sugar examination. Urine samples are also analyzed simultaneously or at the end of one and half hour to detect presence of sugar, if any. A normal person's urine sample does not show a positive Benedict's test and the values of BSL at fasting is 70 mg to 110 mg/dL, 1 hour is approximately 100 mg to 160 mg/dL but never beyond 180 mg/dL and 2 hour is less than 130 mg/dL. By 2.5 hours the BSL reaches back to fasting level as seen in the GTT curve (Fig. 45.1).

However, in latent diabetics at least one of the urine samples shows a positive Benedict's test. O-GTT should not be done in patients of frank diabetes.

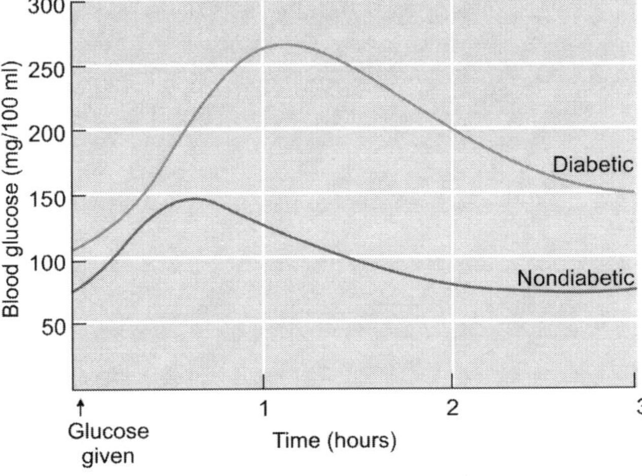

Fig. 45.1 Glucose tolerance test curve

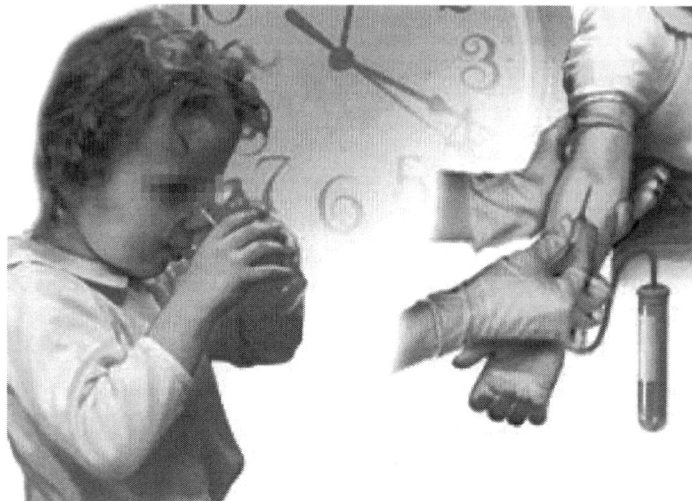

Fig. 45.2 Oral glucose tolerance test

Viva Voce

Q1. Why do we need to maintain a normal fasting blood sugar level?
Q2. Name the methods used for estimation of blood sugar.
Q3. Why has the O-toluidine method been discarded?
Q4. What is the advantage of the enzymatic method over the O-toluidine method of blood sugar estimation?
Q5. Name the different conditions of hyperglycemia.
Q6. What is glycosuria?
Q7. When should we perform the glucose tolerance test?
Q8. Why should we use NaF along with oxalate or EDTA while collecting blood for sugar estimation?
Q9. What is the BSL in O-GTT at 1 hour?
Q10. What is the significance of O-GTT?

CHAPTER

46

Total Protein and A:G Ratio

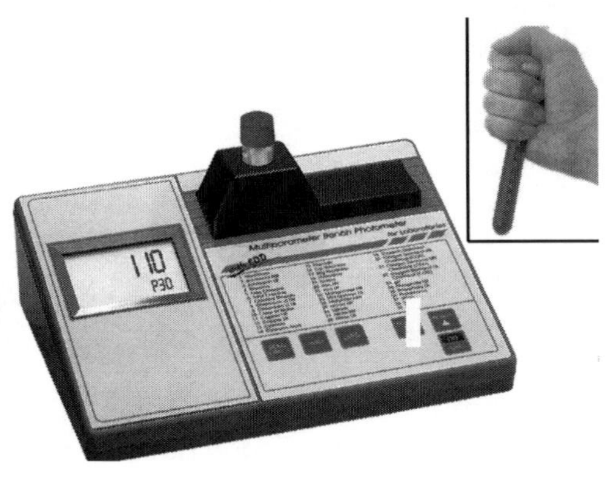

Chapter Framework

Albumin and globulin are the two major classes of proteins in serum. Albumin is synthesized in the liver. Its function includes regulation and distribution of extracellular fluid, transportation of various hormones, vitamins and trace elements.

Globulin constitute several proteins that are separated into four distinct bands (α1, α2, b and g-globulin) on electrophoresis. They perform series of functions which include transportation and distribution of extra cellular fluid, transportation of various hormones, vitamins and trace elements. Serum proteins get altered in a number of clinical conditions and thus accurate measurement of serum protein is important for diagnosis as well as prognosis of these conditions.

Estimation of Total Protein by Biuret Method

Reagents

1. Biuret reagent containing $CuSO_4$, sodium potassium tartrate, potassium iodide and NaOH.
2. Standard protein solution containing 6 g/100 mL of bovine albumin in water.

Principle

Cupric ions form chelates with the peptide bonds of proteins in an alkaline medium. Sodium potassium tartrates keep the cupric ions in solution. The intensity of the violet color formed is proportional to the protein concentration of the sample.

Procedure

Take 3 test tubes and label them as 'blank', 'standard' and 'test'. Now pipette into them as shown in the table:

	Blank	*Standard*	*Test*
Biuret reagent	5 mL	5 mL	5 mL
Standard protein	-	100 µL	-
Serum	-	-	100 µL

Mix and allow standing for 30 minutes. Now read the optical densities of unknown and standard against reagent blank at 540 nm/green filter.

Calculation

$$\text{Serum total protein} = \frac{OD_{test} \times 6}{OD_{std}}$$

Normal Values and its Significance

The normal serum total protein ranges from 6 gm to 8 g/100 mL. The serum total protein values may be increased in dehydration, shock, chronic infections like tuberculosis, alcoholism, leukemia, liver diseases, etc. Serum proteins are reduced in conditions of malnutrition, severe burns, in pregnancy due to loss proteinuria, in some renal diseases like nephrotic syndrome, acute and chronic glomerulonephritis.

Estimation of Albumin by BCG Method

Reagents

1. Bromocresolgreen (BCG) dye
2. Normal saline
3. Standard albumin solution (4 g/mL).

Principle

Among the serum proteins only albumin binds with BCG at pH 4.2. This binding produces a change in the color of BCG which is then measured colorimetrically. The intensity of the color produced is proportional to the concentration of albumin in the sample.

Reaction

$$\text{Albu min} + \underset{\text{Yellow}}{\text{BCG}} \xrightarrow{\text{pH}} \text{Blue} - \text{green complexes}$$

Procedure

Take three test tubes and label them as 'blank', 'standard' and 'test'. Now pipette into each of them as shown in the table:

	Blank	*Standard*	*Test*
BCG reagent	5 mL	5 mL	5 mL
Albumin standard	-	200 µL	-
Serum (dilute)	-	-	200 µL

Incubate for 10 minutes at room temperature and read at 530 nm or green filter.

Calculation

$$\text{Serum albumin} = \frac{OD_{test} - OD_{blank}}{OD_{std} - OD_{blank}} \times \text{Standard albumin concentration}$$

Normal Values and Significance

Serum albumin normal value ranges from 3.5 to 5 g/100 mL. The serum albumin is raised in dehydration, congestive heart failure, glucocorticoid excess, etc. Reduced levels of serum albumin are seen in malnutrition, liver dysfunction, burns, nephrotic syndrome, protein losing enteropathy, etc.

Serum Globulin

Since colorimetric measurement of albumin is much simpler than that of globulin the concentration of total protein and albumin are estimated in serum and globulin is obtained by difference.
Serum globulin = Serum total protein – S Albumin (g/dL)

$$A/G\ \text{ratio} = \frac{\text{Serum albumin concentration}}{\text{Serum globulin concentration}}$$

Normal Value and its Significance

The normal serum globulin ranges from 2.5–3.5 g/100 mL. Raised serum globulin is observed in autoimmune conditions like systemic lupus or collagen disease, rheumatoid arthritis, biliary cirrhosis, multiple myeloma, leukemia, etc. Reduced serum globulins are seen in hypogammaglobulinemia, acute hemolytic anemia, liver dysfunction. A/G ratio normally ranges between 1.2 and 2.5. High A:G ratio is seen in hypothyroidism, hypogammaglobulinemia and reversed A:G ratio is seen in kwashiorkor, liver dysfunction.

Viva voce

Q1. What is the function of plasma proteins?
Q2. Name the major plasma proteins.
Q3. The estimation of total proteins is based on the principle of which test?
Q4. Name the important conditions leading to hypoproteinemia.

Q5. Name the dye used for estimation of serum albumin.
Q6. Why is the serum albumin level reduced in nephrotic syndrome?
Q7. A reversal of A:G ratio may be observed in ....
Q8. Serum albumin is found to be raised in which conditions?
Q9. Name the different electrophoretic bands of globulin.
Q10. What is the normal A:G ratio range?

CHAPTER

47

Serum Urea

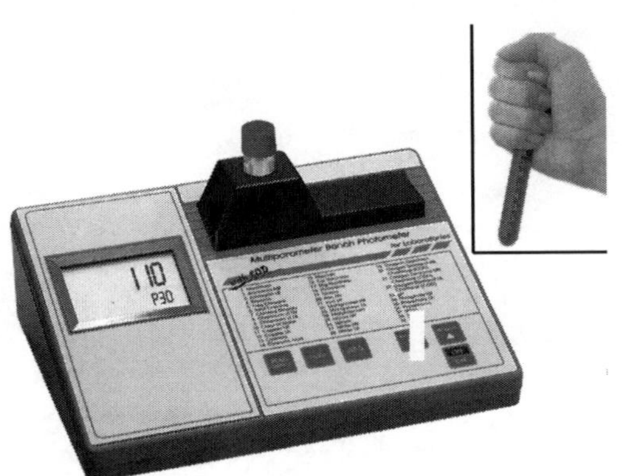

Chapter Framework

Urea is the main end product of protein catabolism. It is synthesized in liver by urea cycle and excreted through urine.

There are several methods for estimation of urea in serum, of these Berthelot method is most widely used for the estimation of serum urea.

Estimation of Serum Urea by Berthelot Method

Principle

The enzyme urease breakdown urea into ammonia and CO_2 in alkaline medium. NH_3 liberated from the breakdown of urea reacts with hypochlorite to form indophenol. Sodium hydroxide converts the indophenol to blue colored product. This reaction is catalyzed by the presence of nitroprusside. The intensity of color produced by the reaction is directly proportional to the concentration of urea in the sample.

$$\text{Urea} + H_2O \xrightarrow{\text{urease}} 2NH_2 + CO_2$$

NH_3 + Hypochlorite sodium → 2, 2-Dicarbonyl + Nitropusside + Indophenol

Reagents

1. Buffered urease solution
2. WR – 1 – Phenol nitroprusside solution
3. WR – 2 – Hypochlorite solution
4. Urea standard—40 mg/dL.

Procedure

Take 3 test tubes and mark them as blank, standard and test. Bring all the reagents to room temperature and proceed as follows:

Reagent	*Blank*	*Standard*	*Test*
Step-I Buffered urease	0.2 mL	0.2 mL	0.2 mL
Standard urea solution	-	20 µl	-
Sample/serum	-	-	20 µL
Mix well and incubate at 37°C for 5 min			
Step-II WR – 1 WR – 2	 5 mL 5 mL	 5 mL 5 mL	 5 mL 5 mL

Calculation

$$\text{Serum Urea (mg/dL)} = \frac{OD_{test}}{OD_{std}} \times 40$$

Normal Value and its Significance

The normal serum-urea concentration varies between 20 mg to 45 mg/dL in normal persons. This value is raised in certain clinical conditions particularly in renal diseases like acute and chronic glomerulonephritis, pyelonephritis, nephrosclerosis, renal carcinoma, etc. Dehydration and shock also raise the serum-urea concentration due to decreased blood volume. Hematemesis and increased tissue breakdown are few additional causes of hyperuremia (due to increased protein catabolism). Raised serum-urea concentration causes symptoms like nausea, vomiting and if not treated for a long-time brain dysfunction and coma.

Serum-urea concentration is reduced in liver disorders as liver is the site of urea synthesis and any functional defect of the liver would compromise its ability to form urea.

Estimation of serum-urea concentration is thus a very significant test in patients of renal or liver disorders.

Viva voce

Q1. Urea is the product of catabolism of ....

Q2. Where is urea synthesized?

Q3. The estimation of urea is done by which method?

Q4. What is the normal serum-urea concentration level?

Q5. Name the different conditions where serum-urea concentration increases.

CHAPTER

48

Serum Creatinine

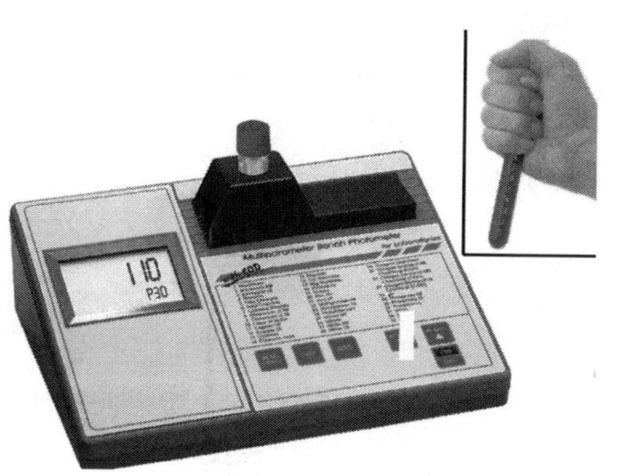

Chapter Framework

- Estimation of Serum Creatinine (by Jaffe's method)
  - Reagents
  - Principle
  - Procedure
  - Calculation
  - Normal Values and its Significance
  - Estimation of Urinary Creatinine

Creatinine is a waste product of muscle metabolism, its level is a reflection of body muscle mass. Serum creatinine level remains constant and within normal range in normal functioning kidneys. Serum creatinine is used to test the functioning of the kidneys.

Estimation of Serum Creatinine (By Jaffe's Method)

Reagents

1. Sodium tungstate (10%)
2. Sulfuric acid (2/3 N)
3. Picric acid (0.04 M)
4. Sodium hydroxide (0.75 N)
5. Creatinine standard (0.04 mg/mL).

Principle

Creatinine present in protein-free filtrate of serum reacts with picric acid in alkaline medium, to form an orange-colored creatinine picrate. The intensity of the color is a measure of amount of creatinine in serum.

Procedure

Label three test tubes and add the reactants as follows:

	Blank (B) mL	*Standard (S) mL*	*Unknown (U) mL*
Serum	-	-	1.0
Standard	-	1.0	-
Distilled water	4.0	3.0	3.0
Sodium tungstate	2.0	2.0	2.0
Sulfuric acid (2/3 N)	2.0	2.0	2.0

Keep the tubes at room temperature for 10 minutes and filter the unknown tube contents to get protein-free filtrate.

Prepare another set of three test tubes and label them as blank, standard and test. Now, pipette as follows:

	Blank	*Standard*	*Test*
Filtrate	3 mL	3 mL	3 mL
NaOH	1 mL	1 mL	1 mL
Picric acid	1 mL	1 mL	1 mL

Mix the tube contents well and keep at room temperature for 10 minutes. Now read the optical densities of standard and test against regent blank at 530 nm or green filter.

Calculation

$$\text{Serum creatinine (in mg / dL)} = \frac{OD_{test} - OD_{blank}}{OD_{std} - OD_{blank}} \times 2$$

Normal Values and its Significance

The normal serum creatinine ranges from 0.6 to 1.5 mg/dL. The normal value of serum creatinine indicates a normal renal function as, creatinine once filtered at the glomerulus, is neither reabsorbed nor secreted by the renal tubules. Thus, estimation of serum creatinine gives an idea of the renal function. A raised serum creatinine is observed in renal diseases like glomerulonephritis, renal failure, pyelonephritis, etc. It is also raised in muscular dystrophies due to muscle damage, in hepatorenal syndrome, eclampsia and pre-eclampsia. The serum creatinine is reduced in persons with short stature due to the smaller muscle mass and in myasthenia gravis.

Estimation of Urinary Creatinine

Urinary creatinine can be measured by the colorimetric method, using the same method as for serum estimations. However, the urine sample should be diluted for the estimation. If the daily urinary output is 1 to 2 liters then it should be diluted 1 in 100, and if the volume is less than 1 liter then the dilution should be greater. The dilution factor should be multiplied during calculations.

Viva voce

Q1. Creatinine is produced due to ....
Q2. What does the normal serum-creatinine level indicate?
Q3. Name the method for estimation of serum creatinine.
Q4. Why do males have higher normal serum creatinine as compared to females?
Q5. Name the conditions when serum creatinine is reduced.

CHAPTER

49

Serum Lipid Profile

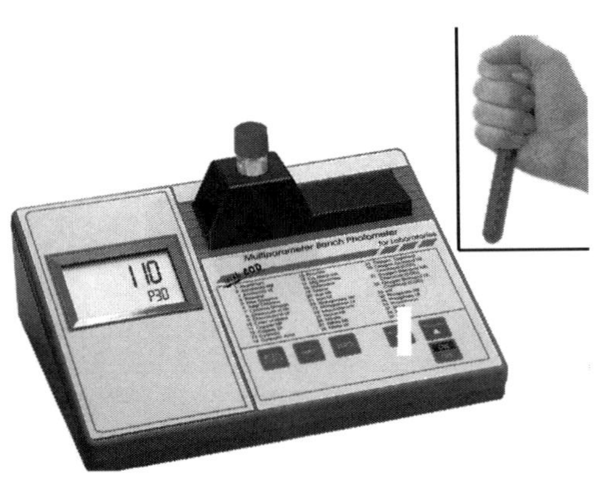

Chapter Framework

- Estimation of Serum Cholesterol (Enzymatic Method)
  - Method: Cholesterol Oxidase Peroxidase Enzymatic
  - Principle
  - Calculation
  - Normal Values
- Estimation of High Density Lipoprotein Cholesterol
  - Method: Magnesium–phosphotungstic acid Precipitation
  - Calculation
  - Normal Values
- Estimation of Triglycerides
  - Principle
  - Calculation
  - Normal Values
- Low Density Lipoprotein Cholesterol
  - Normal Values
  - Clinical Interpretations

The major lipids, present in plasma are cholesterol and its esters, triglycerides, phospholipids and fatty acids. Lipids have to be transported in plasma from one tissue to another. There are different mechanisms that control the transport of lipids from tissues into plasma and the uptake of lipids by the tissues from plasma. Abnormalities of these mechanisms may be associated with different lipid disorders, particularly ischemic heart disease.

There is a positive correlation between risk of developing atherosclerosis and raised serum total cholesterol and LDL cholesterol and a negative one, with HDL-cholesterol.

A lipid profile consists of estimation of the following:

1. Serum total cholesterol
2. Serum triglycerides

3. Lipoprotein analysis including:
   - HDL cholesterol
   - LDL cholesterol
   - VLDL.

Estimation of Serum Cholesterol (Enzymatic Method)

Method: Cholesterol Oxidase Peroxidase Enzymatic (Allain CC et al. 1974)

Reagents

- Working enzyme reagent—The working enzyme reagent consists of cholesterol esterase (CHE), cholesterol oxidase (CHO), peroxidase (POD), 4-amino-anti-pyrine, stabilizers/surfactant.
- Standard cholesterol = 200 mg/dL.

Principle

The cholesterol esters are hydrolyzed to free cholesterol by cholesterol esterase (CHE), cholesterol and free fatty acids are produced. The cholesterol is then oxidized by cholesterol oxidase (CHO) to cholest-4-en-3-one with simultaneous production of H_2O_2. The H_2O_2 reacts with 4-aminoantipyrine and phenol to yield a red quinoneimine dye with maximum absorbance at 505 nm.

a. Cholesterol esters + Cholesterol + Fatty acids
b. Cholesterol + O_2 Cholest-4-en-3-one + H_2O_2
c. H_2O_2 + 4-aminoantipyrine + phenol ⟶ Quinoneimine dye + $4H_2O$.

The intensity of color produced is directly proportional to the concentration of total cholesterol in the sample.

Procedure

Three test tubes were taken and marked as B, S and T for blank, standard and test. Pipetted into the test tubes.

Reagent	*Blank*	*Standard*	*Test*
Working enzyme solution (mL)	1.0	1.0	1.0
Standard (mL)	–	0.01	–
Serum (mL)	–	–	0.01

Mixed well and incubated the assay mixture for 10 minutes at 37°C. Read absorbance of test and standard at 505 nm against reagent blank.

Calculation

$$\text{Total cholesterol (mg / dL)} = \frac{\text{Absorbance of test}}{\text{Absorbance of standard}} \times 200$$

Normal Values

Desirable cholesterol	<200 mg/dL
Borderline cholesterol	= 200 mg to 240 mg/dL
High cholesterol	>240 mg/dL.

Estimation of HDLc

Method: Magnesium–Phosphotungstic Acid Precipitation (Gordon T et al. 1977)

HDL cholesterol precipitating reagent is used in conjunction with cholesterol reagent for enzymatic determination of HDL–cholesterol in serum or plasma.

Components of Precipitating Reagents

1. Phosphotungstic acid
2. $MgCl_2$

Principle

High density lipoprotein is separated from other protein fractions by treating serum with phosphotungstic acid and magnesium chloride. HDL remains in solution while all other lipoprotein fractions are precipitated. Centrifugation separates HDL fractions as clear supernatant and cholesterol content of this supernatant is estimated by enzymatic method.

Serum/Plasma + Phosphotungstic acid ⟶ Supernatant + Precipitate
(HDL) (LDL, VLDL, etc.)

Precipitation Procedure

Centrifuge tube was taken and marked as T for test. Pipetted into the centrifuge tube.

Reagent	*Test*
Sample (mL)	0.2
Precipitating reagent (mL)	0.2

Mixed well and centrifuged at 3500 rpm to 4000 rpm for 10 minutes. Separated the clear supernatant immediately and determined cholesterol content. Three test tubes were taken and marked as B, S and T for blank, standard and test and pipetted into the test tubes.

Reagent	*Blank*	*Standard*	*Test*
Working solution (mL)	1.0	1.0	1.0
Standard (mL)	–	0.05	–
Supernatant (mL)	–	–	0.05

Mixed well and incubated the assay mixture for 10 minutes at 37°C and read absorbance of test and standard against blank at 505 nm.

Calculation

$$\text{Serum HDL cholesterol} = \frac{\text{Absorbance of test (mg / dL)}}{\text{Absorbance of standard}} \times 100$$

Normal Values

HDL Cholesterol (mg/dL)
Females = 40 mg to 70 mg/dL
Males = 40 mg to 65 mg/dL.

Estimation of Triglycerides

Method

Lipases/Glycerol Kinases/Glycerol Phosphate Oxidases/Peroxidases Enzymatic (Foosati P et al. 1982).

Reagents

1. Working enzyme solution—It consists of lipase, glycerol kinase, glycerol phosphate oxidase, peroxidase, ATP, chromogen, activators and stabilizers and phosphate buffer (pH 6.8).
2. Triglyceride standard—200 mg/dL.

Principle

Triglycerides are hydrolyzed by lipoprotein lipase (LPL) into glycerol and free fatty acids. The glycerol is converted by glycerol kinase (GK) into glycerol-3-phosphate. Glycerol-3-phosphate is oxidized by glycerol phosphate oxidase (GPO) into dihydroxyacetone phosphate (DHAP) and H_2O_2. In the presence of peroxidase (POD), H_2O_2 oxidizes phenolic chromogen to a red colored compound.

i. Triglycerides $\xrightarrow{\text{LPL}}$ Fatty acid + Glycerol
ii. Glycerol + ATP $\xrightarrow{\text{GK}}$ Glycerol-3-phosphate + ADP
iii. Glycerol-3-phosphate + O_2 $\xrightarrow{\text{GPO}}$ DHAP + H_2O_2
iv. H_2O_2 + Phenolic chromogen $\xrightarrow{\text{POD}}$ Red-colored compound.

Procedure

Three test tubes were taken and marked as B, S and T for blank, standard, and test. Pipetted into the test tubes.

Reagent	*Blank*	*Standard*	*Test*
Working solution (mL)	1.0	1.0	1.0
Standard (mL)	–	0.01	–
Sample (mL)	–	–	0.01

Mixed well and incubated the assay mixture for 10 minutes at 37°C. Read the absorbance of test and standard against reagent blank at 510 nm.

Calculation

$$\text{Triglycerides} = \frac{\text{Absorbance of test}}{\text{Absorbance of standard}} \times 200$$

Normal Values

Triglycerides—Up to 170 mg/dL.

Very Low Density Lipoprotein Cholesterol

The values of very low density lipoprotein cholesterol (VLDLc) can be determined using the Friedewald's Equation.

$$\text{VLDLc (mg / dL)} = \frac{\text{Triglycerides}}{5}$$

Normal Values

VLDLc < 40 (mg/dL).

Low Density Lipoprotein Cholesterol

The values of low density lipoprotein cholesterol (LDLc) can be calculated, if the values of triglycerides are known by using Friedewald's Equations.

$$\frac{\text{LDL cholesterol}}{\text{(mg / dL)}} = \text{Total cholesterol} + \text{HDLc} + \frac{\text{Triglycerides}}{5}$$

Normal Values

LDLc < 130 mg/dL.

Limitations of Friedewald's Equations:

1. The equations are not valid for triglyceride concentrations greater than 400 mg/dL.
2. The equations give fairly accurate values of VLDL and LDLc for cholesterol less than 400 mg/dL.

Clinical Interpretations

Serum lipid profile is an important blood test performed in the modern day clinical biochemistry laboratory. Serum cholesterol is raised in diabetes mellitus, hypothyroidism, obstructive jaundice, nephrotic syndrome, etc. Raised serum cholesterol increases the tendency of atherosclerosis and the diseases associated with it like—Hypertension, stroke and heart disease. Hypocholesterolemia is observed in hyperthyroidism, anemia, intestinal obstruction, etc. Raised serum triglycerides have been reported in hypothyroidism, diabetes mellitus, alcoholic abuse, cigarette smoking, drugs like—Oral contraceptives, corticosteroids. Hypotriglyceridemia is observed in malnutrition, intestinal obstruction, and hyperthyroidism. Serum HDLc is characteristically raised due to vigorous physical exercise, insulin treatment and is reduced in diabetes mellitus, hypothyroidism, obesity, lack of exercise, and some inherited diseases like—Tangier's disease. HDLc is also termed as the serum good cholesterol as it scavenges the bad cholesterol (LDLc) from the tissues and transports it to the liver to be finally excreted in bile—'reverse cholesterol transport'. The evaluation of serum lipid profile can be made more efficient in assessing the risk of CVDs by calculating the ratios like—Total cholesterol/HDLc and LDLc/HDLc.

Viva voce

Q1. Name the different lipid fractions included in lipid profile.
Q2. Name the lipid fractions of lipid profile that are estimated in laboratory by chemical analysis.
Q3. Give the Friedewald's equation for estimation of LDLc and VLDL.
Q4. Estimation of HDLc is done by which method?
Q5. Why is the serum HDLc level in women higher?
Q6. Name the good and the bad cholesterol.
Q7. Name the cardio protective lipid fraction.
Q8. Name the conditions of hypercholesterolemia.
Q9. Hypercholesterolemia of hypothyroidism is due to ....
Q10. Hypocholesterolemia of hyperthyroidism is due to ....
Q11. The CVD risk can be better evaluated using the ....

CHAPTER

50

Estimation of Sugar in Urine (Benedict's Quantitative Method)

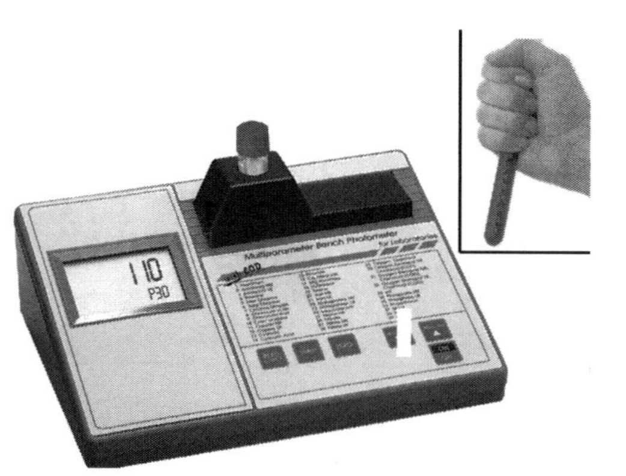

Chapter Framework

- Principle
  - Reagents
  - Procedure
  - Observation
  - Calculation

The quantity of glucose present in urine generally averages about 140 mg per 24 hour specimen. This amount is sufficiently small to escape detection by usual qualitative methods of glucose determination.

Glucose gets excreted in urine in detectable amount in certain conditions known as glycosuria. Glycosuria may be either benign or pathological and its importance is to distinguish between these two types. Persistent glycosuria may indicate diabetes mellitus—A disorder in which the amount of sugar may rise as high as 10%. The quantitative methods for the estimation of sugars in urine enable us to determine the severity of this disorder as well as to follow its course under treatment. The commonly used method for urine glucose analysis is the one described by Benedict as given below:

Principle

Benedict's quantitative reagent is used for estimation of glucose in urine. This reagent contains potassium thiocyanate as well as copper sulfate. In the presence of potassium thiocyanate a white precipitate of cuprous thiocyanate is formed, instead of usual red precipitate of cuprous oxide. Small amount of potassium ferrocyanide present in this reagent also aids in keeping cuprous oxide in solution. As the precipitated form is white, the loss of blue tinge in the solution indicates complete reduction of copper. The alkali used is sodium carbonate instead of sodium hydroxide since it is less likely to cause destruction of a small amount of sugar. The solution also has the great advantage of being stable for independent length of time.

Reagents

1. Benedict's quantitative reagent
2. Sodium carbonate powder
3. Urine sample.

Procedure

Carefully perform Benedict's qualitative tests of urine sample, to determine the approximate concentration of glucose in urine. Then dilute the urine sample according to observation and fill it in the burette.

Take 10 mL of the Benedict's quantitative reagent by a pipette in a conical flask and add 5 mL water. Add approximately 2 grams of sodium carbonate powder and heat the contents till boiling. As soon as the contents begin to boil, lower the flame and titrate with urine sample. The end point is indicated by disappearance of the blue/green color. Keep the contents boiling throughout the titration.

Observation

No.	*Initial burette reading (a)*	*Final burette reading (b)*	*Differences (a – b)*
1.			
2.			
3.			
Mean			

Calculation

Ten millilter of Benedict's quantitative reagent is reduced by 0.02 g of glucose. If X mL of sample is required to reduce 10 mL of Benedict's quantitative reagent, then X mL of urine contain 0.02 g of glucose.

$$\text{Therefore, 100 mL of diluted urine will contain} = \frac{20 \times 100 \text{ mg}}{X}$$

$$\text{Glucose in undiluted 100 mL urine} = \frac{20 \times 100 \times D \text{ mg}}{X}$$

where, D is the dilution fraction.

$$= \frac{20 \times 100 \times D \text{ g}}{X}$$

$$= \frac{2D \text{ g} / 100 \text{ mL}}{X}$$

Besides this, the O-toluidine method may also be used for more accurate results after appropriate dilution of the urine.

Viva voce

Q1. Why is detectable amount of sugar not present in normal urine?
Q2. How is the approximate concentration of sugar in urine determined?
Q3. What is the renal threshold?
Q4. Why are the contents of titration boiled throughout the process?
Q5. Which other method can be used?

Part D

Urine Analysis

- Analysis of Normal Urine
- Analysis of Abnormal/Pathological Urine

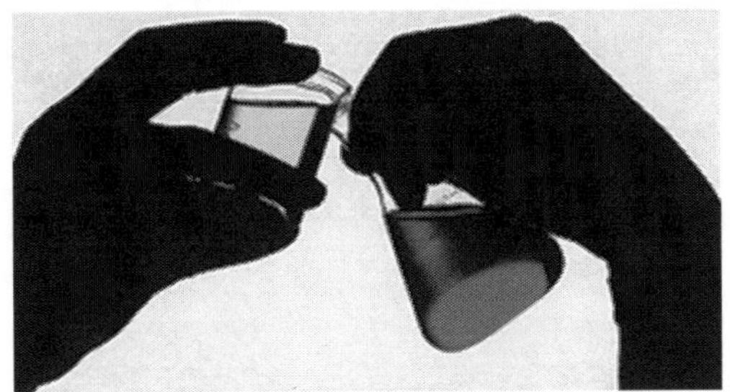

It is rightly said that the urine is mirror of the health of a person. It not only gives us a complete picture of healthy urinary system but the health of a person in totality. Urine analysis is a vast section in a clinical laboratory, including the physical examination, i.e. the color, volume, odor, etc. of the urine sample. Microscopic examination, i.e. observing the presence of various cells, casts, crystals, etc. in the urine and the biochemical analysis of the urine sample. However, here we'd be discussing briefly the biochemical analysis of normal and abnormal urine.

CHAPTER

51

Analysis of Normal Urine

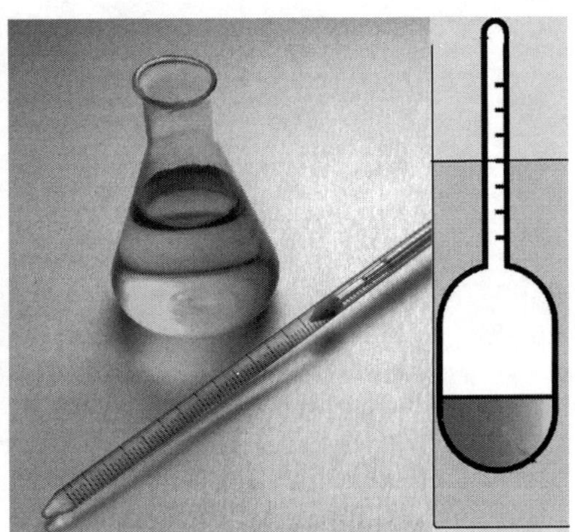

Chapter Framework

- General Characteristics
- Test for Organic Constituents
  - Tests for Urea
  - Tests for Creatinine
  - Tests for Uric Acid
- Test for Inorganic Constituents
  - Test for Chloride
  - Test for Sulfate
  - Test for Phosphate
  - Test for Calcium

Main function of kidney is formation of urine for the excretion of various metabolic waste products formed in body. The process of urine formation basically involves 2 steps:

1. Glomerular filtration
2. Reabsorption and secretion in renal tubule.

Glomerular filtration: It is a passive process that results in formation of ultrafiltrate of blood. All the constituents of plasma less than about molecular weight 10,000 are passed into filtrate, therefore the glomerular filtrate is almost similar in composition to plasma.

Reabsorption and secretion in renal tubules: It involves following processes in different segments of renal tubules:

a. *Selective reabsorption*—In proximal convoluted tubules (PCT) selective reabsorption of important components like glucose, amino acids, etc. occurs by special carriers present in the PCT.
b. *Na^+ reabsorption*—8% by PCT, 10% gets reabsorbed distal convolute tubule (DCT), 2 to 3% by collecting tubule (CT), remaining 2% excreted in urine.
c. *K^+ transport*—K^+ is completely filtered at the glomerulus. It is the only plasma electrolyte that is both reabsorbed and secreted in renal tubules. Almost all the filtered K^+ is actively reabsorbed by PCT. Most of the K^+ produced in urine is due to secretion of K^+ in DCT. This process regulated by aldosterone.

d. *HCO_3^- reabsorption*—Approximately 90% of the filtered HCO_3^- is reabsorbed in PCT and remaining is reabsorbed by DCT and CT.
e. *H^+ secretion*—This occurs by active transport and is coupled to Na^+ reabsorption approximately 85% of total H^+ secretion occurs in PCT and 10% in DCT and remaining 5% in CT.
f. *Cl^- transport*—Cl– reabsorption is inversely related to HCO_3^- reabsorption.
g. *Water reabsorption*—There is passive reabsorption of water (75%–80%) in PCT and loop of Henley, another 5 to 10% of the filtered water is removed under the influence of ADH another 10 to 12% filtered water is reabsorbed in DCT and CT.

General Characteristics

Volume

The daily output of urine usually is 1 to 2 liters. Under certain physiological circumstances it may increase to 2.5 liters. Normally, it depends upon intake, diet and environmental temperature, etc.

a. *Polyuria*—The output of urine is >2 liters/day. It could be due to high fluid intake, spicy food, tea, and coffee and alcohol consumption. Pathologically the volume of urine is observed to be increased in—Diabetes insipidus, diabetes mellitus, chronic renal failure (Fig. 51.1).
b. *Oliguria*—When the output of urine is below 500 mL/day but above 50 mL/day is called as oliguria. Common causes for oliguria are fever, diarrhea, vomiting, acute glomerulonephritis.
c. *Anuria*—It is a condition when the daily output of urine is below 50 mL/day. Common causes of anuria are severe shock, renal stone obstruction.

Appearance

Normal urine is clear and transparent when freshly voided. On standing, it may become turbid due to precipitation of nucleoproteins and mucoproteins and due to precipitation of PO_4^{-3} is normally noted in urine passed after a heavy meal. This is due to alkaline tide. Urine obtained 2 to 3 hours after meal is normally free form turbidity. A permanently turbid urine arises from pathological conditions like-Presence of pus cells, casts, etc. in urinary tract infection or presence of chyle.

Color

Normal color of urine in amber yellow. Color of urine is mainly due to urochrome. Depth of the color being dependent on density of urine. Certain abnormal constituent in drugs, when excreted in urine may impart different color to urine.

Odor

Freshly passed urine has faint aromatic odor due to presence of minute amount of certain volatile organic acids. When urine undergoes decomposition due to bacterial activity there is alkaline fermentation and a very unpleasant ammoniacal odor is evolved. A fruity odor of acetone is typical of ketone bodies. Certain foods and drugs may also produce abnormal odors.

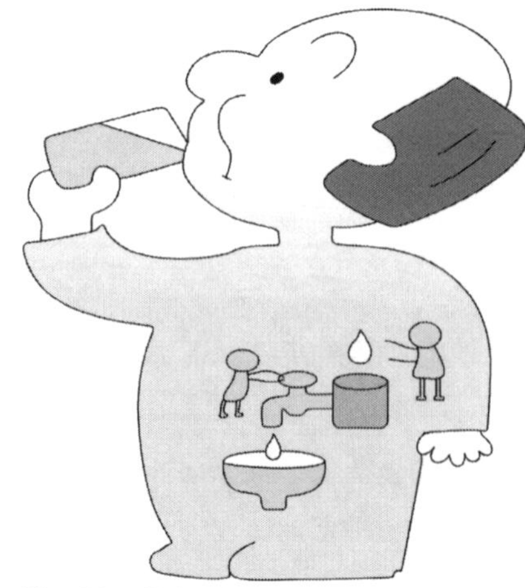

Fig. 51.1 Polyuria

Specific Gravity

The specific gravity of urine of normal individual varies between 1.015 and 1.025. Following copious water drinking, the specific gravity may fall to 1.003 or lower where as in case of excessive perspiration it may rise as high as 1.040. In acute nephritis, the urine is concentrated and has a high specific gravity whereas in chronic nephritis reverse condition prevails. In diabetes mellitus, the volume of urine is large and specific gravity high owing to sugar that is present in the urine.

Determination of Specific Gravity

Fill 3/4 of cylinder with the given urine and gently float urinometer in it (Fig. 16.2). The urinometer should not touch the side of cylinder. Note the reading on the stem of the urinometer ordinarily. The reading in urinometer represents second and third decimal places of specific gravity. Thus, a reading 20 recorded as 1.020.

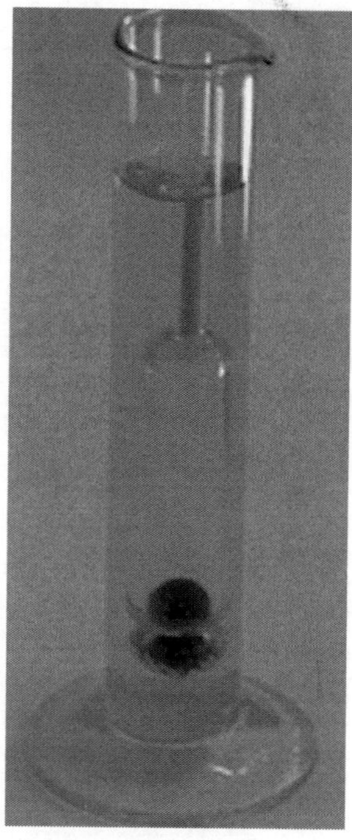

Fig. 51.2 Urinometer

Temperature Correction

Note the temperature of specimen. The urinometer is calibrated at 15°C. For every 3°C above 15°C add 0.001 and for every 3°C fall of temperature reduce 0.001.

Urine composition (Fig. 51.3)

The chief constituents of normal urine:

1. Water—it constitutes about 95% of urine.
2. Inorganic components—PO_4^{-3}, SO_4^{-2}, Na^+, K^+, Cl^-, Ca^{++}, Mg^{+2}, NH_4^+, Fe^{+2}, HCO_3^-, Zn^{+2} and NO_3^- in traces.
3. Organic components—urea, uric acid and creatinine.

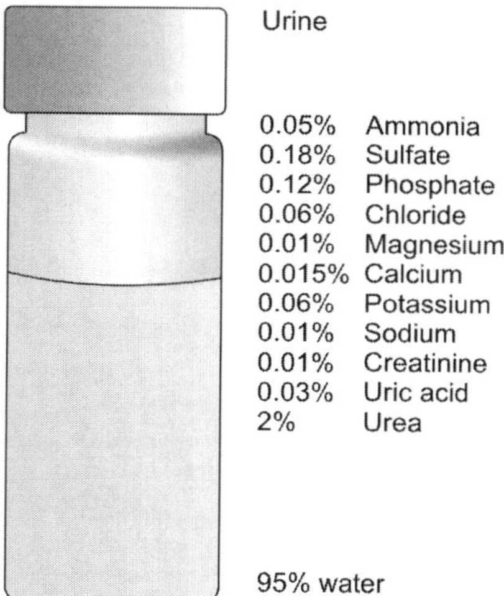

Fig. 51.3 Composition of urine

Test for Organic Constituents

Tests for Urea

Urease Test

Principle

Urea in presence of urease and H_2O gives CO_2 and NH_4^+. The pink color is given by NH_3.

Procedure

Take a pinch of jack bean meal in a test tube containing urine sample and add few drops of phenolphthalein in urine. Keep at 37°C and see the color changes to pink in about 10 minutes to 15 minutes.

Hypobromide Test

Procedure

Take 5 mL of urine. Add a drop of Na hypobromide. Marked effervescence of N_2 gas is observed.

$NH_2CONH_2 + 3\ NaOBr + 2\ NaOH \longrightarrow 3NaBr + N_2\uparrow + Na_2CO_3 + 3H_2O$

Tests for Creatinine

Jaffe's Test

Principle

Creatinine forms creatinine picrate in alkaline medium and develop deep orange color.

Procedure

Take 3 mL of urine. Add 1 mL of picric acid. Color changes from yellow to orange showing the presence of creatinine.

Tests for Uric Acid

Murexide Test

Take a small pinch of uric acid in a clean and dry porcelain dish. Add 3 drops of concentrated HNO_3 and heat to evaporation. Cool it, red deposits remain. Now add 2 drops of NH_3 purplish red color appears which indicates formation for murexide.

Test for Inorganic Constituents

For testing the major inorganic constituents in urine, following reagents are used:

- $AgNO_3$
- $BaCl_2$
- Ammonium molybdate
- Ammonium oxalate.

The urine sample (2 ml) is taken in a test tube and the inorganic ions are tested by adding the suitable reagent (few drops) as shown in the reactions below.

1. Test for Cl–
   Sample + $AgNO_3$ white ppt (AgCl).

2. Test for SO_4^{-2}
   Sample + $BaCl_2$ white ppt ($BaSO_4$).
3. Test for PO_4^{-3}
   Sample + ammonium molybdate + drops of HNO_3 ⟶ canary yellow ppt. (Phosphoammonium molybdate)
4. Test for Ca^{+2}
   Sample + ammonium oxalate ⟶ white ppt (Calcium oxalate).

Viva voce

Q1. What is the site of urine formation?
Q2. Normal urine has a pH ....
Q3. Normal person excretes how much urine?
Q4. What are the major organic constituents of urine?
Q5. How is the presence of urea detected in urine?
Q6. Which test is used for the detection of creatinine and what is its clinical application?
Q7. Which test is used for the detection of uric acid?
Q8. Uric acid is the product of metabolism of ....
Q9. Name the major inorganic components of urine.
Q10. What gives the urine its typical color?
Q11. Polyuria is observed in diabetes mellitus, why?
Q12. Name conditions of oliguria.
Q13. What is the normal specific gravity of urine?
Q14. Why is temperature correction necessary for calculating the correct value of specific gravity?

CHAPTER

52

Analysis of Abnormal/Pathological Urine

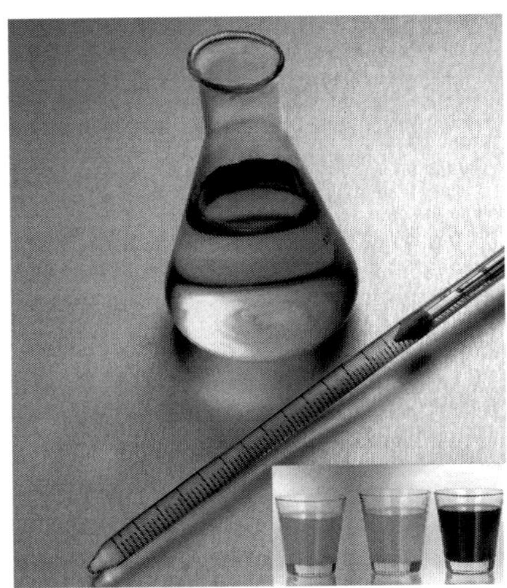

Chapter Framework

- Proteins
- Detection of Proteins in Urine
- Detection of Sugar in Urine
  - True Glycosuria
  - Renal Glycosuria
  - Alimentary Glycosuria
- Detection of Ketone Bodies
- Detection of Bile Pigments and Bile Salts
- Detection of Blood

Urine is said to be pathological when it contains abnormal constituents is detectable amounts. The abnormal constituents in pathological urine are:

- Proteins
- Sugar
- Ketone bodies
- Bile salts and pigments
- Blood.

Proteins

The presence of protein in urine is known proteinuria. The proteins commonly found in urine are albumin and globulin. Proteinuria may be divided in:

Functional Proteinuria

This is not associated with any organic disease usually. It is temporary and harmless. It may occur after severe exercise, after a cold bath and in pregnancy.

Organic Proteinuria

This is due to some definite organic disease. It may be divided into pre-renal, renal and postrenal depending upon the site of the disease.

Prerenal

In this condition the cause of proteinuria lies outside the excretory system. It may be seen in cardiac failure, liver disease and collagen diseases.

Renal

The cause of proteinuria lies in the kidneys. Generally glomerular damage from any cause resulting in increased glomerular permeability may lead to proteinuria. The common causes are acute and chronic glomerulo nephritis, nephrotic syndrome, cancer of kidneys, etc.

Postrenal

It may be caused due to traumatic lesions involving pelvis of the kidney, ureters, urinary bladder, prostate or urethra.

Sometimes a peculiar protein 'Bence Jones' is present in urine. When urine is heated, the Bence Jones proteins get precipitated between 40°C and 60°C and redissolved on further heating at 100°C. The precipitate reappears again on cooling to 40°C to 60°C. It is believed to be derived from immunoglobulin. It is commonly seen in multiple myeloma and sometimes in leukemia.

Detection of Proteins in Urine

The major proteins present in urine are albumin and globulin. These are heat coaguable proteins and are easily precipitated by alkaloidal reagents and concentrated acids. Thus the major tests performed for detection of proteins are:

Sulfosalicylic Acid Test

Take 3 mL of urine sample. Add sulfosalicylic acid drop by drop, mixing after each addition. A white precipitate appears indicating protein is present.

Heat Coagulation Test

Fill the test tube 2/3rd with urine solution. Hold the test tube at its bottom, incline it slightly. Now heat the upper portion of solution, 1 drop of 1% acetic acid and heat again, a dense coagulum is formed in the upper part of the solution. The test is given by heat coaguable protein.

Heller's Nitric Acid Test

Take 3 mL of urine sample in a test tube. Now add equal volume of concentrated HNO_3 slowly into the urine sample. A white ring of acid metaproteins will be observed at the junction of the 2 liquids.

Detection of Sugar in Urine

The principal sugar present in the urine is glucose. Glucose is present even in normal urine but its concentration is too low to be detected by ordinary test. The presence of detectable amount of carbohydrate in urine is called glycosuria. The most common cause of glycosuria are:

True Glycosuria

In this condition there is a disorder affecting the carbohydrate metabolism leading to hyperglycemia and eventually glycosuria.

- Diabetes mellitus
- Endocrinal disorders such as hyperpituitarism, hyperthyroidism, Cushing's syndrome.

Renal Glycosuria

In this condition the capacity of renal tubules to reabsorb glucose is subnormal, so the glucose filtered is not reabsorbed.

Alimentary Glycosuria

This condition may be observed in some normal persons when glucose is present in urine after excessive dietary consumption of carbohydrates.

Sometimes reducing carbohydrates other than glucose may be present in urine, e.g. lactose in lactation, galactose in congenital galactosemia, fructose in an inherited metabolic disorder, L-xylulose-in essential pentosuria, etc.

Benedict's Test

Take 5 ml of Benedict's solution in a test tube and add 8 drops of urine sample in it. Boil for 2 minutes. The development of precipitate gives an idea of percentage of sugar present in urine (Fig. 52.1).

- Blue—No sugar
- Green—0.5% sugar
- Yellow—1% sugar
- Orange—1.5% sugar
- Red—>2% sugar.

Detection of Ketone Bodies

Acetoacetate, β-hydroxy butyrate and acetone are collectively termed as ketone bodies. They are found normally in very small quantities in urine. They are synthesized at liver from fatty acids oxidation (Ketogenesis). Clinical condition resulting from increased ketone bodies production is termed as 'ketosis'. This occurs when carbohydrate metabolism is impaired and oxidation of fatty acid is increased. Ketosis is commonly observed in severe diabetes mellitus and starvation.

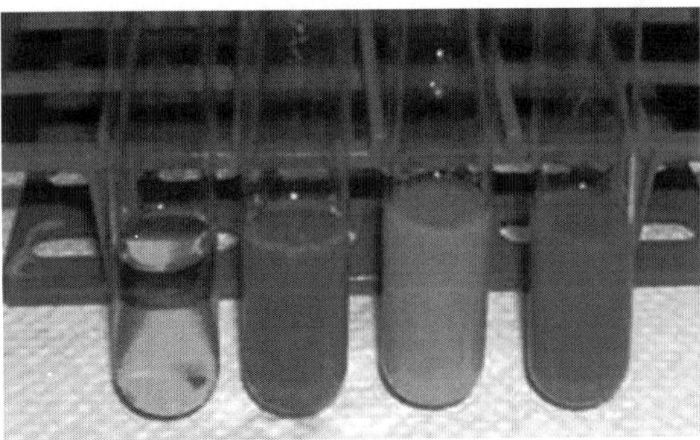

Fig. 52.1 Benedict's test

Adverse effect of ketosis is acidosis metabolic acidosis occurs because ketone bodies are acidic in nature and are excreted as Na salts in urine. This causes a loss of the *alkali reserve* of the body, leading to acidosis. Acidosis is dangerous may result in coma and even death if not treated.

Rothera's Test

Take 5 mL of urine sample in a test tube and saturate it with solid ammonium sulfate. Now add 2 to 3 drop of freshly prepared 5% solution of sodium nitroprusside and 2 mL of ammonia solution. Mix and allow standing for 10 minutes, a permanganate color indicates presence of ketone bodies.

Detection of Bile Pigments and Bile Salts

Bilirubin is major bile pigment in humans. It is formed from the breakdown of heme in RE cells and is released into circulation. This is called unconjugated bilirubin. At liver it gets conjugated with glucuronic acid and is excreted in bile. It appears in urine in hepatocellular and obstructive jaundice.

Bile salts are Na and K glycocholate and taurocholate. They are formed in liver and excreted in bile as bile salts in urine. Bile salts are observed in urine in hepatic disorders, e.g. hepatitis, hepatic and posthepatic jaundice.

Detection of Bile Pigments in Urine by Gmelin's Test

Principle

Bile pigments are oxidized in rapid succession by concentrated HNO_3 to form different oxidation products having different colors.

Procedure

Take 3 mL of concentrated HNO_3 in test tube and add 3 mL of urine sample along the wall of the test tube. Appearance of rings of different colors green, blue, violet, red and reddish yellow in rapid succession occurs at the junction of the liquids. This is due to oxidation of bile pigments.

Detection of Bile Salts in Urine by Hay's Sulfur Test

Principle

The mass of the sulfur flowers (Sulfur powder) is so small that they are unable to penetrate the liquid of high surface tension like water. Bile salts reduce the surface tension of water and thus the sulfur flowers penetrate and sink to the bottom of the solution containing them.

Procedure

Take 10 mL of urine sample in a test tube and gently sprinkle some sulfur flowers on the surface of urine sample. Do not shake the test tube. The sulfur flowers sink to the bottom of the test tube indicating the presence of bile salts.

Detection of Blood

The presence of detectable amount of blood in urine is termed as hematuria. Hematuria has typically presence of intact red blood cells (RBCs). Few RBCs may be present in normal urine too but in undetectable amount. Hematuria is observed in clinical conditions like acute glomerulonephritis, cancer and stone of urinary tract, bleeding disorders like hemophilia and sometimes in leukemia.

The presence of free hemoglobin in urine is called hemoglobinuria. It occurs in hemolytic anemia, typhoid, extensive burns and mismatched blood transfusion.

Benzidine Test

Reagents

- Benzidine
- Hydrogen peroxide

Principle

This test is based upon the peroxidase like activity of hemoglobin. Hemoglobin breaks up hydrogen peroxide into water and nascent oxygen. The nascent oxygen oxidises benzidine into a blue-green-colored complex.

Procedure

Take 3 ml of urine sample. Add 2 to 3 drops of benzidine solution. Now add 2 to 3 drops H_2O_2. Mix the solution well, a blue-green color appears indicating the presence of blood.

Note: *Benzidine is a potent carcinogenic agent therefore the test has been modified such that other chemicals which also get oxidized by nascent oxygen to develop color, are used these days. One such agent is Guaiac resin.*

- Guaiac resin test

  This test is a card test, where guaiac resin is impregnated on to a paper strip. This is kept soaked in H_2O_2. On dipping the strip in a urine sample containing blood, the same reaction occurs and guaiac resin gives a bluish green color indicating the presence of blood.

Viva voce

Q1. What is abnormal urine?
Q2. Name the major abnormalities that may be present in urine.
Q3. How is the presence of sugar in urine detected and why?
Q4. Name the conditions of true glycosuria.
Q5. Why is sugar present in urine in true glycosuria?
Q6. What is the reason behind renal glycosuria?
Q7. Detection of proteins in urine is done using which tests?
Q8. What are the major proteins excreted in urine?
Q9. Why proteins are not present in normal urine?
Q10. What are the proteins excreted in multiple myeloma?
Q11. When do we observe presence of only bile salts in urine and why?
Q12. Bile salts are produced at ....
Q13. Name a condition when both bile pigments and bile salts are present in urine and why?
Q14. The detection of bile salts is done by Hay's test. Name the reagent used and why it is used?
Q15. When do we observe sugar and ketone bodies together in urine and why?
Q16. What is the odor of urine containing ketone bodies?
Q17. Why do ketone bodies cause metabolic acidosis when present in excess?
Q18. What is the difference between hematuria and hemoglobinuria?
Q19. How is the presence of blood in urine detected?
Q20. Why is the Benzidine test modified to a card test?

Part E

Applications of Clinical Biochemistry

- Liver Function Tests
- Renal Function Tests
- Thyroid Function Tests
- Parathyroid Function Tests

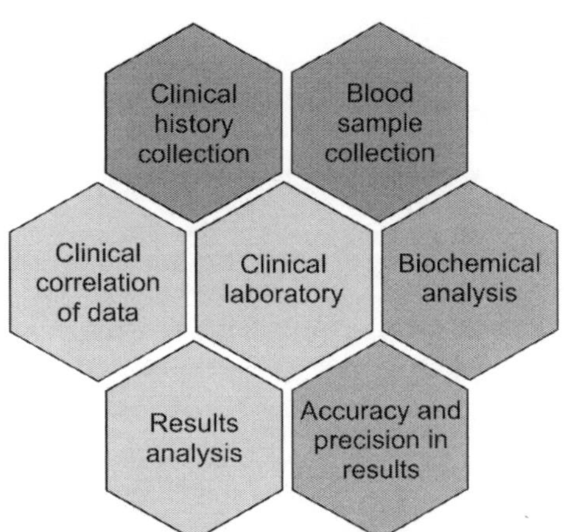

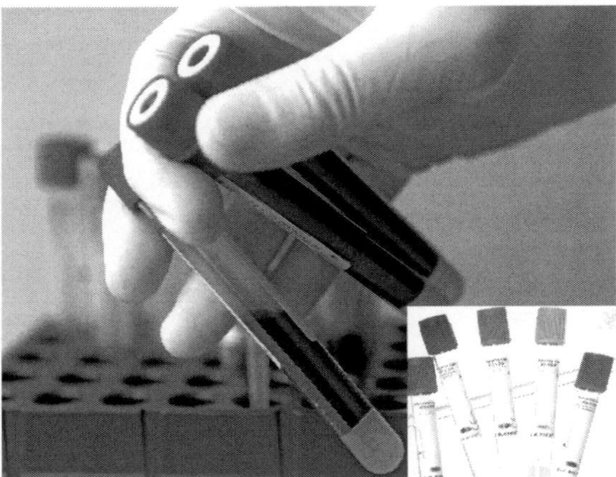

Organ Function Tests

Clinical biochemistry is a founding stone of modern medicine. It is a rapidly growing field. The major focus of clinical biochemistry is the analysis and evaluation of normal biochemical parameters in various body fluids. The normal values are used as reference for comparing the abnormal rise or fall in these values, which may be due to a disease. Thus clinical biochemistry is an important tool in a physician's tool box.

Organ function tests form an important section in the battery of tests that are done in a clinical biochemistry laboratory. These tests give an idea about the normal or abnormal functioning of the organ concerned. The most important organ function tests performed routinely in a clinical biochemistry laboratory are:

1. LFT—To diagnose liver disorders
2. RFT—To diagnose renal disorders
3. TFT—To diagnose thyroid disorders
4. Parathyroid Function Test—To diagnose parathyroid disorders.

There are many more function tests but they are beyond the scope of this book. The knowledge of these basic function tests would give the undergraduate students a vision for the clinical assessment of the patients.

CHAPTER

53

Liver Function Tests

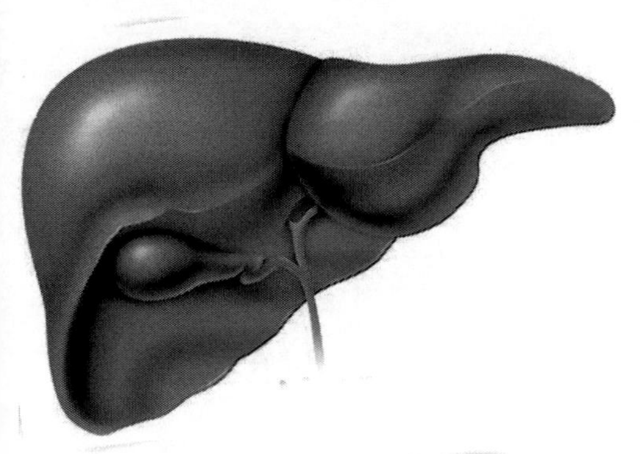

Chapter Framework

Liver is the largest gland in the body and weighs 1.5 kg in an adult. It performs a large number of functions which can be classified as:

1. *Metabolic function:* Liver is the principal site of metabolism of carbohydrates, lipids and proteins. Besides, liver is also involved in the metabolism of vitamins, minerals and nucleic acids.
2. *Secretory function:* Liver is the site of synthesis and secretion of bile.
3. *Excretory function:* Liver gets a very high blood supply. It is the site of removal of certain dyes from the blood and their excretion.
4. *Synthesis of clotting factors:* Liver synthesizes the clotting factors II, VII, IX and X, though in a zymogenic form.
5. *Synthesis of plasma proteins:* Liver synthesizes all the plasma proteins except γ-globulins.
6. *Detoxication:* The Kupffer cells lining the liver sinusoids remove foreign agents from blood by phagocytosis. Liver is also a site of detoxication of drugs and hormones to convert them into less toxic substances.
7. *Storage:* Liver is the site of storage of important vitamins and minerals like vitamin A, D, K and B_{12} and Fe. Liver is also the site of storage of glycogen. This liver glycogen helps regulate the normal blood sugar level.

There are a host of tests that are performed to assess the normal functional capacity of the liver.

The most commonly performed LFTs include blood tests like van dan Berg's test, serum bilirubin, total protein and A:G ratio, enzyme assays of serum transaminases, ALP, g GGT. Some urine tests are also performed like bilirubin and bile salt presence in urine. Tests like flocculation and turbidity tests are not performed these days. Instead, the functional capacity of liver is assessed by testing the excretory capacity of liver, i.e. by giving exogenous compounds like aminopyrine, BSP dyes, etc.

The tests commonly done in a lab for LFT assessment are:

Tests Based on Bilirubin Metabolism

This includes the measurement of serum urinary bilirubin by VD Berg's reagent.

Reagent

- Diazo reagent
- Solution A—Sulfanilic acid in concentrated HCl
- Solution B—Sodium nitrite in water.

Principle

Diazotized sulfanilic acid (VD Berg's reagent) reacts with conjugated bilirubin to give reddish purple color immediately (direct positive) and with unconjugated bilirubin gives a delayed positive reaction. The intensity of the color is proportional to the concentration of bilirubin in the sample and can be measured colorimetrically.

Clinical Interpretations

Bilirubin is seen in urine in obstructive jaundice (VD Berg direct positive) due to presence of conjugated bilirubin. VD Berg test is indirect positive with Hemolytic jaundice serum due to unconjugated bilirubin and VD Berg's test is biphasic positive in hepatocellular jaundice as both conjugated and unconjugated bilirubin are present in blood.

Fecal and Urinary Urobilinogen

Fecal urinary urobilinogen (UBG) depends upon the amount of bilirubin getting reduced to urobilinogen in intestine. This value increases in hemolytic jaundice and decreases in obstructive jaundice. A high fecal urobilinogen is observed in hemolytic and low fecal urobilinogen is seen in obstructive jaundice.

[Normal value 50 mg–250 mg/day]

Similarly, urinary UBG is high in hemolytic jaundice and low in obstructive jaundice.

[Normal value 0.6 mg–4 mg/day]

Tests Based upon Metabolic Function of Liver

Galactose Tolerance Test

Liver is the site of conversion of all monosaccharides other than glucose into glucose. Under a normal functioning liver, the galactose absorbed would be converted into glucose. However in a functionally compromised liver, this would be disrupted and more galactose would be present in the circulating blood and would also be excreted excessively in urine. This test assesses the intrahepatic damage and can distinguish obstructive and nonobstructive jaundice.

Procedure

The test is conducted after an overnight fast, 40 gm of galactose is given dissolved in water orally. Blood samples are collected at ½ hour interval for 2 hours.

Clinical Interpretations

The blood galactose returns to normal in 1 hour in obstructive jaundice and in normal persons and urinary excretion are 3 gm or less. In intrahepatic jaundice the excretion is 4 gm to 5 gm or more.

Test Based on Synthesis of Plasma Proteins

Colorimetric assessment of total protein and A:G ratio (already discussed in chapter No. 46).

Clinical Interpretations

In advanced parenchymal liver diseases, liver function is compromised and A:G ratio is reversed. In obstructive jaundice normal values are seen. Thus, it may help in differential diagnosis of hepatic and obstructive jaundice.

Tests Based on Detoxication Action of Liver

Hippuric acid test is the best known LFT for assessing the detoxifying action of liver. Benzoic acid when given either orally/IV get converted into hippuric acid at liver by its combination with glycine, which is then excreted is urine (normal renal function is desired).

Clinical Interpretations

6 gm of sodium benzoate dissolved in 200 ml water given orally/IV after light breakfast. Hippuric acid is excreted about 3 gm to 3.5 gm normally. Lower amount excreted in acute/chronic liver cell damage.

Tests Based on Excretory Function of Liver

The liver has ability to excrete certain dyes like bromosulfathalein (BSP) when given intravenous.

Clinical Interpretations

In a normal healthy person not more than 5% of the dye injected should be retained at the end of 45 minutes.

However, in liver cell damage, the removal of this dye is much slower so that 40% to 50% dye is still retained circulating in the blood by the end of 45 minutes.

This test is not advisable to obstructive jaundice patients, as it is removed after conjugation along with bile. Any obstruction of biliary tree would obstruct the flow of this dye too.

Another dye used is Rose-Bengal dye. This dye is I^{131} labeled dye.

Tests Based on the Synthesis of Clotting Factors by Liver

Prothrombin time is assessed (normal 10 sec – 16 seconds). The value increases in parenchymatous liver diseases and obstructive jaundice.

PT index can also be calculated

Normal value—70% to 100%

Enzyme Assays

A large number of enzyme assays are done to assess the liver function. The most commonly performed are:

- SGOT and SGPT
- Alkaline phosphatases
- γ-Glutamyl transpeptidases.

Serum Transaminases

- SGOT (4 IU–17 IU/l)
- SGPT (3 IU–15 IU/l).

Transaminases are extremely useful in assessing parenchymal liver diseases like—Acute hepatitis, cirrhosis of liver, toxic hepatitis. Out of the 2 transaminases, SGPT is more specific as SGOT levels tend to be raised in Myocardial infarction too.

Alkaline Phosphatases

Normal Value of ALP—3 KÅ–13 KÅ units/100 mL (23 IU–92 IU/L)

This is very useful for differentiating the hepatic and posthepatic jaundice, as the values of Alkaline phosphatases (ALP) are fairly higher in the latter case (>35 kA/100 ml)

Several other important enzyme assays include γ-GT, LDH, cholin esterase, 5-nucleotides, etc.

Viva voce

Q1. What are the major liver functions?
Q2. Name the LFTs based on the bilirubin metabolism.
Q3. Which is the test that helps assess the detoxicating properties of liver?
Q4. Why is the VD Berg's test biphasic positive in hepatocellular jaundice?
Q5. The synthetic function of liver is assessed by ....
Q6. The plasma protein which is not synthesized at liver is ....
Q7. What is prothrombin Index?
Q8. When is the prothrombin index increased?
Q9. How to assess the detoxicating function of liver?
Q10. Which serum transaminase is more specific for liver disorders?

CHAPTER

54

Renal Function Tests

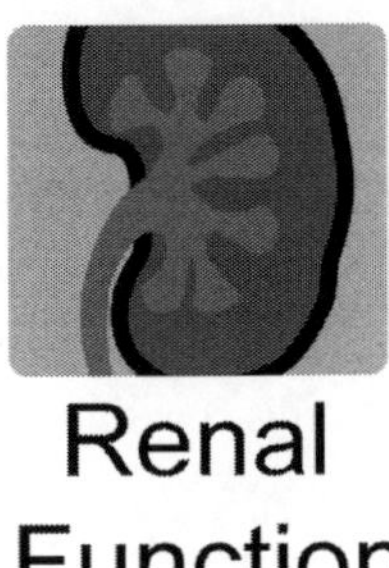

Renal Function

Chapter Framework

- Test for Assessment of Glomerular Function
  - Clearance Tests
  - Salient Features for Substance Suitable for Measuring GFR
  - Clinical interpretations
- Tests for Measuring Renal Plasma flow
  - Para-amino Hippurate Test
  - Clinical Interpretations
- Tests for Tubular Function
- Phenolfsullon-phathalein Test
- Kidney Imaging
- Kidney Biopsy

The kidneys are bean-shaped organs, each about the size of a fist. The functional unit in the kidney is the nephron. Kidneys perform many important functions. The various function performed by the kidneys are:

- The kidneys remove wastes and water from the blood to form urine.
- Excretion of nonprotein nitrogenous substances such as urea, creatinine and uric acid.
- Regulation of water, electrolyte and acid-base balance.
- Production of hormones, e.g. erythropoietin, renin and calcitriol.
- Health professionals use the term "renal function" to talk about how efficiently the kidneys filter blood. Healthy people with two normally functioning kidneys have 100% of their kidney function. Small or mild damage to the kidneys deteriorates the kidney function as much as 30% to 40% —would rarely be noticeable. Assessment of renal function is required for:
  - Finding out the extent of damage in renal disease.
  - Monitoring the progress of renal disease.
  - Monitoring the dose and adjusting the dose of drugs that are excreted via kidneys.

In order to assess the renal function a number of tests have been devised which give information regarding:

- Renal blood flow

  - Glomerular filtration rate (GFR)
  - Renal tubular function
  - Urinary output.

Thus the RFTs can be divided into:

- Urine analysis
  - Physical examination
  - Chemical examination
  - Microscopic examination

  (Already discussed in Chapter 51).
- Test for assessment of glomerular function
  - Clearance tests
  - Blood urea and creatinine estimation (see Chapters 47 and 48)
  - Proteinuria and Hematuria (see Chapter 52).
- Tests for measuring renal plasma flow [RPF]
  - Para-amino hippurate test.
- Test for assessment of tubular function
  - Urine concentration test
  - Urine dilution test
  - Acid load test
  - Phenolsulfonpthalein test (PSP)

Test for Assessment of Glomerular Function

Clearance Tests

Clearance can be defined as the volume of plasma completely cleared of a substance per minute by the kidneys. It is expressed as ml/minute. Clearance helps to measure the glomerular filtration rate (GFR). Measurement of GFR provides the most useful index for assessing the severity of renal damage.

$$\text{Clearance} = \frac{\text{mg of substance excreted per minute}}{\text{mg of substance per mL of plasma}}$$

$$C = U \times V / P$$

where,

U is concentration of substance in urine

V is volume of urine in mL excreted per minute

P is concentration of substance in plasma.

The substance used for estimation of clearance should be such that it is neither reabsorbed nor secreted in the renal tubules and should freely filter out through the glomerulus.

Salient Features for Substance Suitable for Measuring GFR

- Should be freely filtered at glomerulus
- Once filtered should not reabsorbed by the renal tubules
- Should be nontoxic

- Should not be metabolized in the body
- Should not be stored in the body
- Should be easy to measure in blood and urine
- Substances commonly used for measuring GFR
- Exogenous—Inulin
- Endogenous—Creatinine and urea.

Normal Value

- Urea clearance:
  Maximum urea clearance = 75 mL/min
  Standard urea clearance = 54 mL/min
- Creatinine clearance = 95 mL to 105 mL/min.

Procedure

An accurate 24 hours urine sample is collected (7 am on first day to 7 am next day). Total volume is measured. Blood sample is collected for serum creatinine.

Clinical Interpretations

A reduced creatinine clearance is the most sensitive indicator of reduced GFR due to acute/chronic renal damage. Creatinine clearance is also influenced by other prerenal, renal and postrenal conditions. The importance of creatinine clearance is in early detection of functional impairment of kidneys, without overt signs and symptoms. Clearance upto 75% of the average value indicates adequate renal function.

Tests for Measuring Renal Plasma Flow

Para-amino Hippurate Test

Para-amino hippurate (PAH) is completely removed from the blood by kidneys in a single circulation. This is due to the fact that PAH is both filtered and actively secreted by the kidneys. Thus, PAH clearance gives an idea about the renal blood/plasma flow.

Procedure

3 mL of 20% PAH in saline (250 mL) is infused at a rate of 20 mL/min. Followed by 14 mL of 20% PAH in saline (500 mL) infused at a rate of 4 mL/min. Urinary and blood PAH are measured as in clearance test. PAH clearance is equal to RPF.

Clinical Interpretations

Normal healthy adults have a RPF of 600 mL/min. It increases in hypertension and decreases in glomerulonephritis.

Tests for Tubular Function

Assessment of the concentrating and diluting capacity of the kidney is done by measuring the osmolality and specific gravity of urine. These tests provide for the most sensitive means of detecting early impairment in renal function.

Urine Concentration Test

- Fluid intake is withheld for 15 hours.
- First urine sample midstream is collected in the morning and osmolality and specific gravity measured. Under normal tubular function osmolality is 850 mOsm/kg or more and specific gravity 1.025. If the specific gravity or osmolality do not show these values then there is some defect in renal concentrating ability either due to (i) Tubular defect or (ii) Defective or decreased secretion of antidiuretic hormone (ADH).

Urine Dilution Test

In this test, after emptying the bladder, 1000 ml to 1200 ml of water is given to patient and urine samples collected for next 4 hours at 1 hour interval.

- Normal response—Specific gravity less than 1.005.
- Defective renal tubules—Defective concentration of urine, concentration remains constant irrespective of excess fluid intake.
- Decrease urine output due to cardiac failure.

Acid Load Test

It is done for diagnosis of the renal tubular acidosis which may occur due to:

- Defective H^+ secretion in distal convoluted tubules (DCT) inherited/acquired.
- Decreased capacity to reabsorb HCO_3^- in proximal convoluted tubules (PCT).
- Impaired HCO_3^- reabsorption due to aldosterone deficiency.

Test Procedure

Ammonium sulfate is given orally in a Gelatin capsule 100 mg/kg body weight.

Acidification of urine occurs as kidneys will absorb HCO_3^- filtered at glomerulus and excrete H^+.

- Normal response—Urine pH falls below 5.5 in at least one sample.
- In renaltubular acidosis—Urine pH ranges from 5.7 to 7.0. No acidification of urine occurs—No H^+ secreted leading to metabolic acidosis.

Phenolsulfonphthalein Test

Phenolsulfonphthalein (PSP) is nontoxic and is excreted exclusively by the kidneys.

Test Procedure

Intravenous injection of 6 mg PSP in saline is given. Urine samples are collected at 15 min, 30 min, 60 min and 120 min.

Normal Response

15 min—25% or more PSP excreted
1 hour—40% to 60% PSP excreted
2 hour—70% to 75% PSP excreted.

Abnormal Response

Less than 23% excreted during first 15 min, however, 2 hours excretion may be normal.

Kidney Imaging

Methods of kidney imaging—Taking pictures of the kidneys—Include ultrasound, computerized tomography (CT) scan, and magnetic resonance imaging (MRI). These tools are most helpful in finding unusual growths or blockages to the flow of urine.

Kidney Biopsy

A doctor may want to examine a tiny piece of kidney tissue with a microscope.

However, the latter two techniques are beyond the scope of this book.

Viva voce

Q1. The RFTs give information about ....
Q2. The renal plasma flow is assessed by which test?
Q3. GFR can be assessed by which test?
Q4. Name the metabolite produced within the body that can be used for assessing the GFR.
Q5. Tubular function can be assessed by which RFTs?
Q6. An abnormally high specific gravity of urine during urine dilution test can be seen in which disease?
Q7. Name the dye used for assessing the tubular function of the kidneys and why?

CHAPTER

55

Thyroid Function Tests

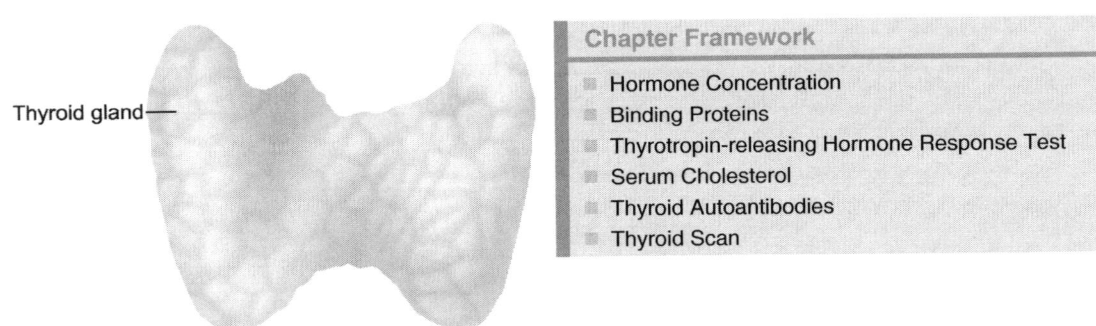

Chapter Framework

- Hormone Concentration
- Binding Proteins
- Thyrotropin-releasing Hormone Response Test
- Serum Cholesterol
- Thyroid Autoantibodies
- Thyroid Scan

Thyroid is an endocrine gland located in the neck region, around the trachea. It is a butterfly-shaped gland with 4 lobes. The thyroid gland secretes 2 very important hormones—Triiodothyronine (T_3) and Tetraiodothyronine (T_4) or thyroxine. Both the hormones are formed by the iodination of tyrosine. These hormones play significant role in regulation of basal metabolism, normal growth, development and tissue differentiation. Besides, these hormones also play important role in the regulation of intermediary metabolism of carbohydrates, lipids and proteins.

The secretion of thyroid hormones is under the control of the anterior pituitary hormone—Thyroid-stimulating hormone (TSH), which in-turn is under the control of hypothalamic thyrotropin-releasing hormone (TRH).

The disorders of thyroid are quite common in the general population. Both hypo- and hyperthyroidism occur with increased frequency in the adult population. A battery of biochemical tests is employed in the diagnosis of these thyroid disorders. The most commonly performed TFTs in a clinical biochemistry laboratory are:

Hormone Concentration

The estimation of thyroid hormones (T_3 and T_4) and anterior pituitary hormone TSH is routinely done for the diagnosis of thyroid disorders.

The evaluation of the T_3, T_4 and TSH is done by ELISA or RIA techniques. In primary hypothyroidism, the serum T_3, T_4 are reduced and TSH is raised. In primary hyperthyroidism, the serum T_3, T_4 are raised and TSH is reduced.

In case of secondary hypothyroidism the serum TSH is also reduced along with low T_3 and T_4 due to defect in the pituitary. Similarly in secondary hyperthyroidism TSH is raised along with T_3 and T_4 due to resistance to feedback inhibition caused by a defective pituitary.

Binding Proteins

The thyroid hormones are transported in the blood bound to transport proteins—Thyroxine binding globulin (TBG) and Thyroxine binding prealbumin (TBPA). Any alterations in the levels of these proteins would cause a change in the circulating levels of free T_3 [FT_3] and Free T_4 [FT_4].These proteins are increased in response to estrogens, as in pregnancy, so the number of binding sites is increased. This would decrease FT_3 and FT_4. Conversely in nephrotic syndrome the loss of TBG in urine causes a decrease in the number of binding sites, leading to raised FT_3 and FT_4.

This increase or decrease in FT_3 and FT_4 can be evaluated using a resin which also has affinity for T_3 and T_4.

In case of hypothyroidism, the patients' serum is incubated with radiolabeled T_3 and resin. The amount of radiolabeled T_3 bound to resin would be proportional to the amount of unlabeled hormone (T_3) in the serum and inversely proportional to the TBG binding sites. In hypothyroidism there are greater free binding sites of TBG and low T_3 and vice versa in hyperthyroidism.

Some drugs like salicylates and phenytoin also bind on TBG reducing the number of free sites for the T_3 and T_4 thus increasing FT_3 and FT_4.

Thyrotropin-releasing Hormone Response Test

Thyrotropin-releasing hormone (TRH) stimulates the anterior pituitary for secretion of TSH. TSH in turn stimulates the thyroid gland for secretion of T_3 and T_4. An abnormal response to TRH may be observed in–

Hyperthyroidism—The high T_4 levels negative feedback effect on anterior pituitary is far too strong than the stimulant effect of TRH. Thus an abnormal TRH response is seen.

Hypothyroidism—In primary hypothyroidism, there is a low T_3 and T_4, stimulating anterior pituitary for TSH secretion. This causes an exaggerated response to TRH at the anterior pituitary.

Hypopituitarism—Due to a defect with the pituitary itself, there may be no response to TRH by the pituitary.

Serum Cholesterol

Thyroid hormones increase both synthesis and degradation of cholesterol. Therefore in hyperthyroidism the serum cholesterol drops increased due to degradation. Hypercholesterolemia is seen in hypothyroidism due to reduced degradation of cholesterol. Hypercholesterolemia is not a condition exclusively indicating hypothyroidism. There are many other clinical states characterized by hypercholesterolemia. However, serum cholesterol estimation in thyroid disorders can help to see the efficacy of the therapy given.

Thyroid Autoantibodies

The most common thyroid disorder is Hashimoto's thyroiditis and Graves' disease. Both of these are autoimmune diseases caused by production of autoantibodies—Thyroid-stimulating Ig

(TSIg)—Graves' disease. These bind to TSH receptors and stimulate the gland uncontrolled—hyperthyroidism.

In Hashimoto's thyroiditis, autoantibodies are seen against thyroglobulin, microsomes and nucleus. They cause cell destruction and hypothyroidism.

Nowadays, hypo- or hyperthyroid conditions are clinically established by the detection of these antibodies.

Thyroid Scan

Thyroid scan can be done by using radiolabeled iodine. A high concentration of radiolabeled iodine would be seen in hyperthyroidism and vice versa in hypothyroidism.

Viva voce

Q1. Name the hormones secreted by the thyroid gland.

Q2. The secretion of thyroid hormones is regulated by .... from pituitary and from hypothalamus.

Q3. The TFTs help in the diagnosis of .... and ....

Q4. Serum T_3, T_4 and TSH are reduced in secondary hypothyroidism. Why?

Q5. Name the transport proteins of thyroid hormones.

Q6. Name the drugs that may increase the serum FT_3 and FT_4 and why?

Q7. Why is serum cholesterol increased in hypothyroidism and decreased in hyperthyroidism?

Q8. When is the TRH response exaggerated and why?

Q9. Name the autoimmune thyroid disorders.

Q10. What is used in thyroid scan?

CHAPTER

56

Parathyroid Function Tests

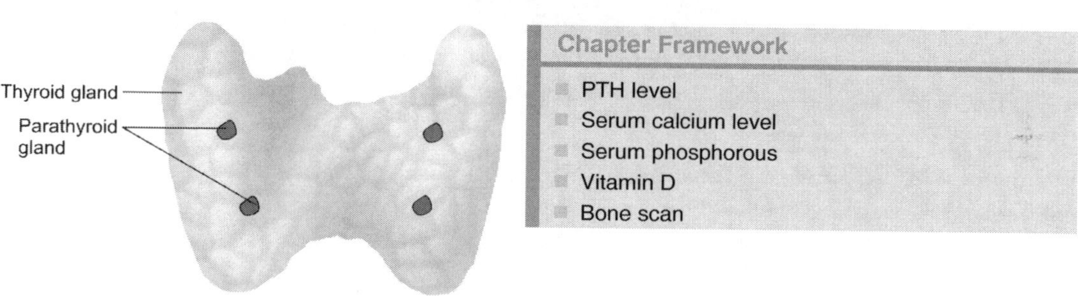

The parathyroid gland is an endocrine gland that is present embedded in the thyroid lobes. There are 2 pairs of parathyroid glands present. These glands secrete the parathormone or the parathyroid hormone (PTH). The PTH is a hormone that principally involved in the maintenance of normal serum calcium level. This hormone increases the reabsorption of filtered calcium and inhibits reabsorption of phosphorus at the DCT of kidneys, increasing the serum calcium. At the bones, PTH increases the osteoclastic activity, causing the bones to dissolve and adds up to the serum calcium.

Disorders of parathyroid are namely hypo- and hyperparathyroidism. The diagnosis of these disorders can be done by employing a set of biochemical tests. The important tests performed as parathyroid function tests are:

1. PTH level (ELISA/RIA)
2. Serum calcium level (Titration)
3. Serum phosphorus level (Colorimetrically)
4. Serum vitamin D level (Chromatography/RIA)
5. Bone scan.

PTH level

Normally for evaluating the parathyroid status, serum parathyroid hormone related protein (discovered in 1987) is measured. The PTHrP is generally measured using immunoassays. PTHrP is unstable in serum and plasma at 4°C, so the sample should be collected in the presence of protease inhibitors and EDTA. Plasma should then be immediately separated and frozen.

The normal reference range of PTHrP is 1.5 pmol 2.5 pmol/L. High values are seen in hyperparathyroidism and low in hypoparathyroidism.

Serum Calcium Level

Serum calcium can be estimated by titration. The method is termed as the *Clark and Collip* method.

Principle

Serum is treated with ammonium oxalate for precipitating calcium oxalate. The precipitate is washed with ammonia for removal of excess oxalate. Now the precipitate is treated with sulfuric acid to convert calcium oxalate into oxalic acid. The latter is then titrated with standard potassium permanganate.

The normal serum calcium level ranges within 9 mg to 11 mg/dL. The level of serum calcium rises in hyperparathyroidism and reduces in hypoparathyroidism.

Serum Phosphorus

Serum phosphorus is measured colorimetrically. The method is named as the *Fiske and Subbarow method.*

Principle

Deproteinized serum is treated with acid molybdate which combines with phosphate to form phosphomolybdic acid. This is then reacted with 1,2,4 -aminonaphthol-sulfonic acid to give a blue colored phosphomolybdic acid. The intensity of the color is measured colorimetrically at a red-filter (680 nm).

The normal serum phosphorus level is 2.5 mg to 4.5 mg/dL for the adults and 4 mg to 6 mg/dL for the children. The serum phosphorus level is raised in hypoparathyroidism and vice-versa in hyperparathyroidism.

Serum Vitamin D

Highly sensitive and specific assays have been devised for the estimation of vitamin D. Most assays of vitamin D require two or three of the following steps:

1. Deproteinization/extraction
2. Purification
3. Quantification.

After deproteinization with acetonitrile, either RIA or high pressure liquid chromatography (HPLC) is used for measurement of the vitamin-D levels.

The specimen of vitamin D is stable at room temperature, however if the estimation is to be delayed the samples (serum) should be frozen.

Normal vitamin D level ranges from 10 mg to 50 mg/mL (25–OH D) and 15 ng to 60 ng/mL (1, 25–OH D).

The levels of vitamin D are found to be raised in hyperparathyroidism and lowered in hypoparathyroidism.

Bone scan

This method is beyond the scope of this book. However, in hyperparathyroidism bone scan would show a rarefied bone due to increased osteoclastic activity.

Viva voce

Q1. What is the function of PTH?
Q2. How is serum PTH level assessed?
Q3. Hypoparathyroidism shows serum calcium level to be ....
Q4. Serum vitamin D levels are found to be raised in hyperparathyroidism. Why?
Q5. What would the bone scan in hyperparathyroidism show?

Part F

Demonstrations

- Analysis of Saliva
- Analysis of Food-Stuffs
- Biochemical Techniques
- Titrable Acidity of Urine
- Nonprotein Nitrogen
- Recent Advances in Clinical Biochemistry
- Preparation of Various Reagents
- Normal Reference Values of Various Biochemical Parameters

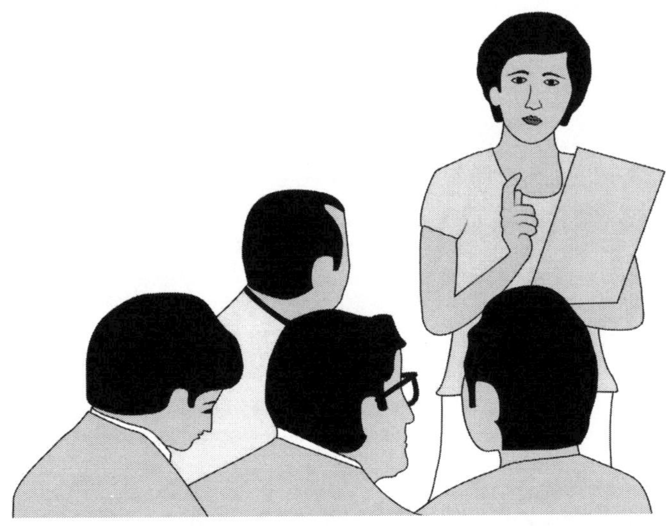

This section includes those biochemical analyses which the undergraduate students would not perform in the laboratory. However, these analyses form an important section for the students to understand the basics of clinical and nutritional biochemistry.

CHAPTER

57

Analysis of Saliva

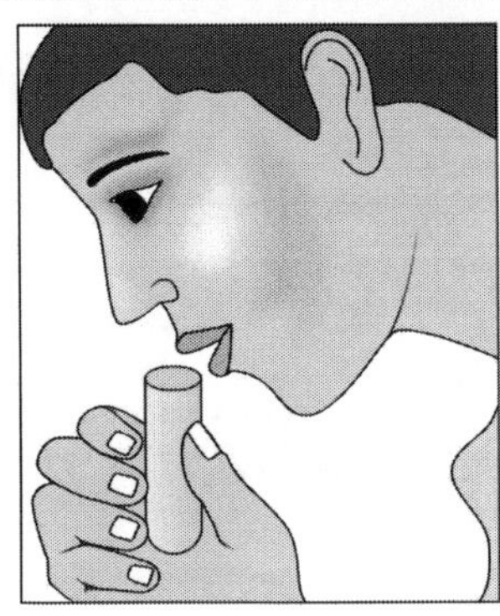

Chapter Framework

- Composition of Saliva
- Analysis of Saliva
- Tests for Organic Constituents
- Tests for Inorganic Constituents

Saliva is a secretion of three pairs of salivary glands—parotid, submaxillary and sublingual glands. It is a very important digestive juice. It plays vital role in:

- Preparing the food for swallowing.
- Sense of taste.
- Digestion of boiled starch by salivary amylase and emulsified lipids (milk fats) by lingual lipase.
- Keeping the buccal cavity rinsed and clean.
- Protective action is seen due to the presence of lysozyme, which kills bacteria.
- Helps in speech.

Composition of Saliva

The composition of saliva is quite variable. It contains:

- 99.5% water
- 0.5% solids.

Of the solids, 60% are organic and 40% are inorganic constituents. The chief *organic constituents* are:

- Mucin
- Enzymes.

Mucin is a mucoprotein. The lubricating property of saliva is mainly due to its mucin content. The main enzymes of saliva are amylase and lysozyme.

Amylase is an amylolytic enzyme whereas lysozyme has an antibacterial activity.

The major *inorganic constituents* are:

- Cations like–Na^+, K^+, Ca^{++}, Mg^{++}.
- Anions like—Thiocyanates (SCN^-), sulfates (SO_4^{-2}), chlorides (Cl^-), phosphates (PO_4^{-3}), and bicarbonates (HCO_3^-).

Analysis of Saliva

Procedure

Collection of Saliva

Rinse your mouth with clean water. Take a mouthful of water and hold it in your mouth for 2 minutes, moving it with your tongue. Now collect the water in a beaker.

Tests for Organic Constituents

Test for Mucin

- Take 5 mL of dilute saliva in a test tube and add 30% acetic acid drop by drop mixing vigorously in between each addition. A sticky precipitate will show the presence of mucin.
- Test for salivary amylase.

Reagents

- Iodine solution
- Starch solution.

Principle

Amylase acts on its substrate starch at its optimum pH (6.8) and optimum temperature (37°C). Starch is successively hydrolyzed into amylodextrin, erythrodextrin, and achrodextrin and maltose. The time required for the conversion of starch into achrodextrin (which gives no color with iodine) is known as the *chromic period*. It is inversely proportional to the concentration of amylase in saliva. The chloride ions present in the saliva are necessary for the activity of the amylase.

Procedure

Take five test tubes and label them from 1–5. Take 3 mL of starch in each of the test tubes. Now add 1 mL of saliva in first test tube, and immediately add 2 drops of iodine solution. A blue color indicates the presence of unhydrolyzed starch.

In the second test tube 1 mL of saliva and add iodine after 15 sec to 20 seconds. A violet color appears, showing the presence of amylodextrin formed by hydrolysis of starch.

In the third test tube add 1 mL of saliva and after about 1 min to 1.5 minute add 2 drops of iodine. A red color appears showing the presence of erythrodextrin.

In the fourth test and fifth test tubes also add 1 mL starch solution and then add 2 drops of iodine after 3 and 4 minutes respectively. There is no color observed in the fourth and fifth test tube, indicating the presence of achrodextrin in fourth and maltose in fifth test tube. Presence of maltose may be confirmed by the Benedict's test. Appearance of dull green-colored precipitate shows the presence of maltose.

Note:

Achromatic point—*The point at which no color develops on adding iodine to a starch—Saliva mixture.*

Chromatic period—*Time required to give achromatic point by a starch saliva mixture.*

Tests for Inorganic Constituents

- Test for Sulfate Ions (SO_4^{-2})
  Take 2 mL dilute saliva and add 1 mL HCl and 1 mL $BaCl_2$. A white precipitate is formed of $BaSO_4$.
- Test for Chloride Ions (Cl^-)
  Take 3 mL dilute saliva and add 2 drops of HNO_3 and few drops of $AgNO_3$. A white precipitate is formed of AgCl.
- Test for Phosphate Ions (PO_4^{-3})
  Take 3 mL dilute saliva and add 1 mL of HNO_3 and 1 mL of ammonium molybdate. A canary yellow precipitate is formed of phospho-ammonium molybdate.

Viva voce

Q1. What percentage of saliva is water?
Q2. What are the major constituents of saliva?
Q3. Name the enzymes of saliva.
Q4. How is amylase estimated?
Q5. What are achromatic and chromatic points?
Q6. Name the inorganic constituents of saliva.
Q7. How can you detect the presence of maltose in a saliva starch mixture?
Q8. Name the antibacterial enzyme of saliva.
Q9. How are the different dextrin molecules presence indicated?
Q10. What are the functions of saliva?

CHAPTER

58

Analysis of Food-Stuffs

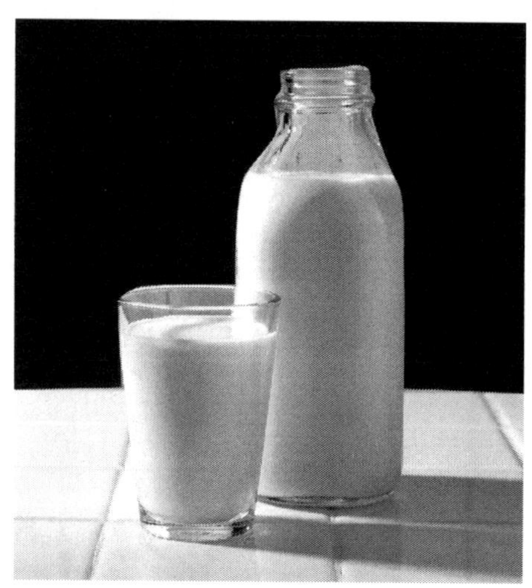

Chapter Framework

- Milk
- Composition
  - Humanization of Cow's milk
  - Pasteurization and Sterilization
- Analysis of Milk
  - Physical Examination of Milk
  - Chemical Examination of Milk

Milk

Milk is a natural food for the infants and a supplementary food for the adults. Milk is a balanced food except that it is deficient in iron and vitamin C. It is the secretion of mammary glands during the period of lactation. Hormone, in particular prolactin, regulates its secretion. Secretion during the earliest phase of the lactation is called as *colostrum.*

Colostrum is viscid yellowish secretion and contains certain essential substances for newborn like immunoglobulin. Colostrum secretion lasts for about a week after the delivery.

Composition

The average concentration of chief solid constituents in the milk of human, cow, buffalo and goat are given in the following table:

Species	*Protein (g%)*	*Fats (g%)*	*Carbohydrates (g%)*	*Ash (g%)*
Human	1.2	3.8	7.0	0.2
Cow	3.3	3.8	4.8	0.7
Buffalo	4.7	7.5	4.8	0.8
Goat	3.4	4.1	4.7	0.8

- *Milk Proteins:* Main protein of milk is casein other proteins are lactoalbumin and lactoglobulin. Casein is conjugated phosphoprotein. Milk contains a salt calcium caseinate. Lactoalbumin is similar to serum albumin. It is an important source of cysteine. Lactoglobulin present in traces provide immunity against various infections. The three proteins are of the high biological value containing all essential amino acids.
- *Milk Fat:* It is mainly present as triglycerides containing variety of fatty acid. Oleic acid and palmitic acid are the predominant fatty acids. Cholesterol and free fatty acids (FFA) are present in small amounts.
- *Milk Carbohydrates:* Lactose is the principal carbohydrate in milk. There is 7% lactose in human milk and 4.88% in cow's milk, glucose and galactose may be present in traces.
- *Minerals of Milk:* Milk is a good source of nearly all the essential minerals like Ca, P, Na, K, Mg, etc. However, it is a poor source of iron.
- *Vitamins:* Milk is rich in vitamin A and B_2 (riboflavin), only small amounts of vitamin C and D is present. Cow's milk is slightly yellow due to high amount of riboflavin.

Humanization of Cow's Milk

Modifying cow's milk in order to bring it to the same standard as to that of human milk is called humanization. It is achieved by diluting cow's milk and supplementing milk with extra lactose. So that cow's milk is at par with human milk.

Pasteurization and Sterilization

When milk is heated for half an hour at 62.5°C all the pathogenic bacteria are killed and the process is called pasteurization. Sterilization of milk is done, when milk is heated 110°C for 15 min.

Analysis of Milk

Physical Examination of Milk

- *Color:* Milk is white in color due to presence of casein and fat.
- *pH:* pH of fresh milk normally lies within 6 to 7.
- *Specific gravity:* Specific gravity of milk is measured with the help of lactometer. Normally, the specific gravity of milk lies between 1.028 to 1.034.

Chemical Examination of Milk

Add 1 test tube full each of milk and water into a small beaker and 1% acetic acid drop by drop till maximum precipitation is obtained. Filter it through Whatman's filter paper.

- Test with precipitate
  - Neumann's test—Dry small amount of precipitate by pressing it with folded filter paper. Perform Neuman's test as shown in Chapter 42. A positive test shows the presence of phosphorus in casein. (Phosphoprotein).
  - Grease-Spot test (as in lipid analysis)

  Test with filtrate:
  - Benedict test—(as in carbohydrate analysis)
    Lactose gives a positive test.

- Osazone test—(as in carbohydrate analysis)
  Cotton puff-shaped crystals of lactose osazone are obtained.
- Test for calcium—(as in urine analysis)
  A white precipitate shows presence of Ca.
- Test for inorganic phosphorus—(as in urine analysis)
  A yellow precipitate shows presence of inorganic phosphorus.
- Heat coagulation test—(as in protein analysis)
  Lactalbumin and lactglobulin gives positive test.
- Color reactions—(as in protein analysis)
  Biuret test, xanthoproteic, Million Nasse's, Aldehyde and lead sulfide test all the test are positive.

Viva voce

Q1. What is colostrum?
Q2. Why is colostrum important for the neonate?
Q3. Which vitamin is lacking in milk?
Q4. What is the amount of lactose in human milk?
Q5. Name the milk proteins.
Q6. How is cow's milk humanized?
Q7. What is sterilization and pasteurization of milk?
Q8. What is precipitated from milk on adding acetic acid?
Q9. Name the phosphoprotein present in milk.
Q10. The canary-yellow precipitate of Neumann's test is the precipitate of what?

CHAPTER

59

Biochemical Techniques

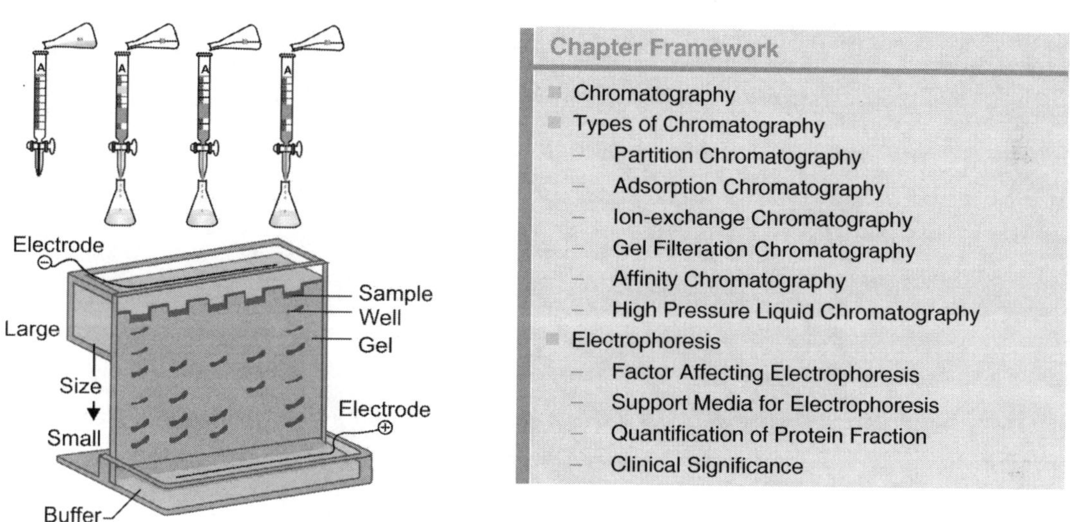

Chapter Framework

- Chromatography
- Types of Chromatography
  - Partition Chromatography
  - Adsorption Chromatography
  - Ion-exchange Chromatography
  - Gel Filteration Chromatography
  - Affinity Chromatography
  - High Pressure Liquid Chromatography
- Electrophoresis
  - Factor Affecting Electrophoresis
  - Support Media for Electrophoresis
  - Quantification of Protein Fraction
  - Clinical Significance

Clinical biochemistry has a very great impact on the human life, as it deals with the biochemical alterations of body constituents in diseases. Human body is essentially made-up of chemical constituents. Maintenance of stipulated levels of metabolites in various circumstances is wonderfully maintained in a healthy individual.

However during disease this may be disturbed. Therefore various diseases can be diagnosed based on the analysis of metabolites—qualitative/quantitative in body fluids like blood, CSF, urine, gastric juice, etc. The analysis is carried out using various instruments and techniques like chromatography, electrophoresis, and colorimetry.

In this chapter, we discuss the principles and procedures of few important biochemical techniques.

Chromatography

Chromatography is one of the most useful and popular tool of biochemistry. The word *'chromatography'* is derived from a Greek word meaning colored writing. It was first used by Russian botanist Mikhail Tswett in 1903 to describe the separation of plant pigments on a column of Alumina.

It is an analytical technique dealing with separation of closely related compounds from a mixture like lipids, proteins, peptides, amino acids, carbohydrate and vitamins, based upon their distribution in two immiscible phases—Stationary and mobile phase.

The mobile phase refers to the mixture of substances (to be separated) dissolved in a liquid or gas. The stationary phase is a porous, solid matrix through which sample content of the mobile phase percolates. The interaction between mobile and stationary phases results in separation of compounds from the mixture. These interactions include the physiochemical principle such adsorption, partition, ion-exchange, molecular sieving and affinity (Fig. 59.1).

Types of Chromatography

A summary of different types of chromatographies is given in Flow chart 59.1.

Partition Chromatography – (Martin and Synge 1941)

In this technique separation is achieved as the constituents have a relative affinity for the substances in the stationary or mobile phase.

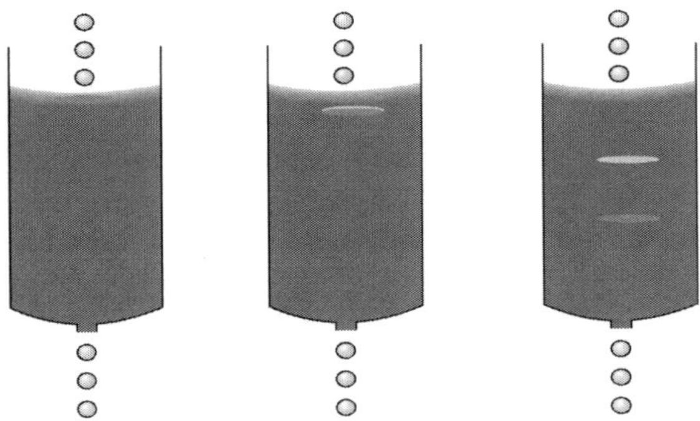

Fig. 59.1 Column chromatography

Flow chart 59.1 Types of chromatography

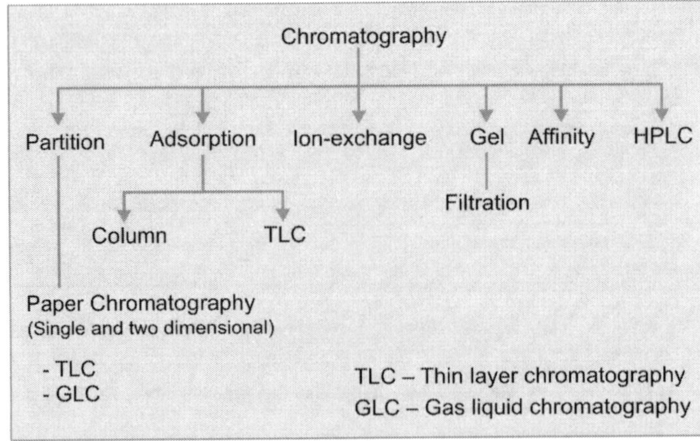

- *Paper chromatography:* In paper chromatography, few drops of solution containing a mixture of compounds to be separated is applied at one end, normally 2 cm above the end of filter paper. (Whatman's No. 1 and 3)

The paper is dried and dipped into a solvents mixture consisting of butanol, acetic acid and water in 4:1:5 ratios (for the separation of amino acids).

The aqueous component of the solvent system binds to the paper and forms the stationary phase. The organic component that migrates on the paper is mobile phase. When the migration of the solvent is upward it is referred to as 'ascending chromatography'. In descending chromatography solvent moves downwards. The rate of migration of molecules depends on the relative solubilities in stationary phase (aqueous) and mobile phase (organic) as seen in Figure 59.2.

After sufficient migration of solvent front, the paper (chromatogram) is removed, dried and developed for identification of specific spot. Ninhydrin which forms purple complex with α-amino acids is frequently used as a coloring reagent. The migration of substance is expressed as Rf value.

$$\text{Rf value} = \frac{\text{Distance traveled by substance}}{\text{Distance traveled by solvent}}$$

Rf = Ratio of fronts

The Rf value is constant for a particular solvent system at a given temperature.

The better separation can be achieved by two dimensional chromatography, i.e. separation in one direction first then in a direction perpendicular to it.

Thin layer chromatography (TLC): The principle of, TLC is same as described in paper chromatography. In place of paper, an inert substances, such as cellulose is employed as supporting material. Cellulose is spread as a thin layer on glass or plastic sheet. The chromatographic separation is comparatively rapid in TLC.

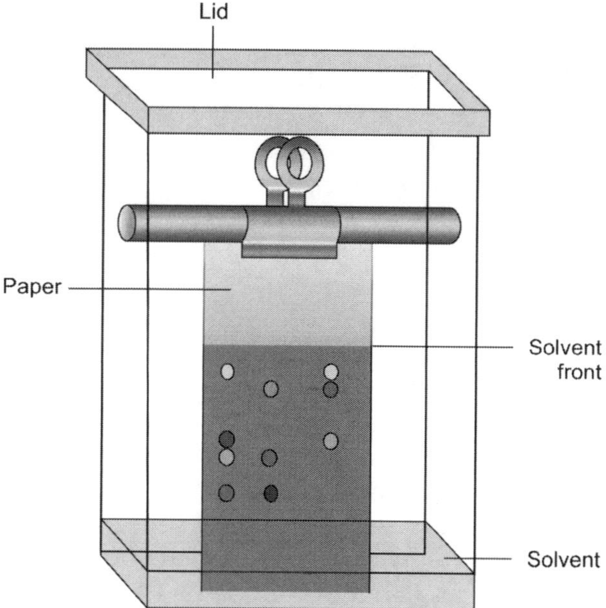

Fig. 59.2: Paper chromatography

Gas liquid chromatography (GLC): This is the method of choice for 'Separation of volatile substance'. In GLC stationary phase is liquid and mobile phase is gas. The stationary liquid phase is supported by a column of inert material such as silica in a long, narrow column and maintained at high temperature around 200°C. A mixture of volatile material is injected into the column along with mobile phase which is an inert gas (Ar, Ne or N_2). The separated compounds can be identified and quantitated by detector. The detector works on principle of ionization and thermal conductivity. GLC is sensitive, rapid, and reliable. It is frequently used for quantitative estimation biological material such as lipids, drugs and vitamins.

Adsorption Chromatography

The adsorbents such as silica gel, alumina, charcoal powder and Ca– hydroxyapatites are packed into a column in glass tube. This serves as a stationary phase. The sample mixture, a solvent is loaded in this column.

The individual components get differentially adsorbed onto adsorbents. The elution is carried out by a buffer system (mobile phase). The individual compounds come out of the column at different rates, which may be separately collected and identified as seen in Figure 59.3.

Ion-exchange Chromatography

In ion-exchange chromatography separation is based upon difference in net charges of protein at a given pH. Individual glass column is filled with insoluble matrix [ion-exchange resin or modified glucose] to which charged groups have been attached.

A matrix with negative groups is called cationic exchange resin. A matrix with positive group is called anionic exchange resin.

If the mixture is added to a cationic exchange resin, ions with greater positive charges bind more tightly to the cationic exchange resin. The components with largest net negative charges will pass through the column before the components with small net negative charge. Thus, the solution moves out at different time and rate at different pH as seen in Figure 59.4.

- The amino acid analysis is based upon this principle.

Gel Filteration Chromatography

The separation of molecule is based on their size, shape and molecular weight. This technique is also referred to as molecular sieve or molecular exclusion chromatography. The apparatus consist of a column packed with sponge-like gel (cross-linked polysaccharide) containing pores. The gel served as molecular sieve for separation of smaller and higher molecules as seen in Figure 59.5. The commercially available gels are G-10, G-85, G-100, P-10, 80, 100.

- The sample is applied to the top of the column and then washed through the bed of the gel particles with water or buffered solution.
- Substances with molecules larger than the largest pores of the swollen beads (above the exclusion limit) are not able to penetrate the gel particles and therefore pass through the bed in the liquid phase outside the particles and emerge from the column first
- Smaller molecules penetrate the particles to varying extents depending upon their shape and size. There is thus a partition of the molecules between the liquid inside the gel particles and that outside. The smaller the molecules, the larger the percentage of liquid within the particles that is available to them.

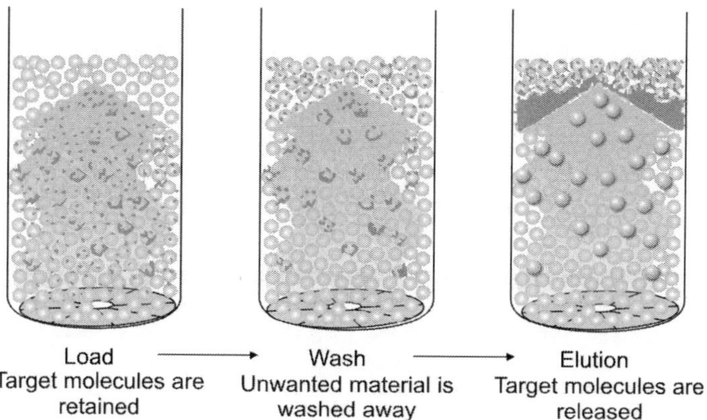

Fig. 59.3 Adsorption chromatography

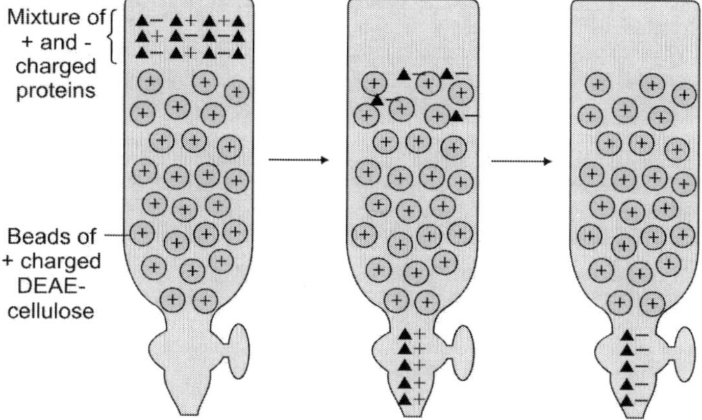

Fig. 59.4 Ion-exchange chromatography

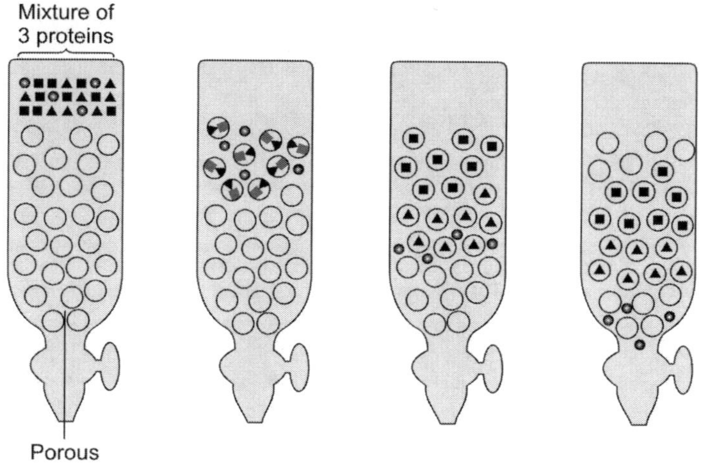

Fig. 59.5 Gel filteration chromatography

- Molecules, therefore, leave the column in the order of decreasing molecular size. The method can be used for approximate determination of molecular weight.

Affinity Chromatography

It is based on the property of specific and noncovalent binding of proteins to other molecules referred to as legends. For instance enzyme binds with legends such as substrate or cofactor as seen in Figure 59.6.

Affinity chromatography is useful for purification of vitamins, enzymes, hormones, receptors and antibodies.

High Pressure Liquid Chromatography

In general chromatographies are slow, with time consuming. Separation can be greatly improved by applying high pressure in the range of 5000 PSL to 10000 PSL (pounds per square inch). Hence, this technique is also referred to as high pressure liquid chromatography.

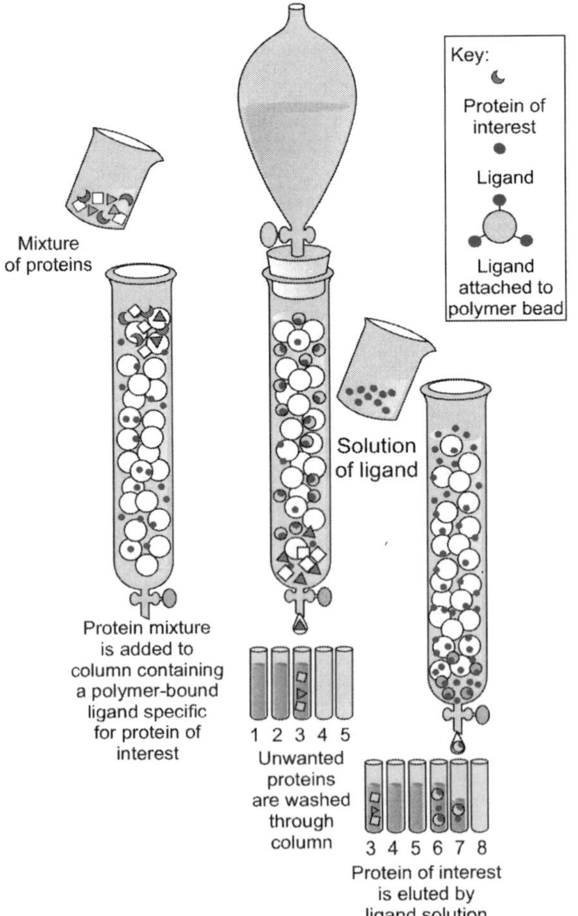

Fig. 59.6 Affinity chromatography

- HPLC requires the use of noncompressible resin filled in strong metal columns.
- The eluents of the column are detected by methods such as UV-absorbance and fluorescence as seen in Figure 59.7.
- It is used for isolation and purification of drugs, vitamins, steroids and diagnosis various amino acid disorders.

Electrophoresis

The movement of charged particles (ion) in an electric field resulting in their migration towards oppositely charged electrodes is called as electrophoresis.

Molecules with net negative charge migrate towards positive electrode/anode and those with net positive charge move towards negative electrode/cathode.

- Electrophoresis is a widely-used analytical technique for the separation of biological molecules such as plasma protein, lipoprotein and immunoglobulin.
- This technique was first used by A. Tiselius in 1937 and named it has moving boundary electrophoresis. He was awarded Nobel Prize in 1948.

Factor Affecting Electrophoresis

- Net charge on particles.
- Mass and shape of the particles.
- The pH of the medium.
- Strength of the electric field/magnitude of current.
- Properties of supporting medium.
- Temperature.

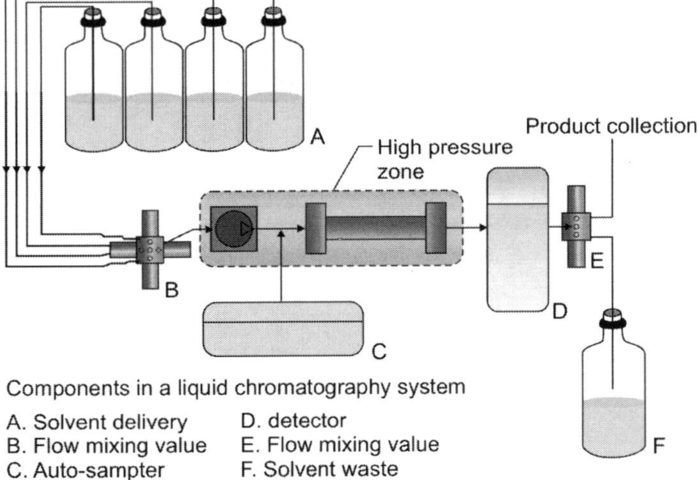

Fig. 59.7 High pressure liquid chromatography (HPLC)

Support Media for Electrophoresis

Commonly inert media is selected for electrophoresis as it has little effect on the substances to be separated examples includes Whatman's filter paper 1 and 3, cellulose acetate, agar gel, polyacrylamide gel.

Cellulose Acetate, Agar Gel and Polyacrylamide Gel Types of Electrophoresis

Among the electrophoresis technique zone electrophoresis, isoelectric focussing and immunoelectrophoresis are important and commonly employed in clinical laboratory.

- *Zone electrophoresis:* It is of 2 types on the basis of inert supporting material:
  - Paper Electrophoresis: The electrophoresis system basically consist of electrophoresis tank holding the buffer and fitted with electrodes as well as a power pack to supply electricity at constant current and voltage. In paper electrophoresis the sample is applied on a strip of filter paper wetted with desired buffer solution. The ends of strip are dipped into the buffer solutions in which electrodes are placed. The electric current is applied to allow the molecules to migrate for sufficient time. The paper is removed, dried and stained with a dye. The colored spots can be identified by comparing with set of standards simultaneously as seen in figure 59.8.

    For the separation of plasma proteins Whatman's no. 1 filter paper, tris buffer (barbitone buffer) at pH 8.6 and stains amido black or bromophenol blue are employed. The plasma proteins are separated into 5 distinct bands—Albumin, α1, α2, β and γ-globulins.
  - Gel Electrophoresis: This technique involves the separation of molecules based on their size in addition to electric charge. The movement of large molecules is slow in gel electrophoresis. Differentiation is much higher in this technique. Thus plasma proteins can be separated into 15 bands. The gels commonly used in gel electrophoresis are agarose, polyacrylamide gel, sodium dodecil sulfate (SDS). Polyacrylamide is employed for determination of molecular weight of proteins.
  - *Isoelectric focussing:* This technique is based on immobilization of molecules at isoelectric pH. During electrophoresis stable pH gradients are set up (gel) covering the pH range to

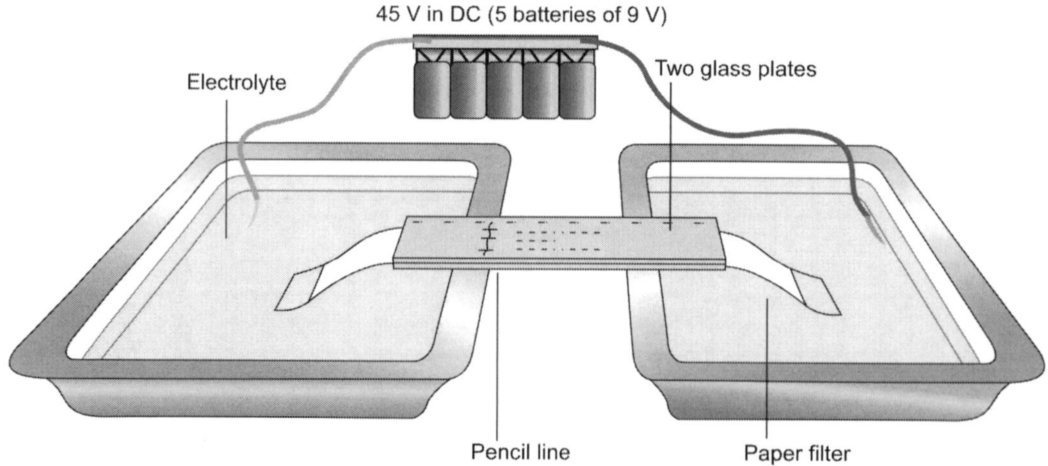

Fig. 59.8 Paper electrophoresis

include isoelectric points of components in mixture. As electrophoresis occurs the molecules migrate to positions corresponding to their isoelectric points, get immobilized and form sharp stationary bands. The gel blocks can be stained and identified by this technique as seen in Figure 59.9. Serum proteins can be separated to as many as 40 bands. This technique is useful for studying isoenzymes and genetic variants of hemoglobin and purification of proteins.

– *Immunoelectrophoresis:* Grabar and William's first devised this technique. It involves combination of principles of electrophoresis and immunological reaction (Ag – Ab).

  This technique is performed on agar or agarose gel on a slide with an antigen well and an antibody through cut on it. The test serum is placed in the antigen well and electrophoresis is carried out for about an hour. Antibody against human serum is then placed in well and diffusion allowed to proceed for 18 to 24 hours.

  The resulting precipitating arcs can be photographed and slides dried, stained and preserved for record as seen in Figure 59.10. Over 30 different proteins can be identified by this method in human serum. This is useful for testing of normal and abnormal proteins in serum and urine.

Quantification of Protein Fraction

Electrophoresis pattern is inserted into automated computerized densitometer and quantitative densitograph is obtained in printer. Thus proteins are automatically quantitated. This instrument does the scanning very fast.

Clinical Significance

Alteration in the normal electrophoretic pattern occurs in certain pathological condition. The common clinical conditions where alterations are seen in Figures 59.11 and 59.12:

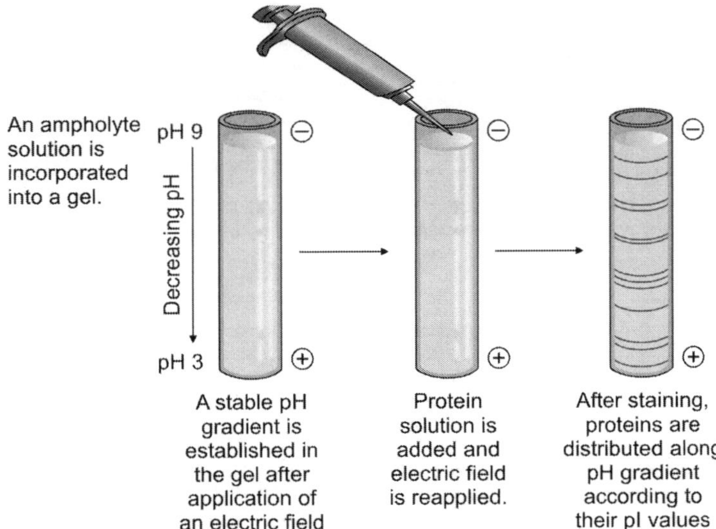

Fig. 59.9 Isoelectric focussing

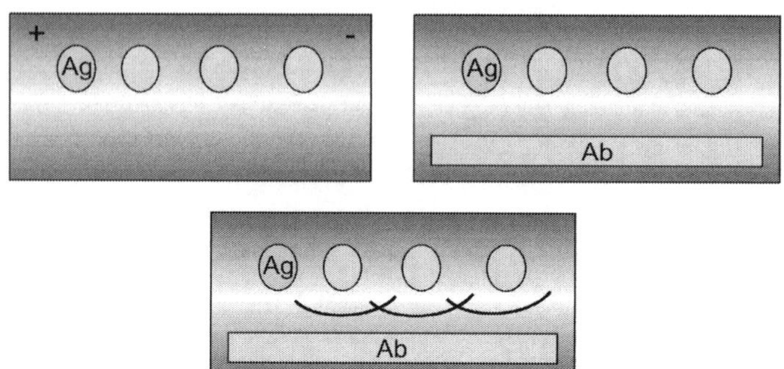

Fig. 59.10 Immunoelectrophoresis

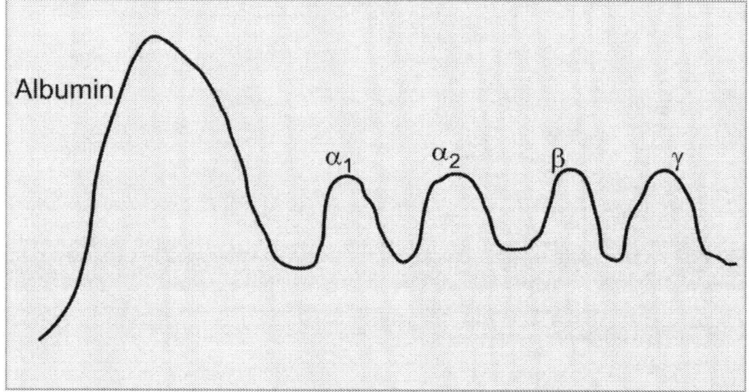

Fig. 59.11 Normal plasma protein electrophoretic pattern

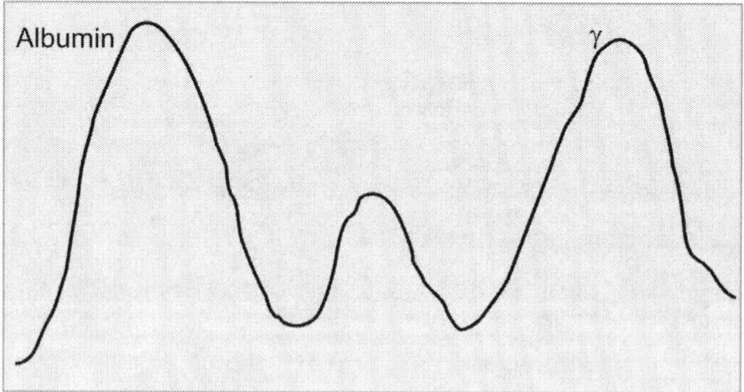

Fig. 59.12 Multiple myeloma plasma protein electrophoretic pattern

- Cirrhosis of liver —Increase globulin
- Nephrotic syndrome —Increase α_2 fraction
- Multiple myeloma —Increase γ fraction
- Agammaglobulinemia —Decrease γ-globulin

Viva voce

Q1. What is the principle of chromatography?
Q2. Name the different types of chromatographies.
Q3. What is the support media used in paper chromatography?
Q4. What is Rf value?
Q5. When is GLC used?
Q6. What is the basis of ion-exchange chromatography?
Q7. How are the molecules with different molecular weight but with similar charges separated by chromatography?
Q8. Name the fastest chromatographic technique and when is it used?
Q9. What is electrophoresis?
Q10. Name the different types of electrophoresis.
Q11. What are the factors regulating the rate of electrophoretic migration?
Q12. Name the various support media of electrophoresis.
Q13. Name the buffer used in paper electrophoresis.
Q14. Paper electrophoresis separates plasma proteins into how many bands?
Q15. Name the support media of gel electrophoresis.
Q16. How many bands of plasma proteins are differentiated in gel electrophoresis?
Q17. What is isoelectric focussing?
Q18. How are the genetic variants of hemoglobin differentiated by electrophoresis?
Q19. What is immunoelectrophoresis?

CHAPTER

60

Titratable Acidity of Urine

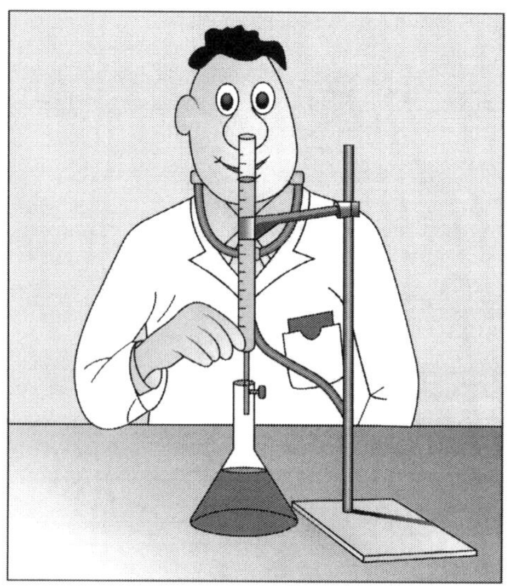

Chapter Framework

- Determination of Titratable Acidity
  - Calculation
  - Normal Values and Clinical Importance

Urine is acidic in pH. Acidification of urine takes place mainly due to the secretion of H^+, due to the presence of other metabolic acids like Acetoacetic acid, and β-hydroxybutyrate in ketosis.

The renal tubular cells secrete H^+ in much the similar way as that by the gastric mucosa, i.e. by activity of carbonic anhydrase. For each H^+ secreted there is an equivalent number of HCO_3^- produced, and a Na^+ is absorbed into the circulation as sodium bicarbonate. The H^+ secreted reacts with three buffer systems present in the proximal convoluted tubules (PCT) and distal convoluted tubules (DCT):

- Bicarbonate (PCT)
- Phosphate (DCT)
- Ammonia (DCT).

The H^+ also react with the ammonia secreted by the tubular cells, produced as a result of action glutaminase enzyme on amino acids.

Determination of Titratable Acidity

Measurement of titratable acidity is done by titration with a suitable volume of urine with 0.05 N NaOH till pH 7.4, using phenol red as an indicator.

Calculation

$$\text{Titrable acidity of urine (mEq / L)} = \frac{0.05\ \text{N NaOH (mL)} \times \text{Volume of 24 hour urine}}{10} \times \frac{1}{20}$$

Normal Values and Clinical Importance

The normal value of titratable acidity ranges between 20 mEq to 30 mEq/L. The value may be as high as 150 mEq/L in diabetic ketoacidosis, as a result of compensatory mechanism for maintaining the blood pH. It is reduced in alkalosis for the same reason.

Viva voce

Q1. What is the titratable acidity of urine?
Q2. What is the site of H^+ secretion in the renal tubules?
Q3. Name the different buffer systems present in the kidneys.
Q4. When is the titratable acidity increased in urine and why?

CHAPTER

61

Nonprotein Nitrogen

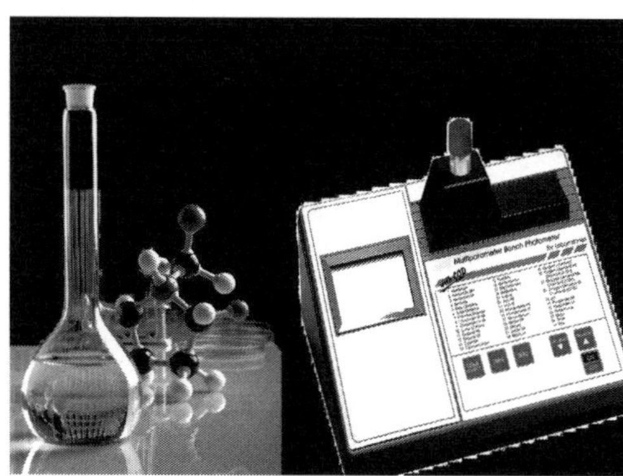

Chapter Framework

- Principle
- Reagent
  - Nessler's Reagent
  - Procedure
  - Normal Values and its Significance

Blood nonprotein nitrogen (NPN) includes the nitrogen present in urea, creatine, creatinine, uric acid, amino acids, glutathione, etc. However, it does not include the nitrogen present in the proteins. Therefore, any estimation of nonprotein nitrogen would require the serum to be first deproteinized. Most of the methods used are a modification of the *Kjeldahl's method.*

Principle

Blood is deproteinized using the tungstic acid. The protein-free filtrate is digested with sulfuric acid and hydrogen peroxide to release ammonia. The ammonia formed is measured by direct nesselerization colorimetrically.

Reagent

10% sodium tungstate.

Sulfuric acid digestion mixture—50% (v/v) H_2SO_4 in water containing 1 g selenium dioxide/100 mL.

Nessler's Reagent

Standard ammonium sulfate solution.

Procedure

Prepare the protein-free filtrate. Pipette 1 mL of this filtrate and 0.2 mL of sulfuric acid digestion mixture into a borosil test tube. Heat very carefully over a small flame until the solution becomes colorless. Continue to heat for another 5 to 10 minutes, then cool it. Now pour this into a 10 mL volumetric cylinder and make the volume up to 6 mL. Add 3 mL of Nessler's reagent, mix and make the volume up to the mark. Now put up a standard, using water and standard ammonium sulfate. Finally read using a colorimeter at 480 nm against water or reagent blank.

Normal Values and its Significance

The normal blood NPN ranges within 25 mg to 50 mg/dL. The range is lower for plasma sample, it is 20 mg to 30 mg/dL. Its value runs parallel to those of blood urea. Thus, the NPN values are high in uremic conditions and low in liver diseases.

Viva voce

Q1. Name the components of blood nonprotein nitrogen.
Q2. Which is the most common method of blood NPN determination?
Q3. Why is the blood deproteinized before estimating NPN?

CHAPTER

62

Recent Advances in Clinical Biochemistry

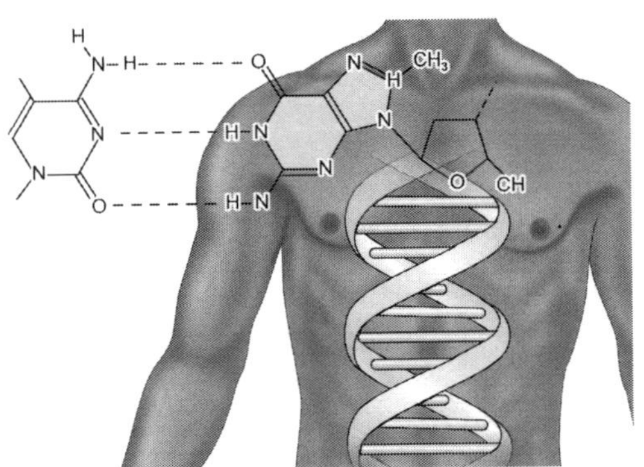

Chapter Framework

The clinical biochemistry laboratory has been the focus of modern diagnostic medicine for a long-time now. This focus has given constant impetus to the modern clinical biochemists as they have come up with newer, more efficient, sensitive and less time consuming techniques. This not only helps in diagnosing but also determining the cause of disease even at genetic level, in tracking the progression of disease and in therapy (gene therapy). These techniques are proving to be the guiding principles in the diagnosis and prognosis of diseases and in drug analysis in present era.

Brief information about the various latest techniques of clinical biochemistry is a must for any student studying biochemistry and moving on in the clinical medical stream/dental stream. This would make the budding doctors/dentists aware of the new advances in this field.

Spectroscopy

The most fundamental spectroscopic technique used in the clinical biochemistry laboratory, governed by the laws of photometry—Colorimetry has already been discussed in detail along with its applications. Here we discuss some more advanced spectroscopic techniques.

There has been a constant effort in laboratory sciences to study matter at the molecular level. The clinical biochemistry laboratory is no exception to this and has developed techniques like NMR spectroscopy, ESR spectroscopy, luminometry, nephlometry, turbidimetry and X-ray spectroscopy. A brief discussion about each of these techniques has been elaborated along with their respective applications. The instrumentation of these techniques has been omitted as it is beyond the scope of this book.

Nuclear Magnetic Resonance/NMR Spectroscopy

The subatomic particles like nucleus, proton and electron have the property of spinning. This spinning generates magnetic field. The magnetic field generated by nucleus, having spin (I) = ½ is called nuclear magnetic field.

This nuclear magnetic field gets split into lower and higher energy levels under the effect of an external magnetic field (EMF) and radiowaves.

At a particular combination of the EMF and radiowaves there occurs resonance and resonance peaks are obtained. This is NMR spectroscopy. The NMR peaks signifies the number of protons in a substance and number of protons giving rise to a single peak.

Applications

Nuclear magnetic resonance (NMR) spectroscopy finds utility in studying protein folding, drug metabolism, detecting tumors, study of membrane dynamics and for identifying amino acid residues at catalytic sites of enzymes.

Electron Spin Resonance/ESR Spectroscopy

This type of spectroscopy is exclusively used for paramagnetic substances. Here the spinning subatomic particle is electron and works on the principle as NMR.

Applications

It finds importance in the study of free radicals and in the diagnosis of diseased tissue based on conformation of free radical.

Luminescence (Flow chart 62.1)

Electrons have a tendency to jump to higher energy levels on excitation and to liberate energy on coming back to their ground level.

When these emit energy in the form of light energy the phenomenon is termed as luminescence.

The components which cause luminescence in each of these techniques are:

Chemiluminescence

It involves oxidation of organic compound like luciferin, luminol, isoluminol, etc. by an oxidant.

Bioluminescence

It is due to enzyme activity of luciferase and aequorin.

Flow chart 62.1 Types of luminescence

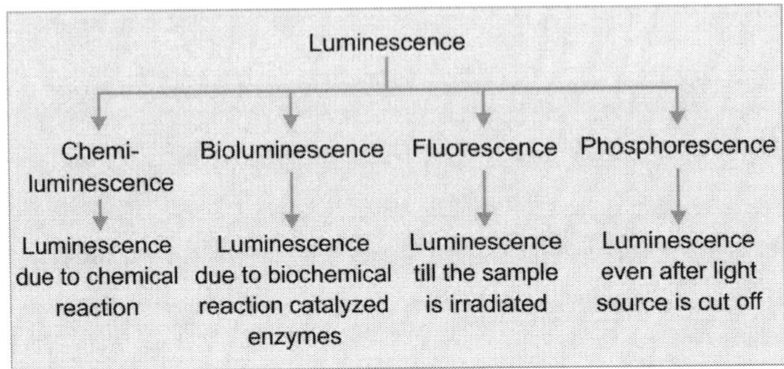

Fluorescence

It occurs due to specific reagent labels used like fluorescein isothiocyanate and β-phycoerythrin.

Applications

The chemi and bioluminescence techniques can make detections up to the limits of attomole to zeptomole.

This makes them highly popular nowadays, with an advent of automation and newer reagents. The luminescence techniques therefore find great utility inquantifying amino acids, conformational studies of enzymes, in immunoassays like—Fluorescence in situ hybridization (FISH), detection of malignant cells, cell sorting and cell counting.

These techniques are 100 to 1000 times more sensitive than absorbance measurements, justifying their current popularity.

Light Scattering Techniques

- Unlike the light emitting techniques, *Nephlometry and Turbidimetry* are light scattering techniques, responsible for analysis of suspensions and turbid solutions.
- In nephlometry, the light scattered by a suspension is measured at right angles to the incident light by a photomultiplier detector.
- In turbidimetry, the light scattered by a turbid solution is measured in at 180°, i.e. in line with the incident light by a photocell.

Choice Between Nephlometry and Turbidimetry

Nephlometry is advantageous as compared to turbidimetry when it comes to sensitivity in measurement of very low concentrations of Ag–Ab reactions.

However, the measurement of light desirable at a right angle necessitated the advent of new instrument nepholmeters, whereas turbidimetric evaluations can be carried out using normal spectrophotometers. Besides, with the synthesis of newer reagents and higher resolution photometric systems, turbidimetric measurements are as competitive/good as nephlometric.

Applications

- These two techniques have been of great utility in the quantification of amino acids, proteins like apoproteins, vitamins and antibiotics in blood.
- These techniques have also been used to determinate molecular weight of biomolecules.

X-ray Spectroscopy

X-ray spectroscopy involves 3 phenomena:

- X-ray absorption
- X-ray diffraction
- X-ray fluorescence.

In all these 3 techniques, the basic requirement is X-rays to be produced (in a Coolidge's tube) and incident on matter. Once incident, the X-rays may be absorbed or diffracted or may cause reemission of X-rays of different wavelength (depending upon the nature and concentration of the substance).

Out of the three techniques, X-ray absorption finds utility in medicine. It is used for detecting fractured bones, for detecting/diagnosing hemorrhages, strokes, and deposits in blood vessels.

The other two techniques are more useful in the industry and agriculture for crystal analysis or trace element detection in fruits and vegetables and to determine amount phosphate in fertilizers.

The laboratory biochemistry took a new leap with the amalgamation of molecular genetics with clinical biochemistry. Today the molecular genetics has progressed phenomenally and is helping in the not just diagnosis of various inherited disorders but also has given hope in the treatment of these diseases by gene therapy.

Today, it is possible to identify, isolate, multiply a particular gene and then store it libraries like books and use it for various purposes like gene therapy, industrial production of various hormones (insulin) and proteins, DNA vaccines, prenatal diagnosis and in medicolegal cases by DNA fingerprinting.

A few important genetic techniques used in the clinical biochemistry laboratories today are:

- Gene identification techniques
  - Southern, northern blotting
  - Microarrays.
- Gene multiplication techniques
  - PCR cell free
  - rDNA within cells.
- Gene storage
  - Genomic libraries.

Gene Identification Techniques

For the use of any gene, it has to be isolated and identified. For this the blotting techniques are used.

Southern blotting — DNA

Northern blotting — RNA

Southern Blotting

It involves the following steps:

1. Extraction of DNA from a tissue and its exposure to site specific restriction end nucleases (cut DNA at particular nucleotide sequences).
2. Gel electrophoresis is done to separate DNA fragments according to size—Larger fragments at the top of the gel and smaller ones at the bottom.
3. DNA is then exposed to strong NaOH solution for denaturation and separation into single strands.

4. Blotting of single-stranded ssDNA on a nitrocellulose membrane. This is called southern Blotting. Now the membrane is baked at 80°C so that ssDNA fragments adhere firmly on to it.
5. Now a radiolabeled small DNA fragment having a nucleotide sequence complimentary to the desired gene to be identified is added, causing its hybridization to the desired gene.
6. Finally, the southern blot is exposed to an X-ray film and the film shows the position of the desired gene. This is called autoradiography (Fig. 62.1).

In northern blotting instead of DNA, mRNA is used mRNA being single-stranded does not need denaturation thus it is omitted. The rest of the procedure is identical to the southern blotting (Fig. 62.2).

In western blotting proteins are identified by the same method.

DNA Microarrays

This is a highly advanced, computerized method used for detecting DNA mutations (abnormal genetic sequence identification). It involves the use of the DNA sample of an individual and a glass slide carrying an oligonucleotide sequence of a mutation. If the individual has the mutated gene, his/her gene gets hybridized to the microarray short DNA sequence. The DNA from the individual may be labelled either radioactively or fluorescent chemical. Thus an abnormal gene can be identified.

Gene Multiplication Techniques

Once the desired gene has been identified and isolated, it can be multiplied. The multiplication of the gene may be carried out either within cells as in rDNA technology or in cell-free media as in polymerase chain reaction (PCR).

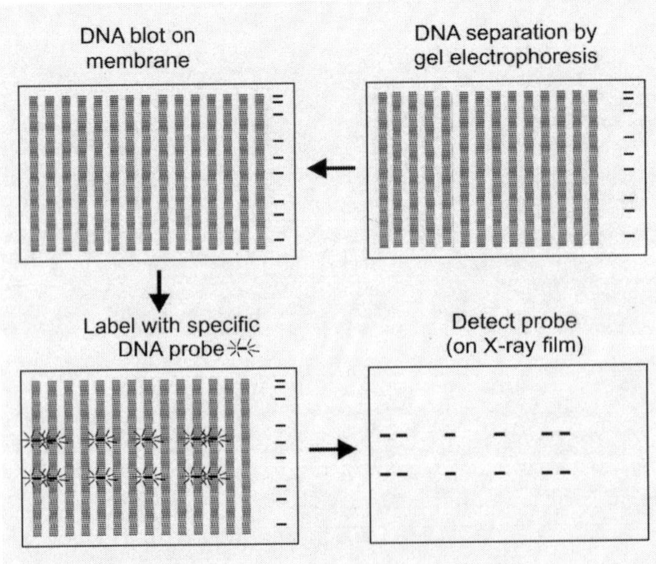

Fig. 62.1 Southern blotting

rDNA Technology

This involves the cloning of a gene by the following steps:

- Generation of DNA fragments by restriction end nucleases.
- Hybridizing the DNA fragments from 2 different sources, creating the recombinant DNA with desired genetic sequence.
- Inserting the rDNA into a vector (plasmid, cosmic YAC, etc.) for carrying the rDNA into a host.
- Finally, the vector containing r-DNA is inserted into a suitable host cell like bacteria or yeast where the rDNA multiply along with the host cell multiplication, giving large quantities of the target DNA sequence. The cloned DNA is selected by nucleic acid hybridization or antibody binding (Fig. 62.3).

Polymerase Chain Reaction

This is a cell-free method of DNA cloning. The process of polymerase chain reaction (PCR) involves the amplification of desired DNA sequences through repeated cycles of DNA synthesis. The preceding DNA molecule acts like a template for new DNA, increasing the number of DNA molecules exponentially. The cycles continue, until all the substrates are used up (Figs 62.4A to C).

- Denaturation of DNA at 95°C to produce ssDNA.
- Annealing of oligonucleotide primers 15 to 20 base pairs in length on both the denatured strands at 55°C.

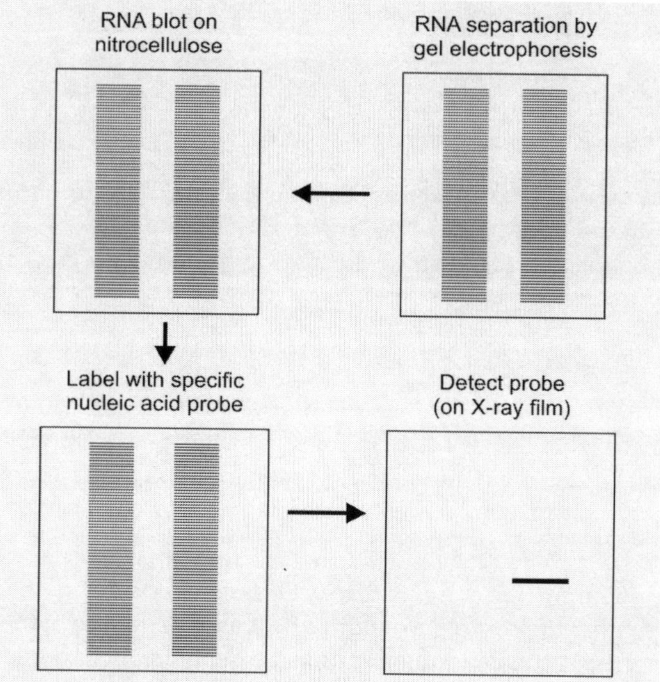

Fig. 62.2 Northern blotting

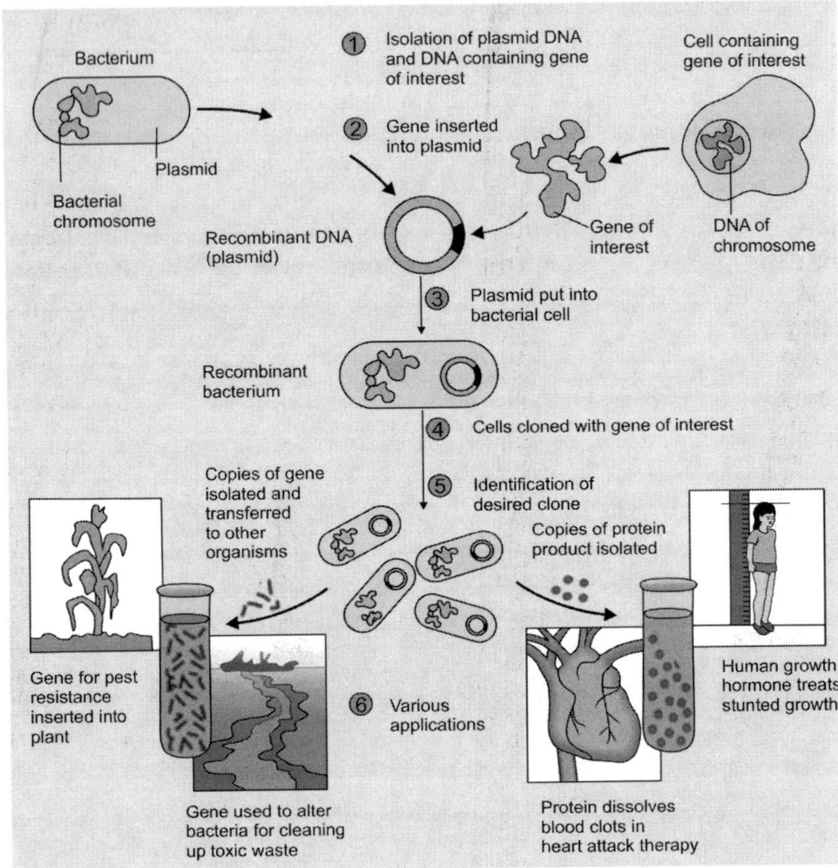

Fig. 62.3 Steps of rDNA technology

- Synthesis of new strands of DNA from both the primers at 72°C using Taq polymerase and various nitrogen bases as dATP, dGTP, dCTP and dTTP.
- The whole cycle is repeated 20–40 times giving are large number of copies of the desired DNA sequence within few hours.

Applications

The amplified DNA finds use in production of important hormones (like insulin) and vaccines (hepatitis B), detecting inherited diseases, in forensic medicine for amplifying DNA of a small sample and in cancer for detecting mutations in oncogenes and tumor suppressor genes.

Gene Storage Techniques

The gene once identified, amplified, isolated, may be stored in DNA libraries for future use.

- These may store either the complete genomic DNA as in genomic libraries.
- These may store specific coding sequences from the genome. Such libraries are prepared from mRNA of the cell, using reverse transcriptase enzyme (RNA-dependent DNA polymerase). These are called cDNA libraries.

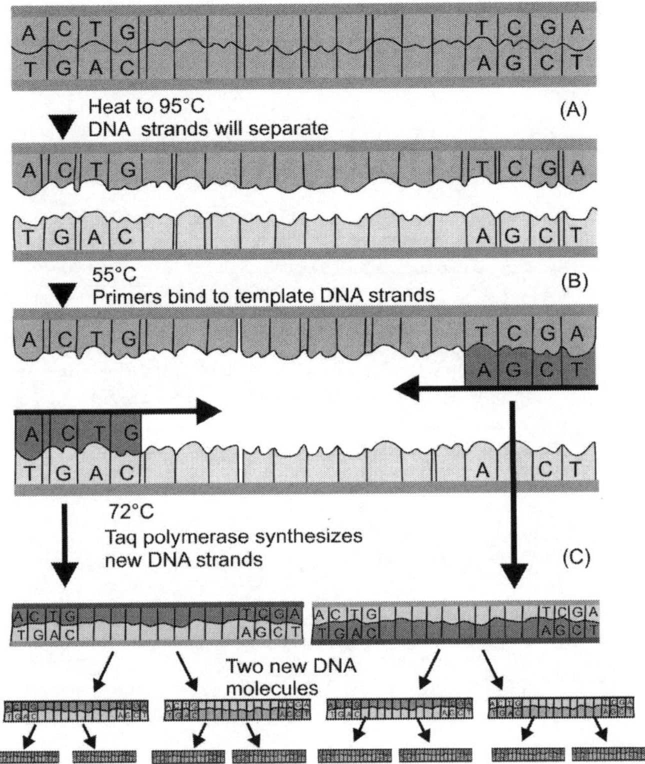

Figs 62.4A to C Steps of PCR

The formation of DNA libraries involves following steps:

- Digesting human DNA by restriction enzyme Sau 3A.
- Inserting DNA fragments into bacteriophage λ.
- Infecting bacterial host cell (*E.coli*) with the phage.

Thus, creating a DNA library for future use.

The genetic laboratory techniques have greatly helped the modern medicine in the diagnosis and therapy of, earlier in curable diseases.

Today the complete human genome map is available owing to these techniques, assuring the human race a very promising and healthy future.

CHAPTER

63

Preparation of Various Reagents

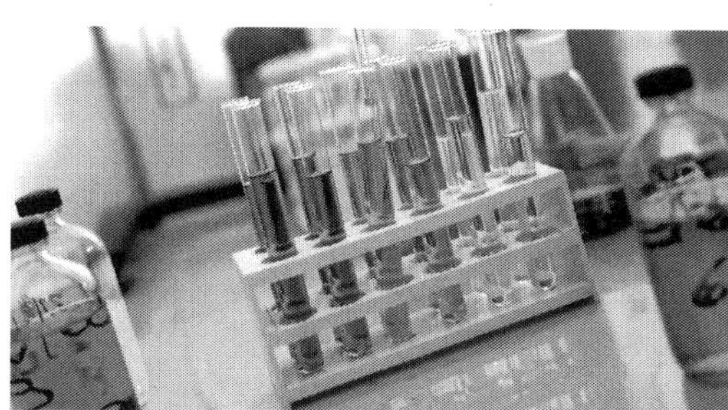

Chapter Framework

- Reagents for Qualitative Analysis
- Reagents for Quantitative Analysis

Reagents for Qualitative Analysis

Acetic acid (1%): Dilute 1 mL glacial acetic acid in 100 mL distilled water.

α-naphthol (5%): Dissolve 500 mg α-naphthol in 100 mL methanol.

Ammonium molybdate (4%): Dissolve 4 g of ammonium molybdate in 100 mL distilled water.

Barfoed's reagent: Dissolve 13.3 g copper acetate in 200 mL distilled water. Add 1.8 mL glacial acid.

Barium chloride (10%): Dissolve 10 g barium in 100 mL distilled water.

Baryta mixture: Add 100 mL supernatant of saturated solution of barium nitrate to 200 mL supernatant solution of saturated barium hydroxide.

Benedict's Qualitative Solution:

Solution A: Dissolve 173 g sodium citrate and 100 g anhydrous sodium carbonate in 800 mL distilled water. Heat and cool the solution.

Solution B: Dissolve 17.3 g of copper sulfate in 100 mL distilled water. Add solution B to solution A with constant stirring, and make up the volume to 100 mL with distilled water.

Benzoic acid (0.25%): Add 2.5 g of benzoic acid to 800 mL distilled water. Heat it to dissolve. Make up the volume to 1000 mL with distilled water in a volumetric flask.

Casein solution: Dissolve 20 g of anhydrous sodium carbonate in 500 mL of distilled water. Dissolve 20 g of pure casein powder in the above sodium carbonate solution and make up the volume to 2,000 mL with distilled water.

Copper acetate (1%): Dissolve 1 g copper acetate in 100 mL distilled water.

Copper sulfate (1%): Dissolve 1 g copper sulfate in 100 mL distilled water.

Dextrin (1%): Take 5 g of dextrin and prepare a thick paste. Boil 400 mL of water in a 1 liter breaker and while boiling add the paste of dextrin into it very slowly and stir it. After cooling, make up the volume to 500 mL.

Formalin (5%): Dilute 4 mL of 40% formaldehyde to 2,000 mL with distilled water.

Fructose solution (1%): Dissolve 25 g fructose in 2,500 mL distilled water.

Gastric juice (artificial sample): 1,000 mL distilled water + 20 mL lactic acid + ~20 mL concentrated hydrochloric acid + 20 g pepsin powder + 500 mL egg white solution. Make up the volume to 2,000 mL.

Gelatin solution (1%): Dissolve 20 g of pure gelatin in distilled water and make up the volume to 2,000 mL with distilled water.

Hydrochloric acid (0.15 N): Dilute 12.6 mL of concentrated hydrochloric acid to 1,000 mL with distilled water.

Iodine stock solution (1.27%, 0.1 N): Add 1.27 g iodine to 3 g potassium iodide crystals and dilute it to 100 mL with distilled water.

Iodine working solution (1:10 dilution): Dilute 200 mL of iodine stock solution to 2,000 mL with distilled water.

Lactose (3%): Dissolve 60 g lactose powder in 2,000 mL distilled water.

Maltose (3%): Dissolve 60 g maltose powder in 2,000 mL distilled water.

Phenylhydrazine buffer for osazone preparation: In a 2 liter conical flask, take 100 g of Phenylhydrazine powder, 350 g of sodium acetate and 120 mL glacial acetic acid in 1,000 mL distilled water. Keep the conical flask in boiling water bath to dissolve this. Make up the volume to 1,500 mL with distilled water.

Seliwanoff's reagent: Dissolve 50 g resorcinol in 33 mL of concentrated hydrochloric acid and dilute it to 100 mL with distilled water.

Sodium carbonate (10%): Dissolve 100 g of carbonate in 1000 mL distilled water in a volumetric flask.

Sodium hydroxide (40%): Dissolve 40 g of sodium hydroxide in 100 mL distilled water.

Sodium hydroxide (0.2 N): Dissolve 16 g sodium hydroxide in 2000 mL distilled water.

Sodium hypobromite: Dilute 10 mL of bromine solution to 1000 mL with 40% sodium hydroxide.

Sodium nitrite solution (1%): Dissolve 20 g of sodium nitrate in 2000 mL distilled water.

Starch (1%): Weigh 20 g of starch (potato starch) amylum and prepare a thick paste. In a 1 liter beaker take 800 mL of water and boil it. While boiling add the paste of starch into the boiling water slowly and stir it. Cool and make the volume to 2000 mL with distilled water.

Sucrose (1%): Dissolve 20 g of sucrose powder in 2,000 mL distilled water.

Sulfosalicylic acid (20%): Dissolve 400 g of sulfosalicylic acid in 2,000 mL distilled water.

Toffer's reagent (0.5%): Dissolve 5 g dimethyl amino azobenzene in 1,000 mL ethyl alcohol.

Reagents for Quantitative Analysis

Creatinine Stock Standard (1 mg/mL)

0.1 N hydrochloric acid: Dissolve 8.66 mL of concentrated hydrochloric acid to 1,000 mL with distilled water.

1 g of creatinine powder is dissolved in 500 mL of 0.1 N hydrochloric acid the volume is made up to 1,000 mL with distilled water.

Working standard (0.04 mg/mL): 4 mL of creatinine stock standard is diluted to 100 mL with distilled water.

Creatinine standard for urine creatinine (0.01 mg/mL): Dilute 1 mL of creatinine stock standard to 100 mL with distilled water.

Proteins

Stock standard (1 g/100 mL): Dissolve 2 g of bovine albumin powder in 200 mL normal saline.

Working standard (0.005 g /mL or 5 mg/mL): Dilute 50 mL of protein stock standard to 100 mL with normal saline.

Standard for CSF proteins (1 mg/mL): Dilute 10 mL of stock standard to 100 mL with normal saline.

Sodium Hydroxide (0.5 N)

Dissolve 40 g of sodium hydroxide in 200 mL distilled water in a volumetric flask.

Sodium Phosphotungstate (for HDLc)

Dissolve 40 g of phosphotungstic acid in 500 mL of distilled water. Adjust the pH of the solution by adding 1 N NaOH to 6.7. Now dilute the reagent to 1000 mL with distilled water.

Sugar

Stock standard (1 g/100 mL or 10 mg/mL): Dissolve 5 g pure glucose powder in 250 mL of 0.25% benzoic acid. This standard is also used for the determination of serum amylase.

Preparation of benzoic acid (0.25%): Add 2.5 g of benzoic acid in 800 mL distilled water. Heat to dissolve. Make up the volume to 1 liter with distilled water in a volumetric flask.

Triglyceride (200 mg/100 ml): Add 200 mg of triolein to 100 mL of isopropanol.

Urea

Stock standard (300 mg/100 mL):

Solution A—1.5 sodium benzoate + 500 mL distilled water + 0.7 mL concentrated sulfuric acid. Make the volume to 1000 mL with distilled water.

Solution B: Dissolve 644 mg of urea powder in 100 mL solution A.

Working standard (3 mg/100 mL): Dilute 1 mL of urea stock standard to 10 mL with distilled water.

Uric Acid

Stock standard (1 mg/mL): *Solution A*—1 g of lithium carbonate is dissolved in 100 mL of distilled water.

Solution B: Dissolve 100 g of uric acid in 100 mL of solution A.

*Working standard (*0.01 mg/mL): Dilute 1 mL of stock standard to 100 mL with distilled water.

BCG Reagent

Solution A: Dissolve 8.85 g succinic acid 1 g sodium hydroxide in 1000 mL distilled water.

Solution B: Dissolve 120 mg bromocresol green + 1 g sodium hydroxide in 100 mL distilled water.

Mix solution A and B together. Check the pH; it should be between 3.8 and 4.2. Make the volume to 1,000 mL with distilled water. Preserve this solution in brown bottle.

Biuret Reagent (Stock)

Dissolve 45 g of sodium potassium tartrate in 400 mL of 0.2 N sodium hydroxide. To this add 15 g copper sulfate and mix it with constant stirring. Add 5 g potassium iodide and make the volume to 1000 mL with 0.2 N sodium hydroxide.

Biuret Reagent (Working)

Dilute 200 mL of stock biuret reagent with 0.2 N NaOH to 1000 mL. Add 5 g of potassium iodide.

Tungstic Acid (Diluted)

Add 50 mL of 10% sodium tungstate to 50 mL of 2/3 N sulfuric acid. Dilute the mixture to 800 mL with distilled water. Add a few drops of phosphoric acid as preservative.

CHAPTER

64

Normal Reference Values of Various Biochemical Parameters

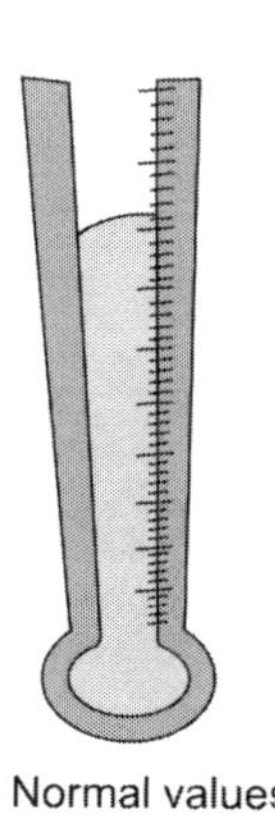

Normal values

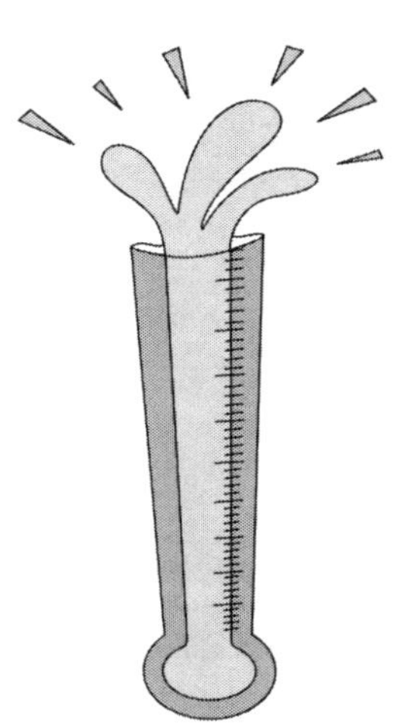

High values

Parameter	*Normal Range*	
Ammonia	Plasma	40–80 µg/dL Enzy method
Bilirubin—Total	Serum	0.2–1 mg/dL
Direct	Serum	<0.4 mg/dL
Indirect	Serum	<0.6 mg/dL
Calcium	Serum	9–11 mg/dL
Chlorides	Serum	95–103 mEq/L
Cholesterol—Total	Serum	150–200 mg/dL
HDL	Serum	30–60 mg/dL
Copper— Male Female	 Serum Serum	 70–140 µg/dL 80–155 µg/dL
Ferritin— Male Female	 Serum Serum	 15–200 ng/dL 12–150 ng/dL
Glucose	CSF	50–80 mg/dL

Contd...

Contd...

Glucose:		
Enzymatic method	Plasma	65–100 mg/dL
Hemoglobin— Male Female	 Whole blood Whole blood	 14–16 g/dL 13–15 g/dL
Insulin	Serum	6–25 μU/ml
Iodine	Serum	4–10 μg/dL
Phospholipids Phosphorus (Children)	Serum	200–275 mg/dL
Phosphorous (Adult)	Serum	3.5–4 mg/dL
Potassium	Serum	2.5–5 mEq/L
Proteins CSF	Serum	15–45 mg/dL
Proteins—Total	Serum	6–8 g/dL
Albumin	Serum	3.5–5 gm/dL
Globulin	Serum	2.5–3.5 gm/dL
Fibrinogen	Serum	200–400 mg/dL
Sodium	Serum	136–145 mEq/dL
Thyroid-stimulating hormone (TSH)	Serum	5–10 μU/mL
Thyroxine, total T4	Serum	5–12 μg/dL
Triiodothyronine T3	Serum	110–180 ng/dL
Triglycerides Male Female	 Serum Serum	 50–200 mg/dL 40–50 mg/dL
Urea	Whole blood	20–40 mg/dL
Blood urea nitrogen (BUN)	Whole blood	5–15 mg/dL
Uric acid	Serum	3.5–7 mg/dL
Vitamin A	Serum	15–60 μg/dL
Vitamin C	Plasma	0.6–1.6 mg/dL
Zinc	Serum	50–150 μg/dL
Acid phosphatase	Serum	1–4 KA Units/dL
Alkaline phosphatase	Serum	1–13
Amylase	Serum	80–180 Somogyi U/dL
Creatine kinase	Serum	10–50 IU/L
Gamma GT	Serum	5–40 IU/L
Lactate dehydrogenase	Serum	50–200 IU/L
Lactate dehydrogenase isoenzymes LDH1	 Serum	 17–27%

Contd...

Contd...

LDH2	Serum	27–37%
LDH3	Serum	18–25%
LDH4	Serum	3–8%
LDH5	Serum	0–5%
Lipase	Serum	0.5–1.5 IU/L
SGOT (Aspartate transaminase) AST	Serum	5–35 IU/L
SGPT (Alanine transaminase) ALT	Plasma	5–30 IU/L
Albumin	Serum	<80 mg/24 h
Calcium	Urine	100–240 mg/24 h
Chloride	Urine	140–250 mEq/24 h
Copper	Urine	0–50 μg/24 h
Creatinine	Urine	1–2 g/24 h
Creatinine clearance — Male Female	Urine	 85–125 mL/min 75–115 mL/min
Magnesium	Urine	6.0–85 mEq/24 h
Oxalic acid	Urine	20–40 g/24 h
Phosphorus	Urine	0.9–1.3 g/24 h
Potassium	Urine	40–80 mEq/24 h
Urea	Urine	15–30 g/24 h
Uric acid	Urine	200–500 mg/24 h
VMA (3-methoxy-4-hydroxymandelic acid)	Urine	1.5–7.5 g/24 h
Zinc	Urine	0.15–1.2 g/24 h

Glossary

A

Absorption (absorbere = to swallow down): The movement of water and of substances dissolved in water into a cell, tissue or organism.

Absorption spectrum: The range of photons that a given atom or molecule is capable of absorbing, depending on the electron energy levels available in the atom or molecule.

Acetylcholine (ACh): The most important of the numerous chemical neurotransmitters responsible for the passing of nerve impulses across synaptic junctions. It is found both in the brain and in the peripheral nervous system.

Acetylcholinesterase: An enzyme found in cholinergic synapses and that removes the left over acetylcholine from the synaptic cleft at the neuromuscular junction after the last impulse. It is one of the fastest acting enzymes in the vertebrate body.

Acetyl-coenzyme A (Acetyl-CoA): A two-carbon water-soluble organic acid whose hydroxyl group has been replaced with coenzyme A; common to the metabolism of all major types of food, forming a step leading to the Krebs cycle.

Acid: Any substance that dissociates to form H^+ ions (protons) when dissolved in water.

Acidosis: A body condition in which there is excessive acidity in body fluids, normally regulated by the kidney; opposite of alkalosis.

Activation: The process by which the regulatory protein binds to DNA and turns on the transcription of specific genes.

Activation energy ($\Delta G\neq$): Extra energy that must be possessed by atoms or molecules in addition to their ground-state energy in order to undergo a particular chemical reaction.

Adenine: It is a purine component of nucleic acids and nucleotides. Adenine always forms complementary base-paring with thymine.

Adenosine: Consists of an adenine base attached to a ribose sugar.

Adenosine phosphates: A group of organic phosphates including adenosine monophosphate (AMP), adenosine diphosphate (ADP) and adenosine triphosphate (ATP). They function in phosphate transfer in the cell, particularly in the transfer of the high-energy phosphate bonds of ADP and ATP. ATP is the most directly utilizable source of energy of the cell.

Adenylation: In cells; the transfer of an adenyl moiety from ATP to another molecule. Some enzymes are regulated by reversible adenylylation.

Adenyl cyclase: An enzyme which catalyzes the formation of cyclic AMP from ATP by the removal of pyrophosphate.

Adipocyte: A fat cell; cell that is specialized for storing triacylglycerols and for releasing them to the blood in the form of fatty acids and glycerol as required.

Adipose tissue: A fatty connective tissue, the matrix of which contains large, closely-packed, fat filled cells; occurs either round the liver and kidneys where it stores energy, or in the dermis of the skin where it stimulates the body from heat loss.

Adrenalin (ad = above; renal = kidney): Hormone released by chromaffin cells (in the medulla of adrenal gland) and by some neurons in response to stress. It prepares the body for emergency action leading to "fight or flight" responses, which include increased heart rate, blood pressure and blood sugar levels, widening of the pupils, and erection of the hair.

Adsorption: The adhesion (attachment), in a very thin layer, of the molecules of gases, dissolved substances, or liquids to the surfaces of solid bodies with which they are in contact. In physical adsorption, molecules are held by van der Waal's forces of attraction; in chemical adsorption, there is exchange or sharing of electrons.

Aerobic (aer = air + bios = life): Oxygen requiring.

Aerobic pathway: A metabolic pathway, at least one step of which is an oxidation/reduction reaction that depends on oxygen gas as an electron acceptor. It includes the citric acid cycle and pyruvate oxidation.

Aglycon: The nonsugar part of a glycoside.

Albinism: The inability to produce melanin. Albinism is a recessive mutation, but mutations in several different gene can result in this phenotype.

Alkaloid: A small but complex organic substance in which at least one nitrogen is part of a ring, having strong basic properties, e.g. Caffeine, nicotine, cocaine, morphine, colchicine, quinine and strychnine.

Alkalosis: A body condition in which there is excessive alkalinity in body fluids; opposite of acidosis.

Allele: Two or more different forms of the same gene are termed as allelic genes.

Allergen: Any antigenic substance that initiates a strong immune response in a particular individual.

Allergy: The overreaction of the immune response of the body to minute traces of foreign substances (antigens). The reaction is usually visible in the form of rashes, itching, breathing difficulties etc.

Allosteric enzyme: Multi subunit enzyme that has a physically distinct allosteric site and a catalytic site. Allosteric site binds an allosteric modifier and catalytic site is for the susbtrate to bind.

Allosteric interaction (allos = other + stereos = shape): The interaction of an allosteric enzyme with is allosteric modifier that causes a change in the structure of the enzyme to either facilitate or inhibit the binding of its substrate.

Allozyme: Distinct allelic forms of an enzyme that can be physically separated by electrophoresis.

Alpha-cell (α-cell): A cell in the islets of Langerhans that produces the hormone glucagon, which causes liver cells to release stored glucose and fat cells to breakdown triglycerides.

Alpha-helix (α-helix): Common structural motif of proteins in which a linear sequence of amino acids folds into a right-handed helix, which are stabilized by internal hydrogen bonds between backbone atoms.

Alzheimer's disease: A type of dementia seen in the elderly, probably resulting from a deficiency of acetylcholine, which leads to degeneration and death of neurons.

Aminopeptidase: An enzyme that catalyzes the sequential hydrolysis of amino acids in a polypeptide chain from the N-terminal.

Aminotransferases: Enzymes that catalyze the transfer of amino groups from α-amino to α- keto acids; also called transaminases.

Amphipathic: For a molecule, the property of having both hydrophilic and hydrophobic proteins. Usually, one end or side of the molecule is hydrophilic and the other end or side is hydrophobic.

Ampholyte: A substance whose molecules have both acidic and basic groups.

Amphoteric: A chemical that can act both as an acid and as a base, e.g. Amino acids.

Anion: A negatively charged ion that is attracted to the anode during electrolysis.

Anticodon: A three-nucleotide sequence at the end of a transfer RNA (tRNA) molecule, that is complementary to the three-nucleotide codon on a messenger RNA (mRNA) molecule.

Antimetabolite: A substance that is a structural analogue of a normal metabolite or otherwise resembles it and that interferes with the utilization of the metabolite by the cell.

Antiparallel: Refers to two strands running in opposite direction parallel to each other as the two strands of DNA or in β-pleated sheets of proteins.

Apoenzyme: The basic or protein part of a holoenzyme.

Aqueous: Pertaining to water, as in an aqueous solution.

Aromatic: Refers to a molecule that contains carbon atoms in a ring, linked through alternating single and double bonds. Often a molecule related to benzene.

Atrophy (a = not + trophe = nourishment): Wasting or the reduction in size of an organism or tissue mass, often after disuse.

B

Bactericide: A substance causing death to bacteria; for example, an antibiotic.

Bacteriophage (bakterion = little rod + phagein = to eat): A type of virus that infects and destroys bacterial cells and often replicate within them; extensively used in virus and DNA studies. Also called a phage.

Barbiturate: Any ureide such as amytal, seconal, phenobarbital etc; have depressant effect on the central nervous system (CNS), usually producing sleep.

Basal: Situated near the base. The basal surface of a cell is opposite the apical surface.

Base: Any substance that combines with H^+ ions (protons) present in a solution and thereby increasing the number of hydroxyl ions.

Benign: Nonmalignant, as in a growth.

Bile pigments: The pigments secreted in bile, bilirubin and biliverdin, which result from the breakdown of hemoglobin in red blood corpuscles, giving the bile its coloration which in turn affects the color of the feces.

Bile salts: The sodium salts secreted in bile, sodium taurocholate and sodium glycocholate, which greatly lower surface tension and are important in emulsifying fats.

Bioluminescence: The emission of light from living organisms as a result of internal oxidative changes.

Biotic: Pertaining to living organisms.

Buffer: A chemical substance which has the capacity to bond to H^+ ions, removing them from solution when their concentration begins to rise and releasing H^+ ions when their concentration begins to fall. In this way, buffers stabilize the pH of biological solutions and are thus important in maintaining homeostasis.

C

Calciferol: Vitamin D_2, a fat-soluble anti-rachitic vitamin.

Calcitonin (calcem = lime): A polypeptide hormone, secreted by both thyroid and parathyroid glands, that lowers the calcium content of the blood.

Calmodulin: An ubiquitous protein that is activated when it binds to calcium ions (Ca^{2+}); calmodulin activates enzymes in membranes; as much as 2% of the plasma membrane may be calmodulin.

Calorie, Cal (calorie = heat): A unit of heat which is equal to 1,000 calories. One Calorie (capital "C") is the amount of energy in the form of heat required to raise the temperature of 1 kilogram of water by 1°C.

calorie, cal (calorie = heat): Also a unit of heat which is equal to 1/1,000 = 0.001 Calories. One calorie (small "c") is the amount of heat energy required to raise the temperature of 1 gram (1 cm^3) of water by 1°C. Used as a unit of energy content or output, but now largely superseded by the S.I. unit joule (1 cal = 4.12 J).

Carcinogen (karkinos = a crab, symbolizing cancerous growth + –gen = producing): An agent, such as a chemical or a form of radiation, that causes cancer.

Carcinoma (karkinos = a crab): A malignant growth from epithelial tissues that cover the body surface and line the intestine and other internal organs; the most common form of human cancer; carcinomas account for about 90% of malignant tumors.

Carrier protein: Membrane transport protein that binds to a solute and transports it across the membrane by undergoing a series of conformational changes.

Chaperone: A protein that helps other proteins avoid misfolding pathways that produce inactive or aggregated states.

Cistron: The smallest unit of DNA that must be intact to code for the amino acid sequence of a polypeptide; thus, the coding part of a gene, minus 5′ and 3′ untranslated sequences and regulatory elements.

Clathrin: A protein that assembles into a polyhedral cage on the cytoplasmic side of a membrane so as to form a clathrin-coated pit, which buds off to form a clathrin-coated vesicle.

Colloid: A mixture of two substances which are immiscible, but where the particles of one are too small to settle out, and so remain suspended indefinitely; colloids are common in cells; colloid particles measure between 0.000001 to 0.0001 mm in diameter; does not diffuse through cell membranes; a liquid colloid is called a sol, and a solid colloid, a gel.

Concentration gradient: The concentration difference of a substance as a function of distance. In a cell, a greater concentration of its molecules in one region than in another.

Configuration: The spatial arrangement of an organic molecule that is conferred by the presence of either (a) double bonds, around which there is no freedom of rotation, or (b) chiral centers, around which substituent groups are arranged in a specific sequence. Configurational isomers cannot be interconverted without breaking one or more covalent bonds.

Conformation: The spatial arrangement of substituent groups that are free to assume different positions in space, without breaking any bonds, because of the freedom of bond rotation.

Conjugate acid-base pair: A proton donor and its corresponding deprotonated species.

Constitutive enzyme: An enzyme that is made all the time at a constant rate, unaffected by inducers.

Cyclic AMP, cAMP: A second messenger within cells that is generated from ATP in response to hormonal stimulation of cell-surface receptors; cAMP acts as a signalling molecule by activating A-kinase; it is hydrolyzed to AMP by phosphodiesterase.

Carnitine: A low-molecular-weight lysine derivative or betaine that shuttles fatty acids through the inner mitochondrial membrane to the matrix. The fatty acyl moiety is transferred from CoA to carnitine for transit through the membrane and is then transferred back to CoA; the carnitine released on the matrix side of the membrane is shuffled back for reuse.

Carotenoids: A group of yellow/orange fat-soluble accessory pigments that are derived from isoprene units linked together.

Complementary DNA, cDNA: DNA that is made by reverse-transcribing mRNA into its DNA complement and therefore lacking the introns that are present in genomic DNA; used to determine the amino acid sequence of a protein by DNA sequencing or to make the protein in large quantities by cloning followed by expression; the collection of vector-cloned cDNA fragments of an organism are its cDNA library.

Cytochromes: Colored heme-containing metalloproteins that serve as electron carriers during cellular respiration, photosynthesis, and other oxidation–reduction reactions; usually designated as cytochromes a, b, and c.

D

Deficiency disease: Any condition exhibiting abnormalities produced by lack of a particular component in the diet of animals and plants; examples include beriberi (due to deficiency of vitamin B1), scurvy (vitamin C), rickets (vitamin D) and kwashiorkor (proteins).

Degenerate Code: A code in which one amino acid is specified by more than one codon.

Diabetes insipidus (diabetes, a siphon, from dia = through + be nai = to go; insipidus = tasteless): A metabolic disorder resulting due to the failure of the pituitary to secrete antidiuretic hormone (ADH); characterized by an increase in the amount of urine excreted (polyuria) and an increased thirst (polydipsia).

Diabetes mellitus (mellitus = honeyed): A metabolic disease resulting from insulin deficiency; characterized by a failure in glucose transport from the blood into cells at normal glucose concentrations, with the result excess sugar appears in the blood and urine, associated with thirst and loss of body weight; more common than diabetes insipidus.

Disease: An abnormality of an animal or plant caused by a pathogenic organism that affects performance of the vital functions and usually gives diagnostic symptoms.

Differential centrifugation: Separation of cell organelles or other particles of different size by their rates of sedimentation in a centrifugal field.

Dyspepsia (dys = bad + peptos = cooked): Deranged digestion.

E

E0 values: A numerical series indicative of the redox potential of molecules; protons are accepted by a molecule from any other molecule with a more positive E0 value.

Edema: A swelling of the body tissues caused by the capillary blood vessels passing out water into the surrounding tissues, and so increasing the intercellular fluid content; in old English, also spelt as oedema.

Electrochemical gradient: Driving force that causes an ion to move across a membrane due to the combined influence of a difference in its concentration on the two sides of the membrane and the electrical charge difference across the membrane.

Electrolyte: A compound with ionic bonds, forming ions and capable of transmitting electric current in solution.

Electron acceptor: An atom or molecule that receives electrons readily (and thereby becoming reduced) in an oxidation–reduction reaction.

Electron carrier: A protein, such as a flavoproteins or a cytochrome, that can reversibly gain and lose electrons; functions in the transfer of an electron from a donor molecule to an acceptor molecule.

Electron donor: A molecule that readily gives up electrons (and thereby becoming oxidized) in an oxidation–reduction reaction.

Electrophoresis: Movement of charged solutes in response to an electric field; a technique often used to separate mixtures of ions, proteins, or nucleic acids.

Elongation factors: Specific nonribosomal proteins required for the addition of amino acids to growing polypeptide chains on ribosomes.

Encephalitis (enkephalos = brain, from en = in + kephale = head + –itis = inflammation): Inflammation of the brain.

Endemic: Refers to organisms or disease whose occurrence is limited to a particular geographical area.

Endergonic reaction (endon = within + ergon = work): A chemical reaction that requires an input of energy before it can proceed (that is, for which ΔG is positive); endergonic reactions never occur spontaneously; compare exergonic reaction.

Endocytosis (endon = within + kytos = cell): The process by which the plasma membrane invaginates and forms vesicles (endosomes) whose contents from outside of the cell can be brought into the cell.

Endonuclease: An enzyme that hydrolyzes the interior phosphodiester bonds of a nucleic acid; that is, it acts at points other than the terminal bonds.

Energy charge: The fractional degree to which the ATP/ADP/AMP system is filled with high energy phosphate groups.

Epidemic: The occurrence of many cases of a disease within an area.

Epiphysis: The ossified part of the end of a mammalian limb bone or vertebra which, during growth, is separated by a plate of cartilage from the rest of the ossified bone. When growth is complete, the epiphysis fuses with the rest of the bone.

Epithelium (epi = on + thele = nipple): A thin layer of cells forming a tissue that covers the internal and external surfaces of the body.

Equilibrium: The state of a system in which no further net change is occurring; the free energy is at a minimum.

Equilibrium constant (Keq): A ratio of forward and reverse rate constants for a reaction and equal to the association constant; a constant characteristic for each chemical reaction.

Exergonic reaction (ex = out + ergon = work): A chemical reaction that proceeds with the release of free energy (that is, for which ΔG is negative); exergonic reactions occur .spontaneously; compare endergonic reaction.

Exocytosis: An active process in which vesicles containing excretory or secretory materials are actively carried to the periphery of the cell, and released to the outside when the vesicle membrane fuses with the cell membrane; opposite of endocytosis.

F

Feedback inhibition: A regulatory mechanism in which a biochemical pathway is regulated by the amount of the product that the pathway produces; also known as end-product inhibition.

Fermentation (fermentum = ferment): A process by which energy is obtained from organic compounds without the use of oxygen as an electron acceptor; yields lactate, ethanol, or some other simple product.

Ferritin: A conjugated, electron-dense protein concerned in the absorption of iron through the intestinal mucosa; serves as a storage protein for iron in the liver and spleen.

Fibrosis (fibra = a fiber): Formation of scar tissues.

First-order reaction: A reaction in which the rate of reaction is directly proportional to the concentration of one of the reactants, either product or substrate.

Flatulence (flatus = a blowing): Excess of gas in the digestive tract.

Flavin nucleotides: Nucleotide coenzymes (FMN and FAD) containing riboflavin.

Flavin-linked dehydrogenases: Dehydrogenases requiring one of the riboflavin coenzymes, FMN or FAD.

Flavoprotein: An enzyme containing a flavin nucleotide as a tightly bound prosthetic group; acts as an intermediate carrier in respiratory chains between dehydrogenases and cytochromes.

Flocculation: The formation of jelly-like masses of coagulated material.

Fluorescence: The property of giving out light when molecules are excited by incident light; emitted light is always of a shorter wavelength than the incident light.

G

G proteins: A large family of heterotrimeric proteins that are important intermediaries in cell signaling pathways. Usually activated by the binding of a hormone or other signaling ligand to seven-pass transmembrane receptor protein. They are called G proteins because binding of GTP and GDP is essential for their functioning.

Galactosemia: A rare inborn error of metabolism in which the breast-fed human infant is literally poisoned by mother's milk. The affected infants are unable to metabolize the milk sugar galactose, which normally is converted to glucose ready for oxidation and the release of energy. Instead, affected infants store the galactose in various tissues including the brain, resulting in severe malnutrition along with mental retardation.

Gene (genos = birth, race): The basic unit of heredity. A sequence of DNA nucleotides on a chromosome that codes for a polypeptide or RNA molecule and thus determines of an individual's inherited traits.

Gene amplification: A process in which many copies are made of some genes at one time, while other genes are not replicated. The replicated genes enable enhanced manufacture of product in a short time.

Gene bank: A collection of clones containing all the genes of a particular organism.

Gene cloning: The technique of genetic engineering in which specific genes are excised from host DNA, inserted into a vector plasmid and introduced into a host cell, which then divides to produce many copies (clones) of the transferred gene.

Gene splicing: The enzymatic attachment of one gene, or part of a gene, to another; also called splicing.

Genetic code: The "language" of the genes. The set of triplet code words in DNA (or mRNA) that code for the amino acids of proteins. Of the 64 possible codons, 61 are the codes for amino acids, and the remaining being termination codons that are not translated.

Genetic engineering: A collective term for the techniques of transferring genes from one organism to another and multiplying them; synonymous with recombinant DNA technology.

Genome (genos = offspring + oma = abstract group): Total genetic information encoded in a cell or an organism, or a virus.

Genomic library: The set of fragments of an organism's genome that are cloned in a virus or bacterial plasmid.

Genotype (genos = offspring + typos = form): The genetic constitution of an organism, as distinct from its physical (or visible) characteristics actually developed during its life history, or phenotype; also used to refer to the set of alleles at a single gene locus; compare phenotype.

Glycan: Another term for polysaccharide; a polymer of monosaccharide units joined by glycosidic bonds.

Ground state: The normal, stable form of an atom or molecule; as distinct from the excited state.

H

Half-life: The time required for the disappearance or decay of one-half of a given component in a system. Half-lives vary from isotope to isotope, some being less than a millionth of a second and some more than a million years; symbol, T1/2; also called half-time.

Heat-labile: Destroyable by heat.

Hierarchy (hieros = sacred + archos = leader): Refers to a graded system of classification in which each step of category includes all those below it; especially the Linnean hierarchy used in classification of organisms.

Helix: Anything of a spiral shape; in biology, it refers to the shape of DNA molecules, which occur as double helices.

Heme: A complex organic ring structure, called a protoporphyrin, to which an iron atom is bound; occurs in cytochromes of all organisms and in the hemoglobin of animals; also spelt as haem.

Heme protein: A protein containing a heme as a prosthetic group.

Hemicellulose: Primarily a cell wall polysaccharide of variable composition and structure; less complex than cellulose and easily hydrolysable to simple sugars; hemicellulose that is secreted by plants is also called a gum.

Hemorrhage (haima = blood + rhegnunai= to break): An escape of blood from the blood vessels, due to a wound or disease.

Henderson–Hasselbalch equation: An equation relating the pH, pKa, and the ratio of the concentrations of the proton-acceptor (A–) and proton-donor (HA) species in a solution. Alternatively, it is a formula for calculating the pH of a buffer solution.

Heterogeneous nuclear RNA (hn RNA): The pool of primary RNA transcripts in the nucleus which are of various, usually large sizes. It is, in fact, the immediate product of transcription in an eukaryote, containing both introns and exons; also known as pre-mRNA.

High-energy bond: A covalent bond that has a low activation energy and is broken easily and which on hydrolysis releases an unusually large amount of free energy (>-7.6kcal/mol) under the conditions existing in a cell.

Homologous proteins: Proteins having sequences and functions similar in different species, for example, the hemoglobins.

Hydrophobic interactions: The association of nonpolar groups, or compounds, with each other in aqueous systems, driven by the tendency of the surrounding water molecules to seek their most stable (disordered) state.

Hyperchromic effect: The large increase in light absorption at 260 nm occurring as a doublehelical DNA is melted (unwound).

Hyperplasia: An increase in tissue mass caused by an increase in cell number.

Hypertonic (hyper = above + tonos = tension): Refers to the solution surrounding a cell that has a sufficiently high concentration of solutes to cause water to move out of the cell due to osmosis.

Hypotonic (hypo = under + tonos = tension): Refers to the solution surrounding a cell that has a sufficiently low concentration of solutes to cause water to move into the cell due to osmosis.

I

In vitro (Latin, for "in glass"): A term used by biochemists to describe a process taking place in an isolated cell-free extract. Also used by cell biologists to refer to cells growing in culture usually taken in glass equipments, as opposed to in an organism (in vivo).

In vivo (Latin, for "in life"): Refers to a process taking place in an intact (i.e. living) cell or an organism, as opposed to in a culture (in vitro).

Induced fit: A change in the conformation of an enzyme in response to substrate binding that renders the enzyme catalytically active.

Inducer: A signal molecule that, when bound to a regulatory protein, produces an increase in the expression of a given gene. It is an environmental agent that triggers transcription from an operon.

Inducible enzyme: An enzyme that is produced in response to the presence of its inducer.

Informational macromolecules: Biomolecules containing information in the form of specific sequences of different monomers; for example, many proteins, lipids, polysaccharides and nucleic acids.

Inhibitor: A chemical whose binding alters the shape of a protein and shuts off enzyme activity.

Innate (innatus = born): Describing a characteristic based partly or wholly on inherited gene differences.

Interferon: A class of glycoproteins produced naturally in virus-infected cells that inhibits viral multiplication.

Intron (intra = within): A noncoding sequence of nucleotides within a eukaryotic gene that is transcribed into an mRNA molecule but is then excised by RNA splicing before the gene is translated. These untranslated regions of DNA make up the bulk of most eukaryotic genes; also called as intervening sequence.

Ion channel: An integral membrane protein that provides for the regulated transport of a specific ion or ions, across a membrane.

Ion exchange resin: A polymericresin that contains fixed charged groups; used in chromatographic columns to separate ionic compounds.

Ionic bond: A noncovalent bond formed between two ions, one with a positive charge and the other with a negative charge, as a result of the attraction of opposite electrical charges.

Ionization: The process of spontaneous ion formation.

Ionizing radiation: A type of radiation such as x-rays and gamma-rays which cause loss of electrons from some organic molecules, thus making them more reactive.

Ionophore: A small hydrophobic molecule that binds one or more metal ions and is capable of diffusing across a membrane, carrying the bound ion.

Iron–sulfur center (Fe–S center): A prosthetic group of certain redox proteins involved in electron transfers; Fe_2^+ and Fe_3^+ is bound to inorganic sulfur and to cysteine groups in the protein.

Isothermal: Occurring at constant temperature.

Isotonic (isos = equal + tonos = tension): Refers to the solution surrounding a cell that has the same concentration of solutes as in the cell.

J

Jaundice (jaunice = yellowness): Condition characterized by yellowness of the skin and mucous membranes and the secretion of bile pigments in the urine, turning it dark yellowish.

K

Karyotype (karyon = kernel + typos = stamp or print): Full set of chromosomes of a cell arranged with respect to size, shape and number.

Keto–enol tautomerism: A type of tautomerism that occurs in ketones as the result of the migration of a hydrogen atom from an alkyl group to the carbonyl group.

Ketogenic amino acids: Amino acids with carbon skeletons that can serve as precursors of the ketone bodies.

Ketone: An organic molecule containing a carbonyl group linked to two alkyl groups.

Ketone bodies: Water-soluble fuels normally exported by the liver but overproduced during fasting or in untreated diabetes mellitus; acetoacetate, D-β-hydroxybutyrate and acetone common examples.

Ketonuria (ketone = variant of a acetone, from acetum = vinegar + ouron = urine): The presence of ketone bodies in the urine.

Ketose: A simple monosaccharide in which the carbonyl group occurs within the chain and, hence, represents a ketone group, e.g. Fructose; compare aldose.

L

Lac operon: A cluster of genes encoding 3 proteins that bacteria use to obtain energy from the sugar lactose.

Lagging strand: One of the two newly-made strands of DNA found at a replication fork. The lagging strand is synthesized in the direction opposite to that in which the replication fork moves and is made in discontinuous lengths that are later joined covalently.

Leader sequence: A short, noncoding sequence of DNA, immediately upstream from the beginning of a gene, that is transcribed into RNA; also called signal sequence.

Leading strand: One of the two newly-made strands of DNA found at a replication fork. The leading strand is synthesized in the same direction in which the replication fork moves and is made by continuous synthesis in the 5′ to 3′ direction.

Lesion: A localized area of diseased tissue.

Lineweaver–Burk equation: An algebraic transform of the Michaelis-Menten equation, allowing determination of Vmax and Km by extrapolation of [S] to infinity.

Linkage: The condition of having genes on the same chromosome (linked); alleles of genes that are linked tend to be inherited together; the greater the linkage, the lower the frequency of recombination between the two loci.

Lysozyme: An enzyme that breaksdown bacterial cell walls and provides protection against bacterial invasion in the skin, mucous membranes and many body fluids.

M

Macromolecule (macros = large + moliculus = a little mass): A large molecule having a molecular weight in the range of a few thousand to many millions; refers specifically to polysaccharides, proteins, enzymes, lipids, and nucleic acids.

Malaise: A general feeling of illness.

Malignant (malignus = of an evil nature): Describes tumors and tumor cells that are invasive and/or able to undergo metasis; a malignant tumor is a cancer.

Membrane protein: Protein that is normally closely associated with a cell membrane.

Membrane transport: Movement of molecules across a membrane via a specific membrane protein (a transporter).

Metabolic pathway: The sequence of enzymatic reactions followed in the formation of one substrate from another.

Metabolic rate: The rate at which an organism carries out metabolism, and which is closely linked to temperature. The relationship between metabolic rate and temperture can be expressed in terms of a value called Q10.

Metabolic waste: Any waste substance that is produced during the metabolism of an organism, such as nitrogen in the form of urea.

Metabolism (metabole = change): The entire set of enzyme-catalyzed transformations of organic molecules in living cells; the sum total of all the processes involved in the building up and tearing down of protoplasm; the synthetic or building up processes constitute the anabolic phase of metabolism and the degradative or tearing down processes, the catabolic phase. A special energy-carrying molecule called ATP is involved in these processes.

Metabolite: A chemical intermediate in the enzyme catalyzed reactions of metabolism.

Metalloprotein: A protein having a metal ion as its prosthetic group.

Metaplasia: The transformation of a tissue to another form.

Molar solution: One mole of solute dissolved in water to give a total volume of 1,000 mL.

Mole: A mole is the amount of a substance, in grams, that equals the combined atomic mass of all the atoms in a molecule of that substance.

Mole, mol (moles = mass): The atomic weight of a substance, expressed in grams. One mole of any substance is defined as the mass of 6.0222×10^{23} atoms.

Monochromatic light: Light consisting of vibrations of the same or nearly the same frequency; light of one color.

Mutagen (mutare = to change): A chemical capable of damaging DNA, thus causing mutation.

Mutant (mutare= to change): A mutated gene. An organism carrying a gene that has undergone a mutation.

Mutarotation: The change in specific rotation of a pyranose or furanose sugar or glycoside accompanying the equilibration of its α- and β- anomeric forms.

Mutases: Enzymes that catalyze the transposition of functional groups.

N

Native conformation: The biologically-active conformation of a macromolecule.

Nausea (nausia = sea-sickness, from naus = a ship): Feeling of sickness.

Negative feedback: Regulation of a biochemical pathway achieved when a reaction product inhibits an earlier step in the pathway.

Neonatal: (of newborn offspring, particularly human) the first month of independent life.

Nick: A single-stranded cut or break in a DNA molecule; nicking of DNA may form part of a DNA repair mechanism, as occurs after damage caused by ultraviolet light.

Noncovalent bond: A chemical bond in which, in contrast to a covalent bond, no electrons are shared. Noncovalent bonds are relatively weak but they can sum together to produce strong, highly specific interactions between molecules.

Nonheme iron proteins: Proteins containing iron but no porphyrin groups; usually acting in oxidation–reduction reactions.

Nonhistone proteins: Proteins associated with chromosomes that are not histones. For example, they may be enzymes involved in DNA replication or structural components of the chromatin.

Nonpolar molecules: Molecules or groups that are poorly soluble in water (i.e. hydrophobic); lack any asymmetric accumulation of positive or negative charge; also called as apolar molecules.

Nucleophile: An electron-rich group with a strong tendency to donate electrons to an electron deficient nucleus (electrophile); the entering reactant in a bimolecular substitution reaction.

Nutrient: A substance derived from outside a cell and providing it with energy and structural material.

O

Oligomer (oligos = few, little): A short polymer, usually consisting (in a cell) of amino acids (oligopeptide), sugars (oligosaccharide), or nucleotides (oligonucleotide); the definition of "short" is somewhat arbitrary, but usually less than 50 subunits.

Operator: A short region of DNA in a bacterial chromosome that interacts with a repressor protein to control the expression (transcription) of adjaent gene(s).

Operon (operis = work): In bacterial chromosome, a group of contiguous functionally-related genes that are transcribed into a single mRNA molecule; although a common mode of gene regulation in prokaryotes, it is rare in eukaryotes except fungi.

Opsin: A protein that occurs in rodes and cones of the retina of the eye, which forms visual pigments rhodopsin and conopsin.

Optical activity: The capacity of a substance to rotate the plane of plane-polarized light.

Optimum pH: The characteristic pH at which an enzyme has maximal catalytic activity.

Osteoblast (osteon = bone + blastos = bud): A bone-forming cell.

Osteocyte (osteon = bone + kytos = hollow vessel): A mature osteoblast.

Oxidizing agent: The acceptor of electrons in an oxidation–reduction reaction; also called oxidant.

Oxidoreductase: One of a group of enzymes that catalyzes oxidation–reduction reactions.

Oxygenases: Enzymes that catalyze the incorporation of oxygen into a substrate reactions in which oxygen is introduced into an acceptor molecule.

P

Pain: A conscious sensation produced in the brain and stimulated by pain receptors in, for example, the skin; pain has a protective function and often produces a reflex action in response.

Palindrome: A segment of duplex DNA with a nucleotide sequence that is identical to its complementary strand when each is read in the same chemical direction; for example, TGAC in the following DNA segment:

5' XXX TGAC XXX 3'

3' XXX CAGT XXX 5'

Papain: A proteolytic enzyme obtained from the juice of the green fruit of the papaya or papaw tree (Carica papaw).

Partition coefficient: A constant that expresses the ratio in which a given solute will be partitioned or distributed between two given immiscible liquids at equilibrium.

Perfusion: The passage of a liquid through an organ or tissue.

Phosphocreatine: A compound used in the production of ATP from ADP in muscles, being converted to creatine with the release of inorganic phosphorus.

Photon (photos = light): The elementary particle of light and other electromagnetic radiation.

Photo-oxidation: A chemical reaction occurring as a result of absorption of light in the presence of oxygen.

pK: The negative logarithm of an equilibrium constant.

Placebo: (1) Any inactive substance given to satisfy a patient's psychological need for medication. (2) A control in an experiment to test the effect of a drug.

Pleated sheet: The side-by-side hydrogen-bonded arrangement of polypeptide chains in the extended β-conformation.

Poly-A tail: A chain of adenylic acid molecules that is added to a molecule of RNA immediately after it has been transcribed and cleaved from its DNA template.

Polydipsia (polys many + dipsa = thirst): Increased thirst.

Polyuria (polys = many + ouron = urine): Increased urine output.

Primary transcript: The immediate RNA product of transcription before any posttranscriptional processing reactions.

Primase: An enzyme that catalyzes the formation of RNA oligonucleotides used as primers by DNA polymerase.

Primer: A short oligomer (of sugars or nucleotides, for example) to which an enzyme adds additional monomeric subunits.

Prion: An infectious agent that contains protein but no nucleic acid.

Probe: In genetic research, a fragment of labeled (radioactively or chemically labeled) DNA or RNA, containing a nucleotide sequence complementary to a gene or genomic sequence that one wishes to detect in a hybridization experiment.

Protein kinase: Enzyme that transfers the terminal phosphate group of ATP to a specific amino acid of a target protein.

Protein targeting: The process by which newly synthesized proteins are sorted and transported to their proper locations in the cell.

Proton acceptor: An anionic compound capable of accepting a proton from a proton donor, that is, a base.

Proton donor: The donor of a proton in an acid–base reaction, that is, an acid.

Q

Quaternary structure: The three-dimensional structure of a multi-subunit protein; particularly the manner in which the subunits fit together.

Quinone: Any of the various compounds derived from benzene.

R

R group: (1) Formally, an abbreviation denoting any alkyl group (2) Occasionally, used in a more general sense to denote virtually any organic substituent, such as a methyl group, a hydroxyl group, or a monosaccharide.

Racemic mixture: An equimolar mixture of the D and L stereoisomers of an optically-active compound.

Radical: (1) A functional group of atoms recurring as part of various different molecules. (2) An atom or group of atoms possessing an unpaired electron; also called a free radical.

Radioimmunoassay (RIA): A sensitive and quantitative method for detecting trace amounts of a biomolecule, based on its capacity to displace a radioactive form of the molecule from combination with its specific antibody.

Redox pair: An electron donor and its corresponding oxidized form; for example, NADH and NAD^+.

Redox potential: A quantitative measurement of the willingness of an electron carrier to act as a reducing or oxidizing agent. Redox potential is measured in volts; the more negative the value, the better the carrier will act as a reducing agent. Thus, in an electron transport system the carriers are arranged in order of increasing redox potentials (negative to positive).

Reducing agent: The electron donor in an oxidation–reduction reaction; also called reductant.

Restriction fragment: A segment of double-stranded DNA produced by the action of a restriction endonuclease on a larger DNA.

Retinoblastoma: A childhood cancer of the retina.

RNA splicing: The trimming of larger primary RNA transcripts, in the nucleus, into smaller, coding sequences that are exported into the cytosol. Alternatively, a process in which intron sequences are excised from RNA molecules in the nucleus during formation of mRNA. Synonymous with RNA processing.

S

S-adenosylmethionine (adoMet): An enzymatic cofactor involved in methyl group transfers.

Salvage pathway: Synthesis of a biomolecule (such as a nucleotide) from intermediates in the degradative pathway for the biomolecule; a recycling pathway, as distinct from a de novo pathway.

Satellite DNA: DNA consisting of multiple tandem repeats of very short, simple nucleotide sequences; makes up 10% to 20% of genome of higher eukaryotes; usually identifiable by its unusual nucleotide composition; most often associated with the centromeric region; satellite DNA is not transcribed and has no known function.

Second messenger: A small effector molecule that is formed in or released into the cytosol in response to an extracellular signal (first messenger) such as a hormone; helps to relay the signal to the interior of the cell; examples include cAMP, IP_3/Ca_2^+.

Second order reaction: A reaction in which 2 reactant molecules must come together for the reaction to occur. The reaction is called second order because the reaction rate depends on the square of reactant concentration (for 2 molecules of the same reactant) or on the product of 2 reactant concentrations (for 2 different reactants).

Sedimentation coefficient: A physical constant specifying the rate of sedimentation of a particle in a centrifugal field under specified conditions.

Senescence: The process of growing old which occurs in all species and is characterized by a gradual slowing down of metabolism and breakdown of tissues, often accompanied by endocrinal changes.

SI units: Those units of measurement forming the *Systeme International d'Unites*, consisting of the metre, kilogram, second, mole, kelvin, ampere, candela and katal.

Symport: A form of cotransport in which a membrane carrier protein transports two solute species across the membrane in the same direction.

T

Tachycardia (tachys = fast + kardia = heart): Rapid beating of the heart.

TATA box: Consensus sequence in the promoter region of many eukaryotic genes that binds a general transcription factor and hence specifies the position where transcription is initiated.

Tautomers (tauto = same, meros = part): A term coined by Laar in 1225; structural isomers that differ in the location of their hydrogens and double bonds; aldehydes, ketones and other carbonyl compounds such as esters exhibit tautomerism.

Thioester bond: A high-energy bond formed by a condensation reaction between an acid (acyl) group and a thiol (–SH) group; present in acetyl- CoA and many enzyme–substrate complexes.

Thiols: A class of organic compounds of the general formula, RSH, with sulfur attached directly to carbon. They are the sulfur analogues of alcohols, containing SH instead of OH groups. Formely called mercaptans.

Threshold: The lowest value of any stimulus, signal, or agency that results in a specified effect or response, e.g. threshold frequency. Below the threshold value, there is no response despite the application of a stimulus.

Transition State: A structure that forms transiently, in the course of a chemical reaction and has the highest free-energy of any reaction intermediate; a rate-limiting step in the reaction.

U

Ubiquinol: The reduced form of ubiquinone; ubiquinol donates electrons to cytochrome b in the electron transport chain.

Ubiquinone: A lipid-soluble quinone; ubiquinone accepts electrons from electron donors like NADH and from the oxidation of fatty acids; also called coenzyme Q.

Ubiquitin: A small, highly conserved protein present in all eukaryotic cells that becomes covalently attached to lysines of other proteins. Attachment of a chain of ubiquitones tags a protein for intracellular proteolytic destruction in a proteasome.

Uniport: A transport system that carries only one solute, as distinct from cotransport.

V

Vasoconstriction: A narrowing of the blood vessels, often in response to cold, which through a contraction of involuntary muscles in the walls of the vessels brought about by a stimulus from the sympathetic nervous system.

Vasodilation: The expansion of blood vessels by relaxation of muscles, mainly controlled by the sympathetic nervous system.

Viral vector: A virus DNA altered so that it can act as a vector for recombinant DNA.

Virion: A complete virus particle outside its host cell.

Virulence: The collective properties of an organism that render it pathogenic to another one, the host.

W

Western blotting: A technique by which proteins are separated and immobilized on a paper sheet and then analyzed, usually by means of a labeled antibody.

Wild type: The normal unmutated form of an organism; the form found in nature (in the wild); wild type alleles are usually given a 'plus' symbol.

X

X-ray crystallography: A technique for determining the three-dimensional arrangement of atoms in a molecule, based on the diffraction pattern of x-rays passing through a crystal of the molecule.

Z

Zero-order reaction: A chemical reaction in which the rate is independent of the concentration of the reactants.

Zwitterion ('ions of both kind'): A dipolar ion, with spatially separated positive and negative charges.

Zymogen: An inactive precursor of an enzyme, particularly by those concerned with protein digestion; for example, pepsinogen, the precursor of pepsin and trypsinogen, the precursor of trypsin; zymogens require activation energy to become functional.

Index

Page numbers followed by *f* refer to figure and *t* refer to table

A

B

C

D

E

F

G

H

I

J

K

L

M

N

O

P

Q

R

S

T

U

V

W

X

Y

Z